Advanced
RESPIRATORY
THERAPIST *Exam Guide*

**The Complete Resource for the Written Registry
and Clinical Simulation Exams**

Advanced
RESPIRATORY
THERAPIST *Exam Guide*

The Complete Resource for the Written Registry and Clinical Simulation Exams

third edition

JAMES R. SILLS, MEd, CPFT, RRT
Director, Respiratory Care Program
Rock Valley College
Rockford, Illinois

Original illustrations by
Sandra Hogan, Rock Valley College, Rockford, Illinois

MOSBY

ELSEVIER

11830 Westline Industrial Drive
St. Louis, Missouri 63146

ADVANCED RESPIRATORY THERAPIST EXAM GUIDE: ISBN-13: 978-0-323-02825-7
THE COMPLETE RESOURCE FOR THE WRITTEN   ISBN-10: 0-323-02825-X
REGISTRY AND CLINICAL SIMULATION EXAMS, THIRD
EDITION
Copyright © 2006, 2002, 1995 by Mosby, Inc., an affiliate of Elsevier Inc.

Notice

Knowledge and best practice in this field are constantly changing. As new research and experience broaden our knowledge, changes in practice, treatment, and drug therapy may become necessary or appropriate. Readers are advised to check the most current information provided (i) on procedures featured or (ii) by the manufacturer of each product to be administered, to verify the recommended dose or formula, the method and duration of administration, and contraindications. It is the responsibility of the practitioner, relying on his or her own experience and knowledge of the patient, to make diagnoses, to determine dosages and the best treatment for each individual patient, and to take all appropriate safety precautions. To the fullest extent of the law, neither the Publisher nor the Author assumes any liability for any injury and/or damage to persons or property arising out or related to any use of the material contained in this book.

The Publisher

ISBN-13: 978-0-323-02825-7
ISBN-10: 0-323-02825-X

Managing Editor: *Mindy Hutchinson*
Senior Developmental Editor: *Melissa K. Boyle*
Publishing Services Manager: *Melissa Lastarria*
Senior Project Manager: *Joy Moore*
Design Manager: *Bill Drone*

Working together to grow
libraries in developing countries

www.elsevier.com | www.bookaid.org | www.sabre.org

ELSEVIER   BOOK AID International   Sabre Foundation

Printed in the United States of America

Last digit is the print number: 9 8 7 6 5 4 3 2 1

This book is dedicated to my wife,
Deb,
and our children,
Rachael *and* **David,**
who make my life full and complete;
the memory of our first dog **Amber;**
our new dog, **Abby,** *who takes me for long walks;*
my **Mom** *and the memory of my* **Dad;**
and
Carl Hammond,
who taught me respiratory care.

Words to live by:
The journey of 1000 miles begins with a single step.
Confucius

Hope for the best but plan for the worst.

Reviewers

SINDEE KALMINSON KARPEL, MPA, RRT, AE-C
Clinical Coordinator
Cardiovascular Technology and Respiratory Care
  Programs
Edison Community College
Fort Myers, Florida

STEPHEN MICKLES, EdS, RRT
Program Director
Respiratory Care Program
St. Petersburg College
Pinellas Park, Florida

DENNIS R. WISSING, PhD, RRT, CPFT
Professor and Program Coordinator
Department of Cardiopulmonary Science
Louisiana State University Health Sciences Center
Shreveport, Louisiana

Foreword

Advanced Respiratory Therapist Exam Guide, Third Edition, is a wonderful—and must-have—resource for all graduates of respiratory care programs who are preparing for the National Board for Respiratory Care (NBRC) Written Registry Examination and Clinical Simulation Examination. In addition to the clear and precise presentation of the essential knowledge, skills, and professional attributes required by the NBRC examinations, the third edition of this textbook provides the following new and important features.

This new and outstanding exam guide text covers all the items listed as testable on the most recent NBRC Written Registry Exam and Clinical Simulation Exam content outlines. In additions, all the items no longer tested by the NBRC have been eliminated, numerous items have been updated, and new items have been added—especially in the new chapter on hyperinflation therapy. All of the postchapter questions have been updated, and a rationale is given for each question. Finally, the actual NBRC content outlines for the Written Registry Exam and Clinical Simulation Exam are included as appendices in this new *Advanced Respiratory Therapist Exam Guide* book.

Updated and current content is also provided in the Written Registry Exam pretest, posttest, and the 10 clinical simulation problems, which are provided on the CD-ROM bound into the back of the text. This computer-based testing format is an important resource that gives the student two separate opportunities to practice for the actual Written Registry Examination. A rationale is provided for each correct and incorrect answer, and a rationale is presented for every option in the 10 clinical simulation problems.

Once again, Jim Sills has created a very useful and important resource for students of respiratory therapy to successfully navigate the NBRC Written Registry Exam and Clinical Simulation Exam. Similar to how my past second-year students have found the earlier editions, I am confident that my future students will find *Advanced Respiratory Therapy Exam Guide,* Third Edition, to be a must-have resource!

Terry Des Jardins, MEd, RRT
Department of Respiratory Care Director
Professor Emeritus
Parkland College
Champaign, Illinois

Preface

Advanced Respiratory Therapist Exam Guide, Third Edition, has been updated to cover all items listed as testable by the National Board for Respiratory Care (NBRC) for the Written Registry Examination and Clinical Simulation Examination to earn the Registered Respiratory Therapist (RRT) credential. In August 2003, the NBRC published the RRT Examination Matrix, which detailed everything testable on the Written Registry Examination. In February 2005, the NBRC published the CSE Examination Outline, which detailed everything testable on the Clinical Simulation Examination. Both of these content outlines are printed here in their entirety so that the exam taker may compare what the NBRC has provided and my attempt to cover those items in this book. Whether a student is preparing for the Written Registry Examination or the Clinical Simulation Examination, this book should cover all items.

Based on these two NBRC content outlines, this book has been changed in the following ways: (1) new items have been added and discussed, (2) items that will no longer be tested have been deleted, (3) chapter "Exam Hints" have been updated to reflect the most commonly found question areas, (4) the end-of-chapter Self-Study Questions have been revised as necessary, (5) the pretest and posttest for the Written Registry Exam on the CD-ROM have been revised, and (6) the 10 patient scenarios for the practice Clinical Simulation Exam on the CD-ROM have been revised. It is my sincere hope that these revisions will help the exam taker to better focus on the key factors that will lead to successfully passing the NBRC's Written Registry Examination and Clinical Simulation Examination to earn the RRT credential.

James R. Sills, MEd, CPFT, RRT

Introduction

INTRODUCTION AND RECOMMENDATIONS FOR EXAM SUCCESS

This book was written to cover every testable item that could be found on the National Board for Respiratory Care (NBRC) Written Registry Examination and Clinical Simulation Examination. In August 2003, the NBRC published the *RRT Examination Matrix,* which detailed everything testable on the Written Registry Examination. In February 2005, the NBRC published the *CSE Examination Outline,* which covered everything testable on the Clinical Simulation Examination. Both of these content outlines are printed in this book and available from the NBRC at its website. Every item listed on these two content outlines is discussed in this book.

"Exam Hints" within the chapters point out commonly tested items. Self-assessment questions are included at the end of each chapter. The results of the Written Registry Exam pretest and posttest will help you analyze your strengths and weaknesses. It is recommended that the Written Registry Exam pretest on the enclosed CD-ROM be taken and analyzed before beginning the text and studying. After studying, take the Written Registry Examination posttest and Clinical Simulation Examination on the enclosed CD-ROM. Both Written Registry Examination sample tests are designed to follow the format, question styles, difficulty levels, and relative weight of tested areas as the real exam. The 10 Clinical Simulation Examination problems are the same mix of patient scenarios as seen on the actual exam.

The text includes bold topic headings followed by two codes. The **first code** will be either WRE for items found on the Written Registry Exam *and* Clinical Simulation Exam Written *or* CSE for items found only on the Clinical Simulation Exam. The first (in parentheses) is the NBRC code for that subject found in the two previously listed NBRC detailed content outlines. My choice of words for topic headings is a paraphrasing of the NBRC's. Occasionally a heading appears without an NBRC code after it. These headings were added to help you understand what the NBRC is testing for. Some discussion of pathologic processes is included in the general discussion of each chapter as they relate to the treatment or procedure that the respiratory therapist performs. It is recommended that you study the major types of adult and infant disease states and abnormal conditions.

The **second code** [in brackets] is the NBRC code for the difficulty level of the questions on the Written Registry Exam that will be used to test your understanding of the material. *R* stands for Recall, *Ap* stands for Application, and *An* stands for Analysis. You will find that the NBRC asks questions at these three different levels of difficulty. The NBRC does not provide a difficulty code for items tested on the Clinical Simulation Exam. Be prepared for any difficulty level in the 10 patient scenarios.

WRITTEN REGISTRY EXAMINATION

The Written Registry Examination is made up of *100 tested questions.* (However, the NBRC also includes 15 extra questions that are being pretested for future versions of the examination. *Therefore, you will answer a total of 115 questions.* These pretested questions are not scored as part of your exam, but, because you will not know which questions are real and which are being pretested, answer all questions to the best of your ability.) The examination is offered in a computer-based testing format through the Internet. You cannot bring a calculator or any other type of test aid device with you. A pencil and blank piece of paper is provided for making notes and calculations.

Make sure that you follow all commands on the computer screens so that you do not make any mistakes. You will have 2 hours to complete the examination. Pace yourself to be at about question 60 after 1 hour and question 115 after 2 hours. If you have difficulty with a question, make a note of it and move on. Go back to these near the end of the second hour. Do not leave any questions unanswered. A passing score is listed as 70% or higher (at least 70 correct questions). However, you can get less than 70 correct and still pass because the Application and Analysis questions are weighted more heavily than the Recall questions (see the following). Those who pass the exam (and the Clinical Simulation Examination) are awarded the Registered Respiratory Therapist (RRT) credential by the National Board for Respiratory Care.

The actual content of a given examination is a closely guarded secret. The NBRC usually maintains several exams at a given time, with others in production. Old exams are retired. Not everyone will be taking the same exam even at the same test site. The best way to prepare is to know the types of things that may be tested and how the test is constructed. There are three difficulty levels to the questions:

Recall [R]

Recall refers to remembering factual information that was previously learned. "Identify" is a commonly used action verb in this type of question. You may be asked to identify specific facts, terms, methods, procedures, principles, or concepts. Prepare for this type of question by studying the full range of factual information, equations, and so on that are seen in respiratory care practice. These types of questions are on the lowest order of difficulty. You either know the answer or you do not; there is little to ponder more deeply. It is very important to have a solid understanding of the factual basis of respiratory care to do well in this and the next two categories of questions.

Application [Ap]

Application refers to being able to use factual information in real clinical situations that may be new to you. "Apply," "classify," and "calculate" are commonly used action verbs in this type of question. You may be asked to apply laws, theories, concepts, and/or principles to new, practical clinical situations. Calculations may have to be performed. Charts and graphs, such as seen in pulmonary function testing, may need to be used. This type of question is on a higher order of difficulty than the Recall [R] type. Critical thinking must be applied to the factual information to answer these questions.

Analysis [An]

Analysis refers to being able to separate a patient care problem into its component parts or elements to evaluate the relationship of the parts or elements to the whole problem. "Evaluate," "compare," "contrast," "revise," and "select" are commonly used action verbs in this type of question. You may be questioned about revising a patient care plan or evaluating therapy. This type of question requires the highest level of critical thinking. You may have to recall previously learned information, apply it to a patient care situation, and make a judgment as to the best way to care for the patient.

You will find that the NBRC uses two different types of questions on the exam in the following three ways.

One Best Answer

This type of question has a stem (the question) followed by four possible answers coded A, B, C, and D. You must select the best answer from among those presented. Only one is clearly best even though other possible answers may be good. Carefully read the stem to make sure that you do not misunderstand the clear intent of the question.

Controversial issues may be questioned. The use of "should" in the stem will clue you in to the need to select the answer that would be selected by the majority of practitioners.

Some questions may be worded in such a way that you will need to exclude a false answer. In other words, three answers are correct and one is incorrect. The use of "except" will clue you in to this type of question. Other phrases to pay attention to include the following: "What is the *first* thing . . .," "What is the *most* important thing . . .," and "What is the *least* important thing. . . ."

Multiple True-False

This type of question has a stem (the question) followed by four or five possible answers coded with Roman numerals I, II, III, IV, and V; four combinations of the answers, coded by letters A, B, C, and D, follow. The stem may ask you to include all true statements or all false statements in the final answer. You must select the letter that represents the correct combination of answers.

No controversial answers should be offered. They are all either clearly correct or incorrect. That is the key to selecting the best answer. Read each possible answer as separate from the others. It is suggested that you mark each possible answer as true or false. Even if you are not sure of every option you should be able to determine the best answer.

Situational Sets

These are seen on the Entry Level Examination only. They have been replaced with the Clinical Simulation Examination for advanced practitioners.

Suggestions for Preparing for the Written Registry Examination

1. Pace yourself so that you have enough time to get through the 115 total questions before the 2-hour time limit is reached. You should be at about question 60 in 1 hour. Make a note on your blank paper on any difficult questions that you skip or want to go back to. You can also "bookmark" any questions you want to come back to later. The computer-based test will prompt you if any questions have been skipped. Come back to them at the end of the test time. Do not leave any blank questions. You will not be penalized for guessing on the last few questions if you are running out of time.
2. Completely read each question. Determine what it is that you are really being asked. Look for qualifying words such as "not," "except," "most," "least desirable," "undesirable," and so forth.
3. Separate the important information from that which is not important. Many questions contain patient information and data on blood gases, pulmonary function, hemodynamics, ventilator settings, and so on. Disregard what does not pertain to the question being asked. Interpret the important data.

4. Do not read beyond the question. Resist the temptation to "psych out" what you think the question writer wants. Use only what is given to you.
5. Carefully read every answer that is offered.
6. In one best answer (multiple-choice) questions, pick the best answer that is offered. The answer that you might like best may not be offered. Regardless, you must pick from among those that are offered.
7. In multiple true-false (multiple-multiple choice) questions, use the following strategy: (1) Find an option that you know to be incorrect and cross off any of the answers that contain it; (2) find an option that you know to be correct and cross off any answers that do not contain it; (3) find the remaining answer, which must be correct.
8. Again, answer every question. There is no penalty for guessing incorrectly.
9. Take a practice Written Registry Examination under actual testing conditions. Evaluate your strengths and weaknesses and spend more time studying your weak areas. The CD-ROM with this book contains a computer-based pretest and posttest formatted like the actual examination. Other exams are available through the Internet from the NBRC. The NBRC's address is included at the end of this Introduction.

Relative Weights of the Various Tested Areas on the Written Registry Exam

I have attempted to analyze the content of each of the 100 questions on the available Written Registry Examinations covering the content of the 2003 examination content outline. Each question has been matched to one of the chapters in this book, listed in Table 1. The numbers of questions and percentages are averages and may not be followed exactly on all versions of the examination. However, the relative weights can offer solid guidance as to what content is relatively more important or less important. Study time can be spent accordingly.

The content of chapters 1, 3, 4, and 5 must be thoroughly understood. This information is questioned directly and also incorporated into questions that cover all the other chapters. The content in Chapter 15, "Mechanical Ventilation of the Adult," is the most heavily questioned of all the chapters. You *must* understand mechanical ventilation to do well on the Written Registry Exam and the Clinical Simulation Exam.

CLINICAL SIMULATION EXAMINATION

The Clinical Simulation Examination (CSE) is composed of *10 broad-based patient problems.* They are designed to evaluate how well the exam taker is able to gather information,

TABLE 1 Examination Content Found in Each Chapter	
Chapter	Question Numbers/Percentage of the Examination Content
1. Patient Assessment	15
2. Infection Control	1
3. Blood Gas Analysis and Monitoring	5
4. Pulmonary Function Testing	4
5. Advanced Cardiopulmonary Monitoring	3
6. Oxygen and Medical Gas Therapy	7
7. Hyperinflation Therapy	2
8. Humidity and Aerosol Therapy	2
9. Pharmacology	6
10. Bronchopulmonary Hygiene Therapy	3
11. Cardiac Monitoring and Cardiopulmonary Resuscitation	5
12. Airway Management	6
13. Suctioning the Airway	3
14. Intermittent Positive-Pressure Breathing (IPPB)	2
15. Mechanical Ventilation of the Adult	23
16. Mechanical Ventilation of the Neonate	2
17. Home Care and Pulmonary Rehabilitation	5
18. Special Procedures	6
Pathology	1
TOTAL	100

BOX 1   The Mix of 10 Problems Found on the Clinical Simulation Examination

1. Two adult patients with chronic obstructive pulmonary disease (COPD). These patients could have chronic bronchitis, emphysema, and/or asthma. Areas of focus on the simulation include, but are not limited to, pre- and postoperative evaluation, critical care management, mechanical ventilation, pulmonary function testing, home care, rehabilitation, and infection control.
2. One or two adult patients with trauma. These patients could have chest, head, or skeletal injuries; surface burns; smoke inhalation, carbon monoxide poisoning; or hypothermia.
3. One or two adult patients with cardiovascular disease. These patients could have congestive heart failure, coronary artery disease, myocardial infarction, valvular heart disease, or cardiac surgery.
4. One or two adult patients with neurologic or neuromuscular diseases. These patients could have myasthenia gravis, Guillain-Barré syndrome, tetanus, muscular dystrophy, cerebrovascular accident (stroke), or drug overdosage.
5. One pediatric patient. This patient could have epiglottitis, laryngotracheobronchitis (croup), bronchiolitis, asthma, cystic fibrosis, foreign body aspiration, toxic substance ingestion, or bronchopulmonary dysplasia.
6. One neonatal patient. This patient could require care in the delivery room; need resuscitation; or have infant apnea, meconium aspiration, respiratory distress syndrome, or a congenital heart defect.
7. The *possible* miscellaneous category could involve one adult patient with a medical or surgical problem. This could include head, neck, or thoracic surgery; obesity-hypoventilation syndrome; or acquired immunodeficiency syndrome (AIDS).

---

evaluate it, and make clinical decisions that relate to simulated real patient situations. This test does *not* look at the recollection of simple facts. Box 1 lists the types of patient care problems that will be seen. In addition, the CSE will include one additional simulated patient problem that is being evaluated for possible inclusion on a future exam. You will have a *total of 11 patient problems* on the exam. Because you cannot tell which scenario is being pretested, approach each one seriously.

The computer-based examination process is unique. Each clinical simulation problem is designed to flow in the same manner in which actual patient data is delivered and care decisions are made. Therefore, the problems are designed in a branching logic format. This means that there may be more than one way to solve them. To some extent, you choose your own path; however, only one path is best. There may be one or two that are acceptable. There may be another one or two that are unacceptable. The exam taker is allowed 4 hours to complete the exam, which works out to about 20 minutes per problem.

There are three components to the clinical simulation problem: (1) the scenario, (2) the information-gathering sections, and (3) the decision-making sections. Each is discussed in turn.

Scenario

The scenario establishes the setting for the patient and for you as the respiratory therapist. Typically, it includes the type of hospital, where the patient is within the hospital, and the time of day. General information about the patient, such as name, age, and sex; some general presenting conditions; and a brief history of the illness or event, is given. Your role as a respiratory therapist is described. You may have to gather more information or may need to make a clinical decision. Determine if the situation is an emergency. If it is, you will have to take immediate steps

to help the patient. (The exam taker should assume that any and all services needed to give optimal care are available in any of the patient scenarios.)

Information-Gathering Sections

Usually, the respiratory therapist is directed to gather more information. A list of about 15 to 20 parameters from which to choose—for example, vital signs, blood gases, pulmonary function tests, various laboratory studies, and so forth—will be available. You will be instructed to select as many as you believe are important based on what you know at that point in time. Obviously, you should not select information that is unnecessarily risky or irrelevant or that delays important care. Select the desired information. The computer screen will then reveal the data. Interpret the data to make the proper decisions in the next section. When you have finished gathering and interpreting the data, you will be directed to go to a decision-making section. Typically there are two to four information-gathering steps in each clinical simulation problem.

Decision-Making Sections

It is now required that you make a decision on the best care for the patient based on the information that you have at this point in time. Usually you are instructed to "choose only one" from about four to eight options. One of the choices is best, one or two may be acceptable, and the others are not acceptable. Select the option and the computer will reveal the answer. Usually it will say "Physician agrees. Done" or something to that effect. One or more of the available answers will reveal "Physician disagrees. Make another selection in this section" when it is exposed. This may or may not mean that a bad choice was made. It is possible that the author of the scenario simply does not want to follow that particular course of action.

Occasionally, you will be directed to "select as many as indicated" for the situation with which you are dealing. This involves a scenario in which proper care includes several procedures being done simultaneously with a patient. Again, select the options, and the computer will reveal the answer.

Whether you are directed to make one or several decisions, when finished, you will be instructed to go to a new area. This usually takes you to another information-gathering section. You will now need to evaluate how the patient responded to your earlier decision(s). You will then need to make one or more patient care decisions. Typically, there are 8 to 10 decision-making steps in each clinical simulation pattern. This pattern of information gathering and decision making repeats itself until the problem is ended. You will then go on to the next problem until all 10 have been completed. See Table 2 for how this unique examination is scored.

Each problem is individually scored for information gathering and decision making based on the judgment of the problem author and the examination committee. The scores in these two areas on all 11 problems are totaled to give two final scores. Both the information-gathering and decision-making areas must be passed to pass the examination. The examination committee determines the two required scores to pass the Clinical Simulation Examination. These scores may vary from exam to exam, but a score of at least 65% on both exam areas is needed to pass the Clinical Simulation Examination.

Suggestions for Preparing for the Clinical Simulation Examination

Things you should do:

1. Carefully follow all directions. If instructed to make only one choice, make only one.
2. Read the scenario to understand the patient's situation and what you are required to do. Is this an emergency? If it is, you will want to gather only the most vital information needed to make a patient care decision. Quick action will be required to decide on the best care to give. If it is not an emergency, a more thorough gathering of data is called for. Then a more well-considered decision for patient care can be made.
3. Know the rules for the initiation and changing of mechanical ventilation parameters. Use 10 mL/kg of ideal body weight for the initial tidal volume setting. Make adjustments from there based on arterial blood gas results.
4. Thoroughly read all options. For information-gathering sections, make a list of each desirable option on your paper before making your choices. Choose all the options that will give you important information. You will be penalized for skipping over important data and also for making dangerous or wasteful choices. When you are sure of your selections, reveal them all and then review and interpret them. Avoid the temptation to reveal and interpret one piece of data at a time. You may mistakenly decide not to gather some important information later.
5. Try to visualize yourself in the real situation as described. Do what you would do on the job. Make the best choice(s) that you can based on what you know at this point. This is true for both information-gathering and decision-making sections. It may be necessary to go back over past information or choices.
6. It is recommended that you make a map on your paper of where you have been for each of the 11 problems. This will help you keep track of past choices.
7. Pace yourself to get through all 11 problems in the 4-hour time limit. That gives you about 20 minutes per problem. For example, you should be finishing your third problem after 1 hour. Unlike on the Written Registry Exam, you should *not* rush ahead at the end and pick just anything. You will be penalized for incorrect choices.

TABLE 2	Scoring of the Clinical Simulation Problem and Examination
All the options selected on each problem are scored on the following scale. The score is based on how appropriate it is to the condition of the patient at the time it was selected.	
Score	**Score Rationale**
+3	Critically important for good patient care. It is necessary for prompt, proper care. Omitting it would result in the patient being seriously harmed from delays in care, pain, cost, and increased chance of morbidity and/or mortality.
+2	Very important for good patient care.
+1	Helpful for good patient care.
0	Neither helpful nor harmful to patient care.
−1	Somewhat counterproductive to good patient care.
−2	Quite counterproductive to good patient care.
−3	Extremely counterproductive to good patient care. Detrimental to prompt, proper care. Its inclusion will result in the patient being seriously harmed from delays in care, pain, cost, and increased chance of morbidity and/or mortality.

8. Take a practice Clinical Simulation Examination. Ten practice patient simulations are offered on the CD-ROM with this book. Others are available by the Internet from the NBRC.

Things you should avoid:

1. Do not try to jump ahead in the problem or guess what the author is leading to. With the branching logic format, there are several possible pathways. Work only with what you know now and from the past.

2. Try not to become flustered if you are faced with a scenario you have never experienced at work. Imagine what you would do if faced with this problem and go from there. Also, do not become frustrated if the choice that you prefer is not available. There is more than one way to take care of a patient's problems. Make your next best choice and move on.

3. Do not make changes in patient care unless they are needed. If a patient is stable with acceptable arterial blood gas values and vital signs, be content to leave the patient as he or she is.

4. Do not get flustered by patient complications or equipment problems. They do not mean that you did anything wrong! They are meant to test your ability to solve problems.

5. Do not select everything in the information-gathering section. You will lose points by choosing unimportant, time-consuming, unnecessarily expensive, or dangerous procedures.

6. Avoid selecting new or unusual procedures that you are not familiar with—jet ventilation, for example. You will lower your score if you do not know how to operate the equipment properly.

7. Do not misinterpret the data you are given. Avoid assumptions about things that are not spelled out for you.

SUMMARY—GENERAL SUGGESTIONS FOR EITHER EXAMINATION

1. Take the Written Registry Exam pretest included in the CD-ROM that accompanies this book. Evaluate your results to find your strengths and weaknesses.

2. Begin studying about 2 months before the exam. Pace yourself so that everything can be covered in the time that you have. Avoid "cramming" a few days before the examination; these tests demand more than the simple recall of facts.

3. Study the most important and heavily tested areas first. Work down to the less important ones.

4. Focus on the areas where you are weakest, especially if they are heavily tested.

5. Take the Written Registry Exam posttest and Clinical Simulation Exam included on the CD-ROM.

6. If it is necessary to travel out of your hometown to take the exam, arrive at the city where the test will be given the evening before the exam. Make a practice drive from your motel to the test site and see where you will park. Check the time required to get there and add more for the morning traffic.

7. Have a good dinner. Avoid alcohol, even if you are nervous, to keep a clear head in the morning.

8. Do not cram for the exam back at the motel. Unfortunately, if you are not prepared by now, a few more hours will not really help. If necessary, brush up on only a few test areas.

9. Set the alarm to get you up in plenty of time to be ready. Get a good night's sleep. Avoid sleeping pills.

10. Eat a good breakfast to get you through to lunch. Minimize caffeine. You will have plenty of adrenaline running through your system to keep you awake while taking the test!

11. Attempt to relax with the self-confidence that comes from knowing that you are well prepared.

IMPORTANT ADDRESSES AND PHONE NUMBERS

For information on the examination processes, taking a practice exam, scheduling an exam date and location (linking to Applied Measurement Professionals), and getting a copy of the exam detailed content outlines, contact:

National Board for Respiratory Care
8310 Nieman Road
Lenexa, KS 66214-1579
Telephone: (913) 599-4200
Fax: (913) 541-0156
E-mail: nbrc-info@nbrc.org
Internet address: http://www.nbrc.org

For information on examination sites and to schedule an exam, contact:

Applied Measurement Professionals
8310 Nieman Road
Lenexa, KS 66214-1579
Telephone: (913) 541-0400
Fax: (913) 541-0156
Internet address: http://www.goAMP.com

For information on accredited respiratory care educational programs, contact:

Committee on Accreditation for Respiratory Care
1248 Harwood Road
Bedford, TX 76021-4244
Telephone: (817) 283-2835
Fax: (817) 354-8519
Internet address: http://www.coarc.com

For information on state credentialing requirements, contact:

American Association for Respiratory Care
9425 N. MacArthur Boulevard
Suite 100
Irving, TX 75063-4706
Telephone: (972) 243-AARC (2272)
Fax: (972) 484-2720
E-mail: info@aarc.org
Internet address: http://www.aarc.org

Contents

1 Patient Assessment and Care Management

Note 1: The National Board for Respiratory Care (NBRC) has released the *RRT Examination Matrix* (covering the testable items on the Written Registry Exam) and the *CSE Examination Matrix* (covering the testable items on the Clinical Simulation Exam). Turn to the appendices at the back of this book for both publications in their original format. This book is intended to cover all of the testable items in these two publications. This chapter (and all others) uses the abbreviation "WRE" for the coded items testable on the Written Registry Exam *and* the Clinical Simulation Exam. The listed difficulty (R, Recall; Ap, Application; An, Analysis) relates to the question difficulty on the Written Registry Exam. The abbreviation "CSE" will be used for the coded items testable *only* on the Clinical Simulation Exam. Because no question difficulty level is given for this exam, be prepared for anything.

Note 2: A review of the most recent Written Registry Examinations has shown an average of 15 questions (15% of the exam) that cover patient assessment and care management. Of these 15 questions, an average of 11 cover patient assessment and an average of 4 cover care management. Typically, nine of the patient-assessment questions deal with adult patients. The remaining two patient-assessment questions deal with neonatal or pediatric patients. The Clinical Simulation Exam is comprehensive and may include everything that should be known or performed by an advanced level respiratory therapist.

Note 3: The Written Registry Exam has shown an average of one question (1% of the exam) that directly covers a cardiopulmonary pathology issue. It is beyond the scope of this book to cover all of the cardiopulmonary diseases and conditions that befall patients whom respiratory therapists may care for. It is recommended that asthma, chronic obstructive pulmonary disease (COPD; emphysema or chronic bronchitis or both), pneumonia, pneumothorax, flail chest, congestive heart failure with pulmonary edema, myasthenia gravis, Guillain-Barré syndrome, head (brain) injury with increased intracranial pressure, pediatric croup and epiglottitis, infant respiratory distress syndrome, acute (adult) respiratory distress syndrome (ARDS), and smoke inhalation with carbon monoxide poisoning be studied. Some limited discussion of these topics is covered in this book. The Written Registry Exam will frequently ask questions about the respiratory therapy procedures that patients with these types of problems are receiving. In addition, the 10 Clinical Simulation Exam scenarios are built around the care of patients with these types of diseases and conditions. See Box 1 in the Introduction.

PART 1. PATIENT ASSESSMENT

MODULE A

Review the patient's chart for the following data and recommend the following diagnostic procedures based on current information

Note: The following discussion involves noninvasive, bedside activities that apply to adults in most respiratory care settings. Some assessment items have been placed in later chapters because they are procedure specific. Topics that relate to neonates and children are included in Module H.

1. **Review the patient's history: present illness, admission notes, diagnosis, progress notes, do not resuscitate orders, and respiratory care orders (WRE code: IA1) [Difficulty: Ap, An]**
   a. Patient history

Review the complete initial patient history and note the following:

1. Date of history taking
2. Patient data: name, age, sex, race, and occupation
3. Primary complaints
4. Secondary complaints
5. Present illness history and symptoms
6. Family history
7. Medical history of cardiopulmonary disease(s)

After the medical history is completed, the patient should be placed into one of the following four categories. Refer to Table 1-1 for examples of each category.

1. Crisis/acute onset of illness
2. Intermittent but repeated illness
3. Progressive worsening
4. Mixed patterns/multiple problems

It is important to obtain a *brief* history before beginning therapeutic procedures. Determine how the patient has been doing since the last treatment. Has there been a change in dyspnea, cough and secretions, chest pain, and so on? This will help guide therapy as effectively as possible.

TABLE 1-1 Patient Illness Categories

Category	Examples
Crisis/acute onset of illness	Trauma, heart attack, allergic reaction, aspiration of a foreign body, pneumothorax, pulmonary embolism, and some pneumonias
Intermittent but repeated illness	Asthma, chronic bronchitis, congestive heart failure, angina pectoris, myasthenia gravis, and some pneumonias
Progressive worsening	Congestive heart failure, chronic bronchitis, emphysema, and upper respiratory tract infection leading to bronchitis or pneumonia
Mixed patterns/ multiple problems	Chronic obstructive pulmonary disease and cystic fibrosis complicated by multiple problems, mucous plugging, or infection; mixes of congestive heart failure and chronic lung disease; mixes of neuromuscular and lung disease; mixes of renal failure and congestive heart failure with chronic lung disease

b. Do not resuscitate status

The physician and patient and family should determine the patient's cardiopulmonary resuscitation status. A patient with a terminal condition, such as end-stage COPD, will often choose not to be resuscitated. If it has been determined that the patient does not want to be resuscitated, his or her do not resuscitate (DNR) status should be clearly posted in the chart and in the patient's room. All members of the health care team should be aware of the patient's decision.

c. Current respiratory care orders

Physician orders must have the patient's name, date, time, complete and proper orders for each therapeutic procedure, and the physician's signature. Verbal orders from the physician to the nurse or respiratory therapist must follow hospital guidelines and include the preceding information. Incomplete, improper, or questionable orders must be confirmed by calling the physician for clarification or correction.

d. Progress notes

Review the physician's, nurse's, and respiratory therapist's patient progress notes before seeing the patient and beginning the therapeutic procedure. Look for any cardiopulmonary or other organ-system changes that will have an impact on the patient's ability to take the treatment. You may need to revise the therapy, get different equipment, or seek help. Check for new patient care orders if the physician notes a change in the patient's care plan.

2. Review the results of the patient's physical examination and vital signs (WRE code: IA2) [Difficulty: An]

Review the results of the physical examinations performed by physicians, nurses, and respiratory therapists. Review the following organ systems:

1. Pulmonary
2. Cardiovascular
3. Neuromuscular
4. Renal

3. Review the results of the patient's serum electrolyte levels and other blood chemistries (WRE code: IA3) [Difficulty: Ap, An]

The serum (blood) electrolytes are commonly measured in most patients as they are being admitted to the hospital and as needed after that. This is to determine whether they are within the normal ranges listed in Table 1-2. Any abnormality should be promptly corrected so that the patient's nervous system, muscle function, and cellular processes can be optimized. Diet and a number of medications have effects on the various electrolytes. Most abnormalities can be corrected by dietary adjustments or, if necessary, by oral or intravenous supplement.

1. Potassium (K^+)

    Potassium is the most important electrolyte to monitor because of its effect on general nerve function and cardiac function. Hyperkalemia is a high blood level of potassium that causes the following electrocardiographic (ECG) changes: high, peaked T waves and depressed S-T segments, widening QRS complex, and bradycardia. Hypokalemia is a low blood level and will

TABLE 1-2 Normal Serum Electrolyte and Glucose Levels

NORMAL ELECTROLYTE VALUES*	
Chloride (Cl^-)	95–106 mEq/L
Potassium (K^+)	3.5–5.5 mEq/L
Sodium (Na^+)	135–145 mEq/L
Calcium (Ca^{++})	4.5–5.5 mEq/L
Bicarbonate (HCO_3^-)	22–25 mEq/L
NORMAL GLUCOSE VALUES*	
Serum or plasma	70–110 mg/100 mL (dL)
Whole blood	60–100 mg/100 mL (dL)

* These values may vary somewhat among references.

cause the following ECG changes: flat or inverted T waves, depression of the S-T segments, premature ventricular contractions (PVCs), and ventricular fibrillation (if severe enough). Chapter 11 offers a more complete discussion of ECG interpretation.

Exam Hint

Hypokalemia may be caused by the use of diuretic medications such as furosemide (Lasix). Signs of hypokalemia include the cardiac rhythm disturbances noted previously and muscle weakness. In addition, a metabolic alkalosis is found when interpreting the results of an arterial blood gas analysis. Be prepared to recommend the administration of potassium if the serum level is low.

---

2. Chloride (Cl^-)
   Hyperchloremia is a high blood level of chloride that causes a significant prolongation of the ST segment and the QT interval on the ECG. Hypochloremia is a low blood level that causes the QT interval to be shortened and perhaps widens and rounds off the T waves on the ECG.
3. Sodium (Na^+)
   Hypernatremia is a high blood level of sodium that might be seen in a patient who is dehydrated or has been given excessive amounts of sodium intravenously. Hyponatremia is a low blood level that might be seen in a patient who has lost many gastrointestinal secretions because of vomiting, nasogastric tube drainage, or diarrhea.
4. Bicarbonate (HCO_3^-)
   Altered bicarbonate levels are commonly seen in patients with pulmonary conditions. The kidneys of patients with a chronically elevated $PaCO_2$ typically retain bicarbonate to moderate the respiratory acidosis caused by the elevated carbon dioxide level. Conversely, the kidneys of patients with a chronically decreased $PaCO_2$ level excrete bicarbonate to moderate the respiratory alkalosis caused by the decreased $PaCO_2$ level.
5. Calcium (Ca^{++})
   Hypercalcemia is an elevated level of calcium that may be associated with patients taking diuretics. ECG changes associated with an increased calcium level include a shortened QT interval and widened and rounded T waves. Hypocalcemia is a decreased level of calcium. ECG changes include a lengthening of the ST segment and the QT interval.
6. Glucose
   The blood glucose level is important to monitor because it directly relates to how much sugar is available to the patient for energy for daily activities. The normal values are listed in Table 1-2. Hypoglycemia is a low blood level of glucose; it can mean that the patient is malnourished. Hyperglycemia is a high blood level that can indicate that the patient has diabetes mellitus, has Cushing's disease, or is being treated with corticosteroids. More-specific testing must be done to prove the diagnosis.

4. Review the patient's urinalysis (WRE code: IA3) [Difficulty: Ap, An]

A urine sample is routinely taken from every patient admitted to the hospital, pregnant women, and presurgical patients. Much information about the functioning of the kidneys and other metabolic processes can be gathered from the urinalysis results. A urinalysis also is done for diagnostic purposes in patients with abdominal or back pain, hematuria, and chronic renal disease. Table 1-3 lists the normal findings found in a urinalysis. Any abnormal findings should be further investigated to discover the cause.

5. Review the results of the patient's complete blood count (WRE code: IA3) [Difficulty: Ap, An]

A complete blood count (CBC) is routinely done on all hospitalized patients and patients being seen for a variety of illnesses and for routine physical examinations. The red blood cell (RBC or erythrocyte) count, white blood cell (WBC or leukocyte) count, and differential (Diff) provide a great deal of information about the hematologic system and many other organ systems.

The key normal RBC count values are listed in Table 1-4. The hemoglobin and hematocrit values are important because they directly relate to the patient's oxygen-carrying capacity. Decreased hemoglobin and hematocrit values indicate that the patient is anemic. An anemic patient has less oxygen-carrying capacity, which places more stress on the heart during exercise. Hypoxemia resulting from a cardiopulmonary abnormality places this patient at great risk. A transfusion is indicated if the hematocrit is below what the physician considers to be a clinically safe level.

TABLE 1-3	Normal Urinalysis Results
Test Item	**Normal Value**
Appearance	Clear
Color	Amber yellow
pH	4.6–8.0 (average 6.0)
Specific gravity	Adult: 1.005–1.030 (usually 1.010–1.025)
	Newborn: 1.001–1.020
White blood cells	0–4
Red blood cells	0–2

TABLE 1-4	Normal Hemoglobin, Hematocrit, and Red Blood Cell Counts for Adults and Children		
	Adult*	Infant*	Child*
HEMOGLOBIN (in g/100 mL [g/dL])			
Female	12.0–16.0	12.2–20.0	11.2–13.4
Male	13.5–18.0	Same	Same
HEMATOCRIT (in mL/100 mL [mL/dL])			
Female	38%–47%		
Male	40%–54%		
RED BLOOD CELL COUNT (in millions/mL)			
Female	4.2–5.4	5.0–5.1	4.6–4.8
Male	4.6–6.2	Same	Same

* These values may vary somewhat among references.

Increased numbers of circulating erythrocytes indicate that the patient has polycythemia. When this is seen as a response to chronic hypoxemia from COPD, cyanotic congenital heart disease, or another disorder, it is labeled *secondary polycythemia*. This patient is at added risk because the thickened blood causes an increased afterload against which the heart must pump. These patients also are more prone to blood clots. Supplemental oxygen or other clinical treatment to increase the PaO_2 to at least 55 to 60 torr will, over time, result in the erythrocyte and hematocrit levels returning to normal.

The key normal leukocyte count and differential are listed in Table 1-5. A normal leukocyte count and differential count reveals two things about the patient. First, no active bacterial infection is present. Second, the patient has the ability to produce the normal number and variety of WBCs to combat an infection.

A mild to moderate increase in the leukocyte count is called leukocytosis. It is seen as a WBC count of 11,000 to 17,000 per cubic millimeter (mm^3). Usually the higher the count, the more severe the infection. A WBC count of

more than 17,000/mm^3 is seen in patients with severe sepsis, miliary tuberculosis, and other overwhelming infections. An extreme shift to the left in the differential count means a significant increase in the number of neutrophils. This is usually seen when a patient has an acute, severe bacterial infection. Exceptions to this are patients who are elderly, have acquired immunodeficiency syndrome (AIDS), or have other immunodeficiencies. They may have an infection but show only a mildly elevated WBC count.

Leukopenia is a low absolute WBC count of 3000 to 5000/mm^3 or less. An acute viral infection can cause a mild to moderate decrease in the neutrophil count. The patient who has a low WBC count is at great risk of bacterial or other infections.

6. Review the patient's coagulation study results (WRE code: IA3) [Difficulty: Ap, An]

Coagulation studies are routinely done on many hospitalized patients, those who are to have surgery, or if a blood-clotting disorder is known or suspected. Additionally, many medications speed or slow clotting time (so-called blood thinners). It is important to review a patient's coagulation studies before drawing a blood sample or performing a procedure that may lead to bleeding. Table 1-6 lists normal coagulation study results. If the patient's clotting time is increased, he or she is at risk of bleeding. Be prepared to apply pressure to a blood-sampling site (especially if arterial) longer than expected.

7. Gram stain results, culture results, and antibiotic sensitivity results

a. Recommend a Gram stain and culture-and-sensitivity study (WRE code: IA3) [Difficulty: Ap, An]

Whenever an infection is suspected, it is important to obtain a sample of fluid or tissue from the site in question. This patient material is tested for possible bacterial infection by a Gram stain and culture-and-sensitivity (C & S) study. Whenever bronchitis or pneumonia is suspected, it is important to obtain a mucus or sputum sample for evaluation. A sample of mucus suctioned from the lungs should

TABLE 1-5	White Blood Cell and Differential Counts
WHITE BLOOD CELL COUNT (mm^3)*	
Adult	4500–11,000
Infant and child	9000–33,000
DIFFERENTIAL COUNT*	
Segmented neutrophil	40%–75%
Lymphocytes	20%–45%
Monocytes	2%–10%
Eosinophils	0%–6%
Bands	0%–6%
Basophils	0%–1%

* These values may vary somewhat among references.

TABLE 1-6	Normal Coagulation Study Results	
Test Name	Normal Value	Critical Value
Bleeding time	1–9 min	>15 min
Prothrombin time (PT or Pro-time)	11.0–12.5 sec; 85%–100%	>20 sec
Partial thromboplastin time (PTT)	60–70 sec	>100 sec
Activated partial thromboplastin time (APTT)	30–40 sec	>70 sec

show only pulmonary organisms. Sputum is the mix of mucus from the lungs and saliva from the mouth; therefore the organisms that are found in it may have come from either place. If the patient has pleural fluid, that also must be sampled. Often a blood sample also is taken to look for evidence of a septicemia.

b. Review the patient's Gram stain results, culture results, and antibiotic sensitivity results (WRE code: IA3) [Difficulty: Ap, An]

The first step in the microbial analysis of sputum, mucus, and so on is a Gram stain. It is a special staining process to colorize bacteria into one of two groups. Gram$^+$ (g$^+$) bacteria are stained violet. The most common types of bacteria that cause bronchitis and pneumonia are g$^+$. In general, penicillin or related drugs and sulfa-type antibiotics kill these bacteria. Gram$^-$ (g$^-$) bacteria are stained pink. These organisms, unfortunately, are found in many of the sickest and weakest patients. Often the only way to kill these bacteria is with a specific antibiotic to which they have been proven sensitive. So-called *broad-spectrum antibiotics*, such as tetracycline, may also be used.

After the sample of fluid or tissue is Gram stained, a C & S test is performed. Culturing involves actively growing the organism(s) to determine what they are. A sensitivity test is the act of exposing the cultured organisms to a variety of antimicrobial drugs. The goal is to find which drug(s) kill the pathogen most effectively. The patient is then treated with that antibiotic. It may take 1 to 3 days to get the C & S results back.

Viruses cannot be identified by Gram stain. The Ziehl-Neelsen stain has been widely used to identify the *Mycobacterium tuberculosis* (TB) organism. Other pathogens, such as protozoa and fungi, need specialized stains for identification. Fungi and *M. tuberculosis* may take 6 to 8 weeks to culture.

8. Review the patient's pleural fluid study results (WRE code: IA3) [Difficulty: Ap, An]

If a patient has had a thoracentesis procedure to remove pleural fluid, the fluid is sent to the laboratory for further analysis. The fluid may turn out to be watery, bloody, infected, or lymphatic. See Chapter 18 for a complete discussion of the types of pleural fluids.

MODULE B
Radiographic imaging

1. Review the patient's imaging findings (WRE code: IA6) [Difficulty: Ap, An]

Look for the results of radiographs (x-rays) of the chest or upper airway, computed tomography (CT) scans, positron emission tomography (PET) scans, ventilation/perfusion ($\dot{V}/\dot{Q}$) scans, angiograms, barium swallow, and magnetic resonance image (MRI) studies. If possible, view these results to gain a better understanding of the patient's condition.

2. Recommend radiographic and other imaging studies (WRE code: IC1) [Difficulty: Ap, An]

A *chest radiograph* should be recommended in the following situations:

a. After an endotracheal or tracheostomy tube has been placed or repositioned
b. After the jugular/subclavian route has been used to insert a central venous pressure (CVP) or pulmonary artery (Swan-Ganz) catheter
c. After a chest tube has been placed in the pleural space to remove air or fluids
d. Hemoptysis (bloody sputum)
e. A sudden deleterious change is noted in the patient's cardiopulmonary condition
f. The balloon on the pulmonary artery (Swan-Ganz) catheter has been inflated for a prolonged period, and a pulmonary infarct is suspected
g. A pneumothorax is suspected

> **Exam Hint**
>
> **E**xpect to see at least one question in which the respiratory therapist should recommend a chest radiograph to rule out or confirm a pneumothorax. Signs and symptoms that the patient may have a pneumothorax include the following: sudden chest pain with an increase in dyspnea and shortness of breath (SOB), absent breath sounds over a lung field, tracheal deviation and heart sounds shifted to the side opposite the pneumothorax, asymmetrical chest movement, hyperresonant percussion noted over the pneumothorax, sudden increase in peak pressure or plateau pressure or both on the patient's ventilator, or air in the soft tissues, or a combination of these. Also be prepared for questions related to recommendation of a chest radiograph to check the placement of an endotracheal tube or to check for a foreign body obstructing the upper airway or a bronchus.

An *upper airway radiograph* (anterior or lateral or both) should be recommended in a patient who presents with indications of upper airway obstruction. This can include:

a. Aspirated foreign body
b. Laryngeal edema
c. Laryngeal tumor
d. Laryngotracheal bronchitis (LTB or croup) versus epiglottitis (see Module H for more information)

A *CT scan* provides a more detailed image than a conventional radiograph. It is able to identify abnormalities of the lungs and mediastinum. Indications include, but are not limited to, the following:

a. Tumor
b. Hematoma
c. Abscess and cyst
d. Pleural effusion
e. Aortic or other vascular abnormalities (after intravenous contrast material is given)

A *PET scan* procedure involves a radioactive substance being either inhaled or given intravenously. As the radioactive substance breaks down in the target organ, it emits a positron (a positive electron). When the positron combines with an electron, they annihilate each other with the release of two gamma rays. Detectors outside the body identify the origin of the gamma rays and can then determine the functioning and metabolism of the target organ. Indications for a PET scan include, but are not limited to, the following:

a. Determining the regional metabolism of the heart and brain.
b. Measuring the size of a myocardial infarction.
c. Measuring the effects of treatment on a cancerous tumor.
d. Determining pulmonary perfusion or ventilation.

A *ventilation/perfusion* ($\dot{V}/\dot{Q}$) *scan* is used to identify where air moves into the lungs during breathing and blood flows through the lungs. A ventilation scan ($\dot{V}$ scan) is performed to verify or refute the clinical suspicion that a patient has an area of the lung(s) that is underventilated. Abnormal ventilation is seen in the case of a bronchial obstruction from a tumor or foreign body or an alveolar problem such as atelectasis, consolidation, or emphysema. Radioactive xenon (^{133}Xe) is mixed with oxygen and inhaled to show the lung fields. A special scanner is used to "pick up" the radioactivity through the chest wall. Areas of normal ventilation can be compared with underventilated areas.

A perfusion scan ($\dot{Q}$ scan) is performed to verify or refute the clinical suspicion that a patient has an area of pulmonary circulation that is underperfused. Abnormal perfusion is seen in the case of a pulmonary embolism, tumor, or vascular problem such as pulmonary hypertension. Radioactive technetium (^{99m}Tc) is injected into the patient's venous system, where it is filtered out by the pulmonary circulation. As previously described, a special scanner is used to pick up the radioactivity through the chest wall. Areas of normal perfusion can be compared with underperfused areas. The ventilation scan and perfusion scan tests can be done singly or as a set.

Comparing the ventilation and perfusion results side by side enables the physician to look for areas of mismatching. Normally, ventilation and perfusion match fairly closely and result in a 1:1 mix of air and blood at the alveolar capillary membrane. A pulmonary embolism results in a $\dot{V}/\dot{Q}$ ratio of 2 (or greater):1 (or less) because normal ventilation is present and perfusion is reduced or absent. An obstructed airway with resulting atelectasis results in a $\dot{V}/\dot{Q}$ ratio of 1 (or less):2 (or greater) because ventilation is reduced or absent, and perfusion is normal.

An *angiogram* involves the placement of a catheter into an artery or vein. Commonly a radioactive dye is injected so that the flow of blood through the vessel can be observed. If a blockage is found, a balloon at the tip of the catheter may be inflated (balloon angioplasty) to flatten the blockage. Indications for an angiogram include, but are not limited to, the following:

a. Check blood flow through the carotid arteries and into the brain.
b. Check blood flow through the coronary arteries and the chambers of the heart.
c. Check blood flow through the pulmonary arteries when perfusion study results are inconclusive.
d. Perform a procedure to remove a blockage from an artery. This could include balloon angioplasty, laser atherectomy, or embolectomy.

A *barium swallow (esophagogram)* enables a radiographic image to be taken of the esophagus, stomach, and small intestine. Indications for a barium swallow include, but are not limited to, the following:

a. Dysphagia
b. Noncardiac chest pain
c. Painful swallowing and swallowing abnormalities
d. Gastroesophageal reflux

An *MRI scan* provides images of body organs without the use of radioactive materials. The images are created when the powerful magnet of the MRI is turned on and off and affects the way that hydrogen atoms align within the body. A limitation of the MRI is that the patient cannot have any metallic implants. In addition, most mechanical ventilators cannot be used during an MRI because the magnetic field will interfere with the unit. Indications for an MRI include, but are not limited to, the following:

a. Imaging the head, spinal cord, and surrounding structures.
b. Imaging the heart and great vessels.
c. Imaging the kidneys, liver, and other organs.

3. Review the chest radiograph film to determine the quality of the imaging. (WRE code: IB6a) [Difficulty: R, Ap]
a. Patient identification

It is standard practice for the patient's name and identification number to be incorporated into the chest radiograph film (chest x-ray film).

b. Patient positioning

The patient will be positioned between the x-ray machine and the film cassette so that the electromagnetic (x-ray) radiation will penetrate the patient's body, hit the film, and provide the desired view of the internal organs. See Fig. 1-1 for the most common radiographic projections used with patients having cardiopulmonary problems. Examples of some of these positions are shown in this chapter.

If possible, the patient should be moved to the radiography department, and the chest radiograph should be taken from the *posterior to anterior (posteroanterior, P-A, or PA) position*. The patient's chest is placed against the film cassette with the shoulders rolled forward. Because x-rays penetrate from back to front, the size of the heart is close to normal. Normally the patient is instructed to take in and hold a deep breath. This reveals more clearly the lung fields, heart, and other structures. This may be contrasted with a chest radiograph taken after the patient has exhaled completely. If the patient has been correctly positioned perpendicular to the film cassette, the x-ray image will show the clavicle bones to be symmetrical.

If a "portable" chest radiograph must be taken because the patient is too ill to be moved from his or her bed, the *anterior to posterior (anteroposterior, A-P, or AP) position* must be used. The x-rays penetrate the body from front to back. This should be noted in the chart because this view of the organs shows the heart's size to be larger than that in a PA radiograph.

The standard *lateral view* is taken with the patient standing upright with both arms raised above the head and the left side against the film cassette. This is done because the heart is left of center in the chest. A lateral view is used to see behind the heart and hemidiaphragms. It can be combined with an AP or a PA view to

Radiographic Projection	Explanation	Graphic Demonstration
AP (anteroposterior)	The anterior surface of the body is closest to the x-ray source with the posterior body surface closest to the film. The x-ray beam enters the anterior surface and exits the posterior surface to strike the film forming the radographic image.	
PA (posteroanterior)	The posterior surface of the body is closest to the x-ray source with the anterior body surface closest to the film. The x-ray beam enters the posterior surface and exits the anterior surface to strike the film forming the radiographic image.	
Lateral	So named for the side of the body closest to the film, that is, a left lateral projection is obtained with the patient's left side closest to the film and the x-ray beam enters the right side to obtain the radiograph	
Oblique	A position in which the patient's body part is rotated so that it does not produce either an AP/PA or lateral projection. RAO (right PA oblique): The patient's right side is rotated towards the film. LAO (left PA oblique): The patient's left side is rotated toward the film. RPO (right AP oblique): The patient's right posterior side is rotated toward the film. LPO (left AP oblique): The patient's left posterior side is rotated toward the film.	
Lateral decubitus	Patient is positioned lying on either the right or the left side; the x-ray beam is directed parallel to the floor and perpendicular to the film. The patient can also be placed in a ventral or dorsal position. (Patient shown is on right side.)	
Lordotic	Patient is postured in an AP orientation, filted back away from the vetrical; the x-ray beam is directed with a cephalic angulation, that is, the x-ray beam is directed toward the head.	

Fig. 1-1 Common radiographic projections of the chest to evaluate the heart and lungs. *(From DiPietro JS, Mustard MN: Clinical guide for respiratory care practitioners, Norwalk, Conn, 1987, Appleton & Lange.)*

localize lesions within the chest. This view also is used to measure the patient's anterior-to-posterior chest diameter. This is often enlarged in patients with air trapping from emphysema.

The *oblique position* provides a third angle for viewing the internal chest structures. This is especially helpful when the physician is checking the heart borders, mediastinal structures, hilar structures, and lung masses.

The *lateral decubitus position* enables fluid within the pleural space to be viewed. As little as 25 to 50 mL of fluid can be detected in the adult as it flows to the horizontal position. An air/fluid level in a lung cavity (cyst) also can be evaluated by the shifting of the fluid line by gravity. The *dorsal decubitus position* is used to help identify a small pneumothorax in an infant.

The *lordotic (apical lordodic) position* is used when it is necessary to view the upper lung fields without the clavicles and first and second ribs obscuring them. The apices, right middle lobe, and lingula can be clearly seen.

Make sure, when viewing any chest radiograph, that you are looking at the film correctly. That is, the film should be viewed as if you were looking directly at the patient's chest. For example, in a PA or AP film, if you reached out your right hand, you would touch the image of the patient's left shoulder. To help with correct viewing, the film should show the letter L over the patient's left shoulder (on your right as you look at the film). Note that sometimes the film will show the letter R over the patient's right shoulder (on your left as you look at the film).

c. Exposure

It is the radiologic technologist's responsibility to expose the patient to x-rays for a long enough period to acquire the proper exposure of the internal organs. In all chest radiograph positions, the patient must take and hold a deep breath without moving as the picture is taken. If the patient is on a mechanical ventilator when an AP chest radiograph is performed, a sigh breath should be delivered and held by the respiratory therapist to inflate the lungs fully.

It must be understood that the image seen on a chest x-ray film is the negative or reverse image of the densities of the structures within the chest. When viewing an x-ray film, a range of shadings will be seen progressing from white to black. *Radiopaque* items are very dense. They will absorb most x-rays, preventing them from striking the film, and therefore appear white on the film. *Radiolucent* items have little density. They will absorb few x-rays, allowing them to strike the film, and therefore appear dark on the film. Altogether, four densities are seen on a chest radiograph:

Air: Because air is the least dense substance, it blocks very few x-rays; most hit the film in the cassette. This causes the film to turn black. Notice that the film around the patient's body is completely black. Because the normal lungs are air filled with little tissue, they appear almost black. Normally some lung-tissue markings can be seen as wispy white shadows. Air in the stomach or intestine will also appear dark compared with the surrounding tissues.

Tissue: The tissues of the lungs, heart, diaphragm, breasts, etc., will partially block the x-rays. This results in white shadows of varying opacity depending on the density of the tissues. For example, the heart will appear as a fairly solid white organ. Fluid also will partially block x-rays. A pleural effusion will be seen as a white shadow around the lung(s).

Bone: The calcium in bone makes it dense enough to block most x-ray penetration, so the ribs, clavicles, and vertebrae will be seen as fairly solid white lines. Broken ribs can be easily identified by the misalignment of their shadows.

Metallic: Bullets, wire sutures, metal plates, artificial heart valves, and coins will completely block all x-ray penetration. This will result in a sharply outlined white shadow. Medical devices like an endotracheal or tracheostomy tube, nasogastric tube, or heart catheter contain materials that completely block x-rays. Therefore these radiopaque items can be easily seen within the patient on a chest radiograph.

When the radiograph is done with proper penetration and exposure, the intervertebral spaces of the spinal column are just visible. If the film is underexposed (the overall color of the film and body tissues is too white), the carina or an internal catheter may not be seen. If the film is overexposed (the overall color of the film and body tissues is too black), the air-filled lung fields will be too black. It may not be possible to detect a pneumothorax.

4. Recommend and review the patient's chest radiograph film to evaluate and monitor the patient's response to respiratory care procedures (WRE code: IIIE1) [Difficulty: An]

A chest radiograph should be taken whenever a significant change occurs in the patient's cardiopulmonary condition or whenever an invasive thoracic procedure (chest-tube insertion, endotracheal intubation, pulmonary artery catheter placement) is performed.

5. Look for the presence of, or any changes in, pneumothorax, subcutaneous emphysema, or any other extrapulmonary air (WRE code: IB6c) [Difficulty: An]

Free air that leaks into the interstitial spaces of the lung or body cavities is abnormal in any patient. Causes for an air leak include barotrauma/volutrauma (alveolar rupture related to the use of a mechanical ventilator), a ruptured bleb (congenital or acquired blister on the visceral pleura), puncture wound through the chest wall, and needle puncture through the pleural space during the insertion of a CVP or pulmonary artery catheter via the subclavian or jugular vein. Once air under pressure is forced through a bronchial or alveolar tear into the interstitial tissues, it tends to follow the path of least resistance. This may result in air being found in any of the following areas singly or in combination.

Pneumothorax is air in the pleural space. The lung tends to collapse toward the hilum. A pneumothorax is identified on the chest radiograph as an area of black, indicating air that surrounds the collapsed lung. No lung markings are visible in the air-filled space, and the edge of the lung can be seen (Fig. 1-2). If the air is under sufficient pressure to shift the lung and mediastinal structures to the opposite side, it is called a *tension pneumothorax*. This is a serious condition that can lead to the death of the patient if it is not quickly identified and treated. A pleural chest tube is always placed into the affected side to remove the air so that the lung can re-expand.

Subcutaneous emphysema is air found in the soft tissues such as the skin, axilla, shoulder, neck, or breast of the affected side. In extreme cases, the air forces its way into skin and soft tissues throughout the body. Scattered dark areas (air pockets) appear in the various soft tissues on the chest radiograph (Fig. 1-3).

Fig. 1-3 Frontal radiograph of a neonate showing subcutaneous emphysema in the shoulders and neck area. Other abnormal air in the patient's chest includes a pneumomediastinum, which outlines the right lobe of the thymus gland *(arrow)*, and a left anterior pneumothorax. *(From Carlo C:* Neonatal respiratory care, *St Louis, 1988, Mosby.)*

The following are other locations where free air can be found: *Pneumomediastinum* is air in the mediastinal space (see Fig. 1-3). *Pneumopericardium* is air in the pericardial space (Fig. 1-4). Both of these conditions can be very serious. A cardiac tamponade is created if the pressure around the heart is great enough to interfere with its function. *Pneumoperitoneum* is air in the peritoneal space. This condition can be dangerous in an infant if a large enough volume of air is below the diaphragm and its movement is limited. *Pulmonary interstitial emphysema (PIE)* is air that has disseminated throughout the interstitial spaces of the injured lung(s). The lungs appear "bubbly" on the chest radiograph image (see Fig. 1-4). The air may further leak into any of the previously listed locations. PIE is most commonly seen in infants with infant respiratory distress syndrome (RDS) who require mechanical ventilation (MV).

6. Look for the presence of, or any changes in, mediastinal shift (WRE code: IB6f) [Difficulty: An]

The mediastinum is the area between the lungs that contains the heart and great vessels, trachea, hilar structures, and esophagus. In the neonate, the heart and other mediastinal structures should be approximately in the center of the chest, with the left ventricle to the left of center. In the adult, the majority of the heart and mediastinal structures should be left of center in the chest. A shift of the mediastinum (and heart) is abnormal, as shown by several conditions in Figs. 1-2 and 1-5.

Fig. 1-2 Frontal radiograph of an adult male with a left-sided tension pneumothorax. The edge of the collapsed lung is shown *(arrows)*. Note how the mediastinum is shifted to the right, the right lung is compressed, and the left hemidiaphragm is depressed. *(From DesJardins TR:* Clinical manifestations of respiratory disease, *ed 2, St Louis, 1990, Mosby.)*

Fig. 1-4 Frontal radiograph of a neonate showing a pneumopericardium that resulted from pulmonary interstitial emphysema. Note the dark outline of air around the heart. Chest tubes have been placed to remove air from around the heart and the right pleural space from an earlier pneumothorax. An endotracheal tube also is seen. *(From Koff PB, Eitzman DV, Neu J: Neonatal and pediatric respiratory care, St Louis, 1988, Mosby.)*

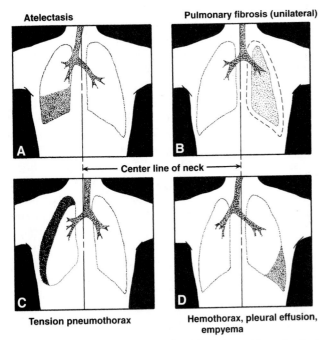

Fig. 1-5 Conditions causing tracheal deviation and mediastinal shift (simulated chest radiograph findings). *A,* Unilateral atelectasis with tracheal deviation *toward* the affected lung. *B,* Unilateral pulmonary fibrosis with tracheal deviation *toward* the affected lung. *C,* Tension pneumothorax with tracheal deviation *away* from the affected lung. *D,* Pleural fluid with tracheal deviation *away* from the affected lung. The normal lung expands more than the abnormal lung during inspiration. *(From Sills JR: Respiratory care certification guide, St Louis, 1991, Mosby.)*

Either atelectasis or pulmonary fibrosis, if unilateral and great enough, will result in a shift *toward* the problem area. Tension pneumothorax will result in a shift *away* from the problem area. Fluid in the pleural space, if great enough, will result in a shift *away* from the problem area.

7. Look for the position of chest tubes, nasogastric and/or feeding tubes, a pacemaker, a pulmonary artery catheter, a central venous pressure catheter, or another catheter (WRE code: IB6d) [Difficulty: R, Ap, An]

All medical devices placed into the body are made of radiopaque material. They can be seen on a chest radiograph as a white object or line.

Chest tubes are placed to remove any abnormal collection of air or fluid from the thoracic cavity so that the function of the heart and lungs will return to normal. A pleural chest tube is placed to remove air or fluid from the pleural space (see Fig. 1-4). The insertion site and depth of insertion of the tube depend on the patient's disorder. (See Chapter 18 for more discussion on the placement of pleural chest tubes.)

A mediastinal or pericardial chest tube is placed to remove air or fluid from either of these spaces (see Figs. 1-4 and 1-6). Cardiac tamponade can result from the pressure of either air or fluid compressing the heart. Most postoperative open-heart surgery patients have one or more mediastinal chest tubes in place for several days to remove any blood from around the heart. The insertion site is below the sternum, and the tube(s) are placed posterior to the heart in the pericardial or mediastinal space or both.

A nasogastric tube appears as a white line on the chest radiograph from the patient's nose or mouth through the esophagus and into the stomach (on the left side below the diaphragm). A feeding tube may be placed as a nasogastric tube or surgically placed through the abdominal wall and into the stomach or small intestine. A white line on the radiograph shows its position.

A cardiac pacemaker is placed in two ways. An external pacemaker is identified on the chest radiograph by the long electrode leads that run through a vein in the right arm, through the superior vena cava, and into the right ventricle. The battery and control unit of an internal pacemaker are placed under the skin below a clavicle. The electrode leads run through the superior vena cava into the right ventricle.

The various venous catheters (pulmonary artery catheter, CVP catheter, umbilical artery catheter [UAC], and umbilical vein catheter [UVC]) should be seen on the chest radiograph from their insertion points to their end points. (See Figs. 1-6 and 1-7 for the placement of several catheters).

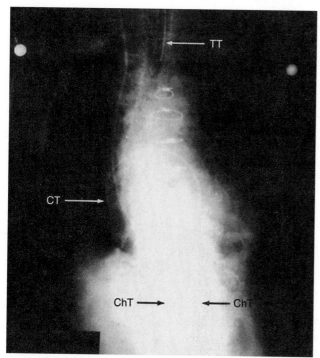

Fig. 1-6 Frontal radiograph of an adult postoperative open-heart surgery patient with several medically necessary devices. A properly placed pulmonary artery (Swan-Ganz) catheter is noted to loop through the right side of the heart and out into the right pulmonary artery. The catheter tip is marked CT. Other foreign bodies include a properly placed endotracheal tube marked TT, sternal wire sutures, ECG chest leads on each shoulder, and pericardial chest tubes marked ChT. *(From Sheldon RL, Wilkins RL: Clinical application of the chest radiograph. In Wilkins RL, Sheldon RL, Krider SJ, editors: Clinical assessment in respiratory care, ed 2, St Louis, 1990, Mosby.)*

8. Look for the presence of, or any changes in, pulmonary infiltrates or consolidation (WRE code: IB6c) [Difficulty: An]

A pulmonary infiltrate occurs when blood plasma (water) passes from the pulmonary vascular bed into the lung tissues. Usually this fluid moves into the lung because the alveolar capillary membrane is damaged. On a chest radiograph, an infiltrate often appears as a faint white blurring of the lung and other associated structures.

A consolidation is a filling of the alveoli with fluid from an infiltrate, aspirated vomitus, blood, or water. It is often segmental or lobar. Consolidation is noticed on the chest radiograph as a dense white shadow because fluid has replaced the air. The mediastinum and heart will be seen in their normal locations. Fig. 1-8 shows the PA and lateral chest radiograph indicating consolidation in each of the segments of both lungs. Air bronchograms also may be noticed on a radiograph film that reveals consolidation.

9. Look for the presence of, or any changes in, atelectasis (WRE code: IB6b) [Difficulty: An]

Atelectasis is the collapse of alveoli; no air is found in them. This problem is commonly seen postoperatively in the lower lobes of patients who have had abdominal or thoracic surgery and do not breathe deeply because of pain. The radiograph of atelectasis shows an increase in lung markings and a decrease in the lung volumes. If one-sided, the mediastinum may shift toward the affected side (see Fig. 1-5, *A*). If bilateral, the mediastinum will be properly located. If severe enough, the lungs will appear a uniform white (Fig. 1-9).

10. Look for the positions of, or any changes in, the hemidiaphragms (WRE code: IB6f) [Difficulty: An]

The normal infant's and adult's AP or PA chest radiograph reveals a domed shape to the hemidiaphragms, with the edges turning down to acute costophrenic angles. A lateral chest radiograph reveals the same domed shape with the edges turning down to acute costophrenic angles. The edges of the hemidiaphragms should be smooth without any unusual dips or peaks. The following conditions result in one hemidiaphragm being positioned abnormally: unilateral atelectasis, pleural fluid, tension pneumothorax, or check-valve bronchial obstruction (see Figs. 1-2 and 1-5). Asthma and COPD result in both hemidiaphragms being depressed (Figs. 1-10 and 1-11). An improvement in the patient's condition should result in a return of the hemidiaphragm(s) to closer to normal position.

11. Look for the presence of, or any changes in, hyperinflation (WRE code: IB6f) [Difficulty: An]

Hyperinflation is an excessive amount of air in one or both lungs. The specific chest radiograph findings, to some degree, depend on the underlying condition that causes the hyperinflation. Unilateral hyperinflation is caused by a check-valve obstruction from a foreign body or airway tumor. At first glance, a tension pneumothorax appears as unilateral lung hyperinflation. Remember that with this condition, the chest is hyperinflated, and the lung is collapsed (see Fig. 1-2).

In the adult with asthma, bronchitis, and emphysema (COPD) or newborn with meconium aspiration, both lungs are overinflated, and both hemidiaphragms are depressed (see Figs. 1-10 and 1-11). Other radiographic findings include widened intercostal spaces; hyperlucent lung fields; a small, vertical heart; a small cardiothoracic diameter; and decreased vascularity of peripheral areas of the lungs with enlarged hilar vessels. The lateral chest radiographic findings in the COPD patient are the same, and they include anterior bowing of the sternum, increased retrosternal air space, and kyphosis.

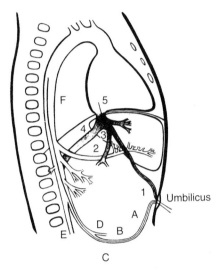

Fig. 1-7 Lateral radiograph and drawing of the internal vascular structures of an infant with an umbilical artery catheter (UAC) and umbilical vein catheter (UVC) in place. The UAC passes through the umbilicus, umbilical artery (*A*), hypogastric artery (*B*), internal iliac artery (*C*), common iliac artery (*D*), abdominal aorta (*E*), to the thoracic aorta (*F*). The umbilical vein catheter passes through the umbilicus, umbilical vein (*1*), portal vein (*2*), ductus venosus (*3*), inferior vena cava (*4*), to the right atrium (*5*). Other medical devices include an endotracheal tube and ECG leads. *(From Sheldon RL, Wilkins RL: Clinical application of the chest radiograph. In Wilkins RL, Sheldon RL, Krider SJ, editors:* Clinical assessment in respiratory care, *ed 2, St Louis, 1990, Mosby.)*

12. Look for the presence of, or any changes in, pleural fluid (WRE code: IB6f) [Difficulty: An]

Pleural fluid is typically shown on a PA or AP film as obscuring the costophrenic angle. This is because gravity tends to draw the fluid to the lowest level. Often this results in an obscuring or blunting of the costophrenic angle of the affected side (Fig. 1-12). In some cases, an air/fluid level is seen within the intrapleural space. The term *meniscus* is used to describe the upward curve seen in the fluid part of this intrapleural air/fluid level. Small amounts of fluid can sometimes be better visualized by taking a lateral decubitus radiograph. If the fluid is able to move freely in the pleural space, it will shift in a few minutes to the lower side (Fig. 1-13). An empyema that is loculated (fixed) by adhesions will not move when the patient lies on his or her side. If large amounts of fluid are removed by a thoracentesis procedure, a chest radiograph should be taken to confirm the removal of fluid, the re-expansion of the lung, and that a pneumothorax did not result.

13. Look for the presence of, or any changes in, pulmonary edema (WRE code: IB6f) [Difficulty: An]

Pulmonary edema is watery fluid (plasma) that has leaked out of the pulmonary capillary bed into the interstitial spaces and alveoli. It is most commonly caused by left ventricular failure (also known as congestive heart failure), but also can be the result of fluid overload, pulmonary capillary damage, or decreased osmotic pressure in the blood from a low level of protein.

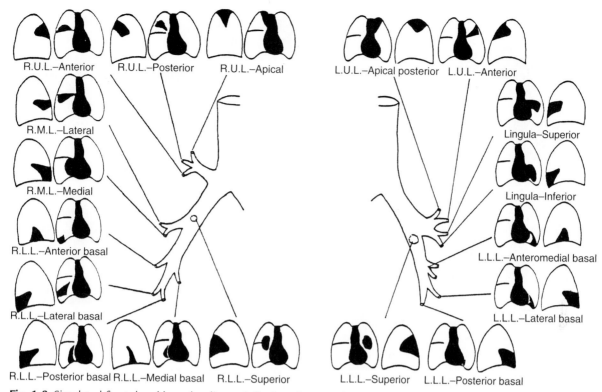

R.U.L.–Anterior   R.U.L.–Posterior   R.U.L.–Apical

R.M.L.–Lateral

R.M.L.–Medial

R.L.L.–Anterior basal

R.L.L.–Lateral basal

R.L.L.–Posterior basal   R.L.L.–Medial basal   R.L.L.–Superior

L.U.L.–Apical posterior   L.U.L.–Anterior

Lingula–Superior

Lingula–Inferior

L.L.L.–Anteromedial basal

L.L.L.–Lateral basal

L.L.L.–Superior   L.L.L.–Posterior basal

Fig. 1-8 Simulated frontal and lateral radiograph findings for consolidation in the various segments of both lungs. L.L.L., Left lower lobe; L.U.L., left upper lobe; R.L.L., right lower lobe; R.M.L., right middle lobe; R.U.L., right upper lobe. *(From Cherniack RM, Cherniack L: Respiration in health and disease, ed 3, Philadelphia, 1983, WB Saunders.)*

Fig. 1-9 Frontal radiograph of a neonate with severe atelectasis from infant respiratory distress syndrome (RDS). Also note the right pleural chest tube and wires to various monitoring systems. *(From Des Jardins TR: Clinical manifestations of respiratory disease, ed 2, St Louis, 1990, Mosby.)*

Fig. 1-10 Frontal radiograph of an adult with advanced chronic obstructive pulmonary disease (COPD). Both lungs are overinflated and hyperlucent. The ribs are spread more widely than normal. Often these patients have a cardiothoracic ratio that is smaller than normal because the heart is elongated and the lateral chest diameter is increased. *(From Sheldon RL, Wilkins RL: Clinical application of the chest radiograph. In Wilkins RL, Sheldon RL, Krider SJ, editors: Clinical assessment in respiratory care, ed 2, St Louis, 1990, Mosby.)*

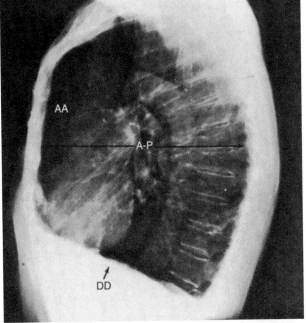

Fig. 1-11 Lateral radiograph of an adult with advanced chronic obstructive pulmonary disease. Note the characteristic shape of a "barrel chest" from the overinflated lungs. The anteroposterior (AP) diameter of the chest is increased. *AA* marks an increased anterior airspace between the heart and sternum. The angle of the manubrium and body of the sternum is more obtuse than normal. *DD* marks depressed hemidiaphragms that are flattened. *(From Sheldon RL, Wilkins RL: Clinical application of the chest radiograph. In Wilkins RL, Sheldon RL, Krider SJ, editors: Clinical assessment in respiratory care, ed 2, St Louis, 1990, Mosby.)*

Fig. 1-12 Frontal radiograph of an adult showing a small pleural effusion in the right chest. Note how the costophrenic angle and hemidiaphragm are obscured by the white shadow of fluid. *(From Sheldon RL, Wilkins RL: Clinical application of the chest radiograph. In Wilkins RL, Sheldon RL, Krider SJ, editors: Clinical assessment in respiratory care, ed 2, St Louis, 1990, Mosby.)*

Fig. 1-13 Lateral decubitus radiograph of an adult showing the shift of a small pleural effusion to the now-dependent part of the pleural space. The layer of fluid is marked by *arrows*. *(From Sheldon RL, Wilkins RL: Clinical application of the chest radiograph. In Wilkins RL, Sheldon RL, Krider SJ, editors: Clinical assessment in respiratory care, ed 2, St Louis, 1990, Mosby.)*

Pulmonary edema appears on a PA or AP chest radiograph as fluffy, white infiltrates in either or both lung fields. These tend to be seen more extensively in the lower lobes as a result of gravity pulling the fluid to the basilar vessels, where it leaks out. If the root cause is left ventricular failure, the vessels in the hila also will be engorged and the left ventricle enlarged (Fig. 1-14). A worsening problem will result in more fluid leaking into the lungs and the appearance of more white infiltrates on succeeding chest radiographs. Once the problem is corrected, the lungs will return to normal as the fluid is reabsorbed and removed.

14. Look for the presence and position of any foreign bodies (WRE code: IB6e) [Difficulty: An]

A foreign body is anything that is not naturally found in the chest. Metallic objects (e.g., bullets or swallowed or aspirated coins or metal buttons) are easily noticed because they completely block any x-ray penetration through the chest and are clearly outlined on the film as solid, white shadows (Fig. 1-15). Nonmetallic foreign objects (such as plastic pieces from toys and foods such as peanuts) are much more difficult to identify because they have about the same densities as normal body tissues. Determining the exact location of a foreign body may require taking PA, lateral, and oblique chest radiographs. Lung volumes can be compared by taking inspiratory and expiratory films. A CT scan may be the most successful method of finding a nonmetallic foreign body.

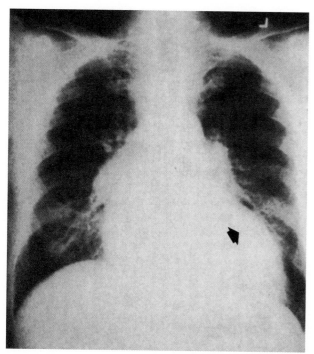

Fig. 1-14 Frontal radiograph of an adult showing pulmonary edema, increased pulmonary vascular markings, and enlarged left ventricle. The cardiothoracic diameter is increased, with the *arrow* showing where the border of the left ventricle should normally be seen. *(From Des Jardins TR:* Clinical manifestations of respiratory disease, *ed 2, St Louis, 1990, Mosby.)*

15. Check the chest radiograph for the size and patency of the patient's major airways (WRE code: IB6f) [Difficulty: An]

The trachea and both the right and left mainstem bronchi should be seen on a properly taken chest radiograph film. They appear as straight, dark air columns in contrast with the white shadows of the various surrounding tissues. A white shadow within the airway may be a foreign body or a tumor. A lung tumor that presses on an airway causes the airway to narrow or be occluded.

16. Check the chest radiograph for the position of the patient's endotracheal or tracheostomy tube (WRE code: IB6b) [Difficulty: An]

The distal ends of these tubes should be seen within the lumen of the trachea and about midway between the larynx and the tracheal bifurcation to the right and left mainstem bronchi (see Figs. 1-4 and 1-6 for endotracheal tube placement). The proximal end of the tracheostomy tube (or transtracheal oxygen catheter) is seen on the film coming out of the surgical insertion site in the suprasternal notch. The distal end should be centered within the trachea above the carina (see Fig. 1-6). All of these tubes are made of a radiopaque material or have a line of radiopaque material imbedded into them so that they can be easily seen on the radiograph.

Care must be taken not to push the endotracheal tube deeper into a bronchus, usually the right, or to pull it out. The tracheostomy tube and transtracheal oxygen catheter are less likely to be displaced if they are properly cared for. Take another radiograph to check the position of any of these tubes if clinical evidence suggests that a position may have changed.

17. Check the chest radiograph for a sign that the cuff on the endotracheal or tracheostomy tube is overinflated (CSE code: IB7c)

A properly inflated cuff fills the space between the tube and the patient's trachea so that an airtight seal is made. If the cuff is overinflated, it places excessive pressure on the trachea. This can cause it to dilate and be seen as a wider dark area than the rest of the tracheal air column. If this is noticed, the cuff pressure should be measured. Excessive pressure should be reduced to a safer level.

> **Exam Hint**
>
> **P**ast exams have had at least one question that requires the identification of the cause of an abnormal chest radiograph. Typically the question refers to a patient who has a pneumothorax or pleural effusion. In addition, expect a question that requires the identification of the location of an endotracheal tube or the tip of a CVP catheter or pulmonary artery catheter. The National Board for Respiratory Care (NBRC) sometimes uses the term *radiograph* in examination questions rather than *x-ray*.

MODULE C
Interview the patient

1. What is the patient's level of consciousness or sedation? (WRE code: IB4a) [Difficulty: An]

One common way to evaluate a patient's level of consciousness is to categorize him or her as alert, stuporous, semicomatose, or comatose as follows.

a. Alert

This is the normal mental state. The patient is conscious or can be fully awakened from sleep by calling his or her name. The patient can voluntarily ask logical questions and answer questions logically. The conversation is relevant to the topic under discussion. The patient's movements and actions are willful and purposeful.

b. Stuporous or lethargic

The patient is sleepy or seems to be in a trance. He or she can be aroused to respond with willful, purposeful movements

Fig. 1-15 Foreign-body obstruction in an 18-month-old girl. *A,* Frontal radiograph with the solid white disk of a coin clearly seen in the hypopharynx. *B,* Lateral view of the chest with the edge of the coin seen as a solid white line. *(From Hunter TB, Bragg DG: Radiologic guide to medical devices and foreign bodies, St Louis, 1994, Mosby.)*

and actions, but the patient may be slow. The patient may not respond to questions in a totally appropriate way.

c. Semicomatose

The patient does not perform requested movements or actions. The patient will not answer questions in an appropriate way. He or she will respond defensively to pain. For example, if the right arm is pinched, it will be withdrawn. Posturing of semicomatose patients includes the following:

1. Decerebrate: legs are extended; arms are extended and rotated either inward or outward.
2. Decorticate: legs are extended; arms are flexed, and the forearms may be rotated either inward or outward.
3. Opisthotonic: legs, arms, and neck are extended, and the body is arched forward.

d. Comatose or coma

The patient has no spontaneous, oriented responses to the environment. Pain causes no defensive movement, but an increase in the heart and respiratory rates may occur.

Another common way to evaluate a patient's level of consciousness is to make use of the Glasgow Coma Scale

(GCS). With this scale of 3 to 15, the larger the total number, the more normal the patient. A score of 15 is achieved in a patient normally awake and alert; a score of 3 is found in an unresponsive patient. See Table 1-7 for details of the scale.

2. Is the patient oriented to time, place, and person? (WRE code: IB4a) [Difficulty: An]

Time refers to the patient knowing the calendar date, the day of the week, and the time of day. Ask the patient, "Do you know what day of the week it is? Do you know what the date is?" (The patient must be able to see a calendar.), "Do you know what time it is?" (The patient must be able to see a clock.). If the patient can answer these questions, he or she is oriented to time. If not, inform and show him or her. Tell the patient that you will return at a certain time. Ask the same questions when you return.

Place refers to the patient knowing where he or she is located (hospital, nursing care unit, extended care facility, home, etc.). Ask the patient, "Do you know where you are?" If the patient knows, he or she is oriented to place. If not, inform the patient of the location. Tell the patient

TABLE 1-7 Glasgow Coma Scale

Test Parameter	Response	Score*
EYES		
Open	Spontaneously	4
	To verbal command	3
	To pain	2
	No response	1
BEST MOTOR RESPONSE		
To verbal command	Obeys command	6
Moves arms to	Localizes pain	5
painful stimulus	Flexion—withdrawal	4
of knuckles	Flexion—abnormal movement	3
against sternum	(decorticate rigidity)	
	Extension—abnormal movement (decerebrate rigidity)	2
	No response	1
BEST VERBAL RESPONSE (MAY AROUSE BY PAINFUL STIMULUS IF NECESSARY)		
	Oriented and converses	5
	Disoriented and converses	4
	Inappropriate words used	3
	Incomprehensible sounds	2
	No response	1

From *Apache II: A severity of disease classification system,* ICU Research Unit, Washington, DC; product information from Upjohn, Kalamazoo, Mich.
*The total is obtained by adding the scores in all three areas. The range is 3 to 15.

that you will return at a certain time. Ask the same question when you return.

Person refers to the patient knowing his or her own name, address, and telephone number. The patient also should know the names of obviously important people. Ask the patient, "Do you know who the president (or the physician) is?" If not, inform the patient. Tell the patient who you are and what your job is. When you return for your next treatment, ask the patient if he remembers who you are and what you do. If the patient remembers who the president (or the physician) is and your name or job, he is oriented to person.

Orienting the stuporous/lethargic patient to person, place, and time may encourage him or her to cooperate more in his or her care. Pain-relieving and sedative drugs, stroke, injury to or edema of the brain, and other illnesses may cause disorientation to person, place, or time.

3. What is the patient's emotional state? (RWE code: IB4a) [Difficulty: An]

Acute illness or injury with great pain may result in some patients feeling fear, anxiety, or panic. Because of these feelings, the patient may be unable to concentrate closely on what you are telling him or her. This can result in

directions not being understood or followed. It is important to tell the patient that you are there to help and need the patient to calm down so that you can help.

Chronic illness has been approached by a number of authors from varying points of view. Table 1-8 gives a presentation of a patient's reaction to chronic illness. Substitute "respiratory therapists" for "nurses" as needed.

A patient's statements and actions that indicate the *disbelief* stage of adaptation include the following:
a. "I don't have (fill in the disease or condition)."
b. "There is nothing really wrong with me."
c. "The laboratory results are wrong."
d. "The equipment is faulty."
e. "The doctor/nurse/therapist is incompetent."
f. Refusal to take medications.
g. Refusal to take treatments or follow other physician orders.

A patient's statements and actions that indicate the *developing awareness* state of adaptation include the following:
a. "The doctor/nurse/therapist doesn't know what he or she is doing."
b. "It's all their fault."
c. "Why is this happening to me?"
d. The patient is angry about his or her illness.
e. The patient may strike out verbally or physically at staff members.
f. Some patients who do not get angry will withdraw into a depression and wish to be left alone.

A patient's statements and actions that indicate that he or she is progressing from the *reorganization* to the *successful adaptation* stage include the following:
a. "I'll never be able to do that again." (Fill in the activity.)
b. "I have to get on with my life."
c. "At least I'm still alive and can do this for myself."
d. The patient may be sad and cry often.
e. The patient may invent a nickname for his or her defect or diseased body part.
f. The patient accepts the disability and focuses on his or her abilities.
g. The patient works with family and others in planning for the future.

4. What is the patient's ability to cooperate? (WRE code: IB4a) [Difficulty: An]

You should be able to judge the patient's ability to cooperate. It should be based on his or her responses to your questions on level of consciousness; orientation to time, place, and person; and emotional state. An alert patient should be able to understand and follow directions. He or she should be able to take an effective treatment or cooperate in a procedure. Conversely, if the patient truly refuses the treatment or procedure, it should not be forced. Contact the patient's nurse or physician about the refusal. The physician must then decide what to do.

TABLE 1-8	Teaching-Learning Process in Adaptation to Chronic Illness		
Stages of Adaptation	Patient's Behavior	Nurse's Behavior	Nurse's Facilitation of the Teaching-Learning Process
Disbelief	Denies threatening condition to protect self and conserve energy; refuses to accept diagnosis; may claim to have something else; may behave so as to avoid the issue; may seem to accept diagnosis but avoids feelings about it	Allows patient to deny illness as he or she needs to; functions as noncritical listener; accepts patient's statements of how he or she feels; helps clarify patient's statements; does not point out reality	Orients all teaching to the present, not to tomorrow or next week; teaches as he or she does other nursing activities; assesses patient's level of anxiety; assures patient that he or she is safe and being observed carefully; explains all procedures and activities to the patient; gives clear, concise explanations; coordinates activities to include rest periods
Developing awareness	Uses anger as a defense against being dependent and against guilt about being sick	Listens to patient's expressions of anger and recognizes them for what they are; explores own feelings about illness and helplessness; does not argue with patient; gives dependable care with an attitude that it is necessary	Does not give anxious patient long lists of facts; continues development of trust and rapport through good physical care; orients teaching to present; explains symptoms, care, and treatment in terms of the fact that they are necessary now; does not mention long-range care needs
Reorganization	Accepts increased dependence and reorganizes relationships with significant others; members of patient's family may also use denial while they adapt to what patient's illness means to them	Establishes climate in which family and friends can express feelings about patient's illness; does not solve patient's problems but helps build communication so that patient and family can work together to solve problems	Assures family that patient is all right and safe; uses clear, concise explanations; does not argue about need for care
Resolution	Acknowledges changes seen in self; identifies with others with same problem	Encourages expression of feelings, including crying; understands own feelings of loss	Brings groups of patients with same illness together for group discussions; has a recovered person visit patient; teaches patient what he or she wants to learn (or perceives he or she needs to learn) first
Identity change	Defines self as an individual who has undergone change and is now different; "There are limits to my life because I have a disease"	Understands own feelings about patient becoming independent again	Realizes that as patient's own perceived needs are met, more mature (more progressive) needs will surface; is prepared to answer patient's questions as they arise
Successful adaptation	Can live comfortably or resignedly with himself as a person who has a specific condition	Initiates closure of nurse-patient relationship	Has helped develop a relationship with the patient in which the nurse is a guide with whom the patient can consult when he or she wishes

From Kenner CV, Guzzetta CE, Dossey BM: *Critical care nursing: body—mind—spirit*, Boston, 1981, Little, Brown.

An alert but panicked, fearful, or anxious patient may be unable to cooperate fully until he or she is calmed by understanding who you are, what you are there to do, and why the treatment or procedure is important. Try to reassure the patient to improve cooperation.

If the patient appears alert but does not follow what you are saying, check to see whether he or she is deaf or does not speak English. An effective way to communicate must be found. Writing materials, a picture board, or a sign-language interpreter is needed to communicate with a deaf patient. A native-language translator will be needed to communicate with a patient who does not speak English.

The stuporous/very lethargic patient may be aroused by talking more loudly or by gentle shaking. He or she may or may not be able to cooperate fully. The practitioner may have to modify the treatment plan or how it is administered to compensate for the patient's lack of cooperation.

Pain relievers and sedatives may make a normally alert patient seem stuporous. If the patient has not been medicated, check with the nurse or physician to see what may have recently changed in the patient's condition.

A semicomatose patient may present the greatest problems in providing treatment or performing a procedure. These patients do not cooperate in any way but are unlikely to fight treatment either. In addition, some of their involuntary body posturings make correct positioning impossible. You must modify your equipment or procedure to accommodate the patient's inability to cooperate.

5. Does the patient complain of dyspnea or orthopnea or both? (WRE code: IB4b) [Difficulty: An]

Dyspnea is the patient's subjective feeling of shortness of breath (SOB) or labored breathing. This is normal after vigorous exercise but abnormal in a resting patient. Orthopnea is the condition in which a patient must sit erect or stand to breathe comfortably. Lying flat causes dyspnea.

Table 1-9 classifies the degrees of dyspnea, and Table 1-10 lists different kinds of dyspnea, including orthopnea. Only class I is normal dyspnea (on severe exertion). Classes II to V are progressively severe and limiting for the patient. Any orthopnea is abnormal, and the more the patient must sit up to breathe, the more limited the patient.

The following are examples of questions to ask in evaluating dyspnea:
a. How far can you walk before you feel short of breath?
b. How many flights of stairs can you climb before you experience SOB?
c. How far can you walk when walking as fast as your spouse?

d. Is there anything you do that makes the SOB *worse*?
e. Is there anything you do that makes the SOB *better*?
f. How long does the SOB last after you stop to rest?
g. Is the SOB worse at any particular time of the *day*?
h. Is the SOB worse at any particular time of the *year*?

The following are examples of questions to ask in evaluating orthopnea:
a. Do you wake up at night with SOB?
b. Does your nighttime SOB get better after you sit up on the side of your bed or in a chair?
c. Do you get SOB when lying down to take a nap?
d. Do you use extra pillows behind your head and back to help you not get SOB at night or during a nap?
e. How many pillows do you need to keep you from getting SOB at night or when taking a nap?

Dyspnea, like pain, is based on the patient's level of discomfort. Some patients may complain of dyspnea, whereas others may not. The therapist can get an impression of the patient's dyspnea by how many words can be spoken continuously. A patient with severe dyspnea cannot complete even a short sentence on a single breath.

6. What is the patient's sputum production like? (WRE code: IB4b) [Difficulty: An]
a. Time of maximal and minimal expectoration

Interview the patient to determine the following:
1. Time of maximal expectoration. Ask the patient, "When do you cough up the most? For example, is it in the morning; after eating spicy foods; after a breathing treatment; after smoking, work, or other exposure to dusts; etc."
2. Time of minimal expectoration. Ask the patient, "When do you cough up the least? For example, during certain nonallergic seasons of the year, after a breathing treatment, after consuming milk or milk products, etc."

b. Quantity

Some practitioners prefer to know of a specific amount such as a teaspoon, tablespoon, 10 mL, and so on. Others

TABLE 1-9 Severity of Dyspnea in Evaluating Permanent Impairment				
Class I	Class II	Class III	Class IV	Class V
Dyspnea only on severe exertion ("appropriate" dyspnea)	Can keep pace with person of same age and body build on the level without breathlessness but not on hills or stairs	Can walk a mile at own pace without dyspnea but cannot keep pace on the level with a normal person	Dyspnea present after walking about 100 yd on the level or on climbing one flight of stairs	Dyspnea on even less activity or at rest

From Burton GG: Practical physical diagnosis in respiratory care. In Burton GG, Hodgkin JE, editors: *Respiratory care: a guide to clinical practice*, ed 2, Philadelphia, 1984, Lippincott.

TABLE 1-10	Causes of Dyspnea Related to Preferred Body Position	
Kind of Dyspnea	**Clinical Correlations**
Orthopnea (must sit up to breathe; often occurs at night as paroxysmal nocturnal dyspnea)	Congestive heart failure
Obstructive sleep apnea (periodically stops breathing, particularly when lying on back)	Obesity; obstructive sleep apnea syndromes
Emphysematous habitus	COPD
Platypnea	Pleural effusion; dyspnea associated with various body positions
Orthodeoxia	Pulmonary fibrosis; dyspnea improved when patient is lying flat

COPD, Chronic obstructive pulmonary disease.
From Burton GG: Patient assessment procedures. In Barnes TA, editor: *Respiratory care practice*, Chicago, 1990, Mosby.

prefer to use subjective measures such as "a little" or "a lot." Interview the patient to determine the following:

1. How does the quantity of sputum relate to the times of maximal and minimal expectoration and the patient's lifestyle? Ask the patient, "Is there anything that you do that increases or decreases the amount you cough out?" For example, the patient states that he coughs up 20 mL after breathing treatments but can cough up nothing after eating a bowl of ice cream.
2. Does the amount coughed up change in a cyclical way? Ask the patient, "Do you cough up the most in the mornings or at night? Is there a work or lifestyle habit that changes how much you cough up? Is there a seasonal allergic condition that influences your asthma and sputum production?"

c. Adhesiveness of the sputum

Interview the patient to determine the following:

1. Are there times of the day or things that you do in the day that seem to result in your secretions becoming thicker or thinner?
2. Do your medications (like acetylcysteine [Mucomyst]) make the secretions easier to cough out?
3. Do some foods make your secretions easier to cough out?

7. What is the patient's work of breathing? (WRE code: IB4b) [Difficulty: An]

Work of breathing (WOB) refers to the patient's subjective feeling of how easy or difficult it is to breathe. A person at rest should feel no difficulty in breathing. During vigorous exercise, a person should be aware that he or she is working harder than normal to breathe. This is to be expected. After recovering from exercise, the work of breathing should again be easy.

Patients with acute or chronic lung disease feel that they are breathing with some difficulty. Because this is a subjective feeling of the patient, it is helpful to have the patient quantify it. Ask the patient to rate his or her WOB on a 1-to-10 scale with 1 being easy breathing and 10 being extremely difficult.

If bronchospasm or secretions have increased, the patient will tell you that his or her WOB has worsened. If medications such as bronchodilators or mucolytics are effective, the patient should feel that his or her breathing is easier.

MODULE D

Use *observation* to determine the patient's complete respiratory condition

1. Evaluate the patient's general appearance (WRE code: IB1a) [Difficulty: An]

Start by quickly inspecting the patient from head to toe, including how he or she is dressed and found in the room. Ideally, this is done without the patient knowing that he or she is being observed. The patient who does not have cardiopulmonary disease should be able to lie flat in bed or on either side without any breathing difficulty. The patient with one-sided lung disease may prefer to lie with the good side down. This might be the case with lobar pneumonia, pleurisy, or broken ribs. The patient with severe airway obstruction, as seen with asthma, bronchitis, or emphysema, tends to sit up in a chair or on the edge of the bed and use locked arms and shoulders for support. This enables the patient to use accessory muscles (Fig. 1-16). The patient with orthopnea will not want to lie down flat because of the resulting SOB. This is commonly seen in patients with congestive heart failure and pulmonary edema.

2. Determine whether the patient is cyanotic (WRE code: IB1a) [Difficulty: An]

Cyanosis is an abnormal blue or ashen gray coloration of the skin and mucous membranes. It is most easily seen in white persons by looking at the lips and nailbeds. It can be seen in darker-pigmented people by looking at the inner portion of the lip, the inner portion of the lower eyelid, and the nailbeds. Commonly, cyanosis is said to be caused by hypoxemia, and that the more bluish a patient's color, the more hypoxemic he or she is. This is often the case, but cyanosis is not an accurate measurement of a patient's oxygenation. To be safe, a patient with cyanosis should have an arterial blood gas sample drawn for Pao_2 measurement or pulse oximetry performed for Spo_2 measurement to evaluate oxygenation.

promptly evaluate the diaphoretic patient's pulse, respiratory rate, blood pressure, and arterial blood gases.

4. Determine whether the patient has nasal flaring (WRE code: IB1a) [Difficulty: An]

Nasal flaring is a dilation of the nares on inspiration. A person breathing comfortably should have little or no nasal flaring. A person who is exercising vigorously may exhibit nasal flaring. It is abnormal to see nasal flaring in a patient who is resting in bed, and it is a sign of increased WOB. The patient is attempting to reduce airway resistance by dilating the nares. Patients of any age have nasal flaring when experiencing increased WOB, but it is most commonly seen in the premature newborn (Fig. 1-17).

Nasal flaring is not specific to any disease or condition. Examples of conditions during which nasal flaring is seen include infant respiratory distress syndrome, acute respiratory distress syndrome, or any condition in which pulmonary compliance is decreased or airway resistance is increased.

5. Determine whether the patient has clubbing of the fingers (WRE code: IB1a) [Difficulty: An]

Clubbing of the fingers (also known as digital clubbing) is an abnormal thickening of the ends of the fingers. It also can occur in the toes. The key finding is an angle of more than 160 degrees between the top of the finger and the nail when seen from the side. Clinically, you will notice both a lateral and an AP thickening of the ends of the fingers (See Fig. 1-18 for a comparison of normal fingers and clubbed fingers). The finger and toenail beds may be cyanotic.

The underlying cause is not completely understood but at least in part seems to be chronic hypoxemia. This results in arteriovenous anastomosis with thickening of the tissues. The list of diseases in which clubbing is seen includes COPD, bronchogenic carcinoma, bronchiectasis, sarcoidosis, and infective endocarditis.

6. Determine whether the patient has peripheral edema (WRE code: IB1a) [Difficulty: An]

Peripheral edema is seen when fluid leaks from the capillary bed into the tissues. It is most commonly seen in the ankles and feet or along the back when the patient is lying supine in bed. The extent of the edema is measured by pressing a finger into the tissues. Normal skin springs back, whereas edematous skin is pitted or depressed. The pitting edema is graded as 1+ for less than ¼-inch (mild), 2+ for ¼- to ½-inch (moderate), and 3+ for ½- to 1-inch (severe) indentation. Obviously, the deeper the pitting, the more peripheral edema the patient has.

Fig. 1-16 Typical posture seen in patients using accessory muscles of respiration. The shoulders are locked so that the accessory muscles can be used more effectively. (**A,** *from Burton GG: Practical physical diagnosis in respiratory care. In Burton GG, Hodgkin JE, editors:* Respiratory care, *ed 2, Philadelphia, 1984, Lippincott.* **B,** *from Barriascout JR: Chest physical therapy and related procedures. In Burton GG, Hodgkin JE, editors:* Respiratory care, *ed 2, Philadelphia, 1984, Lippincott.)*

3. Determine whether the patient is diaphoretic (WRE code: IB1a) [Difficulty: An]

Diaphoresis is profuse sweating. It is normally seen after vigorous exercise. A patient is expected to sweat after a stress test or even an oxygen-assisted walk. Diaphoresis in a patient who is resting in bed should be investigated. When the body is severely stressed, it releases adrenaline into the bloodstream. Diaphoresis is one of many bodily effects caused by the release of the hormone adrenaline. Similar sweating may be seen if a large enough dose of the drug epinephrine is given.

Diaphoresis is a nonspecific sign of serious cardiopulmonary difficulties. It may be seen any time the patient is in shock or hypoxemic. Patients with a myocardial infarct are commonly diaphoretic. The practitioner should

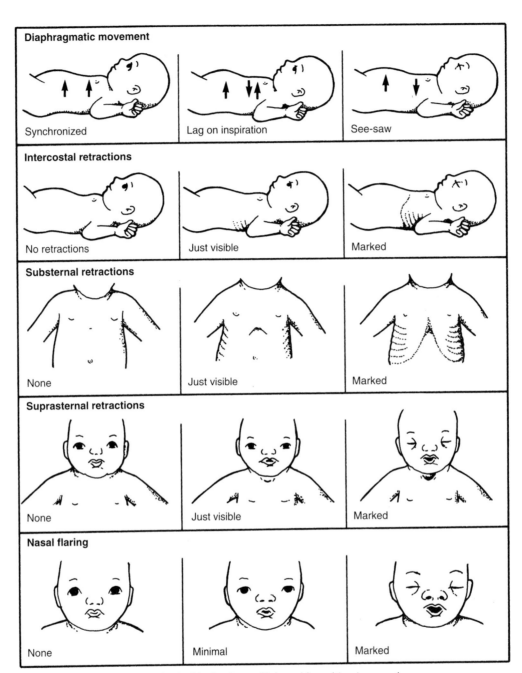

Fig. 1-17 Physical indications of labored breathing in a newborn.

Fig. 1-18 Signs of and test for clubbing. *(From Lehrer S: Understanding lung sounds, Philadelphia, 1984, WB Saunders.)*

Peripheral edema is most commonly seen in patients with congestive heart failure or those who are fluid overloaded. Patients with septicemia often have peripheral edema because the blood-borne pathogen (usually *Staphylococcus*) causes abnormal capillary leakage.

7. Determine the shape (configuration) of the patient's chest (WRE code: IB1a) [Difficulty: An]

The patient should be sitting up straight or standing erect when being examined for chest configuration. Look at the patient from the front, back, and both sides to see the symmetry. (See Fig. 1-19 for the appearance of a normal infant's and adult's chest, barrel chest, funnel chest, pigeon chest, and thoracic kyphoscoliosis). Several variations on curvature of the spine are found. Kyphosis is an exaggerated AP curvature of the upper portion of the spine. Lordosis is an exaggerated AP curvature of the lower portion of the spine. Scoliosis is either a right or left lateral curvature of the spine. Kyphoscoliosis is either a right or left lateral curvature combined with an AP curvature of the spine.

8. Determine whether the patient has asymmetrical chest movement when breathing (WRE code: IB1a) [Difficulty: An]

Normal infants and adults have symmetrical chest movement when breathing at rest or during exercise. All breathing efforts are best observed when the patient is shirtless. In female patients, it may be necessary to observe only the uncovered back to judge chest movement. Any kind of asymmetrical chest movement is abnormal. The asymmetrical movement may result from an abnormality of the chest wall or abdomen or from a pulmonary disorder.

a. Thoracic scoliosis or kyphoscoliosis

(Refer to Fig. 1-19 for the back view of a patient with thoracic scoliosis or kyphoscoliosis.) The scoliosis patient in Fig. 1-19 tends to have more chest movement on the right side because of the right spinal curvature. The left side of the chest and left lung would inflate more than the right if the spine curved to the left. These same findings are seen in a patient with kyphoscoliosis.

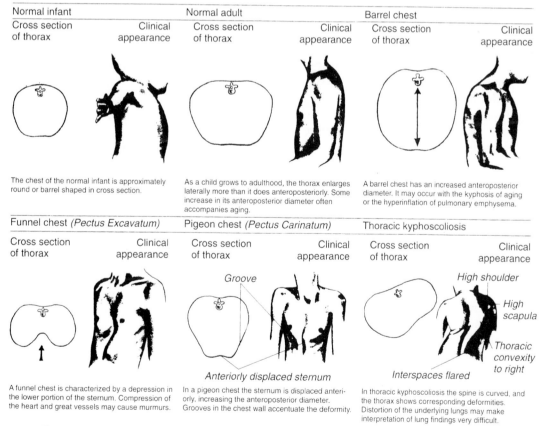

Fig. 1-19 Deformities of the thorax. *(From Bates B: A guide to physical examination and history taking, ed 4, Philadelphia, 1987, Lippincott.)*

b. Flail chest

The flail segment moves in the opposite direction from the rest of the chest (also known as paradoxical movement). That is, with inspiration, the flail segment moves inward while the rest of the chest moves outward, and during expiration, the flail segment moves outward as the rest of the chest moves inward. As the ribs heal, the segment stabilizes and moves with the rest of the chest.

c. Pneumothorax

The side with the collapsed lung does not move as much as the chest wall over the normal lung (see Fig. 1-2).

d. Atelectasis/pneumonia

The side with the atelectasis or pneumonia does not move as much as the chest wall over the normal lung (see Fig. 1-5).

Exam Hint

Frequently a question relates to physical signs that a patient has a pneumothorax. This could include asymmetrical chest movement. The chest wall on the side with the pneumothorax will not move as much as the normal side during breathing.

---

9. Determine whether the patient has intercostal or sternal retractions when breathing (WRE code: IB1a) [Difficulty: An]

Intercostal retractions are noticed when the soft tissues between the ribs are drawn inward during inspiration as the chest wall moves outward. Suprasternal retractions are noticed when the soft tissues *above* the sternum are drawn inward during an inspiration as the chest wall moves outward. Substernal retractions are noticed when the soft tissues *below* the sternum are drawn inward during an inspiration as the chest wall moves outward (see Fig. 1-17).

A person who is breathing at rest should not have any retractions. That same person may have some minor retractions during vigorous exercise. Retractions of any kind are abnormal in any patient of any age who is resting in bed. Retractions are commonly seen in conditions in which airway resistance is increased or lung compliance is decreased. Both increase a patient's WOB. The patient must generate a more negative intrathoracic pressure to breathe, and as a result, the various soft tissues are drawn inward during inspiration. Conditions in which this is seen include infant respiratory distress syndrome, acute respiratory distress syndrome, pulmonary edema, pneumonia, asthma, bronchitis, and emphysema.

10. Determine whether the patient uses accessory muscles when breathing (WRE code: IB1a) [Difficulty: An]

Accessory muscles of respiration should not be needed during passive, resting breathing. They may be used when breathing vigorously during exercise. A dyspneic patient will likely use them even when resting. The accessory muscles of inspiration are the intercostal, scalene, sternocleidomastoid, trapezius, and rhomboid. The abdominal muscles are used during active expiration. The easiest accessory muscles of inspiration to observe in action are the sternocleidomastoids from the front and side of the patient and the trapezius from the back of the patient (Fig. 1-20).

Accessory muscle use in a patient who is resting should make it obvious that the WOB is greatly increased. The finding is not specific for any one condition but is commonly seen in a patient with emphysema (see Fig. 1-16).

11. Determine whether the patient has diaphragmatic movement when breathing (WRE code: IB1a) [Difficulty: An]

Normally, an adult's diaphragm moves downward several centimeters toward the abdomen during inspiration as the chest wall moves outward. This is seen when the abdomen protrudes as its contents are forced forward. The chest and abdomen should rise and fall together during quiet and vigorous breathing efforts. In two conditions, this normal chest and abdominal movement does not occur.

First, patients with emphysema, severe air trapping, and a barrel chest have a diaphragm that is depressed and

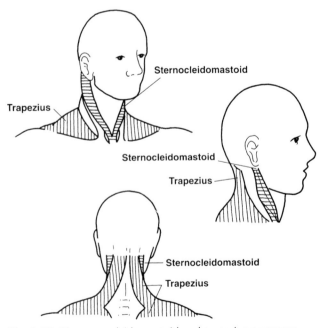

Fig. 1-20 The sternocleidomastoid and trapezius accessory muscles of respiration.

flat rather than domed because of the air that is trapped in the lungs. On inspiration, the diaphragm still contracts but is unable to displace the abdominal contents down to permit air to be drawn into the lungs. These patients do not have the expected abdominal movement during inspiration. These patients use the accessory muscles of inspiration to assist breathing.

Second is any condition in which the airway resistance is increased or lung compliance is decreased. The greater negative intrathoracic pressure needed to draw the tidal volume into the lungs can cause the chest wall to collapse inward as the abdominal contents are displaced outward. The result is a kind of "seesaw" or paradoxical movement relation between the chest wall and abdomen. On inspiration, the chest wall may move inward as the abdomen moves outward. Patients with RDS typically demonstrate this because the premature neonate's rib cage is relatively compliant when compared with stiff lungs (see Fig. 1-17).

12. Determine the patient's breathing pattern (WRE code: IB1a) [Difficulty: An]

The various respiratory patterns can be identified by their characteristic respiratory rate, respiratory cycle, and tidal volume. See Fig. 1-21 for examples of normal and abnormal breathing patterns.

a. Eupnea (normal breathing)

1. Normal respiratory rate for the age of the patient (Table 1-11).
2. Normal respiratory cycle. When timing the flow of air into and out of the lungs, the inspiratory/expiratory (I:E) ratio is about 1:2. A pause of variable time may follow exhalation of the tidal volume. This could change the true I:E ratio from 1:2 to 1:4.
3. Tidal volume is normal for the size of the patient. (See Chapter 4 for calculation of a predicted tidal volume.) Inspiration is achieved without the use of accessory muscles of inspiration; exhalation is passive.
4. A person usually sighs every few minutes; especially when inactive. A sigh breath is typically about 1.5 times as large as a tidal volume. It is thought to help prevent atelectasis. Frequent sighing may indicate a problem.

b. Hypopnea (shallow breathing)

1. Respiratory rate usually somewhat slower than normal.
2. Normal respiratory cycle.
3. Tidal volume decreased for the size of the patient.

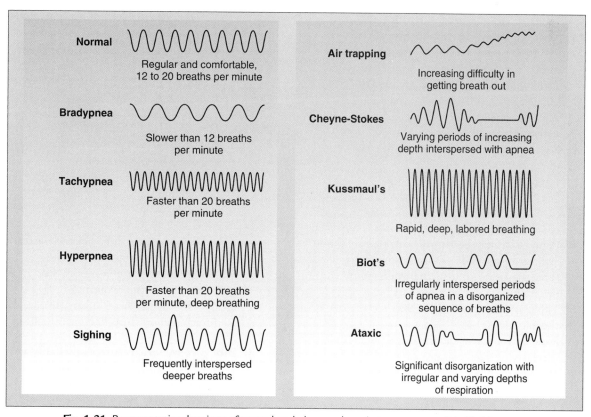

Fig. 1-21 Representative drawings of normal and abnormal respiratory patterns. *(Modified from Seidel HM, Ball JW, Dains JE, et al: Mosby's guide to physical examination, ed 4, St Louis, 1999, Mosby.)*

TABLE 1-11 Normal Resting Respiratory Rates		
Age (Years)	**Male**	**Female**
0–1	31 ± 8	30 ± 6
1–2	26 ± 4	27 ± 4
2–4	25 ± 4	25 ± 3
5–7	22 ± 2	21 ± 2
8–11	19 ± 2	19 ± 2
12–14	19 ± 2	18 ± 2
15–16	17 ± 3	18 ± 3
17–18	16 ± 3	17 ± 3
Older	16 ± 3	17 ± 3

Modified from Eubanks DH, Bone RC: *Comprehensive respiratory care*, ed 2, St Louis, 1990, Mosby.

4. Possible causes: deep sleep, sedation, coma, hypothermia, alkalemia, restrictive lung disease.
5. May be combined with bradypnea.

c. Hyperpnea (deep breathing)

1. Respiratory rate may be normal or somewhat faster.
2. Normal respiratory cycle.
3. Tidal volume increased for the size of the patient.
4. Possible causes: acidemia, fever, pain, fear, anxiety, increased intracranial pressure.
5. May be combined with tachypnea.

d. Bradypnea (slow breathing)

1. Slower-than-normal respiratory rate.
2. Expiration may be longer than normal as a result of a longer pause.
3. Tidal volume may be decreased for the size of the patient.
4. Possible causes: deep sleep, sedation, coma, hypothermia, alkalemia.
5. May be combined with hypopnea.

e. Tachypnea (rapid breathing)

1. Faster than the normal respiratory rate.
2. Inspiration may be faster than normal with the help of inspiratory accessory muscles. Expiration may be shorter than normal, and expiratory accessory muscles may be used to force the air out faster. The pause seen in eupnea is absent. The I:E ratio may be 1:2 or less.
3. Tidal volume may be increased for the size of the patient.
4. Possible causes: acidemia, fever, pain, anxiety, increased intracranial pressure.
5. May be combined with hyperpnea.

f. Obstructed inspiration

1. Normal to slower respiratory rate.
2. Inspiratory time is equal to or longer than expiratory time. Inspiration is aided by use of the inspiratory accessory muscles. Expiration is passive.
3. Tidal volume may be normal or larger or smaller than normal depending on how the patient adapts to the increased WOB. It is most common to see a slower rate with a larger tidal volume.
4. Possible causes: croup, epiglottitis, foreign body aspiration with partial airway obstruction, postextubation laryngeal edema, airway tumor, or airway trauma.

g. Obstructed expiration with or without air trapping

1. Normal to slower respiratory rate.
2. Expiratory time is longer than normal. Accessory muscles of inspiration and expiration may be used.
3. Tidal volume may be normal or decreased for the size of the patient.
4. Possible causes: asthma, emphysema, bronchitis, cystic fibrosis, bronchiectasis, airway tumor, or airway trauma. In severe cases, such as status asthmaticus, incomplete exhalation may cause air trapping.

h. Kussmaul's respiration (rapid, large breaths)

1. Faster-than-normal rate.
2. I:E ratio approaches 1:1. Both inspiratory and expiratory accessory muscles may be used.
3. Tidal volume is increased for the size of the patient.
4. Probable cause: acidemia (pH, 7.2 to 6.95) from diabetic ketoacidosis.

i. Cheyne-Stokes respiration (waxing and waning tidal volumes)

1. The respiratory rate varies from normal to faster and may have short periods of apnea.
2. The respiratory cycle is normal or approximates it, except if the patient has periods of apnea.
3. The tidal volumes increase and decrease over a variable time cycle. A 20-second cycle is fairly common. Periods of apnea may occur between the decreased tidal volumes.
4. Possible causes: head injury, stroke, increased intracranial pressure, or congestive heart failure.

j. Biot's respiration (unpredictably variable)

1. The respiratory rate may be slow with deep breaths or rapid with shallow breaths; sighing is often seen. Periods of apnea will be seen between the periods of breathing.
2. The respiratory cycle varies considerably with periods of apnea.

3. Tidal volume may be larger or smaller than normal.
4. Possible causes: meningitis, head (brain) injury, brain tumor, increased intracranial pressure.

k. Ataxic respiration (unpredictably variable)

1. The respiratory rate varies considerably with abrupt periods of apnea.
2. The respiratory cycle varies considerably with periods of apnea.
3. Tidal volume varies unpredictably between larger and smaller than normal.
4. Possible causes: lesion of the medullary respiratory centers, head (brain) injury, brain tumor, increased intracranial pressure.

l. Apnea (cessation of breathing at the end of exhalation)

1. Apnea that lasts long enough to result in hypoxemia, bradycardia, and hypotension must be treated aggressively. Artificial respiration, with or without supplemental oxygen, must be started immediately.
2. It is important to evaluate the patient's previous breathing pattern to determine the cause of the apnea. Normal breathing followed by apnea could result from a heart attack, stroke, or upper airway obstruction. An abnormal breathing pattern followed by apnea could be the result of worsening of the original problem.
3. Evaluate the previous tidal volume variation for the reasons previously listed.
4. Possible causes: airway obstruction, heart attack, stroke, or head (brain) injury.

13. Determine the kind of cough the patient has (WRE code: IB1b) [Difficulty: An]

a. Normal cough

A normal cough has four parts:
1. A person takes a deep breath.
2. The epiglottis and vocal cords close to keep the air trapped within the lungs.
3. The abdominal and other expiratory muscles contract to increase the air pressure in the lungs.
4. The epiglottis and vocal cords open to allow the compressed air to escape explosively and remove any mucus or foreign matter.

All components must work individually and in a coordinated manner for the patient to have an effective cough. The following are possible variations used by patients who for some reason cannot cough normally.

b. Serial cough

All actions of a normal cough take place, except that the patient performs a series of smaller coughs rather than a single large one. This method of coughing may be used by postoperative patients who have too much abdominal or thoracic pain to cough normally. As the pain lessens, the patient should be able to cough normally.

c. Midinspiratory cough

All actions of a normal cough take place, except that the patient does not take as deep a breath. Patients with emphysema and chronic bronchitis (COPD) sometimes use this to help prevent airway collapse when they cough.

d. Huff cough

Patients with artificial airways use this method. They cannot close their epiglottis and vocal cords, so they can take only a large breath and blow out with as much force as possible. It is still an effective way to remove watery secretions.

e. Assisted cough

This patient needs direct help from the therapist. The patient is given a deep breath by means of intermittent positive pressure breathing (IPPB) machine or manual ventilator. Then the therapist helps the patient blow the air out quickly by pushing on the abdominal area to move the diaphragm up. This procedure is limited to conscious patients with neuromuscular defects who cannot cough effectively on their own.

14. Determine the quantity and characteristics of the patient's sputum (WRE code: IB1b) [Difficulty: An]

a. Quantity

Normally a person is not aware of mucus production. The mucociliary escalator moves mucus toward the throat, where it is unconsciously swallowed. Normally mucus is uninfected and clear or white.

Typically, infections causing bronchitis or pneumonia result in the production of large amounts of mucus. The patient will report coughing and spitting it up. This mix of mucus from the lungs and saliva from the mouth is sputum. Any increase in mucus or sputum production, to the extent that the patient is aware of it, is abnormal.

As mentioned earlier, some practitioners prefer to use subjective measurements of sputum production such as "a little," "medium amount," or "copious." Objective measurements such as a teaspoon, a tablespoon, or 5, 10, or 15 mL, for example, are preferred to quantify production. A marked measuring cup is needed to do this.

Note any changes in the amount of sputum that the patient is producing. This is best done in a timed manner such as production per hour or per shift. It also is wise to correlate sputum production with breathing treatments or other procedures that may increase or decrease its production or clearance.

b. Characteristics

Homogeneity is best determined by letting a sputum sample stand in a test tube for several hours so that it stratifies. This is an important test to perform in the patient with a pulmonary infection. Normal sputum separates into a relatively thin surface layer of gel that floats on a lower layer of water (sol). The patient with a pulmonary infection has more viscous sputum because it contains dead bacterial cells, dead white blood cells, and cellular debris from the infected lung tissues. These cells settle over time to the bottom of a sputum sample and create a third layer of sediment. See Fig. 1-22 for an example of how this layering looks in the sputum from a patient who has a pulmonary infection that eventually clears up. Table 1-12 explains other details on sputum characteristics.

> ### Exam Hint
>
> **U**sually one question requires the therapist to evaluate the patient's sputum. Examples: (1) a change from white or yellow to green indicates pneumonia, (2) a lung abscess is likely when the sputum is green and foul smelling, and (3) pink-tinged bubbly (frothy) secretions are found with pulmonary edema.

15. Determine whether the patient has excessive venous distention (WRE code: IB1a) [Difficulty: An]

The internal jugular vein and external/anterior jugular vein are observed in the normal patient by having him or her lie supine with the head elevated 30 degrees. The crest of the vein column should be seen just above the border of the midclavicle. Make a rough measure of the intravascular volume and CVP by pressing on the veins at the base of the neck. The returning blood should fill the veins and make them distend (Fig. 1-23). When the pressure is released, the veins should return to their previous level of distention just above the level of the midclavicle. Increased venous distention is noted when the veins stand out at a level above the clavicle. This is seen in patients with right heart failure (cor pulmonale), cardiac tamponade, fluid overload, COPD, and when high airway pressures and positive end-expiratory pressure (PEEP) are needed for mechanical ventilation. The more the veins are distended, the more the patient is compromised.

It is not normal for the veins to collapse below the clavicle when the obstructing finger is removed. If this is seen, this patient should then have his or her head laid flat. Normally, when flat, the external jugular vein should be seen as partially distended. If the vein collapses on inspiration, low venous pressure is confirmed, and the patient is probably hypovolemic. This is commonly seen in dehydration, hemorrhage, or increased urine output after the use of diuretics.

16. Determine the patient's capillary refill (WRE code: IB1a) [Difficulty: An]

Capillary refill is the time needed for blood to refill the capillary bed after it has been forced out. The procedure is to pinch the finger or toenail until it blanches and then release the pressure. The pink color of the nailbed should

Infection

Improvement

Normal

1. Gel layer: thicker than normal

2. Sol layer: thinner in ratio to gel layer than normal

3. Cellular debris: dead bacteria, WBCs, other cells

NOTE: The total volume of sputum is greatly increased

1. Gel layer: reducing toward normal

2. Sol layer: returning to normal ratio with gel layer

3. Cellular debris: thinning out as fewer dead cells are being coughed out

1. Gel layer: normal volume

2. Sol layer: normal volume and ratio with the gel layer

NOTE: The total volume of sputum is reduced to normal; also, there is no third layer of cellular debris

Fig. 1-22 Evaluation of the homogeneity of sputum in the infected patient.

TABLE 1-12	Sputum Characteristics			
Sputum Type	**Color**	**Contents**	**Illnesses**	**Odor**
Bloody (hemoptysis)	Red	Blood	Bronchogenic carcinoma; pulmonary hemorrhage; lung abscess; tuberculosis; pulmonary infarction	Typically none
Frothy or bubbly	Clear or pink	Water; plasma proteins; red blood cells	Pulmonary edema	Typically none
Mucoid	Clear or white	Water; complex sugars; glycoproteins; some cellular debris	Asthma; chronic bronchitis	Typically none
Mucopurulent	Light to medium yellow	Decreased water and complex sugars; increased cellular debris and causative organisms (if applicable); organisms are usually aerobes	Chronic and acute bronchitis	Typically none, but may exist depending on organism
Purulent	Dark yellow or green	Decreased water; greatly increased cellular debris and causative organisms that are usually aerobes; complex sugars	Bronchiectasis; lung abscess; pneumonia	Depending on organism, along with clearance of mucus; also may be foul tasting to the patient; odor usually not offensive
Purulent (fetid)	Dark yellow or green	Decreased water; may contain some blood; greatly exaggerated cellular debris and causative organisms that frequently are anaerobes; complex sugars	Bronchiectasis; lung abscess; cystic fibrosis	Offensive odor

From DiPietro JS: *Clinical guide for respiratory care and cardiopulmonary disease,* Acton, Mass, 1998, Copley Custom Publishing.

Fig. 1-23 Evaluating distention of the external jugular vein. These photographs show a patient with right-sided heart failure. Note that the left photograph shows the external jugular vein distended above the level of the clavicle. The right photograph shows how pressing a finger over the external jugular vein results in its further filling with blood and distending. In a normal person, when the pressure is released, the vein should collapse to just above the superior border of the midclavicle. See the text for further discussion. *(From Daily EK, Schroder JS:* Techniques in bedside hemodynamic monitoring, *ed 4, St Louis, 1989, Mosby.)*

return in less than 3 seconds. Any delay in the return to pink color indicates reduced blood flow to the extremities. Cyanotic nailbeds also are seen with reduced blood flow. Examples of conditions that result in a decreased capillary refill include decreased cardiac output, low blood pressure from any cause, and the use of vasopressor medications.

17. Determine whether the patient has muscle wasting (WRE code: IB1a) [Difficulty: An]

Muscle wasting is an abnormal condition of decreased muscle mass. Muscle wasting can be generalized or localized, depending on the underlying cause. Examples of conditions in which muscle wasting is seen include the following.

a. Chronic obstructive pulmonary disease

COPD (emphysema and bronchitis) often results in muscle wasting because the patient is using an unusually large number of calories through the act of breathing. In addition, these patients often do not eat well because a full stomach restricts the movement of the diaphragm and worsens their WOB and SOB. Because of this, they are frequently malnourished or undernourished. Their arms and legs are thin; their shoulder, elbow, and knee joints are prominent; and their ribs are clearly outlined by deep intercostal spaces.

b. Lung cancer

Lung cancer or other cancers usually result in a loss of muscle mass. This is because the growing tumor consumes many calories that are then not available to the normal body tissues. These patients usually also have thin arms and legs with prominent joints during advanced disease.

c. Neurologic injuries

Neurologic injuries, such as transsection of the spinal cord, result in atrophy of the affected muscles. Atrophy of the muscles is a decrease in size resulting from lack of use. This is an unavoidable consequence of the permanent loss of nerve input to the affected muscles. For example, transsection of the spinal cord at the first lumbar vertebra (L1) results in loss of nerve input to the legs. The patient is a paraplegic. In time, the muscles of the legs atrophy; however, if the arms are exercised, they retain normal muscle mass. If the patient has a spinal transsection that results in the loss of nerve input to both the arms and legs (quadriplegia), all of the limbs atrophy.

MODULE E

Measure and record the patient's vital signs (WRE code: IIIE7) [Difficulty: R, AP, AN]

1. Current vital signs

Review the current vital signs in the patient's chart. Compare them with the admission vital signs and what you observe in the patient now. Look for a change in pattern that suggests either a worsening or an improvement in the patient.

2. Temperature

The textbook "normal" oral body temperature is 98.6°F (37°C). It is normal for there to be some range from 96.5°F to 99.5°F (35.8°C to 37.4°C). Make sure the patient has not eaten any hot or cold foods recently or has been smoking before taking an oral temperature.

A rectal or core temperature is commonly taken in very sick patients because it is more accurate and reliable. The normal rectal temperature is 97.5°F to 100.4°F (36.4°C to 38°C). It is normal to see some variance here, but less so than orally. Axillary temperatures are used as a last resort in stable patients. These run 1°F less than oral temperatures and are less accurate and reliable.

The variations in temperature noted depend on the time of day, activity level, and, in women, stage of the menstrual cycle. For example, it is normal to see a lower body temperature when a person is in a deep sleep. An oral temperature of more than 99.4°F or 37.4°C in a patient with a history of respiratory disease indicates a fever. Typically, it can be caused by atelectasis or a pulmonary or systemic infection. Patients are commonly treated to keep the fever below 103°F, if possible. In general, a rectal temperature below 97°F (36°C) is considered hypothermic. In some procedures, such as open-heart surgery, a patient's temperature is lowered to reduce metabolism and oxygen needs. The rectal temperature must be kept above 90°F (32°C) to prevent cardiac dysrhythmias from occurring because of the cold.

3. Respiratory rate

The respiratory rate (f for frequency) is the number of breaths the patient takes in a minute. The number is counted by looking at or feeling the chest or abdominal movements or both. The normal rate varies with age (see Table 1–11). It is assumed that the patient is resting but awake and has a normal temperature and metabolic rate. A respiratory rate that is above or below normal should be a cause for alarm.

Hyperthermia (fever), acidemia, hypoxemia, fear, anxiety, and pain cause a patient to breathe more rapidly. Hypothermia, alkalemia, hyperoxia in the patient breathing on hypoxic drive, sedation, and coma cause a patient to breathe more slowly.

It must be remembered that even in healthy people, considerable variation is found in the respiratory rate. It is best to consider the respiratory rate and the patient's tidal volume and minute volume to have a more complete impression of how the patient is breathing. Carefully measure the respiratory rate of any patient with cardiopulmonary disease or with a respiratory rate outside of the normal range. The rate should be checked as often as needed to monitor the patient's condition.

4. Blood pressure

The blood pressure (BP) is the result of the pumping ability of the left ventricle (made up of the heart rate [HR] and stroke volume), arterial resistance, and blood volume. Normal BP is caused by all three factors being in balance with each other. If one factor is abnormal, the other two have some ability to compensate. For example, if the patient has lost a lot of blood, the body attempts to maintain BP by increasing the arterial resistance and increasing the HR.

Normal BPs: Adults, less than 120/80 mm Hg; infants and children younger than 10 years, more than 60 to 100/20 to 70 mm Hg

As with the other vital signs, some variation of BP is noted among individuals. It is important to know what the patient's normal BP is to compare it with the current value. Carefully measure the BP in any patient who has cardiopulmonary disease or a history of hypotension or hypertension.

Hypotension in the adult is a systolic BP of less than 80 mm Hg. Recommend a BP measurement in any patient who has a history of hypotension, appears to be in shock, has lost a lot of blood, has a weak pulse, shows mental confusion, is unconscious, or has low urine output.

Hypertension in the adult is a systolic BP of 140 mm Hg or greater or a diastolic BP of 90 mm Hg or greater, or both. Carefully measure the BP of any patient with a history of hypertension, bounding pulse, or symptoms of a stroke (mental confusion, headache, and sudden weakness or partial paralysis). Fear, anxiety, and pain also cause the patient's BP to increase temporarily.

5. Heart/pulse rate

The heart/pulse rate (HR) is the number of heartbeats per minute. It can be counted by listening to the heart tones with a stethoscope or by feeling any of the common sites where an artery is easy to locate. Table 1-13 shows the normal pulse rates based on age. It is assumed that the patient is alert but resting when the pulse is counted. Carefully measure the heart/pulse rate in any patient with cardiopulmonary disease or any of the aforementioned conditions for hypotension or hypertension.

TABLE 1-13	Normal Pulse Rates According to Age
Age	**Beats/min**
Birth	70–170
Neonate	120–140
1 year	80–140
2 year	80–130
3 year	80–120
4 year	70–115
Adult	60–100

From Eubanks DH, Bone RC: *Comprehensive respiratory care*, ed 2, St Louis, 1990, Mosby.

MODULE F

Use *palpation* to determine the patient's complete respiratory condition

1. Determine the patient's pulse rate, rhythm, and force (WRE code: IB2a) [Difficulty: An]

The HR is most commonly counted by palpating the following locations: carotid, femoral, radial, and brachial arteries and apical pulse of the heart (Fig. 1-24). The apical pulse is normally located in the area of the left midclavicular line in the fifth intercostal space. The apical pulse is also known as the point of maximal impulse (PMI). The location indicates the apex of the heart (left ventricle). Other arterial sites such as the temporal, dorsalis pedis, and posterior tibial can be used but are more difficult to find. The pulse should be counted for a minimum of 30 seconds; counting for 1 minute provides the most accurate measure of HR.

Palpating a pulse at any of the aforementioned sites reveals the timing between the heartbeats. This rhythm is normally regular in people who are at rest or exercising at a steady level. The rhythm is felt and mentally timed as the pulse rate is counted. The period between beats should be about the same.

The respiratory effort may have some influence on the rhythm. Fairly common in children and sometimes in adults, the heart rhythm and rate increase on inspiration and decrease on expiration. This sinus arrhythmia is not really abnormal. It is caused when the negative intrathoracic pressure during inspiration draws blood more quickly into the thorax and heart. The opposite may be true during mechanical ventilation with a high peak pressure or mean airway pressure. Then the heart rhythm and rate may slow during inspiration and speed up during expiration. In any other case, an irregular rhythm indicates some sort of cardiac problem. An electrocardiogram is needed to help determine the specific cause.

The force of the pulse is an indicator of the strength of the heart's contraction and BP. Normally each heartbeat should be felt with the same amount of force. A "thready" or variable force felt with each heartbeat is usually a sign of heart disease. Atrial fibrillation is an example of an irregular heart rhythm that results in an irregular force. The irregular rate and rhythm cause variable volumes of blood to be pumped with each contraction. A large volume of blood is felt as a strong pulse, whereas a small volume of blood is felt as a weak pulse.

A "bounding" or greater-than-normal force felt with each beat is usually a sign of hypertension. In either case, for safety's sake, BP should be measured and compared with the patient's previous BP to see if a change has occurred.

Fig. 1-24 Determining the position of the apical pulse. **A,** Technique for locating the apical pulse by palpation. **B,** Location of the apical pulse. *(From Eubanks DH, Bone RC:* Comprehensive respiratory care, *ed 2, St Louis, 1990, Mosby.)*

2. Determine whether the patient has asymmetrical chest movements when breathing (WRE code: IB2b) [Difficulty: An]

Normally the lungs and chest move together in symmetry throughout the respiratory cycle. Asymmetrical chest wall movement during inspiration indicates a lung or chest wall problem. If the patient does not have an abnormal chest wall configuration, the problem has to be in the lungs. Less air is getting into the affected lung area(s), so the chest wall does not move out as far as the chest wall over the normal lung. This is a nonspecific finding of lung disease but is also seen in pneumonia, bronchial or lung tumor, and pneumothorax.

The therapist's hands should be placed over the patient's chest to assess for asymmetrical chest movement (Fig. 1-25). The thumbs should touch at the end of expiration. The patient is then instructed to breathe in deeply as asymmetrical movement is looked and felt for. In Fig. 1-25, *A* and *B* show the movement of the anterior apical lobes, *C* and *D* show the movement of the anterior middle and lower lobes, *E* and *F* show the movement in the posterior lower lobes, and *G* and *H* show the movement of the costal margins.

3. Determine whether the patient has tactile fremitus (WRE code: IB2b) [Difficulty: An]

Tactile fremitus is a vibration felt through the chest wall when the patient speaks. Normally, when a sound is created in the larynx, its vibration is carried throughout the tracheobronchial tree to the lung parenchyma and to the chest wall. The intensity of the vibration or its absence gives the practitioner important information on the patient's condition.

Fig. 1-26 shows different methods of detecting tactile fremitus. Some practitioners may prefer to use their fingertips, as in *A* and *B,* whereas others prefer the ulnar edge of the open or closed hand, as in *C* and *D.* The practitioner should feel all areas of the patient's chest for tactile fremitus to detect any variations and should touch the chest over both lung fields to compare their symmetry as well as anterior and posterior differences (see Fig. 1-26, *E* and *F*). Fig. 1-27 shows the posterior and anterior locations for the evaluation of tactile fremitus. Start with the supraclavicular fossae and proceed to alternate intercostal spaces. An attempt must be made to preserve the adult female patient's modesty when evaluating the anterior locations. The patient may be asked to lift the breast for the examiner to palpate beneath it.

The procedure for evaluating tactile fremitus is to have the patient say "99" in a normal voice as the practitioner's fingers or hands are moved from location to location. This procedure also is called *palpation for bronchophony.* The "99" should be spoken at least once for each location to determine any variations. Having the patient speak more loudly or deeply should increase the intensity of the vibrations felt. The intensity of the vibrations directly relates to the density of the underlying lung and chest cavity. Conditions that increase density result in more intense vibrations. Conversely, conditions that decrease density result in less-intense vibrations. Vibrations also are reduced when they are blocked from penetrating through to the surface. See Table 1-14 for conditions that alter tactile fremitus.

4. Determine whether the patient has rhonchial fremitus, indicating secretions in the airway (WRE code: IB2b) [Difficulty: An]

Rhonchial fremitus, also known as *palpable rhonchi,* is a type of tactile fremitus noticed when vibrations from airway secretions can be felt through the chest wall as the patient breathes. They are abnormal because they indicate that the patient has a significant secretion problem. Palpable rhonchi is not detected in a patient with clear airways. Having the patient cough or suctioning the airway to remove secretions results in the reduction or complete elimination of palpable rhonchi. Remember that an airway that is completely occluded by a mucus plug or foreign body will *not* reveal palpable rhonchi

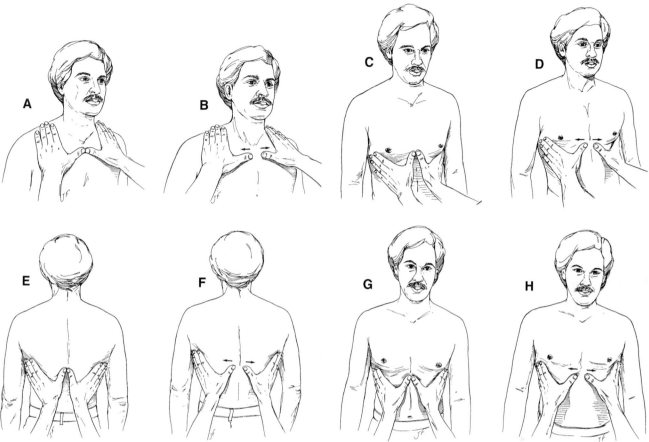

Fig. 1-25 Palpation to access symmetrical chest movements. **A,** Hand position over the apical lobes during expiration. **B,** Apical movement during inspiration. **C,** Hand position over middle and lower lobes during expiration. **D,** Middle and lower lobe movement during inspiration. **E,** Hand position over the posterior middle lobes during expiration. **F,** Movement of the posterior middle lobes during inspiration. **G,** Hand position to check for movement of the costal margins during expiration. **H,** Costal movement during inspiration. *(From Eubanks DH, Bone RC: Comprehensive respiratory care ed 2, St Louis, 1990, Mosby.)*

because no airflow is present. Breath sounds also are absent in this area.

Different methods are available for detecting palpable rhonchi. Some therapists may prefer to use their fingertips, whereas others prefer to use the edge of the open or closed hand. It is important to assess all areas of the patient's chest to detect the exact location(s) of the secretions.

5. Determine whether the patient has crepitus (WRE code: IB2b) [Difficulty: An]

Crepitus (or crepitation) is the sound heard when an area with subcutaneous emphysema is gently pressed. The dry crackling-like sound resembles that of Rice Krispies in milk. A stethoscope can be used to help focus the sound to the exact location. In extreme instances, the unaided ear detects the sound. As the fingers of one hand are sequentially pressed into the affected area, the subcutaneous air is felt to move away from the pressure points.

Subcutaneous emphysema is air under the skin that has leaked from a damaged lung. The skin appears puffy

or edematous and is most commonly seen in the tissues on the side of the leaking lung. The pressurized air dissects through the tissues, following the path of least resistance, and is most likely found under the skin in the axilla, neck, chest wall, and breast. In extreme cases, air is found under the skin throughout the body.

Although not dangerous, crepitus is a serious finding because it indicates that the patient has a pulmonary air leak. It may be accompanied by pneumothorax, pneumomediastinum, or pulmonary interstitial emphysema. A chest radiographic examination should be done immediately if the crepitation is a new finding.

6. Determine whether the patient has any tracheal deviation (WRE code: IB2b) [Difficulty: An]

Normally the trachea is in a midline position within the neck and thorax. The location of the trachea is found by having the patient look straight ahead and gently inserting the index finger into the suprasternal notch of an

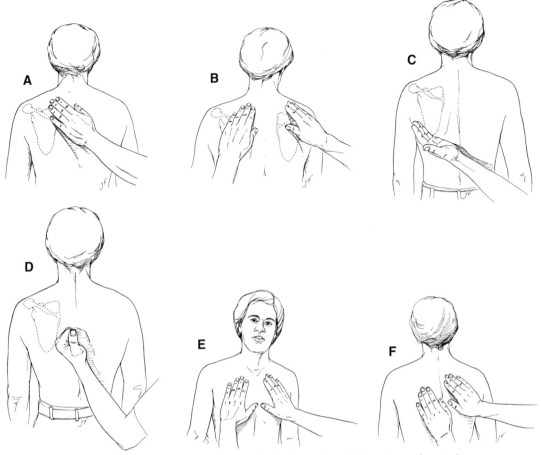

Fig. 1-26 A to **D**, Techniques for feeling tactile fremitus. **E** and **F**, Anterior and posterior placement of the hands to detect tactile fremitus. *(From Eubanks DH, Bone RC:* Comprehensive respiratory care, *ed 2, St Louis, 1990, Mosby.)*

upright or supine patient (Fig. 1-28). The trachea should be detected in midline, with soft tissues on both sides. A trachea that is shifted off to one side is abnormal and can be caused by the following (see Fig. 1-5):

a. Atelectasis, which causes the trachea to be pulled *toward* the affected side
b. Pulmonary fibrosis, which causes the trachea to be pulled *toward* the most affected side

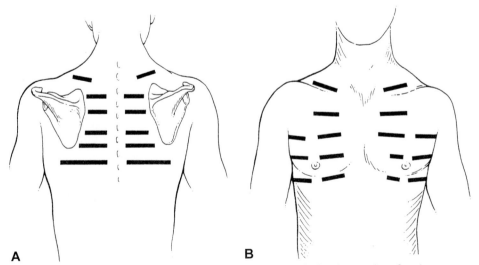

Fig. 1-27 A, Locations on the posterior chest for feeling tactile fremitus and performing percussion. **B**, Locations on the anterior chest for feeling tactile fremitus and performing percussion. *(From Swartz MH:* Textbook of physical diagnosis, *Philadelphia, 1989, WB Saunders.)*

TABLE 1-14	Abnormal Tactile Fremitus
Increased	**Decreased**
UNILATERAL	**UNILATERAL**
Pneumonia	Pneumothorax
Atelectasis	Pleural effusion
Consolidation	Bronchial obstruction
BILATERAL	**BILATERAL**
Pulmonary edema	Thick chest wall (fat or muscle)
Acute respiratory distress syndrome	Chronic obstructive pulmonary disease

c. Tension pneumothorax, which causes the trachea to be pushed *away* from the affected side

d. Hemothorax, pleural effusion, and empyema, which push the trachea *away* from the affected side

Correction of the underlying pulmonary problem results in the trachea returning to its normal midline position.

7. Determine whether the patient has any tenderness (WRE code: IB2b) [Difficulty: An]

Tenderness is an increased local sensation of pain when the chest is gently hit with the ulnar area of the fist. This tapping is done in a symmetrical pattern over the posterior and anterior lung areas and normally should not cause any pain. Intercostal tenderness is felt at the site of an inflamed pleura. Local tenderness and a history of trauma to an area of the chest lead to the conclusion of musculoskeletal pain. A chest radiograph might be indicated to determine whether any ribs have been fractured. The absence of chest wall tenderness should lead to a further investigation as to the cause of the chest pain. Consider angina pectoris (hypoxic heart pain).

A   **B**

Fig. 1-28 A and **B**, Detecting the position of the trachea by pressing the index finger into the suprasternal notch. *(From Eubanks DH, Bone RC:* Comprehensive respiratory care, *ed 2, St Louis, 1990, Mosby.)*

MODULE G

Use *auscultation* to determine the patient's complete respiratory condition

1. Breath sounds

a. Determine whether the patient has bilaterally normal breath sounds (WRE code: IB3a) [Difficulty: An]

Three types of normal breath sounds are found (Fig. 1-29):

1. *Normal* breath sounds also are called *vesicular*. These normal breath sounds are heard over all areas of normally ventilated lungs. Normal breath sounds have been variously described as "leaves rustling" or "like a gentle breeze." These faint sounds are made as air is moved through the small airways of the lungs during the breathing cycle. The inspiratory to expiratory (I:E) ratio is about 3:1. The inspiratory sound is louder than the expiratory sound, and there is no pause between inspiration and expiration.

2. *Bronchial* breath sounds also are called *tracheal*. These normal breath sounds are heard over the trachea and main bronchi. Bronchial breath sounds have been described as being louder, harsher, and higher-pitched than normal. They have a fairly uniform pitch on inspiration and expiration, with a distinct pause in the transition of flow. The I:E ratio is about 1:1.5.

3. *Bronchovesicular* sounds are a cross between bronchial and vesicular. Bronchovesicular sounds are more muffled than bronchial but louder than vesicular and have the same pitch throughout inspiration and expiration. The I:E ratio is about 1:1.

Bronchial and bronchovesicular breath sounds are abnormal if heard in any other areas except those mentioned here. When these sounds are heard over areas that should be normal vesicular, it is a sign of consolidation or atelectasis with a patent airway.

b. Determine whether the patient has abnormal breath sounds (WRE code: IB3a) [Difficulty: An]

This following discussion is limited to variations in normal vesicular breath sounds. The abnormal appearance of bronchial and bronchovesicular breath sounds was discussed earlier.

1. Increased normal vesicular breath sounds

a. Found most often in children and in debilitated adults because their thinner chest walls transmit the sounds better.

b. Increased breath sounds are commonly described as *harsh*.

2. Decreased normal vesicular breath sounds

a. Most commonly caused by a pleural effusion, hemothorax, or empyema because of fluid between the lung and the stethoscope (see Fig. 1-5, *D*).

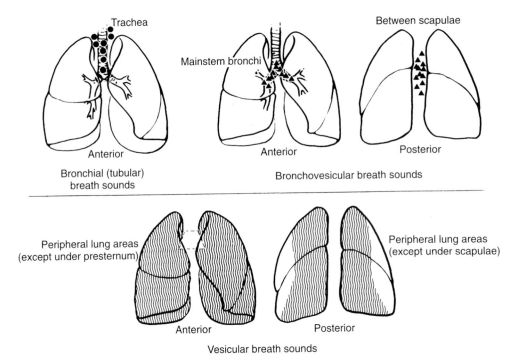

Fig. 1-29 Breath sounds heard over the normal chest. *(From Lehrer S: Understanding lung sounds, Philadelphia, 1984, WB Saunders.)*

b. Pulmonary fibrosis resulting from decreased airflow (see Fig. 1-5, *B*).
c. Emphysema resulting from decreased airflow.
d. Pleural thickening resulting from dampening from the thicker pleural tissues.

3. Absent normal vesicular breath sounds

a. Pneumothorax caused by the lung being forced away from the chest wall (see Fig. 1-5, *C*).
b. Atelectasis (see Fig. 1-5, *A*) or severe bronchospasm results because no air is moving into the alveoli.
c. Endotracheal tube placed into a bronchus instead of the trachea. In this case, the right bronchus is most commonly intubated, so that the breath sounds are absent over the left lung.
d. Large pleural effusion.
e. Obese patient.

4. Unequal normal vesicular breath sounds

a. Pneumonia, consolidation, or atelectasis that decreases airflow into a segment or lobe.
b. Foreign body or tumor in a bronchus that decreases airflow to the distal lung.
c. Spinal or thoracic deformity that reduces airflow to the underlying lung.

The term *adventitious* is used to describe collectively all types of abnormal breath sounds.

5. Wheezing

Wheezing (also known as wheeze and rhonchi) has the following features or characteristics:

a. They are continuous sounds.
b. They are more commonly heard on expiration than inspiration.
c. Low-pitched, polyphonic expiratory wheezing is commonly associated with secretions in the airways. A common term for these sounds is *rhonchi.* Common pulmonary conditions include bronchitis, pneumonia, or any other secretion-causing problem. Coughing or tracheal suctioning often causes these sounds to be modified or eliminated.
d. High-pitched, *monophonic* expiratory sounds are commonly associated with closure of one large airway. This is commonly found with an airway tumor.
e. High-pitched, *polyphonic* expiratory sounds are commonly associated with closure of many small airways. The term *wheeze* is commonly used to describe these sounds caused by bronchospasm in an asthmatic patient. Coughing or tracheal suctioning is unlikely to eliminate these high-pitched sounds. Effective treatment with bronchodilating medications should make the wheezing diminish and vesicular sounds return.

6. Crackles (rales)

Crackles have the following features or characteristics:

a. They are discontinuous sounds.

b. They are more commonly heard on inspiration than expiration.

c. They may be caused by the sudden opening of collapsed airways. Early inspiratory crackles are heard in patients with obstructive lung diseases such as chronic bronchitis, bronchiectasis, asthma, and emphysema. Late inspiratory crackles are heard in patients with atelectasis, pneumonia, pulmonary edema, or fibrosis.

d. They may be caused by air passing through secretions and are heard as a repeated sound during the same phase of the respiratory cycle.

7. Stridor

Stridor is heard as a harsh, monophonic, high-pitched inspiratory sound over the larynx. (It is not the normal tracheal sound.) It has these features or characteristics:

a. Stridor can often be heard without a stethoscope.

b. Common pediatric conditions include acute epiglottitis, laryngotracheobronchitis (croup), and laryngomalacia (congenital stridor).

c. Common adult conditions include postextubation laryngeal edema and a laryngeal tumor.

d. When stridor is heard on inspiration and expiration, it is commonly caused by an aspirated foreign body, tracheal stenosis, or a laryngeal tumor.

8. Friction rub

A friction rub (also known as a *pleural* friction rub) is the sound caused by the rubbing together of the inflamed and adherent visceral and parietal pleura as seen in pleurisy. It is heard through a stethoscope and is described as loud and grating, clicking, or the creaking of old leather. The inspiratory sound frequently is reversed from the expiratory sound as the pleural tissues rub against each other in the opposite direction.

A friction rub is heard most commonly over the lower lung areas. Commonly, the sound is found at the site where the patient complains of pleural pain on breathing. Coughing and suctioning do not affect it. The causes include pulmonary infarct or any pneumonia that leads to an abscess or empyema.

2. Heart sounds

a. Determine whether the patient has normal heart sounds (WRE code: IB3b) [Difficulty: An]

The patient's HR and rhythm can be easily determined by listening at the point of the apical pulse (see Fig. 1-24). Obviously, if a heart sound cannot be detected, the

> ### Exam Hint
>
> Usually at least one question concerns the interpretation of breath sounds or identifying a situation that might cause an abnormal breath sound. Examples include (1) absent breath sounds over an area of pneumothorax; (2) absent breath sounds over the left lung when an endotracheal tube has been misplaced into the right mainstem bronchus; (3) stridor over the larynx of a patient with epiglottitis or laryngeal edema. Remember that severe stridor is a respiratory emergency because the airway may rapidly close completely. The patient is usually intubated to provide a secure airway. (4) Evaluate wheezing in a patient with asthma. Effective medication treatment will result in less wheezing and an improved patient. Ineffective medication treatment will result in less wheezing and a patient who is getting worse.

patient should be assessed for cardiac arrest. Begin cardiopulmonary resuscitation (CPR) if needed.

b. Determine whether the patient has abnormal heart sounds (WRE code: IB3b) [Difficulty: An]
1. Dysrhythmias (arrhythmias)

A steady rhythm has approximately equal amounts of time between ventricular contractions. It is considered normal to have a slight increase in the HR and faster rhythm during an inspiration than during an expiration. This is caused by the increase in blood brought into the chest during the inspiration when the intrathoracic pressure is more negative. The opposite pattern might be seen when a patient is being mechanically ventilated with high peak-airway pressures. This indicates that the venous return to the heart is decreased during a mechanically delivered inspiration.

Any sudden variations in rate and rhythm not related to the respiratory cycle are abnormal. It is difficult to determine the origin of most dysrhythmias (arrhythmias) solely on the basis of their sound patterns; an ECG is indicated. A premature ventricular contraction (PVC) can be noted by the following rhythm characteristics: (1) the heartbeat is premature, and (2) a complete compensatory pause is noted between the PVC and the following normal beat. The complete compensatory pause is the time interval of two normal heartbeats. (See the representative rhythm strip [Fig. 11-36] in Chapter 11.)

3. Determine the patient's blood pressure (WRE code: IB3c) [Difficulty: An]

Measure a BP on any patient to establish a baseline normal value and whenever you think a significant increase or decrease in the BP might be present. The BP should be the same on any arm or leg. However, an arm is typically used. Place the proper cuff around the arm and inflate the cuff pressure above the patient's normal value. Place the diaphragm of the stethoscope over the brachial artery, and slowly let the air out of the cuff. The first distinct sound heard as the blood flows through the artery is the systolic pressure. The last distinct sound heard is the diastolic pressure. Clinical practice is needed to determine BP accurately.

> ## Exam Hint
>
> **A**lthough the NBRC has deleted percussion from the exam content outline, this subject has been tested on recent examinations. Typically, one question relates to an abnormal percussion note. Know that a hyperresonant percussion note is heard over an area of pneumothorax.

Sounds such as hyperresonance are always abnormal when found over lung areas. They indicate that more air than normal is present. Be careful not to confuse hyperresonance associated with a pneumothorax with the normal sound of tympany found over an air-filled stomach. An increase in the density of the underlying lung or related structures results in a dull sound at an abnormal location. This sound is associated with pneumonia, consolidation, or atelectasis when the alveoli are fluid filled or airless; with tumor; and with pleural fluid such as effusion, blood, pus, or chyle. It is normal to hear dullness over the heart and liver.

MODULE H
Neonatal assessment

1. Review the perinatal/neonatal patient's chart for the following data
a. Review the maternal and perinatal/neonatal history and data (WRE code: IA8) [Difficulty: Ap, An]

Perinatal refers to the period toward the end of a pregnancy and for up to 4 weeks after the neonate is born.

1. Antenatal assessment (assessment during the pregnancy)

The medical and personal history of the mother is obviously important because it directly relates to the health of the fetus she is carrying. The mother's age is important because women younger than 16 years and older than 40 years are more likely to have a high-risk pregnancy. This is especially true if a woman older than 40 years is having her first child. *Gravida* is the term that refers to pregnancy; *primigravida* refers to a woman with her first pregnancy. *Para* is the term that refers to the woman delivering a potentially live infant; *primipara/primiparous* refer to a woman's first delivery of an infant. Box 1-1 lists a number of maternal and other factors that can result in the anticipation of a high-risk infant being

---

BOX 1-1   Some Factors Associated with a High-Risk Newborn Infant

MATERNAL FACTORS
Maternal age of younger than 16 or older than
   40 years
Low socioeconomic status
Poor nutrition
Lack of medical care during pregnancy
Smoking, drug, or alcohol abuse
Underweight or overweight
Abnormal fetal growth
Hereditary anomalies
Vaginal bleeding early in pregnancy
Low maternal urinary estriol
Polyhydramnios or oligohydramnios
Toxemia of pregnancy/pre-eclampsia
Previous history of infant(s) with jaundice, respiratory
   distress, or previous premature delivery
Chronic disease
   Hypertension unrelated to pregnancy
   Diabetes mellitus
   Cardiovascular
   Pulmonary
   Anemia
   Renal

LABOR AND DELIVERY/OBSTETRIC FACTORS
Premature rupture of the membranes
Prolonged rupture of the membranes >24 hr
Premature labor (<38 weeks' gestation)
Postmature labor (>42 weeks' gestation)
Rapid or prolonged labor
Prolapsed umbilical cord
Previous or primary cesarean section
Breech or other abnormal presentation
Analgesia and anesthesia

FETAL FACTORS
Multiple births
Meconium in amniotic fluid
Abnormal fetal heart rate or rhythm
Fetal acidosis
Prematurity or postmaturity
Small or large for gestational age
Rh factor sensitization
Congenital malformation
Immature lecithin/sphingomyelin (L/S) ratio or negative
   phosphatidylglycerol (PG) test
Birth trauma

born. It must be noted that about 25% of high-risk infants are born with no indication from the history of any problem.

2. Intrapartum assessment (assessment during labor)

Some of the labor and delivery/obstetric factors that can adversely affect the delivery process include premature labor (less than 38 weeks' gestation), postmature labor (greater than 42 weeks' gestation), prolapsed umbilical cord, and cesarean section. Fetal heart rate (FHR, or fetal heart tones) is usually monitored to determine how the fetus is tolerating the stress of labor and delivery.

FHR should range between 120 and 160 beats/min and is normally variable with the fetus's waking and sleeping periods. The FHR can be measured externally through the mother's abdominal wall. During a contraction of the uterus, the HR commonly slows to near or less than 120 beats/min. This is because of vagus nerve stimulation during the compression of the head into the birth canal (Fig. 1-30, *A*). The HR returns to normal when the contraction is over. This normal decrease and increase in FHR that is related to uterine contractions is called early deceleration or type I dips.

Late deceleration or type II dips are seen when the FHR slows sometime after the contraction begins and does not return to normal until sometime after the contraction is over (see Fig. 1-30, *B*). This is often caused by uteroplacental insufficiency from compression of the vessels in the placenta. It is frequently associated with low Apgar scores and fetal asphyxia and acidosis.

Variable deceleration is seen when the FHR slows and increases in an unpredictable pattern in comparison with the contractions (see Fig. 1-30, *C*). This pattern is more commonly seen than late deceleration and is believed to be caused by compression of the umbilical cord by a body part. During the compression, little or no blood reaches the fetus. It also is often associated with low Apgar scores and fetal asphyxia and acidosis.

With late and variable deceleration, the mother's HR and BP should be monitored. Treatment includes giving the mother supplemental oxygen and placing her in a head-down, left lateral position. If the fetus is thought to be at risk of asphyxia, a cesarean section must be performed.

Other heartbeat irregularities are not related to labor and delivery. Tachycardia of greater than 160 beats/min can be associated with infection, fetal immaturity, congenital heart malformations, and the effects of maternal

Fig. 1-30 Fetal heart rate patterns showing normal early deceleration, abnormal late deceleration, and variable deceleration. *(From Avery GB: Neonatology: pathophysiology and management of the newborn, ed 2, Philadelphia, 1981, JB Lippincott.)*

TABLE 1-15	Normal Newborn Vital Signs	
Characteristic	**Normal Range**	
Heart rate	>120 beats/min	
	<160 beats/min	
Blood pressure	*Systolic*	*Diastolic*
1000–2000 g birth weight	55 mm Hg	30 mm Hg
>3000 g birth weight	65 mm Hg	40 mm Hg
Respiratory rate	30–60 breaths/min	
	Periodic breathing with apneic spells of <10 sec common; should not be associated with bradycardia or cyanosis	
Temperature	Keep abdominal skin temperature at 36.5°C	
	Keep rectal (core) temperature between 35.5° and 37.5°C	

drugs. Bradycardia of less than 120 beats/min and decreased beat-to-beat variability (fixed heart rate) are seen with fetal asphyxia and distress.

3. Postpartum or neonatal assessment

Some of the fetal factors that can adversely affect the newborn include multiple births, meconium in the amniotic fluid, abnormal FHR or rhythm, prematurity or postmaturity, small or large for gestational age, congenital malformation, and birth trauma.

4. Resuscitation and vital signs

All newborns require some level of resuscitation. This is usually limited to suctioning amniotic fluid out of the nose and mouth, drying the skin, providing warmth, and the tactile stimulation that comes from these procedures. Newborns with moderate Apgar scores may need to breathe in some supplemental oxygen until they are more vigorous and ventilating better. The newborn with a low Apgar score requires CPR. Table 1-15 lists the vital signs seen in a normal newborn.

5. Weight

The relation between birth weight and gestational age is important to evaluate. In general, if an infant is between the 10th and 90th percentiles of normal weight for gestational age, the infant is within normal limits. Any infant who is either large or small for gestational age is at increased risk of complications during and after delivery. Large post-term infants and small preterm infants are especially at risk.

b. Review the results of the neonate's lecithin/sphingomyelin ratio test (WRE code: IA8) [Difficulty: Ap, An]

To determine the lung maturity of the fetus, a sample of amniotic fluid must be obtained by an amniocentesis. The maturity of the fetus's lungs can be determined by evaluating three components of surfactant released by the developing alveolar type II cells. Recall that, in a premature neonate without sufficient surfactant in its lungs, infant respiratory distress syndrome (RDS) will probably develop.

The first test of lung maturity is the lecithin/sphingomyelin (L/S) ratio. The test is a comparison of the relative amounts of these two surfactant components. In general, the more lecithin compared with sphingomyelin, the more mature the lungs. Usually a significant increase in the lecithin level occurs at about 35 weeks of gestation. A weakness of the L/S ratio test is that borderline values are difficult to interpret, and false-positive values are sometimes found.

The second test is determining the presence of phosphatidylglycerol (PG) in the amniotic fluid. It appears at about 36 weeks of gestation and increases through the duration of the pregnancy. The laboratory reports PG as either present or absent from the sample of amniotic fluid. Its presence always indicates lung maturity. Table 1-16 gives more information on the interpretation of these two tests.

c. Review the patient's Apgar scores (WRE code: IA8) [Difficulty: Ap, An]

The Apgar scoring system is used in the delivery room to give a general evaluation of how a newborn infant is responding. The following five parameters are judged: HR, respiratory effort, muscle tone, reflex response, and color. Table 1-17 shows how the five parameters are scored on a scale of 0, 1, and 2. The newborn is evaluated

TABLE 1-16	Lecithin/Sphingomyelin (L/S) Ratio and Phosphatidylglycerol (PG) as Markers of Fetal Lung Maturity	
Clinical Finding	**Interpretation**	
L/S ratio 2:1 (2.0) or greater	Mature lungs; less than 5% chance of RDS	
L/S ratio 1.5:1 (1.5)	Transitional lungs; about a 50% chance of RDS	
L/S ratio 1:1 (1.0) or less	Immature lungs; about a 90% chance of RDS	
PG present	Mature lungs	
PG absent	Immature lungs	

RDS, Infant respiratory distress syndrome.

TABLE 1-17 Apgar Scoring Chart			
Sign	**0**	**1**	**2**
Heart rate	Absent	Slow (<100 beats/min)	Over 100
Respiratory effort	Absent	Weak cry, hypoventilation	Good strong cry
Muscle tone	Limp	Some flexion of extremities	Well flexed
Reflex response	No response	Grimace	Cough, sneeze, or cry
Response to catheter in nostril or to other cutaneous stimulation			
Color	Blue, pale	Body pink, extremities blue	Completely pink

From Lough MD, Doershuk CF, Stern RC: *Pediatric respiratory therapy*, ed 3, St Louis, 1985, Mosby.

soon after birth to calculate a 1-minute Apgar score. A 5 minute evaluation and Apgar score also are calculated. The infant is rated as good if the score is 7 to 10, fair if the score is 4 to 6, and poor if the score is 0 to 3. If the 5-minute score is less than 7, the newborn is rescored every 5 minutes up to 20 minutes after the delivery.

d. Review information on the patient's gestational age (Dubowitz score) (WRE code: IA8) [Difficulty: Ap, An]

The Dubowitz score is made up of 11 physical and 10 neurologic criteria that develop at a set rate during gestation. Ballard and co-workers modified the scoring system by simplifying it to six physical and six neurologic criteria. Fig. 1-31 shows the criteria, scoring system, and scale for rating the maturity of the newborn. A score of between 35 and 45 indicates that the infant was born between 38 and 42 weeks of gestation; this is a normal score for a term infant. A premature infant has a score of less than 35, and a post-term infant has a score of greater than 45. The maturity rating scale can be used to give an estimation of gestational age accurate within 2 weeks.

e. Review information on the patient's preductal and postductal oxygenation studies (WRE code: IA8) [Difficulty: Ap, An]

In a normal neonate, the ductus arteriosus closes shortly after birth, causing equal oxygenation of all arterial blood to the body. With persistent pulmonary hypertension of the newborn (PPHN) the ductus arteriosus does not properly close. A diagnostic test for PPHN involves measuring the P_{O_2} in preductal blood and postductal blood. Preductal blood P_{O_2} is measured by a right radial artery sample, pulse oximetry on the right hand, or transcutaneous probe placed on the right arm or right upper chest. Postductal blood P_{O_2} is measured by an umbilical artery sample, pulse oximetry of the left hand or either foot, or transcutaneous probe on the abdomen or either thigh.

A right-to-left shunt indicating PPHN is shown by either (1) a decrease in Sp_{O_2} of greater than 10% from preductal to postductal blood, or (2) a decrease in P_{O_2} of greater than 15 to 20 torr from preductal to postductal

blood. However, it is important to understand that a normal test result does not rule out PPHN.

2. Determine the perinatal or neonatal patient's complete respiratory condition in the following ways by *inspection*

a. Determine the patient's Apgar scores (WRE code: IB1c) [Difficulty: R, Ap, An]

Review the previous information and Table 1-17 as needed. The 1-minute Apgar score is a good index of how the newborn tolerated the delivery process. The 5-minute Apgar score is a good index of how the newborn's cardiopulmonary system is adjusting from fetal to adult conditions. A low 5-minute Apgar score is associated with increased mortality in the first month of life. Survivors have a high risk of mental impairment and cerebral palsy.

> **Exam Hint**
>
> Usually at least one question deals with a newborn's Apgar score. Also be able to determine the score based on the given information. Be able also to interpret the patient's condition based on the Apgar score.

b. Determine the patient's gestational age (Dubowitz score) (WRE code: IB1c) [Difficulty: R, Ap, An]

The descriptions of gestational development for the criteria of physical maturity are listed in Fig. 1-31. As can be seen, more points are earned for each step of gestational development. A term infant will score 3 or 4 points for each of the 12 criteria. The illustrations of gestational development for the criteria of neurologic/neuromuscular maturity can be seen in the figure; however, because the infant must be manipulated to perform the rating, the following descriptions will be helpful.

Posture. The infant should be supine and quiet. Simply observe how the infant positions its arms and legs. The more mature infant will fully flex its elbows, hips, and knees.

Square Window. Flex the hand at the wrist. Exert gentle pressure to have the wrist flex as much as possible. The

Neuromuscular maturity

	−1	0	1	2	3	4	5
Posture							
Square window (wrist)	>90°	90°	60°	45°	30°	0°	
Arm recoil		180°	140°-180°	110°-140°	90°-110°	<90°	
Popliteal angle	180°	160°	140°	120°	100°	90°	<90°
Scarf sign							
Heel to ear							

Physical maturity

Skin	Sticky, friable, transparent	Gelatinous red, translucent	Smooth, pink, visible veins	Superficial peeling and/or rash, few veins	Cracking, pale areas, rare veins	Parchment, deep cracking, no vessels	Leathery, cracked, wrinkled
Lanugo	None	Sparse	Abundant	Thinning	Bald areas	Mostly bald	
Plantar surface	Heel-toe 40-50 mm:−1 <40 mm:−2	>50 mm No crease	Faint red marks	Anterior transverse crease only	Creases ant. 2/3	Creases over entire sole	
Breast	Imperceptible	Barely perceptible	Flat areola, no bud	Stippled areola, 1-2 mm bud	Raised areola, 3-4 mm bud	Full areola, 5-10 mm bud	
Eye/Ear	Lids fused loosely: −1 tightly: −2	Lids open; pinna flat; stays folded	Slightly curved pinna; soft; slow recoil	Well-curved pinna; soft but ready recoil	Formed and firm instant recoil	Thick cartilage ear stiff	
Genitals male	Scrotum flat, smooth	Scrotum empty; faint rugae	Testes in upper canal; rare rugae	Testes descending; few rugae	Testes down; good rugae	Testes pendulous; deep rugae	
Genitals female	Clitoris prominent; labia flat	Prominent clitoris; small labia minora	Prominent clitoris; enlarging minora	Majora and minora equally prominent	Majora large; minora small	Majora cover clitoris and minora	

Maturity rating

score	weeks
−10	20
−5	22
0	24
5	26
10	28
15	30
20	32
25	34
30	36
35	38
40	40
45	42
50	44

Fig. 1-31 The Ballard modification of Dubowitz Gestational Age Assessment. *(From Ballard JL, Khoury JC, Wedig K: New Ballard Score, expanded to include extremely premature infants. J Pediatr 119:417, 1991.)*

more mature infant will have full flexibility of the hand against the forearm.

Arm Recoil. With the infant supine, fully flex the forearms for 5 seconds. Then fully extend the forearms by pulling on the hands. When released, the more mature infant will quickly return its forearms to full flexion.

Popliteal Angle. The infant must lie supine with the pelvis flat on the examining surface. The lower leg is flexed onto the thigh, and the thigh is fully flexed to the abdomen. One hand is used to hold the thigh in the flexed position and the other hand is used to extend the lower leg. The angle between the thigh and lower leg is then measured. The more mature infant will have less joint flexion and a smaller angle.

Scarf Sign. With the infant supine, take one of the infant's hands and extend it as far as possible across the neck toward the opposite shoulder. The infant is scored as follows:

0 = The elbow reaches the opposite anterior axillary line.
1 = The elbow reaches closer to the opposite anterior axillary line than the midline of the chest.
2 = The elbow reaches midway between the opposite anterior axillary line and the midline of the chest.
3 = The elbow reaches the midline of the chest.
4 = The elbow does not reach the midline of the chest.

Heel-to-Ear Maneuver. The infant should be supine on the examining table with the pelvis flat. Take the infant's foot in one hand and move it as near to the head as possible. Do not force it! The more mature infant will have less joint flexibility and will not be as able to move the foot as near the head as a less mature infant.

c. Assess the patient's cardiopulmonary condition by viewing the results of transillumination of the chest (WRE code: IB1c) [Difficulty: R, Ap, An]

Transillumination of the chest is a test performed on a neonate to identify the presence of a pneumothorax. To perform a test for a pneumothorax, the room is darkened and a bright light from a flashlight is placed against the patient's chest. When free air is around the collapsed lung, the light will create a "halo" effect through the thin chest wall of the neonate. This confirms the pneumothorax.

Exam Hint

Know the indication (suspected pneumothorax) and interpretation of the transillumination procedure results.

3. Inspect a lateral neck radiograph to evaluate the following:

NOTE: The following discussion usually applies to a child but also can apply to an adult.

a. Look for the presence of epiglottitis (CSE code: IB8a)

Epiglottitis is an inflammation of the epiglottis and surrounding supraglottic structures. It is a medical emergency and is usually diagnosed on the basis of the history and physical examination and results in the child being intubated. If a lateral neck radiograph is taken of an epiglottitis, it will show a white haziness in the supraglottic area. This is the swollen epiglottis and is sometimes obvious enough to be called the "thumb sign." This is seen when the usually thin epiglottis is swollen and looks like the end of the thumb. It must be emphasized that under no circumstances should the child be laid supine for the neck radiograph. This can result in the swollen epiglottis fatally closing over the opening to the trachea. Allow the child to sit upright in the most comfortable position. (Fig. 1-32

Fig. 1-32 A drawing of the normal upper airway is shown in the middle. Contrast it with **(A)** epiglottitis, and **(B)** laryngotracheobronchitis (croup). *EP,* epiglottis; *SEP,* swollen epiglottis; *STT,* swollen trachea tissue; *TG,* tongue; *TR,* trachea; *VC,* vocal chords. *(From Des Jardins TR: Clinical manifestations of respiratory disease, ed 2, St Louis, 1990, Mosby.)*

Fig. 1-33 Lateral neck radiographs on children showing **(A)** normal upper airway during an inspiration; **(B)** laryngotracheobronchitis (croup) showing haziness of the subglottic trachea from mucosal edema; and **(C)** epiglottitis with a swollen, rounded epiglottis. Areas marked *E* show the epiglottis; areas marked *S* show the subglottic trachea. *(From Williams JL: Radiographic evaluations. In Koff PB, Eitzman DV, Neu J, editors:* Neonatal and pediatric respiratory care, *St Louis, 1988, Mosby.)*

shows the epiglottis, and Fig. 1-33 shows a lateral neck radiograph of the epiglottis. Table 1-18 lists the general history and physical findings for distinguishing between epiglottitis and laryngotracheobronchitis.)

b. Look for the presence of subglottic edema (CSE code: IB7a)

Subglottic edema is an inflammation of the subglottic mucous membranes of the larynx, trachea, and bronchi. This condition also is known as laryngotracheal bronchitis (LTB) and croup. Subglottic edema is usually treated with the inhalation of a cool aerosol in a mist tent and racemic epinephrine for mucosal vasoconstriction. If a lateral neck radiograph of subglottic edema is taken, it will show a white haziness in the subglottic area. This is the swollen laryngeal and tracheal tissue and is sometimes obvious enough to be called the "pencil sign" or "steeple sign." This is seen when the usually blunt end of the trachea at the vocal cords is thinned to a narrow point by the swollen mucous membrane (Fig. 1-32 shows subglottic edema, and Fig. 1-33 shows a lateral neck radiograph image of this problem).

TABLE 1-18	General History and Physical Findings of Laryngotracheobronchitis (LTB) and Epiglottitis	
Clinical Finding	**LTB**	**Epiglottitis**
Age	3–36 mo	2–4 yr
Onset	Slow (24–48 hr)	Abrupt (2–4 hr)
Fever	Absent	Present
Drooling	Absent	Present
Lateral neck radiograph	Haziness in subglottic area	Haziness in supraglottic area
Inspiratory stridor	High pitched and loud	Low pitched and muffled
Hoarseness	Present	Absent
Swallowing difficulty	Absent	Present
White blood cell count	Normal (viral)	Elevated (bacterial)

From Des Jardins TR: *Clinical manifestations and assessment of respiratory disease,* ed 4, St Louis, 2000, Mosby-Year Book.

Exam Hint

A past version of the Clinical Simulation Examination included a problem with a pediatric patient in which the differential diagnosis between croup and epiglottitis had to be made. The care of the patient was then tested.

c. Look for the presence and position of any foreign bodies (WRE code: IB6e) [Difficulty: An]

The history of sudden breathing difficulty, cough, and inspiratory stridor combined with a physical examination of the patient usually points to aspiration. A lateral neck radiograph or PA or AP chest and neck radiograph or both often help to confirm the presence and position of a foreign body. See Fig. 1-15 for an AP chest and neck radiograph image. The clearly seen solid white shape of the foreign body indicates that the object is metallic (a coin).

d. Check the chest radiograph for the size and patency of the patient's major airways (WRE code: IB6f) [Difficulty: An]

Plastic toy pieces and foods such as peanuts are much harder to see on a neck radiograph than are metallic objects because their densities are closer to those found in the body. It is easier to identify obstructing plastic toys or food by looking for a narrowing or distortion of the dark air column of the upper airway and trachea.

Airway narrowing also can be caused by a tumor. This can be either a growth within the lumen of the airway or a growth from outside of the trachea or bronchi that forces it to collapse.

Exam Hint

The Written Registry Exam usually includes two questions about some aspect of fetal, neonatal, or pediatric patient assessment. The Clinical Simulation Exam includes one neonatal and one pediatric patient scenario.

MODULE I

Determine and continue to monitor how the patient responds to the treatment or procedure

1. Determine the patient's vital signs (WRE code: IIIE7) [Difficulty: R, Ap, An]

2. Monitor the patient's heart rhythm (WRE code: IIIE7) [Difficulty: R, Ap, An]

3. Auscultate the patient's breath sounds, and interpret any changes (WRE code: IIIE12) [Difficulty: An]

4. Recommend and review a chest radiograph, as needed, to help determine the patient's condition (WRE code: IIIE1) [Difficulty: An]

5. Look for changes in the patient's sputum production or consistency (WRE code: IIIE5) [Difficulty: An]

6. Recommend the measurement of the patient's electrolytes, hemoglobin, complete blood count, other chemistry values, or a combination of these (CSE code: IA2a)

All of the preceding topics were discussed earlier in this chapter. Review them as necessary. They must be applied to all respiratory care procedures as presented in the following chapters.

7. Evaluate the patient's fluid balance (intake and output) (WRE code: IIIE7) [Difficulty: R, Ap, An]

Fluid intake and output (I and O) should be approximately equal in a normal person with a properly functioning heart and kidneys. Fluid intake includes liquids that the patient drinks or is given by nasogastric tube and intravenous fluids. Output includes urine output and fluid loss from vomiting or the nasogastric tube. Insensible water loss through perspiration and breathing are usually ignored in adults because the amount lost is relatively small and can only be estimated. Insensible water loss can be a risk in the low-birth-weight infant. Prevent this by keeping the infant's environmental temperature within 1°C of its body temperature (neutral thermal environment or NTE). Supplemental oxygen should be humidified.

Any patient who has a history of heart or kidney problems or who has a current serious cardiopulmonary disorder should have intake and output monitored closely. Do this by adding all the patient's intake (oral, intravenous, etc.) and output (urine, blood work, etc.) for each 8-hour shift. See Box 1-2 for the normal adult's values for fluid intake and urine output and Table 1-3 for urine specific gravity and other urinalysis information.

The dehydrated patient will likely show some or all of the following signs and symptoms: tachycardia, hypotension, high urine specific gravity, oliguria (low urine output), low CVP and pulmonary capillary wedge pressure (PCWP) readings, tenting of the skin when pinched, and mental confusion. This patient needs more fluid.

Often a patient with heart or kidney failure will have a decreased output compared with input. This can lead to fluid-overload problems with peripheral or pulmonary edema and heart failure. The patient will likely show some or all of the following signs and symptoms: tachycardia, hypertension, low urine specific gravity, increased urine output, increased CVP and PCWP readings, peripheral edema in the dependent parts of the body, and pulmonary edema with breath sounds revealing crackles/rales. This patient needs to be fluid restricted and sodium restricted. If a patient is given a diuretic medication, the urine output can greatly increase to exceed the intake. Remember that the loss of 1 L of fluid results in the patient losing 1 kg (2.2 pounds) of weight.

BOX 1-2 Fluid Intake and Urine Output for Normal Adults

Normal, minimal daily water requirement for an adult patient is ~1,500–2,000 mL

Average urine output is 0.5–1.0 mL/kg/hr

Polyuria is a urine output of >1500 mL/hr

Oliguria is a urine output of < 400 mL in 24 hr

Anuria is a urine output of < 100 mL in 24 hr

PART 2. CARE MANAGEMENT

MODULE A
Respiratory care plan

1. Assess the patient's learning needs (WRE code: IB5) [Difficulty: Ap, An]

Based on the previously gathered information, the respiratory therapist should be able to determine what the patient understands of his or her condition and what the patient needs to be taught.

a. Age-appropriate teaching

The patient is taught based on his or her age and ability to understand. This is most important with small children. They commonly have these fears when hospitalized:

1. Fear of abandonment (separation anxiety). Small children are afraid of being abandoned in the hospital by their parents.
2. Fear of the unknown. Equipment and procedures must be explained so that the child will not be left to use his or her imagination.
3. Fear of punishment. Children may imagine that their illness is a punishment for doing something wrong.
4. Fear of bodily harm. Explain a procedure so that the child understands what is going to happen.
5. Fear of death. Children who are sick but expected to recover need to understand that they will get better. It is all right for children to feel afraid. Talking about those feelings or fear of death should be encouraged.

b. Language-appropriate teaching

Use nonmedical terms whenever possible. The patient's native language must be used so that he or she will understand the situation. A translator may be needed.

c. Education level

Patients should be taught in a manner and at a level that is matched to their education and knowledge of their medical condition.

d. Prior disease knowledge

The patient should be taught, as needed, about his or her condition.

e. Medication knowledge

The patient should be taught, as needed, about his or her medication(s), including how the medication is to be taken (e.g., metered dose inhaler with spacer).

Exam Hint

Usually one question deals with patient or family teaching. This could involve assessing a patient's or family member's needs, developing a teaching plan, or assessing the patient's or family member's understanding of what was taught.

2. Interview the patient to determine whether any advance directives exist (WRE code: IB4d) [Difficulty: Ap]

An advance directive is an advance declaration by a patient who is so hopelessly and terminally ill that he or she does not wish to be connected to life-support equipment. This statement could preclude the use of a mechanical ventilator, kidney dialysis equipment, cardiac pacemaker, or other means of artificially prolonging life. The advance directive also can declare that the patient does not want to be resuscitated if a cardiac arrest should occur. This is commonly called a "do not resuscitate" (DNR) order and should be clearly noted in the patient's chart. The advance directive legal document should be part of the patient's medical record. The document may also be known as a Living Will in some states. A related legal document is the Durable Power of Attorney for Health Care. This document assigns another person, such as a relative or close friend, the right to make medical decisions when the patient is unable to do so. This can include stopping or withdrawal of medical treatment and the DNR order. Always be sensitive to a patient's feelings about a personal and difficult decision. The patient's emotional state may very well determine readiness for an advance directive. A related issue is the patient's ability to cooperate based on his or her emotional and physical condition.

Exam Hint

Usually one question deals with checking for an advance directive or implementing the patient's wishes.

3. Interview the patient to determine his or her level of pain. (WRE code: IB4a) [Difficulty: An]

It has been shown that unmanaged pain can slow a patient's recovery from trauma or surgery. Because pain is a subjective feeling by the patient, only the patient can determine how severe the pain is. Some patients have a low pain threshold and will report pain sooner at a higher level than will those with a high pain threshold. Therefore the acceptable way to determine pain level is to have the patient rate it. Commonly, the patient is told to self-rate a pain level of 0 when no pain is felt and to assign a number up to a pain level of 10 for the most severe pain possible. Additionally, the patient should be asked to point with one finger to the area with the greatest pain. After the patient is given a pain medication, and it has had time to take effect, the patient is again asked to rate the pain on the 0-to-10 scale. If the patient can tolerate the new pain level, it may not be necessary to give more medication. However, if the pain is still too great, additional medication may be given, if allowed within the physician's orders for pain management.

4. Analyze available information to determine the patient's pathophysiologic state (CSE code: IIIH1)

The limitations of this text prevent an in-depth discussion of the various cardiopulmonary conditions and disorders that befall patients who are cared for by respiratory therapists. However, some discussion of cardiopulmonary conditions is included in the following chapters as the respiratory therapies are presented.

The NBRC has released information on the mix of patient problems that will be found on the 10 Clinical Simulation Examination problems. See Box 1 in the Introduction for this list and the categories of diseases that will be tested. It is highly recommended that a pathology book be reviewed to help offer guidance on how these disease conditions (for example, COPD or asthma or both) are managed.

5. Determine the appropriateness of the prescribed therapy and goals for the identified pathophysiologic state (CSE code: IIIH3)

a. Review the interdisciplinary patient and family care plan (WRE code: IIIH1b) [Difficulty: An]

b. Review the planned therapy to establish the therapeutic plan (WRE code: IIIH1a) [Difficulty: An]

c. Recommend changes in the therapeutic plan if supportive data exist (WRE code: IIIH2) [Difficulty: An]

For the patient to receive the best care possible, the respiratory therapist must know the indications, contraindications, complications, and hazards of the respiratory care procedures the patient will receive. The patient must be assessed before, during, and after the treatment or procedure to determine whether it was effective. The key goal of an appropriate care plan is that the patient's condition be treated in the best way possible. Modifications to the care plan must be made, as needed, as the patient's condition changes.

The respiratory therapist should be a member of the patient care team of the physician, nurse, and others in deciding how best to care for the patient. The following steps are necessary in developing the respiratory care plan for any patient:

1. Determine an expected outcome or goal(s).
2. Develop a plan to achieve success.
3. Decide how to measure whether the goal(s) have been achieved.

4. Plan a timeline to measure the patient's progress.
5. Document the patient's response to care and the final outcome.

When the patient has recovered sufficiently from illness or injury, a discharge plan will be needed to help in the transition to home or a long-term recovery facility. Typically, the discharge plan would include the following:

1. Patient evaluation that determines the patient is ready for discharge. The patient needs to have recovered sufficiently to leave the hospital.
2. Determination of the best place for the patient to go for further recovery and the necessary patient care resources. It must be determined whether the patient can go home or should go to an extended care facility. If the patient is to go home, it must be determined whether the family can provide the necessary care. If not, home care respiratory therapists and nurses must be arranged for.
3. Determination that the patient's financial resources are adequate. If not, social services must be contacted to work with the patient's insurance company or other financial-support agencies.

Exam Hint

Be prepared to use the information from the respiratory care plan to help in making decisions on patient care. Expect questions that relate to what would be the best recommendations for care.

---

d. Conduct disease management education programs (WRE code: IIIH7) [Difficulty: Ap, An]

The most recent Written Registry Exams have had questions that relate to the management and education of the patient with asthma. It also is recommended that the management and education of a patient with COPD be studied. The bibliography includes information on standard references on these two subjects.

e. Stop the treatment or procedure if the patient has an adverse reaction to it. (CSE code: IIIF1)

Patient safety should always be an important consideration during the treatment or procedure. The respiratory therapist should know the complications and hazards of any patient care activity that is performed. These are discussed in the following chapters. Be prepared to stop the treatment or procedure if the patient has an adverse reaction to it. Additionally, be prepared to recommend to the physician that the treatment or procedure be discontinued if it is likely to result in additional adverse reactions.

f. Discontinue treatment based on the patient's response (WRE code: IIIG1e) [Difficulty: An]

Typically three reasons are found for a patient's treatment to be discontinued. First, the patient has recovered and no longer needs the treatment or procedure. It is expensive and wasteful to perform unnecessary treatments. Second, the patient has had an adverse reaction and is likely to have an adverse reaction every time the treatment or procedure is repeated. For example, the patient's BP goes too high whenever he is placed into a head-down position for postural drainage. Third, the patient's condition is terminal, and the patient or responsible family member wants all treatment to be stopped.

MODULE B
Respiratory care protocols

1. **Develop the outcomes of respiratory care protocols (WRE code: IIIH4b) [Difficulty: An]**
2. **Apply respiratory care protocols to patient care situations (WRE code: IIIH6) [Difficulty: Ap]**
3. **Explain planned therapy and goals to the patient in understandable (nonmedical) terms to achieve the best results from the treatment or procedure (WRE code: IIIA6) [Difficulty: An]**
4. **Monitor the outcomes of respiratory care protocols (WRE code: IIIH5) [Difficulty: An]**

Respiratory care protocols are set treatment plans designed to manage certain patient care conditions. They have been developed to improve the quality of patient care by ensuring that the necessary treatment(s) or procedure(s) be delivered as quickly and appropriately as possible. Common respiratory care protocols include oxygen therapy, aerosolized bronchodilator therapy, hyperinflation therapy (incentive spirometry vs. intermittent positive-pressure ventilation), and aspects of mechanical ventilation and weaning. A patient-driven protocol is one in which the patient is appropriately able to take charge of this aspect of his or her care. The respiratory therapist instructs the patient and monitors that the patient is able to perform the care correctly. Examples could include incentive spirometry and bronchodilator therapy by a metered dose inhaler with reservoir unit. A therapist-driven protocol would be one in which the respiratory therapist is responsible for implementing and changing care within the protocol's guidelines. Examples include making ventilator changes to correct arterial blood gas abnormalities and weaning a patient from the ventilator.

The goal of all protocols is to restore the patient's condition to as close to normal as possible. When it is not possible to restore to normal conditions, acceptable conditions must be listed as the target for care. The patient must be evaluated before, during, and after a protocol is used to determine whether improvement has occurred. Based on the results of the patient assessment, the care can be upregulated (increased) or downregulated (decreased). Protocol information is listed, as indicated, in later chapters of this text.

5. Communicate the outcomes of therapy, and change the therapy based on the protocol (WRE code: IIIA5) [Difficulty: An]

Inform the patient's nurse or physician and the supervising therapist if any serious question or problem occurs with the patient. Routine communication should occur as needed between these people and any other caregiver.

> **Exam Hint**
>
> Usually one question deals with the implementation or evaluation of a patient care protocol.

MODULE C
Record in conventional terminology any treatment(s) or procedure(s) performed, including the date, time, frequency of therapy, medication, and ventilatory data

1. **Apply computer technology to document patient management (WRE code: IIIA4a) [Difficulty: Ap]**
2. **Apply computer technology to monitor workload assignments (WRE code: IIIA4b) [Difficulty: Ap]**
3. **Record and evaluate the patient's response to the treatment(s) or procedure(s), including the following:**
   a. **Record and interpret the following: heart rate and rhythm, respiratory rate, blood pressure, body temperature, and pain level (WRE code: IIIA1b, IIIA1c) [Difficulty: An]**
   b. **Record and interpret the patient's breath sounds (WRE code: IIIA1a) [Difficulty: An]**
   c. **Record and interpret the type of cough the patient has and the nature of the sputum (WRE code: IIIA1a) [Difficulty: An]**

See the earlier discussions on these topics. Later chapters will include more specific information based on the treatment being performed.

d. Recheck any math work and make note of incorrect data (WRE code: IIIA2) [Difficulty: An]

Errors made in charting must be corrected by drawing a single mark through the error and writing in the correct information. Some prefer that the error be further clarified by writing in "error" next to it and adding initials. *Never* erase or use any covering material over an error.

Exam Hint

Often one question concerns the proper way to document patient care or how to document a charting error. Remember that a charting error should never be hidden or covered up. Typically the error is identified, the correct information written, and the charting therapist signs his or her name.

---

4. Communicate information relevant to coordinating patient care and discharge planning (e.g., scheduling, avoiding conflicts, and sequencing of therapies) (WRE code: IIIA3) [Difficulty: An]

Common scheduling problems include eating times and when the patient must go to another department such as radiology or physical therapy. Some procedures, such as giving aerosolized medications and performing chest physiotherapy, should be performed before eating.

BIBLIOGRAPHY

Aloan CA, Hill TV, editors: *Respiratory care of the newborn and child,* ed 2, Philadelphia, 1997, Lippincott-Raven.

American Association for Respiratory Care: Clinical practice guideline: discharge planning for the respiratory care patient, *Respir Care* 40:1308, 1995.

Barkauskas VH, Stoltenberg-Allen K, Baumann LC, et al: *Health physical assessment,* St Louis, 1994, Mosby.

Barnes TA, editor: *Core textbook of respiratory care practice,* ed 2, St Louis, 1994, Mosby.

Barnhart SL, Czervinske MP: *Perinatal and pediatric respiratory care,* Philadelphia, 1995, WB Saunders.

Burton GC, Hodgkin JE, Ward JJ, editors: *Respiratory care: a guide to clinical practice,* ed 4, Philadelphia, 1997, Lippincott-Raven.

Carlo C: *Neonatal respiratory care,* St Louis, 1988, Mosby.

Cherniack RM, Cherniack L: *Respiration in health and disease,* ed 3, Philadelphia, 1983, WB Saunders.

Clochesy JM, Breu C, Cardin S, et al, editors: *Critical care nursing,* ed 2, Philadelphia, 1996, WB Saunders.

Daily EK, Schroeder JS: *Techniques in bedside hemodynamic monitoring,* ed 4, St Louis, 1989, Mosby.

Des Jardins TR, Burton GG: *Clinical manifestations and assessment of respiratory disease,* ed 4, St Louis, 2000, Mosby.

DiPietro JS, Mustard MN: *Clinical guide for respiratory care practitioners,* Norwalk, Conn, 1987, Appleton & Lange.

Erickson B: *Heart sounds and murmurs: a practical guide,* ed 3, St Louis, 1997, Mosby.

Eubanks DH, Bone RC: *Comprehensive respiratory care,* St Louis, 1985, Mosby.

Fink JB, Hunt GE, editors: *Clinical practice in respiratory care,* Philadelphia, 1999, Lippincott-Raven.

Hess DR, Kacmarek RM: *Essentials of mechanical ventilation,* New York, 1996, McGraw-Hill.

Hess DR, MacIntyre NR, Mishoe SC, et al, editors: *Respiratory care principles and practice,* Philadelphia, 2002, WB Saunders.

Kacmarek RM, Mack CW, Dimas S: *The essentials of respiratory therapy,* ed 3, St Louis, 1990, Mosby.

Kenner CV, Guzzetta CE, Dossey BM: *Critical care nursing: body-mind-spirit,* Boston, 1981, Little, Brown.

Koff PB, Eitzman DV, Neu J, editors: *Neonatal and pediatric respiratory care,* ed 2, St Louis, 1993, Mosby.

Lehrer S: *Understanding lung sounds,* Philadelphia, 1984, WB Saunders.

Levitsky MG, Cairo JM, Hall SM: *Introduction to respiratory care,* Philadelphia, 1990, WB Saunders.

National Asthma Education Program: *Expert Panel Report 2: guidelines for the diagnosis and management of asthma.* Bethesda, Md, Publication No. 97-4051, April, 1997, National Heart, Lung, and Blood Institute, National Institutes of Health.

National Heart, Lung, and Blood Institute and World Health Organization Global Initiative for Chronic Obstructive Lung Disease (GOLD): Global strategy for the diagnosis, management and prevention of chronic obstructive pulmonary disease: executive Summary, *Am J Respir Crit Care Med* 163(5):1256–1276, 2001.

Oblouk DG: *Hemodynamic monitoring: invasive and noninvasive clinical monitoring,* Philadelphia, 1987, WB Saunders.

Pagana KD, Pagana TJ: *Manual of diagnostic and laboratory tests,* St Louis, 1998, Mosby.

Peters RM: Chest trauma. In Moser KM, Spragg RG, editors: *Respiratory emergencies,* ed 2, St Louis, 1982, Mosby.

Rau JL, Pearce DJ: *Understanding chest radiographs,* Denver, 1984, Multi-Media Publishing.

Scanlan CL, Wilkins RL, Stoller JK, editors: *Egan's fundamentals of respiratory care,* ed 7, St Louis, 1999, Mosby.

Shapiro BA, Kacmarek RM, Cane RD, et al, editors: *Clinical application of respiratory care,* ed 4, St Louis, 1991, Mosby.

Stillwell SB, McCarter RE: *Pocket guide to cardiovascular care,* ed 2, St Louis, 1994, Mosby.

Tilkian AG, Boudreau CM: *Understanding heart sounds and murmurs,* ed 2, Philadelphia, 1984, WB Saunders.

Whitaker K: *Comprehensive perinatal and pediatric respiratory care,* ed 2, Albany, NY, 1997, Delmar.

Wilkins RL, Hodgkin JE, Lopez B: *Lung sounds: a practical guide,* St Louis, 1988, Mosby.

Wilkins RL, Krider SJ, Sheldon RL: *Clinical assessment in respiratory care,* ed 5, St Louis, 2005, Mosby.

Wilkins RL, Stoller JK, Scanlan CL, editors: *Egan's fundamentals of respiratory care,* ed 8, St Louis, 2003, Mosby.

Wyka KA, Mathews PJ, Clark WF, editors: *Foundations of respiratory care,* Albany, NY, 2002, Delmar.

SELF-STUDY QUESTIONS

1. An adult patient with a smoking history has shown an increased anteroposterior diameter and depressed hemidiaphragms on a PA chest radiograph. It is most likely that the patient:
   A. Has pulmonary fibrosis.
   B. Has emphysema.
   C. Would have normal findings if an AP chest radiograph were taken.
   D. Has left ventricular failure.

2. After 2 days of vomiting and diarrhea caused by the flu, a 50-year-old patient is admitted. Her ECG shows five PVCs in 1 minute and flat T waves. What laboratory test would you recommend?
   A. Urinalysis
   B. Arterial blood gas analysis
   C. Electrolytes
   D. Complete blood count

3. A 48-year-old patient with an extensive smoking history usually coughs out about 20 mL of sputum every day. He developed a "chest cold" 4 days ago and has noticed increased shortness of breath and thicker secretions. What should be done at this time?
   A. Have him increase the flow on his home oxygen concentrator.
   B. Get a sputum sample for a culture-and-sensitivity study.
   C. Have him perform a 6-minute walk test.
   D. Perform percussion to determine the hemidiaphragm positions.

4. A recently home-delivered baby is brought in to the Emergency Department by the paramedics. The physician asks you to help evaluate her condition. Normal vital signs for a term newborn include all of the following *except*:
   A. Heart rate of 130/min
   B. Rectal temperature of 36.5°C
   C. Blood pressure of 64/40 mm Hg
   D. Respiratory rate of 20/min

5. You are assisting with the delivery of a high-risk infant. After evaluating the infant, you give it a 1-minute Apgar score of 8 and recommend that the assisting nurse and physician:
   A. Give the infant supplemental oxygen.
   B. Give the mother supplemental oxygen.
   C. Begin bag-mask rescue breathing on the infant.
   D. Give the infant to the mother as soon as possible for bonding.

6. You are called to the Pediatrics Department to help in the evaluation and care of a 4-year-old girl who has been sick with a bad cold for the past 2 days. The nurse shows you a lateral neck radiograph of the child and asks for your opinion. You notice a clear air column through the upper airway but a pointed narrowing of the tracheal air column below the larynx. You tell the nurse that you suspect the child has:
   A. Laryngotracheobronchitis
   B. Aspirated a coin
   C. Epiglottitis
   D. Bilateral upper lobe pneumonia

7. A young adult who had surgery for a deviated nasal septum was accidentally given 2 L of intravenous fluid in 1 hour. Which of the following signs cause you to suspect that the patient is fluid overloaded?
   I. Tachycardia
   II. Bradycardia
   III. High urine specific gravity
   IV. Peripheral edema in the dependent parts of the body
   V. Low urine specific gravity
   A. I, IV, and V
   B. III and IV
   C. I and III
   D. II and V

8. Patients with heart or lung disease commonly have shifting of mediastinal structures. In evaluating cardiopulmonary disease patients, which of the following could result in a mediastinal shift being seen on a chest radiograph?
   I. Right hemothorax
   II. Bilateral lower lobe pneumonia
   III. Left tension pneumothorax
   IV. Right lower lobe atelectasis
   V. Fibrosis of the left lung
   A. III
   B. IV and V
   C. I, II, and III
   D. I, III, IV, and V

9. The radiologist remarks to you during the viewing of a 65-year-old patient's posteroanterior (PA) chest radiograph film that the patient has an enlarged left side of the heart. This indicates to you that:
   A. The patient has an athletic heart.
   B. The patient has a left pleural effusion.
   C. The patient has an abnormal heart.
   D. The patient has a left middle lobe infiltrate.

10. A patient has acute respiratory distress syndrome (ARDS) and is significantly hypoxemic. It is likely that the patient will exhibit all the following except:
    A. A normal respiratory rate
    B. Nasal flaring
    C. Intercostal retractions
    D. Use of accessory muscles of inspiration

11. An adult patient with a history of COPD and left ventricular failure has been hospitalized. A series of diagnostic procedures is being performed.

The preferred radiographic position to minimize distortion of the heart is:
A. Anteroposterior
B. Posteroanterior
C. Lateral
D. Oblique

12. An intubated patient has been moved from the Operating Room to the Intensive Care Unit. Concern is voiced that the endotracheal tube has been moved. What is the best way to determine its location?
    A. Palpate the larynx.
    B. Listen to stomach sounds.
    C. Percuss the patient's chest.
    D. Get a chest radiograph.

13. A 65-year-old patient with repeated episodes of congestive heart failure has a chest radiograph taken. It shows the left costophrenic angle to be blunted and an air/fluid level with a meniscus around the left lower lung area. How should this be interpreted?
    A. Pleural effusion of the left lung
    B. Pulmonary edema of the left lung
    C. Pneumonia of the left lung
    D. Pulmonary embolism of the left lung

14. A 3-day-old newborn is brought into the Emergency Department with her father after they were involved in an automobile accident. The newborn is showing signs of respiratory distress with cyanosis and tachycardia. What test would you recommend to determine whether she has a pneumothorax?
    A. Arterial blood gases
    B. Apgar score
    C. Transillumination
    D. Thoracentesis

15. You have been assisting with the insertion of a flow-directed, balloon-tipped pulmonary artery catheter. After the procedure, a chest radiograph was taken. It would be acceptable to take a mixed-venous blood sample from the catheter if the tip were found in the:

A. Right pulmonary artery
B. Superior vena cava
C. Aortic arch
D. Right ventricle

16. The respiratory therapist has instructed a 16-year-old asthma patient in the proper use of a metered dose inhaler with reservoir and the bronchodilator medication. The patient has shown the proper drug administration and breathing pattern. What should be recommended now?
    A. Continue to administer the treatment because the patient is a minor.
    B. Have the parent administer the treatment because the patient is a minor.
    C. With the parent's permission, begin a patient-driven medication protocol.
    D. Delegate the treatments to a nurse.

17. You are assisting in the delivery of a high-risk neonate. At 1 minute after birth, the following are noted:
    Heart rate is 90 beats/min.
    There is a weak cry.
    Arms and legs show some flexion.
    The baby grimaces when a nasal catheter is inserted into a nostril.
    Extremities are blue with a pink body (acrocyanosis).
    You would give the neonate an Apgar score of:
    A. 3
    B. 5
    C. 7
    D. 9

18. An elderly patient with congestive heart failure has been treated with the diuretic, furosemide (Lasix). Which serum electrolyte is the most important to monitor in this situation?
    A. Potassium
    B. Chloride
    C. Calcium
    D. Sodium

ANSWER KEY

1. **B.** Rationale: Patients with emphysema will usually have chest radiograph findings of increased AP diameter, depressed hemidiaphragms, and widened intercostal spaces that result from enlarged lungs, caused by air trapping. If the patient had pulmonary fibrosis, the lungs would be small rather than enlarged. If the patient had an AP chest radiograph (rather than PA) the lung finding would not be significantly changed. However, the heart size would be enlarged. The reported radiograph findings relate to lung problems,

not heart problems. No report is made of the heart being enlarged or out of position.

2. **C.** Rationale: Severe vomiting and diarrhea can result in the significant loss of fluids and electrolytes. Her cardiac problems are likely the result of this. If an electrolyte abnormality is found, it must be promptly corrected by intravenous replacement. A urinalysis will be helpful for the evaluation of the patient's kidneys but is not needed at this time. An arterial blood gas analysis will be helpful to

determine whether the patient's acid-base balance is altered. However, it is not needed at this time because it will not guide the patient's clinical management. A complete blood count will not reveal any information that will guide the patient's care related to her cardiac arrhythmia.

3. **B.** Rationale: The patient's history plus recent illness and worsening symptoms indicate a pulmonary infection. It is important to get a sputum sample for a culture-and-sensitivity study to determine the infectious organism and the antibiotic to fight it. Although the patient's illness may make him hypoxic, no information suggests that he has a home oxygen concentrator. A 6-minute walk test would cause unnecessary stress on the patient at this time. It will surely make him feel more short of breath. Although it may be interesting to know the position of the patient's hemidiaphragms, this will not help him with the current problem. This procedure can be done later if indicated.

4. **D.** Rationale: A normal term newborn should have a respiratory rate of 30 to 60 beats/min. All of the other listed vital signs are normal for a term newborn. Review Table 1-15 if needed.

5. **D.** Rationale: An Apgar score of 8 (of a maximum of 10) indicates that the newborn is in good condition and can be given to its mother. Review Table 1-17 for the scoring of the five Apgar signs. Because the newborn is in good condition, there is no need to give it or the mother oxygen or to begin bag-mask rescue breathing.

6. **A.** Rationale: Laryngotracheobronchitis (croup) is a swelling of the mucous membrane below the vocal cords (subglottic area). This is often identified by a narrowing of the dark air column below the vocal cords. This pointed narrowing is sometimes referred to as the steeple sign or pencil sign. See Fig. 1-32. If the patient had aspirated a coin, a solid shape would be seen. See Fig. 1-15. In addition, the patient with an aspiration problem has a history of a sudden problem, not being sick for 2 days. Epiglottitis is a swelling of the airway above the vocal cords (supraglottic area). The upper airway radiograph will show haziness in the throat area with a normal tracheal air column. See Fig. 1-33. Bilateral upper lobe pneumonia will appear on a chest radiograph as white shadows over both upper lung fields. The airway should show a normal, dark air column.

7. **A.** Rationale: The young, healthy heart usually responds to a fluid-overload situation by increasing its rate (tachycardia). The excessive intravenous fluid tends to leak out of the capillaries into the tissues in the dependent parts of the body, such as the feet and lower legs. The kidneys quickly put out the extra fluids, and a low urine specific gravity is found. It is highly unlikely that the heart will slow (bradycardia) in a fluid-overload situation. Rather than a high urine specific gravity indicating low urine output, the kidneys put out extra fluid, resulting in a low urine specific gravity.

8. **D.** Rationale: A right hemothorax pushes the mediastinum to the opposite side. A left tension pneumothorax pushes the mediastinum to the opposite side. Right lower lobe atelectasis pulls the mediastinum to the affected side. Fibrosis of the left lung pulls the mediastinum to the affected side. Review Fig. 1-5 if needed. If a patient has bilateral lower lobe pneumonia, both lungs are affected; therefore no shifting of the lungs or the mediastinum would be seen.

9. **C.** Rationale: An enlarged left side of the heart on a 65-year-old patient is abnormal. The patient should be evaluated for left ventricular failure. An athletic heart is not significantly enlarged compared with a normal-sized heart. What makes it athletic is that it can pump more effectively with a higher-than-normal stroke volume. A left pleural effusion is identified by an obscured left costophrenic angle; a pleural air/fluid level may be seen. A left middle lobe infiltrate will have a distinctive shadow over the affected lung area, not the heart. See Fig. 1-8.

10. **A.** Rationale: It is highly unlikely that a patient with ARDS, which results in small and stiff lungs and significant hypoxemia, would be breathing with a normal respiratory rate. A patient with these serious problems will likely show nasal flaring (to reduce airway resistance), intercostal retractions (because of the stiff lungs), and use of accessory muscles of inspiration (to assist the diaphragm in breathing).

11. **B.** Rationale: The posteroanterior (PA) position has the radiographs penetrating from the back to the front of the patient. Because the heart is located behind the sternum, less distortion of its actual size appears on the radiograph. With the anteroposterior (AP) position, the radiographs penetrate from the front to the back of the patient. This results in the heart's shadow being abnormally enlarged on the film. The lateral and oblique chest radiograph views are indicated to help find the location of a tumor or other lung lesion. These views are not that useful in evaluating a patient with COPD and left ventricular failure.

12. **D.** Rationale: It is best to obtain a chest radiograph because the film will show whether the endotracheal tube is within the trachea (or esophagus or a mainstem bronchus) and where the tip of the tube is located within the trachea. Hearing stomach sounds during ventilation will confirm only that the endotracheal tube is in the esophagus. Breath sounds also must be auscultated to confirm whether the tube is

located within the trachea or a main-stem bronchus. Palpation of the larynx can be used during the initial intubation to confirm that the endotracheal tube has entered the trachea. It cannot be used to determine tube tip location within the trachea. Percussion of the patient's chest will not help determine endotracheal tube location. Abnormal sounds can be from a variety of problems.

13. **A.** Rationale: Both the blunting of the left costophrenic angle and the air/fluid level with a meniscus are consistent with a left pleural effusion (fluid in the intrapleural space). The patient's history also confirms this problem. Pulmonary edema or pneumonia of the left lung is seen on the radiograph film as a distinctive shadow within the lung field, not around it. Occasionally a pulmonary embolism results in a fluid leak within the lung and a localized shadow within the lung field, not around it.

14. **C.** Rationale: Transillumination is an easy test for a pneumothorax in a newborn because the chest wall is relatively thin. If a pneumothorax is present, a "halo" of light will shine through the chest wall where the lung is collapsed. Abnormal arterial blood gas results will not be specific to a pneumothorax in this patient. An Apgar score is performed only shortly after a baby has been born to determine how it tolerated the birthing process. A thoracentesis would be performed to remove fluid from around the lung, which has not been shown.

15. **A.** Rationale: A properly placed pulmonary artery (Swan-Ganz) catheter should have its tip located in either the right or left pulmonary artery. See Fig. 1-6 and Chapter 5 for illustrations of this. A central venous pressure catheter (CVP) would be properly located in the superior vena cava. When a patient is going to have the perfusion of the coronary arteries checked, an arterial catheter passes through the aortic arch to reach them. The pulmonary artery catheter passes through the right ventricle to reach the pulmonary arteries.

16. **C.** Rationale: Because the patient is competent and able to perform the procedure, it would be appropriate to begin a patient-driven protocol. The parent(s) should be involved in the care of a minor child. In this case, no need exists for a therapist or nurse to deliver the patient's inhaled medications. Although the parent could be taught to deliver the medication, it is not necessary because the child can do it.

17. **B.** Rationale: See Table 1-17 for the five Apgar signs and how they are scored. In this example, all five signs would be rated at 1 point each for a total score of 5 points.

18. **A.** Rationale: Potassium is the most important electrolyte to monitor for several reasons. First, it affects the functioning of the heart's conduction system. Second, the serum level is relatively low compared with those of the other electrolytes. Third, potassium, in addition to sodium chloride, tends to be lost through the kidneys when a diuretic medication is given. In general, when a patient is given a diuretic medication, all of the serum electrolyte values should be closely watched. Be prepared to recommend the replacement of electrolytes as needed.

2 Infection Control

Note 1: The National Board for Respiratory Care (NBRC) has released the *RRT Examination Matrix* (covering the testable items on the Written Registry Exam) and *CSE Examination Matrix* (covering the testable items on the Clinical Simulation Exam). Both are included in the appendices at the end of this book, which is intended to cover all items listed as testable on these two publications. This chapter (and all others) uses the abbreviation "WRE" for the coded items testable on the Written Registry Exam *and* Clinical Simulation Exam. The abbreviation "CSE" will be used for the coded items testable on *only* the Clinical Simulation Exam.

Note 2: A review of the most recent Written Registry Examinations has shown an average of two questions (2% of the exam) that cover infection control issues. The Clinical Simulation exam is comprehensive and may include everything that should be known or performed by an advanced level respiratory therapist.

MODULE A

Follow established infection-control policies and procedures (e.g., standard precautions) (WRE code: IIID7) [Difficulty: AP]

1. Hand washing or cleansing

Hand washing or cleansing is probably the single most important procedure for reducing the spread of infection. Washing with plain soap and warm tap water is acceptable in most cases. Antimicrobial soap should be used if called for in the infection control protocol. In many institutions, an isopropyl alcohol and skin-softener cleansing agent is used unless the hands are obviously contaminated. When contaminated with body fluids, the hands should be washed. In any case, respiratory therapists should wash or cleanse their hands before and between each patient contact. The following times are recommended:

a. When coming on duty
b. When hands are obviously soiled or after contamination by blood or other patient body fluids
c. Before contact with the face and mouth of patients, especially if the patient has an artificial airway

d. Before setting up equipment or pouring medicines
e. When leaving an isolation area or handling contaminated articles from an isolation area
f. After handling soiled dressings, sputum containers, urinals, bedpans, catheters, etc.
g. After removing patient care gloves
h. After personal use of the toilet
i. After using hands to cover a cough and after blowing or wiping the nose
j. Before eating or serving food
k. On completion of duty

The most common bacterial organisms spread by personal contact are *Staphylococcus aureus*, *Escherichia coli*, and *Streptococcus* species. Suspect personal contact and poor hand cleaning whenever a patient has one of these infections.

Exam Hint

Past examinations have asked about the importance of hand washing and the indications for it to prevent the spread of infection.

2. Standard precautions

Standard (formerly called *universal*) precautions are designed for care of all patients regardless of their diagnosis or presumed infection status. Barriers such as gloves, masks, and other procedures are used to prevent contact with body fluids. This approach to patient care has been adopted because of the concern of health care workers and the public that the human immunodeficiency virus (HIV), hepatitis B, or other deadly pathogens can be spread unknowingly by contact. Box 2-1 includes specific standard precaution guidelines established by the Centers for Disease Control and Prevention (CDC) and the Occupational Safety and Health Administration (OSHA).

3. Respiratory care equipment and procedures

The following guidelines are recommended to minimize the spread of infection by equipment and procedures.

BOX 2-1 Standard Precautions to Prevent the Spread of Infection

EXCLUSION FROM PATIENT CONTACT
Any health care worker with exudative skin lesions should not work in the direct care of patients.

BARRIERS
1. Gloves should be worn under these conditions: during direct contact with blood, body fluids, secretions, mucous membranes, and wounds; when handling all items or surfaces contaminated by blood or body fluids; when performing venipuncture; or when handling intravenous catheters or monitoring devices.
2. Gloves must be changed between patients or if the gloves become torn or punctured, as with a needle-stick injury.
3. Hands should be washed immediately after the gloves are removed; the hands or any other body areas must be washed immediately if contaminated by blood or other body fluid.
4. Masks, eye goggles, or face shields, as well as gowns or aprons, should be worn when a procedure is performed that may lead to the splashing or splattering of blood, secretions, or body fluids.
5. Contaminated masks, goggles, face shields, gowns, and aprons should be removed and disposed of properly.
6. Contaminated worker uniforms should be left at the hospital for cleaning.

NEEDLE AND INSTRUMENT PRECAUTIONS
1. Care should be taken when needles and sharp instruments are handled.
2. Used needles and sharp instruments should be placed into puncture-resistant containers for proper disposal; reusable needles should be placed into a puncture-resistant container for transport.
3. No attempt should be made to manually recap arterial blood gas or other needles, remove them from the syringe, or bend or cut them (needle-covering systems or methods of pushing the needle into a rubber cube are widely used; these require the use of only one hand with no touching of the needle).

PATIENT SPECIMENS
1. Blood and body fluids should be placed into leak-proof, sturdy plastic bags for transportation to the laboratory.
2. The laboratory requisition form should be placed on the outside of this bag.

CARDIOPULMONARY RESUSCITATION
1. Mouth-to-mouth breathing should be avoided even though no evidence exists that saliva transmits human immunodeficiency virus infection.
2. Mouth-to-valve mask resuscitators and manual resuscitators (bag-valve) should be readily available for use in ventilating patients.

Follow the manufacturer's specific guidelines when applicable.
   a. Each patient should have his or her own equipment.
   b. Disposable equipment should be discarded after use.
   c. Reusable equipment should undergo high-level disinfection or be sterilized between patients.
   d. Equipment such as O_2 masks, large-volume nebulizers, and aerosol tubing should be changed every 24 hours.
   e. Ventilator breathing circuits should not be changed more often than every 48 hours and may be used for up to 5 days if a heat-moisture exchanger is used for humidification.
   f. Sterile water should be used for procedures, and the unused portion should be discarded after 24 hours.
   g. Add water to reservoir systems immediately before use.
   h. Discard any unused water in a reservoir system before refilling.
   i. Drain and discard any water collected in tubing; do *not* drain water back into the reservoir.
   j. Medications should be stored under the conditions set by the manufacturer, should be discarded if they appear abnormal, and should be discarded on the expiration date.
   k. Unused portions of medications should be discarded after 24 hours.
   l. Sterile syringes should be used when measuring medications.
   m. Sterile suction catheters should be used and sterile gloves worn whenever the patient's airway is suctioned.

Exam Hint
Past examinations have questioned the types of routine procedures that should be performed to control the spread of infection through respiratory care equipment.

4. Transmission-based precautions
Transmission-based precautions are used for patients known or suspected to be infected or colonized with epidemiologically significant pathogens, which are spread through airborne or droplet transmission or by contact with dry skin or contaminated surfaces. These precautions are used with standard precautions. The following are general guidelines and specific diseases or conditions established by the CDC for the three types of patient isolation categories. Hospitals may establish extra standards and post them at the door to the patient's room.

a. Airborne precautions

Airborne precautions are used in addition to standard precautions for patients with known or suspected illness transmitted by airborne droplet nuclei, including pulmonary tuberculosis (TB), varicella (chickenpox), and rubeola (measles).

1. Room placement

Patients under airborne precautions must be placed in a room with negative airflow and ultraviolet (UV) light capabilities.

2. Gloves and hand washing

Use standard precautions.

3. Respiratory protection

a. If a patient is known or suspected of having TB, a National Institute for Occupational Safety and Health (NIOSH)-approved respirator mask must be worn by all caregivers entering the room.
b. If a patient is known or suspected of having varicella or rubeola, a NIOSH-approved respirator mask must be worn by all *susceptible* caregivers entering the room.

4. Patient transport

a. Transport personnel must wear a NIOSH-approved respirator mask as discussed earlier.
b. The patient must wear an isolation mask while out of his or her room.

5. Patient equipment

Use standard precautions.

b. Droplet precautions

Droplet precautions are used in addition to standard precautions for patients known or suspected of having serious illness transmitted by large-particle droplets such as influenza, invasive *Haemophilus influenzae* (type b), *Neisseria meningitidis* disease including meningococcal bacteremia and meningitis, *Mycoplasma pneumoniae*, and *Bordetella pertussis*.

1. Room placement

A private room is preferred, but patients with the same infection may be placed in the same room.

2. Gloves and hand washing

Use standard precautions.

3. Gown

Use standard precautions.

4. Respiratory protection

a. Use standard precautions.

b. Caregivers must wear an isolation mask if working within 3 feet of the patient.

5. Patient transport

a. Transport personnel must wear an isolation mask if working within 3 feet of the patient.
b. The patient must wear an isolation mask while out of his or her room.

6. Patient equipment

Use standard precautions.

c. Contact precautions

Contact precautions are used in addition to standard precautions for patients known to have or suspected of having epidemiologically important organisms that can be transmitted by direct contact with environmental surfaces, such as patients with diarrhea, inadequately contained wound infections, or localized herpes zoster (shingles).

1. Room placement

A private room is preferred, but patients with the same infection may be placed in the same room.

2. Gloves and hand washing

a. Wear gloves when entering the patient's room.
b. Change gloves after contact with any contaminated item.
c. Remove gloves and wash hands before leaving the patient's room.

3. Gown

a. Wear a gown when entering the patient's room if you anticipate substantial contact with the patient, environmental surfaces, or patient items.
b. Remove the gown and wash hands before leaving the room.

4. Respiratory protection

Use standard precautions.

5. Patient transport

a. Limit transportation of the patient from the room.
b. If transportation is required, caregivers must wear a gown and gloves.

6. Patient equipment

a. Each patient should have his or her own dedicated noncritical equipment (thermometer, commode, blood pressure cuff, sphygmomanometer, stethoscope, etc.).
b. Clean and disinfect all patient care equipment after the patient is discharged.

MODULE B
Decontaminate respiratory care equipment

Decontamination is the process of disassembling, washing (to remove debris), rinsing, and disinfecting or sterilizing used patient care equipment. The process results in the equipment being free of any pathogens so that it can be used with another patient. Obviously, once disinfected, the equipment must be aseptically reassembled and stored for future use.

1. Choose the appropriate agent and method for disinfection and sterilization (WRE code: IIB1) [Difficulty: An]
a. Disinfection

Disinfection is a procedure that significantly reduces the microbial contamination of the equipment that has been processed. All disinfection processes destroy the vegetative form (the cell) of pathogenic organisms, including the vast majority of respiratory system pathogens. However, a few *Bacillus*-type bacteria are difficult to kill because they have a particularly tough cell wall or have spores for reproduction. Spores are analogous to seeds in that they grow into bacteria under the right conditions and are resistant to drying, heat, and many chemicals that kill the bacterial cell. Therefore a spore-forming organism may be able to reproduce itself after the cells have been killed. Obviously, disinfection can be used only on equipment that is *not* contaminated by spore-forming bacteria. Knowing what pathogen has infected the patient, if possible, can determine the appropriate disinfection (or sterilization) method to be used on the contaminated equipment. Some disinfecting agents kill different kinds of organisms, depending on the length of exposure time.

Another consideration in selecting the appropriate disinfection method is how the equipment will be used in patient care. Equipment or instruments that do not directly touch the patient are classified as *noncritical* (low risk of spreading infection) and can undergo low-level disinfection (e.g., an electrocardiograph machine). Low-level disinfectants are agents capable of killing some vegetative bacteria, fungi, and lipophilic viruses. Equipment or instruments that touch surface mucous membranes and the skin but do not penetrate them are listed as *semicritical* and must undergo high-level disinfection (e.g., laryngoscope blades and a bronchoscope). Agents that kill all microorganisms except bacterial spores are classified as *high-level* disinfectants.

A third consideration in choosing the best disinfection method is the type of equipment that requires decontamination. Certain processes and agents can be used only on certain types of equipment. Table 2-1 lists the various ways of disinfecting reusable patient care equipment decontaminated in the hospital.

The fourth consideration to take into account is the location of the patient. The previous discussion relates to patients in the hospital or a long-term care facility. Home care patients will typically not use these methods because of the high costs. Instead, the plastics used in home care medication nebulizers, etc., are usually cleaned as follows:

1. Disassemble as needed.
2. Run hot water from the tap to eliminate as many organisms as possible. Clean the sink.
3. Use hot water to wash the equipment in a detergent solution.
4. Place the equipment into an acetic acid (white vinegar) solution for disinfection. It should soak for 60 minutes. (Grocery store–purchased white vinegar contains 5% acetic acid. However, it may be diluted with three parts of water to get a 1.25% solution.) After use, the acetic acid must be thrown away because it will no longer be effective.
5. After soaking, the equipment should be rinsed in hot water and placed on a clean towel to air dry.

A 1.25% or higher solution is classified as a low-level disinfectant and will kill most vegetative bacteria (including *Pseudomonas aeruginosa*) and some fungi and viruses. However, *Mycobacterium tuberculosis*, nonlipid viruses, and spores will not be killed.

> ### Exam Hint
>
> **E**xpect to see one question about using white vinegar or acetic acid to disinfect equipment in the home. The percentage of acetic acid should not matter.

b. Sterilization

Sterilization is a procedure that destroys all living microbial organisms and renders them unable to reproduce. All sterilization procedures destroy the vegetative forms and spores of all microscopic organisms. Examples of spore-forming bacteria include *Bacillus anthracis* (anthrax), *Clostridium botulinum* (botulism), *C. tetani* (tetanus), and *C. perfringens* (gas gangrene). Any equipment or instruments that penetrate body tissue are listed as "critical" (high risk of spreading infection) and must be sterilized before use on another patient (e.g., a surgical scalpel). As discussed previously, the method of sterilization depends on the type of equipment under consideration. Table 2-2 lists the various methods of sterilization for reusable supplies and patient care equipment decontaminated in the hospital.

2. Disinfect or sterilize respiratory care equipment (WRE code: IIB1) [Difficulty: An]
As previously discussed, the choice of whether to disinfect or sterilize equipment depends on how it is used clinically,

TABLE 2-1	Methods of Disinfection Used in the Hospital Setting						
		Microbes effective against					
Method	Conditions	Bacteria	TB	Spores	Viruses	Fungi	Comments
LOW AND INTERMEDIATE LEVEL DISINFECTION							
Pasteurization	Complete immersion in water heated to 70°C (170°F) for 30 min	Yes	Yes	No	Yes	Yes	Used with rubber and many plastics used in respiratory care, especially those that are sensitive to a high temperature **Avoid use** with any item that cannot be immersed or will be damaged at this temperature
Alcohols (70% ethyl or 90% isopropyl)	Complete immersion for several minutes or pooling of the alcohol on the equipment	Yes	Yes	No	Lipophilic only	Yes	Used with metallic or plastic surfaces of large pieces of equipment that cannot be disinfected by any other means. May also be used with most plastics **Avoid use** with any item that cannot be immersed or will absorb or be damaged by the alcohol
Iodines (iodine or iodophor with 70% ethyl alcohol)	Complete immersion for several minutes or pooling of the solution on the equipment	Yes	Yes	No	Yes	Yes	Used with metallic or plastic surfaces of large pieces of equipment that cannot be disinfected by any other means. May also be used with most plastics **Avoid use** with any item that cannot be immersed or will absorb or be damaged by the alcohol
HIGH LEVEL DISINFECTION: GLUTARALDEHYDE SOLUTIONS							
Alkaline glutaraldehyde (Cidex, Cidex 7, Sporicidin)	Complete immersion for 10 min	Yes	Yes	No	Yes	Yes	Used with rubber and many plastics used in respiratory care, especially those that are heat sensitive. Care must be taken to thoroughly rinse items after disinfection **Avoid use** with any item that cannot be immersed or will absorb the solution
Acid glutaraldehyde (Sonacide)	Complete immersion for 20 min	Yes	Yes	No	Yes	Yes	Used with rubber and many plastics used in respiratory care, especially those that are heat sensitive. Care must be taken to thoroughly rinse items after they have been disinfected **Avoid use** with any item that cannot be immersed or will absorb the solution

TB, Tuberculosis.

TABLE 2-2 Methods of Sterilization

Method	Conditions	Comments
Steam autoclave	Autoclave chamber with an internal steam pressure of 15 lb per sq in, 121°C (250°F), 15 min	Used with glass, cloth, bandages, unsharpened stainless steel instruments **Avoid use** with many plastics used in respiratory care, rubber, dextrose solutions, sharpened stainless steel instruments, electrical devices, or machines
Dry heat	Autoclave chamber at 160°–180°C (320°–356°F), 2 hr use	Used with glass or sharpened stainless steel instruments **Avoid use** with many plastics used in respiratory care, rubber, dextrose solutions, electric devices, or machines
Ethylene oxide gas	Specific guidelines vary depending on the manufacturer of the chamber and the supplies or equipment being sterilized. In general, a gas concentration of 800–1000 mg/L must be kept for 3–4 hr at 50%–100% relative humidity and 49°–57°C (120°–135°F). Great care must be taken to pre-dry all items before gassing and to properly aerate them after sterilization	Used with heat-sensitive and moisture-sensitive items as are many plastics used in respiratory care **Avoid use** with supply pouches or plastic films, such as aluminum foil, nylon, thermoplastic resin (Saran), Mylar, cellophane polyamide, polyester, or other films that are not penetrated by the gas, or with PVC that has been previously sterilized by the manufacturer with gamma radiation
GLUTARALDEHYDE SOLUTIONS		
Alkaline glutaraldehyde (Cidex, Cidex 7, Sporicidin)	Complete immersion. Cidex products for 10 hr; Sporicidin for 6 hr and 45 min	Used with rubber and many plastics in respiratory care, especially those that are heat sensitive; care must be taken to thoroughly rinse items after they have been cleaned **Avoid use** with any item that cannot be immersed or that will absorb the solution
Acid glutaraldehyde (Sonacide)	Complete immersion for 1 hr at 60°C (140°F)	Used with rubber and many plastics used in respiratory care, especially those that are heat sensitive; care must be taken to thoroughly rinse items after they have been cleaned **Avoid use** with any item that cannot be immersed or will absorb the solution

PVC, Polyvinyl chloride.

what type of pathogen is involved, and from what material the equipment is made. Most respiratory pathogens are not spore-formers, so low-level or high-level disinfection is acceptable. Either a glutaraldehyde solution or pasteurization is used in most departments for disinfecting plastic masks, hoses, etc.

Any department that processes its own equipment must have adequate facilities. A "dirty" area must exist where contaminated equipment is brought for disassembly, scrubbing of secretions or blood, and rinsing. Equipment is then placed into either the glutaraldehyde solution or a pasteurizing machine. After that, equipment is taken to a "clean" area to be rinsed, dried, reassembled, and placed into plastic bags for storage. Care must be taken not to recontaminate the equipment during this procedure. Items that must be sterilized are usually just processed through the dirty area before being sent to the central supply department, where the equipment is sterilized based on the criteria shown in Table 2-2.

3. Monitor the sterilization process to ensure its effectiveness (WRE code: IIB1) [Difficulty: An]

The term *surveillance* describes the monitoring of equipment to ensure that the disinfection or sterilization process was successful and that in-use equipment is not a source of patient contamination. Processing (chemical) indicators are used to ensure that disinfection or sterilization was done correctly. Examples include special tapes used to hold the wrapping around packages of equipment being autoclaved or placed into ethylene oxide. These tapes turn color when the autoclave has reached the proper temperature or the correct concentration of ethylene oxide has been reached. The color change shows the user that the package was processed correctly; therefore the package contents are sterile.

Another example is a biologic indicator placed into the wrapped package before sterilization. These biologic indicators are bacterial spores that are killed only if the required conditions are met. For example, the spores of *Bacillus subtilis* are placed onto strips of paper to be killed by ethylene oxide gas. After the equipment and spores have been sent through the sterilization process, the spores are placed into conditions favorable for growth. If no growth occurs, they are dead; therefore no other living organisms survived.

Equipment held in storage or being used in patient care also is randomly sampled for contamination. A sample is taken for culturing of possible organisms in three ways. The first involves wiping a sterile swab onto an equipment surface, and then rubbing it over a plate of growth medium or placing it into a tube of liquid broth. The second is used to check inside lengths of tubing, which necessitates pouring a liquid broth through the tube and into a sterile container. The third involves sampling the aerosol that a nebulizer produces. A hose is usually attached to the outlet of the nebulizer. The other end of the hose is connected to a funnel, which is attached to a culture plate where the droplets impact. In all three examples, the growth of any organism in the growth medium indicates a form of contamination. The laboratory then determines whether the organism is pathogenic. If so, measures must be taken to improve the disinfection or sterilization process.

MODULE C
Biohazardous materials

Make sure that biohazardous materials are properly handled. (WRE code: IIB2) [Difficulty: An]

A respiratory therapist is most likely to come into contact with biohazardous materials that are either infectious waste, body fluids, or needles and syringes. All must be handled and disposed of properly to keep the practitioner and patient safe. Although hospital policies will vary,

infectious waste and body fluids are usually placed into a red bag. The bag is removed from the patient care area and incinerated to ensure that all pathogens are killed.

Needles, syringes, or any sharp objects are placed into a sharps container. It also is red and usually is marked with a biohazard symbol. Every patient room should have a sharps container placed so that used needles and syringes can be easily disposed of. If at all possible, the needle should not be recapped after use. Instead, simply drop the used needle and syringe into the slot on the container. Never force anything into the container or put a finger into it. When full, the sharps container should be sealed closed and removed for proper disposal.

BIBLIOGRAPHY

American Association for Respiratory Care: Guidelines for the prevention of nosocomial infections, *AARTimes,* Dallas, Sept. 1983.

American Respiratory Care Foundation: Guidelines for disinfection of respiratory care equipment used in the home, *Respir Care* 33:801, 1988.

Carter C, Stone MK: Respiratory microbiology, infection, and infection control. In Hess DR, MacIntyre NR, et al, editors: *Respiratory care principles and practice,* Philadelphia, 2002, WB Saunders.

Chatburn RL, Kallstrom TJ, Bajaksouzian S: A comparison of acetic acid with a quaternary ammonium compound for disinfection of hand-held nebulizers. *Respir Care* 33(3):179–187, 1988.

Cidexplus, 28-day solution: Product Insert, Johnson & Johnson Medical, Arlington, Tex.

Eubanks DH, Bone RC: *Comprehensive respiratory care,* ed 2, St Louis, 1990, Mosby.

Fink JB: Infection control and safety. In Fink JB, Hunt GE, editors: *Clinical practice in respiratory care,* Philadelphia, 1999, Lippincott Williams & Wilkins.

Infection control precautions, OSF Saint Anthony Medical Center, Rockford, Ill, 1998.

Meyer R, Scanlan CL: Principles of infection control. In Wilkins RL, Stoller JK, Scanlan CL, editors: *Egan's fundamentals of respiratory care,* ed 8, St Louis, 2003, Mosby.

Pagana KD, Pagana TJ: *Mosby's manual of diagnostic and laboratory tests,* St Louis, 1998, Mosby.

Washington JA: Infectious disease aspects of respiratory therapy. In Burton GG, Hodgkin JE, Ward JJ, editors: *Respiratory care,* ed 4, Philadelphia, 1997, Lippincott-Raven.

SELF-STUDY QUESTIONS

1. A hospitalized patient who recovered from a *Clostridium botulinum* infection received several respiratory care services. How should a nondisposable large-volume nebulizer be sterilized before being reused?
   A. Steam autoclave for 15 minutes.
   B. Soak in glutaraldehyde solution for 10 hours.
   C. Pasteurize for 20 minutes.
   D. Soak in an alcohol solution for 15 minutes.

2. Select all of the following that can be used in the home to reduce the chance of bacterial growth in a small volume nebulizer or other respiratory care equipment.
   I. Soak the equipment in white vinegar.
   II. Put the equipment in the oven, and turn on the broiler for 10 minutes.
   III. Rinse a nebulizer in salt water (normal saline) after each use.

IV. Wash the equipment in hot water with a detergent.
- A. I, IV
- B. I, II
- C. I, III, IV
- D. I, II, III, IV

3. After use of a mechanical ventilator has been discontinued, what is the best method to sterilize the reusable main-flow bacteria filter?
- A. Wrap it and soak it in acetic acid
- B. Pasteurization
- C. Glutaraldehyde soak
- D. Steam autoclaving

4. A batch of respiratory care equipment has gone through the gas sterilization process with ethylene oxide. Routine surveillance of the equipment shows that spores of *Bacillus subtilis* have survived the process. What should be done next?
- A. Use the equipment, because this organism does not cause illness.
- B. Aerate the gas as usual, and put into use.
- C. Resterilize the equipment, and check for death of the spores.
- D. Wipe off the equipment with 70% alcohol to remove the spores from the equipment.

5. A retired home care patient living on a fixed income needs to be able to disinfect her respiratory therapy equipment. Which of the following would be best for her?
- A. Acetic acid
- B. Acid glutaraldehyde
- C. Ethylene oxide system
- D. Warm, soapy water

6. What is the most cost-effective way for a respiratory care department to disinfect large amounts of reusable plastic tubing and oxygen masks?
- A. 70% ethyl alcohol
- B. Steam autoclave
- C. Pasteurization
- D. Dry heat

7. A contaminated Bird Mark 7 intermittent positive-pressure breathing (IPPB) unit must be sterilized before use with another patient. What is the best method?
- A. Pasteurization
- B. Ethylene oxide
- C. 10-hour soak in glutaraldehyde
- D. Steam autoclave

8. A home care company has found that several of its tracheostomy patients have *Escherichia coli* tracheal infections. What is the most likely cause of the infections?
- A. Poor hand-washing technique by their visiting respiratory therapist.
- B. Contaminated tracheostomy tubes from the manufacturer.
- C. Contaminated bottles of sterile water from the manufacturer.
- D. Poor hand-washing technique by the patients' family members.

ANSWER KEY

1. **B.** Rationale: A glutaraldehyde solution soak for 10 hours is the only way listed to sterilize plastic equipment without damaging it. Putting plastic equipment into a steam autoclave causes it to melt and be destroyed. Pasteurization or soaking the equipment in an alcohol solution disinfects but does not sterilize the equipment as needed.

2. **A.** Rationale: A hot-water wash with detergent will remove secretions and other debris from the equipment. Soaking the equipment in white vinegar (acetic acid) will kill many of the microorganisms commonly found on home care equipment. The heat generated in an oven under the broiler will melt plastic used in a small volume nebulizer and other respiratory care equipment. Rinsing the equipment in salt water will not make a significant difference in killing microorganisms. In addition, the dried salt crystals may plug up the capillary tube of a nebulizer.

3. **D.** Rationale: Steam autoclaving is the only method listed that is acceptable to sterilize a ventilator's bacteria filter. Review Table 2-2 if needed. The other three options involve solutions that will damage the filter medium and make the filter useless.

4. **C.** Rationale: The equipment must be resterilized because living spores of *Bacillus subtilis* indicate that the sterilization process was not successful. Other microbes also may have survived. Because of this concern, the equipment should not be used. Aeration of the equipment will not sterilize it, and 70% alcohol will not remove the spores from the equipment or sterilize it.

5. **A.** Rationale: Acetic acid is found in white vinegar. It is inexpensive and available in any grocery store. Realize that acetic acid is not a powerful disinfectant and does not kill most pulmonary pathogens. Acid glutaraldehyde and ethylene oxide systems are too expensive to use in a home. Warm, soapy water can be used to clean secretions from equipment but does not disinfect it.

6. **C.** Rationale: Pasteurization is the least expensive way to disinfect large amounts of the plastic equipment used in respiratory care departments. Steam autoclave and dry heat are used to sterilize, not disinfect,

equipment. In addition, the high temperatures used with these methods melts the plastic tubing and oxygen masks. Seventy percent ethyl alcohol is used only to wipe off the surfaces of large equipment items for disinfection.

7. **B.** Rationale: Ethylene oxide gas should be used on an IPPB machine because it sterilizes the unit without causing any damage. Pasteurization and glutaraldehyde involve solutions that damage the internal structures of any IPPB machine. The heat of steam autoclaving melts any plastic or rubber components of the unit and seriously damages the machine.

8. **A.** Rationale: Poor hand-washing technique is the most common cause of E. coli, Staphylococcus aureus, and Streptococcus bacterial infections. The fact that all infected patients have E. coli infections points to a single person as the cause. In this case, it would most likely be the home respiratory therapist. It is very unlikely that the cause of the infections would be from poor manufacturing processes. These equipment and supply items are all produced and sterilized under very demanding standards. If the patients' family members were the cause of the infections, it is likely that a variety of bacterial infections would be present, not just one.

3

Blood Gas Analysis and Monitoring

Note 1: The National Board for Respiratory Care (NBRC) has released the *RRT Examination Matrix* (covering the testable items on the Written Registry Exam) and the *CSE Examination Matrix* (covering the testable items on the Clinical Simulation Exam). Turn to the appendices at the back of this book for both publications in their original format. This book is intended to cover all of the testable items in these two publications. This chapter (and all others) uses the abbreviation "WRE" for the coded items testable on the Written Registry Exam *and* Clinical Simulation Exam. The listed difficulty (R, Recall; Ap, Application; An, Analysis) relates to the question difficulty on the Written Registry Exam. The abbreviation "CSE" will be used for the coded items testable on *only* the Clinical Simulation Exam. Because no question difficulty level is given for this examination, be prepared for anything.

Note 2: A review of the most recent Written Registry Examinations has shown an average of five questions (5% of the exam) that cover blood gas analysis and monitoring. In addition, arterial blood gas results are often given during oxygen therapy and mechanical ventilation questions. The blood gas results must be interpreted to answer these questions correctly. The Clinical Simulation Exam is comprehensive and may include everything that should be known or performed by an advanced level respiratory therapist.

MODULE A

Make a recommendation to obtain a blood sample for blood gas analysis (WRE code: IC3) [Difficulty: AN]

Blood can be sampled from a systemic artery, pulmonary artery, or "arterialized" capillary to determine a patient's oxygen and carbon dioxide pressures, acid-base status (pH), and related values. As is discussed later, a pulmonary artery sample is taken to learn a patient's mixed venous values, and an "arterialized" capillary sample is taken from a neonate when an arterial sample cannot be obtained. *Arterial blood gas* (ABG) is the term commonly used when discussing drawing a sample of blood from a patient's systemic artery.

There are three broad, general indications for this recommendation:

To check a patient's oxygenation status (Pao_2)

To check a patient's acid-base status (pH)
To check a patient's ventilation status ($Paco_2$)
   Some specific indications follow.

1. Cardiac failure
   a. Congenital defect
   b. Heart attack (myocardial infarct)
   c. Congestive heart failure with or without pulmonary edema

2. Chronic obstructive pulmonary disease
   a. Asthma
   b. Emphysema
   c. Bronchitis
   d. Bronchiectasis

3. Any pneumonia that causes hypoxemia

4. Trauma
   a. Broken ribs
   b. Flail chest
   c. Pneumothorax
   d. Hemothorax
   e. Upper airway trauma

5. Ventilatory failure
   a. Overdosage of sedatives or pain relievers
   b. Stroke or head (brain) injury
   c. Spinal cord injury
   d. Neuromuscular diseases such as myasthenia gravis or Guillain-Barré syndrome

6. Airway obstruction
   a. Foreign-body aspiration
   b. Laryngotracheobronchitis (croup)
   c. Epiglottitis

7. Miscellaneous
   a. Smoke inhalation
   b. Carbon monoxide poisoning
   c. Near drowning
   d. Infant respiratory distress syndrome (RDS)/hyaline membrane disease
   e. Acute respiratory distress syndrome (ARDS)

f. The patient does not have an indwelling arterial line

g. A shunt percentage calculation or alveolar-arterial O_2 pressure difference ($P[A–a]O_2$) calculation must be made

h. Cardiopulmonary resuscitation

MODULE B
Obtain a blood sample

1. Perform quality control procedures for a blood gas sampling device (WRE code: IIC1) [Difficulty: An]

A properly assembled sampling device should not create any problems with obtaining the blood sample. Quality control (QC) procedures for an arterial sampling device and steps that can be taken to correct a problem follow.

a. Get the appropriate blood gas sampler

Obtaining an ABG sample generally involves selecting a prepackaged, sterile blood gas kit that contains the following:

1. A variety of short-bevel needles: 23 or 24 gauge for radial or dorsalis pedis puncture and a 22 gauge for brachial or femoral puncture.
2. 3-mL syringe. Many kits contain a syringe prepared with heparin as an anticoagulant.
3. If needed, liquid sodium or lithium heparin with an appropriate concentration.
4. Alcohol or iodophor (Betadine) wipes to clean the puncture site.

If a blood gas kit is not available, an appropriate individual needle, 3-mL syringe, and liquid sodium or lithium heparin must be obtained. These should be available at any nursing station or from the respiratory care department.

A capillary blood gas (CBG) sample requires the following:

1. Several heparinized glass capillary tubes with a volume of at least 100 μL
2. Metal filing (flea) to place into each capillary tube
3. Plastic caps or clay to seal the tubes
4. Magnet to draw the metal filing back and forth in the tube to mix the blood
5. Lancet to make incision
6. Moist, warm (42°C) cloth or diaper to wrap around the puncture site
7. Sterile cotton balls and bandage to place over the puncture site to aid clotting
8. Isopropyl alcohol swabs (70%) to clean the puncture site
9. Clean gloves to protect the practitioner's hands from any contact with spilled blood

In addition, an ice-water mix in a cup is needed to chill the blood taken by any method.

b. Put the equipment together, make sure that it works properly, and identify and fix any problems

To assemble a blood gas syringe, use sterile technique to screw the selected needle onto the syringe. If the syringe does not contain heparin, it must be added. Do this by aspirating liquid heparin through the needle into the syringe. Coat the inside of the syringe with heparin by tipping the needle up, pulling the plunger back, and pushing the plunger forward to squirt the excess heparin out of the needle. This ensures that the needle and dead space of the needle are filled with heparin, and the inside of the syringe is coated.

Make sure that the needle is tightly screwed onto the syringe. The plunger should easily slide within the barrel of the syringe. A blood clot or debris within the needle plugs it and prevents this. Replace and safely dispose of a needle that is obstructed.

c. Make sure no air bubbles are in the syringe

Air bubbles result in the oxygen level and the pH being too high and the carbon dioxide level being too low. If an air bubble is found in the syringe, tilt it so that the needle is up. The bubble will rise by itself or may be raised by tapping the syringe. Push the plunger into the syringe to eject the air bubble. Cap off the hub of the syringe or needle to prevent air from entering the syringe.

d. Use the proper amount of heparin

This is a concern only when liquid heparin is added to a needle and syringe. Aspirate about 1 mL of 10 mg/mL or 1000 units/mL sodium heparin through the needle into the syringe. Pull the plunger back to coat the inside of the syringe. Push the plunger forward to squirt the excess heparin out through the needle. The values of a 2- to 4-mL sample of blood should not be affected by this concentration. Remember that inadequate heparin can cause the blood sample to clot. Excessive heparin can alter the blood gas values by reducing the pH and the carbon dioxide level and increasing the oxygen level.

e. Promptly cool the blood gas sample

If the sample cannot be analyzed within 10 minutes of being drawn, it should be placed in an ice-water bath. Failure to do so results in the living blood consuming the available oxygen and producing carbon dioxide. Obviously, this results in incorrect measured values.

2. Arterial and umbilical artery line (catheter)
a. Select the appropriate catheter (WRE code: IIA17) [Difficulty: R, Ap, An]

An arterial line is a flexible catheter that is placed into a peripheral artery for the purposes of sampling blood, or continuously monitoring the patient's blood pressure, or both. The blood-sampling procedure is explained in the following discussion. Chapter 5 contains a discussion on blood pressure monitoring and illustrations of how the monitoring system is assembled. The radial artery is the most common site for catheter insertion. Alternate arterial sites may be used if needed.

An adult's radial artery is usually catheterized. To do so, a short needle covered with a flexible plastic catheter (an angiocatheter) is selected. Usually the needle is 23 or 24 gauge. After the angiocatheter is inserted into the artery, the needle is removed, and the catheter is left in the artery.

A newborn with a severe cardiopulmonary problem should have the catheter inserted into either of the umbilical arteries. Usually, a long, flexible umbilical artery catheter (UAC) is placed into the patient and advanced into the aorta. If indicated, this should be done as quickly as possible after birth, before arterial spasm prevents the catheter from being advanced. If the patient weighs more than 1250 g, a 6 French (6Fr) catheter is used; a 3.5Fr catheter is used if the neonate weighs less than 1250 g. Besides obtaining blood samples and monitoring the blood pressure, one can give the newborn glucose or a blood transfusion through the catheter. A neonatal patient also may have the umbilical vein catheterized.

b. Put the equipment together and make sure that it works properly (WRE code: IIA17) [Difficulty: R, Ap, An]

Arterial catheters come as single units in sterile packaging. Additional stopcocks, tubing, flush solution, and an automatic solution drip device are needed. These are discussed in Chapter 5 in some detail.

c. Troubleshoot any problems with the equipment (WRE code: IIA17) [Difficulty: R, Ap, An]

See the discussion in Chapter 5.

3. Obtain a blood sample from an arterial line (WRE code: IB7e and IIIE2b) [Difficulty: An]

The steps for obtaining an arterial blood sample include the following:

1. Tell a conscious adult patient that you are going to take a blood sample from the arterial catheter.
2. Put gloves on both hands.
3. Remove the dead-ender cap from the sample (side) port on the three-way stopcock between the catheter and the intravenous (IV) tubing.
4. Screw a sterile 5- to 10-mL syringe to the sample port for removing the IV solution from the catheter. (A smaller syringe should be used for a neonate.)
5. Turn the stopcock off to the IV tubing (Fig. 3-1).

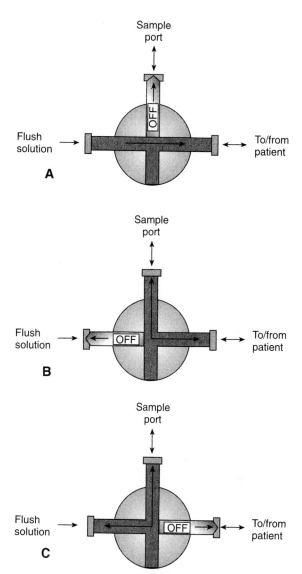

Fig. 3-1 A three-way stopcock for use in an arterial line system. **A,** The normal operating position of the stopcock that allows fluid to flow to the patient (and the blood pressure to be monitored if assembled for continuous blood pressure monitoring). **B,** The stopcock position that allows blood to be withdrawn from the patient through the sample port. The flush solution port is closed. **C,** The stopcock position for flush solution to go to the sample port to clear out any blood. When the stopcock is turned to a 45-degree angle between any two ports, all of the ports are closed. *(From Scanlan CL: Analysis and monitoring of gas exchange. In Scanlan CL, Wilkins RL, Stoller JK, editors: Egan's fundamentals of respiratory care, ed 7, St Louis, 1999, Mosby.)*

6. Pull a waste sample of IV solution and blood into the syringe. (The amount withdrawn and discarded depends on the dead space volume from the tip of the catheter to the side port. Studies indicate that between 2.5 and 6 times this volume should be removed. Typically, this is about 5 mL in an adult and less in a neonate.)

7. Turn the stopcock off to all ports by turning it halfway between any two ports.
8. Attach a preheparinized sterile syringe to the sample port, turn the stopcock open to the syringe, and withdraw about 2 to 3 mL of arterial blood to be analyzed.
9. Turn the stopcock off to all ports by turning it halfway between any two ports.
10. Remove the blood-sample syringe, and cap off the syringe to seal it.
11. Roll the syringe to mix the heparin, and place it into an ice-water bath.
12. Turn the stopcock toward the catheter. Fast flush the IV solution so that any blood left in the sample port is forced out onto a sterile gauze pad.
13. Turn the stopcock toward the sample port so that the IV solution runs into the catheter.
14. Fast flush any blood in the catheter back into the patient.
15. Screw the dead-ender cap onto the sample port.
16. Remove gloves, and properly dispose of them and any other waste materials. Wash your hands.

4. Perform an arterial puncture to obtain a blood sample for analysis (WRE code: IB7e and IIIE2a) [Difficulty: An]

A number of possible variations on the technique exist. The following is a general but thorough listing of the steps and any important related information.

a. Check for a valid physician order.
b. Check the patient's chart for pertinent information on supplemental oxygen being used, bleeding disorders such as hemophilia, and use of anticoagulant medications. It is important to check the patient's clotting time because a hematoma will result in a patient with a slow clotting time if extra time is not spent holding the puncture site.
c. Collect necessary equipment:
   1. Ice water in a cup
   2. A 3-mL glass or plastic syringe
   3. Appropriate needle(s)
   4. Heparin, if needed
   5. 70% isopropyl alcohol or iodophor swabs to clean the puncture site and a sterile 4 × 4-inch gauze pad to hold over the puncture site to aid clotting
   6. A seal for the needle or syringe to prevent room air contamination
   7. Clean gloves to protect the practitioner's hands from any contact with spilled blood
   8. Eyeglasses or goggles
d. Introduce yourself and your department to the patient. Identify the patient. Explain what you are there to do. Gain the patient's confidence so that he or she will offer full cooperation.

e. Select the puncture site. The following choices are listed in order from most to least favorable: radial, brachial, dorsalis pedis, and femoral. If the radial site is selected, try to puncture the left wrist if the patient is right-handed or vice versa.
f. If the radial or pedal sites are selected, the modified Allen's test must be performed to ensure that ade-

Fig. 3-2 The modified Allen's test. **A,** The hand is clenched into a tight fist, and pressure is applied to the radial and ulnar arteries. **B,** The hand is opened (but not fully extended); the palm and fingers are blanched. **C,** Removal of the pressure on the ulnar artery should result in flushing of the entire hand. *(From Shapiro BA, Peruzzi WT, Templin R: Clinical application of blood gases, ed 5, St Louis, 1994, Mosby.)*

quate collateral flow is present in case the artery becomes clotted because of the procedure.

1. Radial artery site. See Fig. 3-2 for the basic procedure. Circulation to the hand is stopped by pressing both the radial and ulnar arteries closed. Releasing the pressure over the ulnar artery should result in the hand flushing within 10 to 15 seconds. This is a positive test result and proves that the ulnar artery has adequate circulation to the hand. If the hand does not flush within 15 seconds of the release of the ulnar artery, the circulation is inadequate, and the radial artery of that wrist must not be punctured. Another site must be evaluated for puncture.

2. Dorsalis pedis artery site. Press down on the dorsalis pedis artery to occlude it. Press on the nail of the great toe so that it blanches. Release the pressure on the nail, and watch for a rapid return of color. This normal test finding confirms that a good blood flow exists through the posterior tibial and lateral plantar arteries. It is safe to draw a sample from the site. A slow return of blood flow indicates poor circulation; another site must be chosen.

g. Prepare the equipment and the puncture site by using sterile technique.

1. If necessary, draw up the heparin solution, flush the syringe with it, and discard the excess.

2. If a radial or brachial site is selected, the joint should be hyperextended with a folded towel to help stabilize it.

3. Clean the site by wiping the area with an alcohol or iodophor swab in a widening spiral motion that starts at the desired puncture site.

4. Put on gloves and goggles.

5. Some prefer to anesthetize the puncture site with a 0.8- to 1.0-mL injection of 2% lidocaine (Xylocaine) into the skin. Others believe that this is unnecessary because the lidocaine injection, itself, will cause pain.

h. Draw the blood sample.

1. Hold the syringe like a pencil. The radial and dorsalis pedis arteries should be entered from a 45-degree angle; the brachial and femoral arteries should be entered from a 90-degree angle (Fig. 3-3). Use the first two fingers of your free hand to palpate the pulse and hold the artery still. The bevel of the needle should be up as it enters the skin.

2. Tell the patient that he or she will "feel a stick."

3. The needle should enter the skin quickly to minimize pain. Carefully advance the needle into the artery. A pulsatile flow is seen with each heartbeat. If unsuccessful, withdraw the needle to the skin, change the angle as needed, and reinsert into the artery.

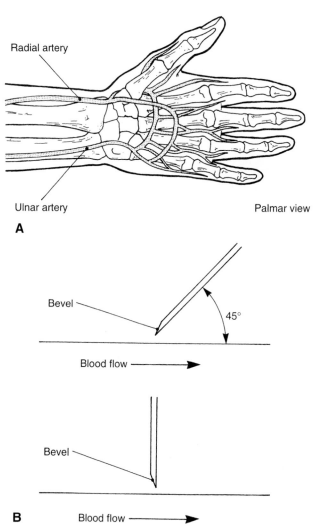

Fig. 3-3 A, Radial arterial position in the lower arm and wrist. **B,** Bevel and needle positioning for radial arterial puncture and other arterial punctures, respectively. *(From Lane EE, Walker JF: Clinical arterial blood gas analysis, St Louis, 1987, Mosby.)*

4. Withdraw about 1 to 2 mL of blood before removing the needle.

5. Press the sterile gauze onto the puncture site for 2 to 5 minutes. Check the site to ensure that clotting has occurred. Hold longer if necessary. An assistant may help with this.

6. While holding the site, seal the syringe or carefully cover the needle.

7. Roll the syringe to mix the heparin, and place the syringe into the ice water. (Failure to put the blood sample in ice water results in a decrease in the Pao_2 value, an increase in the $Paco_2$ value, and a decrease in the pH value.)

8. Label the syringe with the date, time, patient's name, oxygen percentage, and temperature if abnormal. Some departments may also add

the patient's age and the position in which he or she was sitting or lying when the sample was drawn because of the effects they may have on oxygenation.

9. Have the sample analyzed as soon as possible.
10. Properly dispose of gloves and waste materials, and wash your hands.

Exam Hint

Commonly tested areas involve the ABG technique and possible hazards to it. Patient hazards include blood vessel trauma, hematoma, arterial clot formation, arteriospasm, and infected puncture site. In addition, the therapist may receive an accidental needle puncture injury.

5. Perform arterialized capillary blood gas sampling (WRE code: IIIE2c) [Difficulty: R, Ap, An]

Occasionally, a sample of arterialized capillary blood from a patient must be obtained for blood gas analysis. The usual clinical situation is a neonate who has a pulmonary problem that warrants evaluation. However, because of the neonate's small arteries, a sample cannot be drawn. The steps and key points to keep in mind during the sampling procedure follow.

a. Select a highly vascularized and well-perfused site. Usually the heel is selected, but the great toe, earlobe, and finger also are acceptable.

b. Warm the heel (or other site) with a warm towel or heat lamp for about 5 to 10 minutes; 42 °C is ideal. Warming vasodilates the vessels and "arterializes" the capillary blood supply.

c. After warming, unwrap the site, and wipe it with an antiseptic pad.

d. Use a pediatric lance to deeply puncture the outer edge of the heel (Fig. 3-4). Blood should flow freely without squeezing the area. The blood will be "dearterialized" if it is squeezed out with venous blood, and the sample will be useless for blood gas analysis.

e. Insert a preheparinized capillary tube (0.075 to 1.0 mL) deeply into the drop of blood. The blood should easily flow through the tube, and ideally, a second sample tube is filled.

f. Seal both ends of the tubes.

g. Use a magnet to draw the metal filing (flea) back and forth in the tubes to mix the blood.

h. Place the sealed tubes immediately into an ice-water bath.

i. Send the samples to the laboratory for analysis along with the proper paperwork.

Fig. 3-4 Puncture sites on an infant's heel for obtaining an arterialized capillary blood sample. Avoid the posterior tibial artery that runs through the center of the foot. *(From Czervinske MP: Arterial blood gas analysis and other cardiopulmonary monitoring. In Koff PB, Eitzman D, Neu J, editors:* Neonatal and pediatric respiratory care, *ed 2, St Louis, 1993, Mosby.)*

j. Apply pressure to stop the bleeding. Complications include infection, bone spurs, and laceration of the posterior tibial artery.

MODULE C
Analyze blood gas values

1. Point-of-care blood gas analyzer
a. Select the appropriate point-of-care blood gas analyzer (CSE code: IIA10)

A point-of-care (POC) blood gas analyzer can be used as an alternative to a centrally located analyzer. This is especially helpful when a patient is being transported, or when the data are very quickly needed at the bedside. The blood gas values of PaO_2, $PaCO_2$, and pH are typically obtained from either a POC analyzer or a standard blood gas analyzer. These standard units are acceptable for all patient care situations *except* when carbon monoxide poisoning is known or suspected. Neither the POC or standard blood gas analyzer is able to measure carboxyhemoglobin (COHb). A CO-oximeter is needed to measure the patient's level of carboxyhemoglobin in carbon monoxide cases. Some POC analyzers also can measure serum electrolytes and other commonly needed patient values such as hemoglobin and hematocrit.

b. Put the equipment together and make sure that it works properly (CSE code: IIA10)

POC analyzers can be powered through a self-contained battery or by plugging the unit into a standard alternating current electrical outlet. The units have single-use disposable cartridges that include the electrodes and calibration reagents. The following discussion covers the basic principles of operation of the electrodes in POC and standard centrally located analyzers.

pH electrode. The modern pH electrode has existed since the mid-1950s and is usually referred to as the *Sanz electrode* after its principal inventor. The basic principle behind the pH analyzer is its ability to measure the voltage (potential for electrical flow) between two different solutions. This is based on the different hydrogen ion (H^+) concentrations between the solutions that reflect their relative pH values. The reference electrode is immersed in a solution with a pH of 6.840 that fills a glass or plastic chamber. The blood sample, of unknown pH, is placed in a separate measuring chamber called a *cuvette*. These two chambers are separated by a special glass membrane that contains metals and sodium ions (Na^+), thus making it pH sensitive. Both chambers are kept at a stable 37°C

temperature. See Fig. 3-5 for a graphic representation of the pH electrode. When blood or a QC material is introduced into the cuvette, the potential exists for hydrogen ions to replace the sodium ions in the pH-sensitive glass if the two pHs are different. The replacement is proportional to the difference in the two pHs.

PCO₂ electrode. The partial pressure of carbon dioxide (PCO_2) is measured in a modified pH electrode. This was first designed in the mid-1950s by Stowe and further perfected by Severinghaus. Accordingly, these units are now referred to as *Severinghaus,* or sometimes as *Stowe-Severinghaus electrodes.* In Fig. 3-6, the electrode is depicted in cross section. It has a reference half-cell and measuring half-cell that are enclosed within pH-sensitive glass and electrically connected by an electrolyte contact bridge. The blood sample is introduced into a cuvette heated to 37°C.

The principle of operation is based on the amount of CO_2 found in the blood sample that diffuses through the silicon elastic membrane. The CO_2 chemically combines with the bicarbonate solution to change the pH of the solution by the release of H^+. This H^+ change creates a voltage difference between the measuring and reference half-cells that is proportional to the amount of CO_2 found in the patient's blood sample.

Fig. 3-5 Key components of the pH electrode. **A,** A voltage develops across the pH-sensitive glass when a difference exists in the hydrogen ion concentration between the two solutions. **B,** Two separate half-cells are used for the measuring electrode and the reference electrode. **C,** The addition of a KCl contact bridge and voltmeter completes the electrical circuit and enables the pH of the patient's blood sample to be measured. *(From Shapiro BA, Harrison RA, Cane RD, et al: Clinical application of blood gases, ed 4, St Louis, 1989, Mosby.)*

Fig. 3-6 Schematic illustration of the modern P_{CO_2} electrode. (Note that the space between the silicon membrane and the nylon spacer is greatly enlarged for clarity.) *(From Shapiro BA, Harrison RA, Cane RD, et al: Clinical application of blood gases, ed 4, St Louis, 1989, Mosby.)*

Po_2 electrode. This unit is completely different from the others mentioned. It was developed in the late 1950s by Clark and thus is usually called a *Clark electrode.* It is also sometimes known as a *polarographic electrode* because of the basis of its operation. Fig. 3-7 is a drawing of key features of the unit. A phosphate-KCl buffer solution surrounds the silver anode. A thin membrane separates the blood-filled cuvette from direct contact with the electrode but allows oxygen molecules to diffuse slowly through to contact the platinum wire cathode. The whole unit is heated to 37°C. The term *polarographic* comes from the addition of about 0.7 volts to the cathode to make it slightly "polarized" or negative compared with the anode. This is needed to ensure that oxygen is rapidly chemically reduced (that it gains electrons) at the cathode. This creates an electrical current directly proportional to the number of reduced oxygen molecules.

It must be understood that the partial pressure of oxygen (Po_2) being measured is derived from oxygen that is dissolved in the plasma. It does not come from the hemoglobin found in the erythrocytes (red blood cells). The reported value for the saturation of oxygen in the hemoglobin (Sao_2) is calculated by using a mathematical table. Under normal conditions, the calculated Sao_2 value is the same as or close to the true Sao_2 value. Carbon monoxide (CO) poisoning is the only commonly seen clinical situation during which a calculated saturation can be incorrectly high. If carbon

Fig. 3-7 Schematic illustration of the Clark electrode for measuring Po_2. *(From Shapiro BA, Harrison RA, Cane RD, et al: Clinical application of blood gases, ed 4, St Louis, 1989, Mosby.)*

monoxide poisoning is suspected or known, the patient's blood sample should be analyzed on a CO-oximeter unit.

c. Perform quality control procedures for a blood gas analyzer (WRE code: IIC1) [Difficulty: An]

Quality control. QC refers to creating a measurement and documentation system to confirm the accuracy (precision) and reliability of all blood gas measurements. Accuracy or precision means that the measured physiologic values truly reflect the actual physiologic values. Reliability means that a high degree of confidence exists so that the measured values represent the patient's actual physiologic values. Both are critically important if the blood gas results are to be used to make correct clinical decisions.

Quality assurance. Quality assurance refers to the broader concern that the results of the blood gas measurement are not only accurate and reliable but also clinically useful. To help ensure this, the Clinical Laboratory Improvement Amendments of 1988 (CLIA 88) require that the department have written policies and procedures on items including record keeping, equipment maintenance, staff training, and the correction of errors.

Calibration. Calibration is the systematic standardization of the graduations of the blood gas analyzer against known values to ensure consistency. Proper calibration of the electrodes is essential to the accuracy of the blood gas values. Some general calibration steps are discussed later. The manufacturer's guidelines must be followed for the specific steps in calibration.

Quality control materials. A variety of QC materials are available to calibrate the electrodes for Po_2, Pco_2, and pH. Their uses vary. Each of the following materials has its advantages, disadvantages, and limitations. The manufacturer of a particular brand or model of blood gas analyzer may require that a specific type of material be used in its units.

Aqueous buffers are water based and are used to check pH and Pco_2 measurements; they cannot be used to check Po_2 measurements. Commercially prepared gases are used to check Po_2 and Pco_2 measurements; they cannot be used to check pH. The following CO_2 mixes may be used: 0, 5%, 10%, and 12%. The following O_2 mixes may be used: 0, 12%, 20%, 20.95% from room air, 21%, and 100%.

Tonometered liquids are exposed in the laboratory to known oxygen and carbon dioxide gas mixes until the liquids are saturated and have the same partial pressures as the gases. Three types of tonometered liquids are used. First, *human* or *animal serum* or *whole blood.* This is the most accurate method available and is used mainly to obtain Po_2 and Pco_2 levels. Although whole human blood cannot be used for pH, a bovine blood product can be used to obtain all three values. Second, *assayed liquids* are non–water-based liquids that are pretonometered by the manufacturer and are available in sealed glass vials. They can be used to obtain Po_2, Pco_2, and pH. These are very popular because of the advantages of speed and simplicity. Third, *oxygenated fluorocarbon-based emulsions* (perfluorinated compounds) can be used to obtain P_{O_2}, P_{CO_2}, and pH measurements. They are considered as accurate as whole blood without its associated risks.

Levey-Jennings charts. The Levey-Jennings charts (also known as *Shewhart/Levey-Jennings* or *Quality Control [QC] charts*) are used to record the results of each calibration procedure. They are similarly designed with time plotted on the horizontal scale and the analyte (P_{O_2}, P_{CO_2}, or pH) on the vertical scale. The vertical scale for each analyte has a central value for what is normally expected. On both sides of this normal value are standard deviation (SD) points, showing movement away from what is expected. When an analyte electrode is operating within the acceptable limits, it is said to be *in control*. In general, if an analyte is within 2 SDs of the normal value, it is considered to be in control.

An *out-of-control* situation exists whenever a single calibration value or a series of calibration values is outside established limits. A *random error* is an unpredictable aberration in precision that occurs when the QC material is sampled. A *systematic error* shows an accuracy problem and is much more serious. It must be investigated, corrected, and documented. Fig. 3-8 shows an example of both random error and systematic error. Rules have been established for determining whether the error is random or systematic (Table 3-1).

pH electrode. NOTE: These and the following guidelines are based on CLIA standards or widely reported industry standards. The various brands and models of blood gas analyzers may have different frequencies of cali-

TABLE 3-1	Westgard's Rules for Determining When an Analyzer Is Not Functioning Properly
Rule name	**Levey-Jennings chart**
RANDOM ERROR	
1-2 SDs	The measurement is more than 2 SDs but not more than 3 SDs from the mean
1-3 SDs	The measurement is more than 3 SDs from the mean
R*-4 SDs	Two consecutive measurements are 4 SDs or more apart
SYSTEMATIC ERROR	
2-2 SDs	Two consecutive measurements are either 2 SDs above or 2 SDs below the mean
4-1 SDs	Four consecutive measurements are either 1 SD above or 1 SD below the mean
7-trend	Seven consecutive measurements are on only one side of the mean; each measurement is progressively more out of control
10-mean	Ten consecutive measurements are on only one side of the mean

*, Repeat; SDs, standard deviations.
Modified from Lane EE, Walker JF: *Clinical arterial blood gas analysis,* St Louis, 1987, Mosby.

bration requirements, depending on their Food and Drug Administration (FDA)-approved manufacturers' studies.

a. One-point calibration
   1. Should be done before every sample is analyzed if one-point calibration is not automatically performed every 30 minutes

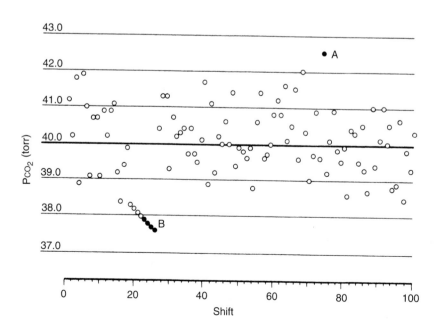

Fig. 3-8 Levey-Jennings quality control chart for Pa_{CO_2}. *Central horizontal line,* Mean value of 40 torr. *Next lower and higher horizontal lines,* One standard deviation (SD) value from the mean. *Second-most-distant lower and higher horizontal lines,* 2 SD values from the mean. *Most distant horizontal lines,* 3 SD values from the mean. *Bottom number scale,* 8-hour work shifts. *Open circles,* Calibration values that are within 2 SDs of the mean value. They are considered to be in control. *Black circles,* Calibration values that are out of control. *A,* A random error; *B,* A systematic error. *(From Shapiro BA, Peruzzi WT, Templin R:* Clinical application of blood gases, *ed 5, St Louis, 1994, Mosby.)*

2. Performed with the near-normal QC material of 7.384 ± 0.005 pH used to set the balance potentiometer
3. Recommended every 30 minutes
4. Should be rechecked after a suspious pH result; the blood sample should then be rerun

b. Two-point calibration
1. Should be done at least once every 8 hours when patient samples are being analyzed
2. Recommended for every 25 patient samples
3. Performed with the slope potentiometer set with a QC material of 6.840 ± 0.005 pH (this is the same pH as the reference electrode solution)
4. Performed with the balance potentiometer set with a QC material of 7.384 ± 0.005 pH

c. Three-point calibration
1. Should be done at least every 6 months on existing equipment
2. Should be done whenever a new electrode is put into use
3. Covers the physiologic range to confirm linearity: QC materials of 6.840 ± 0.005, 7.384 ± 0.005, and 7.874 ± 0.005 pH are used

P_{CO_2} electrode

a. One-point calibration
1. Should be done before every sample is analyzed if one-point calibration is not automatically performed every 30 minutes
2. Performed with 5% ± 0.03% CO_2 used to set the balance potentiometer
3. Recommended every 30 minutes
4. Should be rechecked after a suspicious P_{CO_2} result; the blood sample should then be rerun

The CO_2 can be directly in contact with the electrode, tonometered with an aqueous material or blood, or premixed in aqueous buffers, assayed liquids, or fluorocarbon-based emulsion.

b. Two-point calibration
1. Should be done at least once every 8 hours when patient samples are being analyzed
2. Recommended for every 25 patient samples
3. Performed with 10% ± 0.03% CO_2 to set the slope potentiometer
4. Performed with 5% ± 0.03% CO_2 to set the balance potentiometer

c. Three-point calibration
1. Should be done at least every 6 months on existing equipment
2. Should be done whenever a new electrode is put into use
3. Covers the physiologic range to confirm linearity; three P_{CO_2} values between 0 and 80 mm Hg should be determined
4. Room air or a gas cylinder containing 0 to 0.03% CO_2 can be used to set the 0 point

Exam Hint

Past examinations have required that the following equation be solved. Remember that more than one carbon dioxide percentage can be used. NOTE: The atmospheric pressure of a gas (oxygen, carbon dioxide, etc.) may be listed by the equivalent terms of *torr* or *mm Hg*. For example, a P_{CO_2} of 40 torr is the same as a P_{CO_2} 40 mm Hg. However, it is important to note that on the NBRC exams, the term *torr* is used for gas pressure.

The predicted P_{CO_2} value at a given CO_2 percentage is calculated with this formula:

$$P_{CO_2} = (P_B - P_{H_2O}) \times \% \, CO_2$$

In which P_{CO_2} is the predicted P_{CO_2} in mm Hg or torr; P_B is the barometric pressure at the institution where the analysis is being performed; P_{H_2O} is the water vapor pressure based on the patient's temperature, 47 torr at 37°C/98.6°F; and % CO_2 is the percentage of CO_2 (also listed as F CO_2).

Example for one-point (balance) potentiometer calibration at sea level in which P_{CO_2} is the predicted P_{CO_2} in torr, P_B is 760 torr, P_{H_2O} is 47 torr, and % CO_2 is 5%.

1. $P_{CO_2} = (760 - 47) \times 0.05$
2. $= (713) \times 0.05$
3. $= 35.65$ or 36 torr

Therefore set the P_{CO_2} control at 36 torr.

P_{O_2} electrode

a. One-point calibration
1. Should be done before every sample is analyzed if one-point calibration is not automatically performed every 30 minutes
2. Performed with 12% ± 0.03% O_2 used to set the balance potentiometer; some analyzers are designed to use 20% ± 0.03% O_2 from a gas cylinder or draw room air (20.95% oxygen) into the unit
3. Recommended every 30 minutes
4. Should be rechecked after a suspicious P_{O_2} result; the blood sample should then be rerun

The O_2 can be directly in contact with the electrode, tonometered with an aqueous material or blood, or premixed in aqueous buffers, assayed liquids, or fluorocarbon-based emulsion as discussed.

b. Two-point calibration
1. Should be done at least once every 8 hours when patient samples are being analyzed

2. Should be done whenever readjustment of one-point calibration is greater than 3 torr
3. Recommended for every 25 patient samples
4. Performed with $0 \pm 0.03\% \, O_2$ to set the slope potentiometer
5. Performed with $12\% \pm 0.03\% \, O_2$ to set the balance potentiometer; some analyzers are designed to use $20\% \pm 0.03\% \, O_2$ from a gas cylinder or draw room air (20.95% oxygen) into the unit
c. Three-point calibration
   1. Should be done at least every 6 months on existing equipment
   2. Should be done whenever a new electrode is put into use
   3. Should be done to confirm linearity whenever the P_{O_2} value could be more than 150 torr, assuming that the balance point is set on room oxygen content; the third point should be set on $100\% \pm 0.03\% \, O_2$ from a gas cylinder

Miscellaneous topics

Calibration gas cylinders. For economic reasons, the low-percentage oxygen and carbon dioxide gases are placed together in one cylinder, and the high-percentage oxygen and carbon dioxide gases are placed together in a second cylinder. Box 3-1 summarizes the normal precision of the electrodes discussed and the gases used in their calibration. A cylinder containing 100% oxygen and no carbon dioxide can be used for three-point calibration.

Temperature correction. Temperature correction refers to mathematical adjustment of a patient's P_aO_2, P_aCO_2, and pH values if his or her temperature is not $37°C$. Remember that blood gas analyzers are calibrated at $37°C$ because it is normal body temperature. If the patient has a fever, the oxygen and carbon dioxide partial pressures in the blood will be greater than those found during the blood gas analysis. Conversely, the hypothermic patient will have lower oxygen and carbon dioxide partial pressures in the blood than those found during the blood gas analysis. The pH value will shift in the opposite direction from the P_{CO_2} value. Usually this small shift in values is ignored. However, because some physicians may specify that their patient's blood gases be temperature corrected, the patient's temperature should be listed on the blood gas slip. It is a simple mathematical process to temperature correct the blood gas results. Most modern analyzers perform temperature correction automatically when programmed to do so.

d. Troubleshoot any problems with the point-of-care blood gas analyzer (CSE code: IIA10)

Remember to flush the electrode membrane after each use, if possible, to prevent protein buildup. If protein buildup occurs, the response time is longer than normal. Follow the manufacturer's guidelines to change an electrode membrane as needed. Make sure that no air bubbles are

---

BOX 3-1 Electrode Precision and Calibration Gases

ELECTRODES
pH ± 0.01 unit
P_{CO_2} $\pm 2\%$ (approximately ± 1 mm Hg at 40 torr)
P_{O_2} $\pm 3\%$ (approximately ± 2.5 mm Hg at 80 torr)
If the P_{O_2} is >150 torr, the precision is approximately $\pm 10\%$ unless three-point calibration is performed

CALIBRATION GASES
"Low" gas: $0 \, O_2$ ($+0.03\%$), $5\% \, CO_2$ ($\pm 0.03\%$), balance N_2
"High" gas: 12% or $21\% \, O_2$, $10\% \, CO_2$ (both $\pm 0.03\%$), balance N_2
Suggested three-point gases: $100\% \, O_2$ (-0.03%), $0\% \, CO_2$ ($+0.03\%$)

N_2, Nitrogen; P_{CO_2}, pressure of carbon dioxide; P_{O_2}, pressure of oxygen.

under the membrane or within the tubing through which the blood travels. Rerun the calibration for any of the electrodes and reanalyze the sample if you are suspicious of the result. If the electrode does not calibrate close to the reference buffer solutions or gases, it should not be used.

In a random-error situation, the practitioner likely made a simple error when introducing the material or running the analyzer. Common problems include an air bubble injected into the unit or incomplete flushing of the previous sample. Usually flushing out any residual blood and then carefully injecting more of the current patient blood samples will correct the problem. Run the analyzer again to obtain new patient values or run the same patient sample through another analyzer and compare the two sets of results.

A systematic error usually indicates a problem with the analyzer, QC materials, or processes. Examples of systematic errors include misanalyzed CO_2 or O_2 standards for calibration; contaminated QC materials; or deteriorated oxygen, carbon dioxide, or pH electrode function. Each of these must be investigated until the problem is found and corrected. The unit cannot be used again until after it is proven to work properly and to give accurate results.

e. Perform blood gas analysis (WRE code: IB7f and IIIE3b) [Difficulty: An]

Modern blood gas analyzers are simple to operate. Follow the manufacturer's guidelines for insertion of the blood sample. Perform the specified steps in analysis. Print out the results. Many current units run a self-diagnosis if any problems appear.

2. CO-oximeter

a. Perform quality control procedures on the CO-oximeter (WRE code: IIC1) [Difficulty: An]

The unit is preassembled by the manufacturer. Practical experience with a unit is recommended to understand how to add a patient blood sample and perform calibration duties. (See Fig. 3-9 for a schematic drawing of a CO-oximeter.) A thallium-neon hollow cathode lamp emits light in the infrared-visible range. A device called a monochromator contains four filters and rotates through the light beam. Each filter allows only one specific wavelength to pass through it. These four monochromatic wavelengths correspond to the three isosbestic points, discussed later (shown in Fig. 3-10) and 626.6 nm. This last wavelength is poorly absorbed by all four hemoglobin moieties. It is used to find the maximal difference in absorption so that the relative amounts of the hemoglobin species can be determined.

When a blood sample is placed into the cuvette, the same four wavelengths are passed through it. The amount of absorbance at each wavelength is measured and compared with the absorbance at each wavelength by a reference

Fig. 3-9 CO-oximeter basic components. **A,** Thallium-neon hollow cathode light source. **B,** Lens and mirror. **C,** Monochromator with four specific wavelength filters. **D,** Light-beam splitter that diverts half of the light to the reference detector and half to the cuvette. **E,** Reference wavelength detector. **F,** Patient sample cuvette. **G,** Sample wavelength detector. **H,** Temperature-regulated block set at 37°C. *(From Shapiro BA, Peruzzi WT, Templin R: Clinical application of blood gases, ed 5, St Louis, 1994, Mosby.)*

Fig. 3-10 Spectral analysis of the hemoglobin moieties (species). O_2Hb is oxyhemoglobin, COHb is carboxyhemoglobin, RHb is reduced hemoglobin, and MetHb (METHb) is methemoglobin. Point *A* shows the triple isosbestic point at 548 nm for O_2Hb, COHb, and RHb. Point *B* shows the double isosbestic point at 568 nm for O_2Hb and RHb. Point *C* shows the double isosbestic point at 578 nm for RHb and COHb. A fourth wavelength at 626.6 nm is used for comparison purposes. *(From Shapiro BA, Peruzzi WT, Templin R: Clinical application of blood gases, ed 4, St Louis, 1994, Mosby.)*

sample solution (see the following discussion). The computer integrates the data and calculates the total hemoglobin and amounts of the four hemoglobin moieties.

Total hemoglobin (THb) should be calibrated when the unit is installed, at regular intervals suggested by the manufacturer, after the sample tubing is changed, after the cuvette is disassembled or changed, and whenever a suspicious reading is seen. Calibration is done by filling the cuvette with a special dye produced by the manufacturer and analyzing it by following the prescribed steps.

Routine calibration is done every 30 minutes. The unit obtains and stores absorbance readings at the four different wavelengths from a "blank" solution in the reference detector. When the same blank solution is added to the sample cuvette, the same four wavelengths are measured. Their absorption levels are normally identical. The same procedure is performed after every patient sample is analyzed.

The following are examples of common problems and their solutions:

1. Incomplete hemolysis of the blood sample causes the light to scatter off cell fragments and lipids. Sickle cells (as in sickle cell anemia) are difficult to disrupt and may cause false oxyhemoglobin and carboxyhemoglobin readings if extra time is not taken for hemolysis. Follow manufacturer's guidelines on the procedure for hemolyzing the red blood cells.

2. More than 10% methemoglobin may cause errors in the measurement of all hemoglobin moieties. Sulfhemoglobin also causes false readings. The practitioner may need to gather additional information from the chart or laboratory regarding the patient's levels of these abnormal hemoglobin moieties. CO-oximetry should probably not be performed on blood samples with abnormal levels of methemoglobin or sulfhemoglobin.

3. Intravenous dyes such as methylene blue, Evans blue, and indocyanine green used in various cardiac studies can absorb the same wavelengths of light used to identify the various forms of hemoglobin. The presence of these dyes results in a lower measurement of oxyhemoglobin than is actually present. Check the patient's chart for a record of dyes used. CO-oximetry should probably not be used for blood gas analysis on patients who have these dyes in their systems.

4. Failure to reprogram the analyzer for fetal hemoglobin instead of adult hemoglobin may produce false results. Remember to check the chart for the patient's age. Reprogram the analyzer for fetal hemoglobin for any sample taken from an infant who is only a few weeks old.

5. The presence of lipid particles in the blood causes light scattering and results in a reading that is falsely high in total hemoglobin and percentage of methemoglobin and falsely low in percentage of oxyhemoglobin and percentage of carboxyhemoglobin. Follow the laboratory's guidelines to determine when a patient's blood lipid value is too high for accurate use of the CO-oximeter.

6. Air bubbles or incomplete hemolysis of blood in the cuvette causes an absorbance error. Air bubbles must be flushed out and the blood sample inserted again and reanalyzed. Make sure that all blood samples are hemolyzed according to the manufacturer's guidelines.

7. Blood clots in the sample tubing prevent blood from flowing through to the cuvette. If a sample cannot be inserted into the unit, suspect and check for a blood clot. Remove any clotted tubing, replace it, and confirm that the CO-oximeter is working properly.

b. Perform CO-oximetry/hemoximetry (WRE code: IB7f and IIIE3b) [Difficulty: An]

Most hospitals have a CO-oximeter in addition to a blood gas analyzer. A CO-oximeter should be used to analyze a blood gas sample whenever carbon monoxide poisoning is known or suspected. In addition, a CO-oximeter gives a complete analysis of the relative amounts of the different types of patient hemoglobin.

CO-oximeters also are called *spectrophotometric* oximeters and are the most accurate method available to measure the four different hemoglobin moieties (species or variations in the hemoglobin molecule). These hemoglobin species include the following:

1. Oxyhemoglobin (HbO_2 or O_2Hb), which carries oxygen to the tissues, and reduced hemoglobin (HbR or RHb), which has given up its oxygen and picked up carbon dioxide

2. Carboxyhemoglobin (HbCO or COHb), which is nonfunctional because of the tightness with which carbon monoxide binds to the hemoglobin

3. Methemoglobin (HbMet or MetHb), which is nonfunctional because the Hb molecule is unable to combine reversibly with oxygen

4. Sulfhemoglobin (HbS or SHb), which is similar to the HbMet and is also nonfunctional. In addition, a CO-oximeter can measure the fetal hemoglobin (HbF or FHb) found in a newborn infant instead of adult oxyhemoglobin

Each of these hemoglobin moieties has a unique spectroscopic "fingerprint" of absorbed light-wave frequencies. See Fig. 3-10 for the spectral analysis of the various forms of hemoglobin.

Follow the manufacturer's guidelines on rewarming the blood sample to body temperature, hemolyzing the sample, and inserting it into the measurement cuvette. Failure to do so may result in incorrect patient values.

The principle of operation of a CO-oximeter is the comparison of the relative absorbances of four wavelengths of light by oxyhemoglobin, reduced hemoglobin, and carboxyhemoglobin. This is done by comparing the absorptions at the three isosbestic points (at which the moieties being compared have equal absorption) and a wavelength point at which the greatest difference in absorption between the two moieties is found. By computer integration of the data, the relative proportions of oxyhemoglobin, reduced hemoglobin, and carboxyhemoglobin are determined. If the total is less than 100% of the hemoglobin present, the difference has to be methemoglobin (or, rarely, sulfhemoglobin). The unit then provides data on total hemoglobin; percentages for oxyhemoglobin, reduced hemoglobin, carboxyhemoglobin, and methemoglobin; and total amounts for them in grams per deciliter of blood. Some units also calculate O_2 content.

> ### Exam Hint
>
> **I**f a patient is known to have or suspected of having carbon monoxide poisoning (removed from inside a burning building), a CO-oximeter should be used for blood gas analysis. A standard or POC blood gas analyzer or pulse oximeter should not be used. These instruments cannot detect or measure carboxyhemoglobin.

MODULE D

Interpret blood gas analysis results to determine how the patient is responding to respiratory care

1. Review the chart for any blood gas results (WRE code: IA5) [Difficulty: Ap, An]

Look in the chart for any blood gas results, including arterial, capillary, or mixed venous. Any patient may have had an arterial sample analyzed. A neonate also may have had an arterialized capillary sample analyzed. A patient with a pulmonary artery catheter may have had a mixed venous sample analyzed.

2. Interpret the results of arterial blood gas analysis (WRE code: IB8e and IIIE4) [Difficulty: An]

A number of authors have written extensively on how to interpret ABGs. The system proposed by Shapiro and associates (1994) has been found to be both practical and relatively easy to understand. Most of the following discussion and tables are based on this system. This does not mean that if one has learned another system, he or she is at any disadvantage for taking the National Board of Respiratory Care (NBRC) examination.

> ### Exam Hint
>
> **T**he Written Registry Examination includes specific questions about ABG interpretation. The exam also incorporates blood gas results into other questions that relate to any respiratory care technique or procedure, such as oxygen therapy with a chronic obstructive pulmonary disease (COPD) patient and adjustment of mechanical ventilation. In addition, often a question requires the interpretation of mixed venous blood gases or arterialized capillary blood gases. The examinee must be proficient in all aspects of blood gas interpretation to do well on the advanced NBRC examinations.

Assessment of oxygenation. Hypoxemia or hypoxia can rapidly become life threatening. Table 3-2 shows the normal Pa_{O_2} values for the newborn, child to adult, and the elderly when room air (almost 21% oxygen) is inhaled at sea level. These values decrease progressively as altitude increases. However, under most clinical conditions, this is not a factor unless working in a high-altitude setting.

A general rule is that any patient is seriously hypoxemic if the Pa_{O_2} is less than 60 torr on room air. See Table 3-3 for guidelines on judging the seriousness of hypoxemia. Once hypoxemia is recognized, it must be corrected. The most obvious way to correct hypoxemia is to give supplemental oxygen. The clinician must realize that oxygen alone will not correct the hypoxemia if the patient is hypoventilating (increased Pa_{CO_2}), has heart failure, or

TABLE 3-2	Age-Based Acceptable Levels of Partial Pressure of Oxygen in Arterial Blood (Pa_{O_2}) When Breathing Room Air (21% Oxygen) at Sea Level
Age	**Pa_{O_2}**
NEWBORN	
Acceptable range	40 to 70 torr
CHILD TO ADULT	
Normal	97 torr
Acceptable range	>80 torr
Hypoxemia	<80 torr
OLDER ADULT	
60-year-old	>80 torr
70-year-old	>70 torr
80-year-old	>60 torr
90-year-old	>50 torr

Modified from Shapiro BA, Peruzzi WT, Kozelowski-Templin R: *Clinical application of blood gases,* ed 5, Chicago, 1994, Mosby-Year Book.

TABLE 3-3 Evaluation of Hypoxemia

CONDITIONS: ROOM AIR IS INSPIRED; THE PATIENT IS YOUNGER THAN 60 YEARS[*]

Hypoxemia	Pao_2	Sao_2
Mild	60–79 torr	90%–94%
Moderate	40–59 torr	75%–89%
Severe	<40 torr	<75%

CONDITIONS: SUPPLEMENTAL O_2 IS INSPIRED; THE PATIENT IS YOUNGER THAN 60 YEARS

Hypoxemia	Pao_2
Uncorrected	Less than room air acceptable limit
Corrected	Within room air acceptable limit (<100 torr)
Excessively corrected	>100 torr

[*]Subtract 1 torr of O_2 from limits of mild and moderate hypoxemia for each year older than 60. A Pao_2 of < 40 torr indicates severe hypoxemia in any patient at any age.

Modified from Shapiro BA, Peruzzi WT, Kozelowski-Templin R: *Clinical application of blood gases*, ed 5, Chicago, 1994, Mosby-Year Book.

is unable to carry or make use of the oxygen. In general, try to keep the patient's Pao_2 between 60 and 100 torr.

Shapiro and associates (1994) suggested the following formula, in which Fio_2 is the fraction of inspired oxygen, for determining whether the patient will be hypoxemic on room air: "If Pao_2 is less than $Fio_2 \times 5$, the patient can be assumed to be hypoxemic on room air."

Fig. 3-11 shows a normal oxyhemoglobin dissociation curve. The saturation value is important to know because it shows how much hemoglobin is saturated with oxygen. Several important points of correlation exist between the Sao_2 and the Pao_2. (Calculated saturation values can be misleadingly high if the patient has inhaled carbon monoxide. In this situation, it is best to measure the saturation directly on a CO-oximeter–type blood gas analyzer.)

Fig. 3-12 shows a number of factors that can influence the oxyhemoglobin dissociation curve and how oxygen loads onto and unloads from hemoglobin. In a patient with normal oxygenation, these factors are not clinically significant. However, when the Pao_2 is less than 60 torr and the Sao_2 is less than 90%, these factors can become an important consideration. As can be seen, a left-shifted oxyhemoglobin dissociation curve results in a lower Pao_2 at any given saturation. This results in even less oxygen being delivered to the tissues.

Exam Hint

True shunt or venous admixture leading to ventilation/perfusion mismatching are the two most common clinical findings leading to hypoxemia.

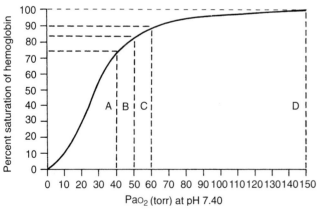

Fig. 3-11 The oxygen (oxyhemoglobin) dissociation curve plots the relation between hemoglobin saturation (y-axis) and plasma Pao_2 (x-axis). *A*, 75% saturation and a Pao_2 of 40 torr are normally seen in venous blood. *B*, 85% saturation and a Pao_2 of 50 torr are the minimal levels that should be allowed in a chronically hypoxemic patient. *C*, 90% saturation and Pao_2 of 60 torr are the minimal levels that should be allowed in an acutely hypoxemic patient. *D*, Hemoglobin in the pulmonary capillaries adjacent to normal alveoli will become 100% saturated when the Pao_2 reaches 150 torr. *(Modified from Lane EE, Walker JF: Clinical arterial blood gas analysis, St Louis, 1987, Mosby.)*

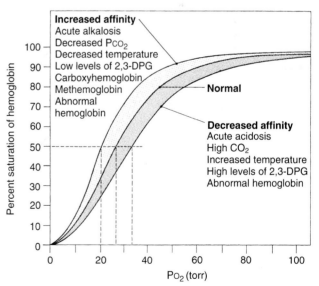

Fig. 3-12 Conditions associated with altered affinity of hemoglobin for O_2. P_{50} is the Pao_2 at which hemoglobin is 50% saturated, normally 26.6 torr. A lower than normal P_{50} represents increased affinity of hemoglobin for O_2; a high P_{50} is seen with decreased affinity. Note that variation from the normal is associated with decreased (low P_{50}) or increased (high P_{50}) availability of O_2 to tissues (*dashed lines*). *Shaded area*, The entire oxyhemoglobin dissociation curve under the same circumstances. *(From Lane EE, Walker JF: Clinical arterial blood gas analysis, St Louis, 1987, Mosby.)*

Assessment of carbon dioxide and pH. The pH is the next important value to interpret because extreme acidemia/acidosis and alkalemia/alkalosis can be life threatening. The carbon dioxide value is important to interpret because it has a direct effect on the pH and indirectly affects the oxygen level. A high or low $PaCO_2$ level, by itself, is not life threatening.

Table 3-4 shows normal values for pH and $PaCO_2$ and the acceptable ranges around the mean or average. Table 3-5 shows the most widely acceptable therapeutic ranges for pH and $PaCO_2$. Values that fall outside of these ranges present a progressively greater risk to the patient.

Table 3-6 shows the definitions of Shapiro and associates for alkalemia and acidemia from a respiratory cause. An acute change in the patient's ventilation causes the following when starting from a $PaCO_2$ of 40 torr:

a. If the $PaCO_2$ increases by 20 torr, the pH decreases by 0.10 units.

b. If the $PaCO_2$ decreases by 10 torr, the pH increases by 0.10 units.

Thus the body can be seen as better able to compensate with metabolic buffers for a respiratory acidosis than a respiratory alkalosis.

Metabolic effects are evaluated by interpreting either the bicarbonate (HCO_3^-) value or base excess/base deficit (BE/BD) value. Both reveal whether any metabolic effect on the pH exists. Normal values are as follows:

a. HCO_3^-: 24 mEq/L

b. BE/BD: 0 mEq/L; ± 1 mEq/L is often listed as the normal range

Values indicating metabolic alkalosis of a primary or secondary nature are as follows:

a. Bicarbonate greater than 24 mEq/L

b. BE greater than 0 or greater than +1 mEq/L

Values indicating metabolic acidosis of a primary or secondary nature are as follows:

a. Bicarbonate less than 24 mEq/L

b. BE less than 0 or greater than −1 mEq/L (i.e., −5mEq/L); some laboratories report this as a BD or negative BE.

Exam Hint

The NBRC uses BE for base excess (regardless of whether it has a positive or negative value) and HCO_3^- for bicarbonate.

Tables 3-7 to 3-9 show definitions of terms and classifications of the various acid-base states. As stated earlier, there are other systems for interpreting blood gases. All are probably satisfactory for interpretation purposes and preparing for the NBRC examinations.

3. Interpret the results of CO-oximetry blood gas analysis (WRE code: IB8e and IIIE4) [Difficulty: An]

The CO-oximeter type blood gas analyzer gives values for oxyhemoglobin (O_2Hb), reduced hemoglobin (RHb), carboxyhemoglobin (COHb), and methemoglobin (MetHb)/sulfhemoglobin (SHb). Each of these hemoglobin moieties can be displayed in terms of grams per deciliter, percentage of the whole, and added together for a total hemoglobin (THb). Table 3-10 shows normal adult hemoglobin values. The amount of carboxyhemoglobin and methemoglobin should be subtracted from the total hemoglobin to find the amount of functional hemoglobin. Any increase in the COHb or MetHb levels above those listed is abnormal and results in even less normal hemoglobin to carry oxygen. The patient with carbon monoxide poisoning is at greatest risk. A COHb level of 30% saturation or greater can be fatal. By subtraction, the O_2Hb (SaO_2) level can be no greater than 70% with a resulting PaO_2 of less than 40 torr.

TABLE 3-4	Normal Laboratory Ranges for Partial Pressure of Carbon Dioxide in Arterial Blood ($PaCO_2$) and pH		
	Mean	**1 SD**	**2 SD**
$PaCO_2$	40.00	38–42 torr	35–45 torr
pH	7.40	7.38–7.42	7.35–7.45

SD, Standard deviation.
Modified from Shapiro BA, Peruzzi WT, Kozelowski-Templin R: *Clinical application of blood gases,* ed 5, Chicago, 1994, Mosby-Year Book.

TABLE 3-5	Acceptable Clinical Ranges for Partial Pressure of Carbon Dioxide in Arterial Blood ($PaCO_2$) and pH
$PaCO_2$	30–50 torr*
pH	7.30–7.50

*This is the range for patients with an acute change. It does not apply to patients with long-standing disease, such as chronic obstructive pulmonary disease. These patients may have $PaCO_2$ values greater than 50 torr.
Modified from Shapiro BA, Peruzzi WT, Kozelowski-Templin R: *Clinical application of blood gases,* ed 5, Chicago, 1994, Mosby-Year Book.

TABLE 3-6	Naming Unacceptable Values for Partial Pressure of CO_2 in Arterial Blood ($PaCO_2$) and pH
$PaCO_2$ > 45 torr	Respiratory acidosis/alveolar hypoventilation/ventilatory failure
pH < 7.35	Acidemia
$PaCO_2$ < 35 torr	Respiratory alkalosis/alveolar hyperventilation
pH > 7.45	Alkalemia

Modified from Shapiro BA, Peruzzi WT, Kozelowski-Templin R: *Clinical application of blood gases,* ed 5, Chicago, 1994, Mosby-Year Book.

TABLE 3-7	Clinical Terminology for Arterial Blood Gas Measurements
Clinical Terminology	**Clinical Findings**
Respiratory acidosis/ alveolar hypoventilation/ ventilatory failure	Pa_{CO_2} > 45 torr
Acute ventilatory failure	Pa_{CO_2} > 45 torr; pH < 7.35
Chronic ventilatory failure	Pa_{CO_2} > 45 torr; pH 7.36–7.40
Respiratory alkalosis/ alveolar hyperventilation	Pa_{CO_2} < 35 torr
Acute alveolar hyperventilation	Pa_{CO_2} < 35 torr; pH > 7.45
Chronic alveolar hyperventilation	Pa_{CO_2} < 35 torr; pH 7.41–7.45
Acidemia	pH < 7.35
Acidosis	Pathophysiologic condition in which the patient has a significant base deficit (plasma bicarbonate below normal)
Alkalemia	pH > 7.45
Alkalosis	Pathophysiologic condition in which the patient has a significant base excess (plasma bicarbonate above normal)

Modified from Shapiro BA, Peruzzi WT, Kozelowski-Templin R: *Clinical application of blood gases,* ed 5, Chicago, 1994, Mosby-Year Book.

TABLE 3-8	Evaluation of Ventilatory and Metabolic Effects on Acid-Base Status

EVALUATION OF Pa_{CO_2}

Pa_{CO_2} > 45 torr	Respiratory acidosis/alveolar hypoventilation/ventilatory failure
Pa_{CO_2} 35–45 torr	Acceptable alveolar ventilation
Pa_{CO_2} < 35 torr	Respiratory alkalosis/alveolar hyperventilation

EVALUATION OF Pa_{CO_2} IN CONJUNCTION WITH pH

Acceptable Alveolar Ventilation (Pa_{CO_2} from 35 to 45 torr)

pH > 7.50	Metabolic alkalosis
pH 7.30–7.50	Acceptable ventilatory and metabolic pH
pH < 7.30	Metabolic acidosis

Alveolar Hypoventilation (Pa_{CO_2} > 45 torr)

pH > 7.50	*Partially compensated* metabolic alkalosis
pH 7.30–7.50	*Chronic* ventilatory failure
pH < 7.30	*Acute* ventilatory failure

Alveolar Hyperventilation (Pa_{CO_2} < 35 torr)

pH > 7.50	*Acute* alveolar hyperventilation
pH 7.40–7.50	*Chronic* alveolar hyperventilation
pH 7.30–7.40	*Compensated* metabolic acidosis
pH < 7.30	*Partially compensated* metabolic acidosis

Pa_{CO_2}, partial pressure of CO_2 in arterial blood.
Some authors use a narrower pH range for these classifications.
Modified from Shapiro BA, Peruzzi WT, Kozelowski-Templin R: *Clinical application of blood gases,* ed 5, Chicago, 1994, Mosby-Year Book.

TABLE 3-9	Primary Blood Gas Classification			
	O_2	pH	Bicarbonate	BE
VENTILATORY IMBALANCE				
Acute alveolar hypoventilation	I	D	N	N
Chronic alveolar hypoventilation	I	N	I	I
Acute alveolar hyperventilation	D	I	N	N
Chronic alveolar hyperventilation	D	N	D	D
METABOLIC IMBALANCE				
Uncompensated acidosis	N	D	D	D
Partially compensated acidosis	D	D	D	D
Uncompensated alkalosis	N	I	I	I
Partially compensated alkalosis	I	I	I	I
Compensated acidosis or alkalosis	I or D	N	I or D	I or D

D, Decreased; I, increased; N, normal range; BE, base excess; Pa_{CO_2}, partial pressure of CO_2 in arterial blood.
Modified from Shapiro BA, Peruzzi WT, Kozelowski-Templin R: *Clinical application of blood gases,* ed 5, Chicago, 1994, Mosby-Year Book.

TABLE 3-10	Normal Hemoglobin Values for Adults
Total hemoglobin (THb)	Men: 13.5–18.0 g/dL Women: 12.0–16.0 g/dL 15.0 g/dL is often listed as an average for both
Oxyhemoglobin	94%–100% of THb (reported as Sa_{O_2} of 94% to 100%
Carboxyhemoglobin	Nonsmokers: <1.5% (0.225 g/dL) of THb Smokers: 1.5%–10% of THb
Methemoglobin	0.5%–3% (0.075–0.45 g/dL) of THb
Oxygen content (arterial sample)	15–23 g/dL

g/dL, Grams per deciliter (sometimes listed as g/100 mL); Sa_{O_2}, O_2 saturation in arterial blood.

EXAMPLE 1

The following example shows how to calculate the amount of functional hemoglobin and saturation for a patient with normal COHb and MetHb levels:

$$
\begin{array}{r}
15.0 \text{ g total Hb} \\
-0.225 \text{ g COHb} \\
\hline
14.775 \text{ g} \\
-0.15 \text{ g MetHb} \\
\hline
14.625 \text{ g functional Hb}
\end{array}
$$

$$\begin{array}{l} \text{100\% potential saturation of O}_2\text{Hb in arterial blood} \\ \underline{-1.5\% \text{ saturation of COHb}} \\ 98.5\% \\ \underline{-1.5\% \text{ saturation MetHb}} \\ 97\% \text{ saturation of arterial blood (Sao}_2 \text{ of 97\%)} \end{array}$$

EXAMPLE 2

The following example is for a patient with an elevated COHb and a normal MetHb level:

$$\begin{array}{l} 15.0 \text{ g total Hb} \\ \underline{-3.0 \text{ g COHb}} \\ 2.0 \text{ g} \\ \underline{-0.15 \text{ g MetHb}} \\ 11.85 \text{ g functional Hb} \end{array}$$

$$\begin{array}{l} \text{100\% potential saturation of O}_2\text{ Hb in arterial blood} \\ \underline{-20\% \text{ saturation of COHb}} \\ 80\% \\ \underline{-1.5\% \text{ saturation of MetHb}} \\ 78.5\% \text{ saturation of arterial blood (Sao}_2 \text{ of 78.5\%)} \end{array}$$

Exam Hint

If a significant difference is found in hemoglobin saturation values between the pulse oximeter, standard or POC analyzer, and a CO-oximeter, suspect that the patient has an elevated CO level. Only the CO-oximeter value will be accurate if the patient has CO poisoning.

4. Mixed venous blood gases

a. Review the patient's chart for mixed venous blood gas results (WRE code: IA5) [Difficulty: Ap, An]

A mixed venous blood sample can be taken from the pulmonary artery of any patient who has a pulmonary artery (Swan-Ganz) catheter. This is a true mixed venous sample and should not be confused with a blood sample taken from an arm vein or other venous site. The symbol $P\bar{v}$ is the prefix for venous blood gas values of oxygen and so forth. In general, a typical patient has mixed venous blood gas values of $S\bar{v}o_2$, 75%; $P\bar{v}o_2$, 40 mm Hg; $P\bar{v}co_2$, 46 mm Hg; and pH 7.35. (Table 3-11 gives details on normal venous blood gas values and their interpretation in patients with cardiovascular disease.)

b. Interpret the results of mixed venous blood gas analysis to evaluate the patient's response to respiratory care (WRE code: IB8e and IIIE4) [Difficulty: An]

In the critically ill patient, it is just as important to measure the mixed venous blood gases as it is to measure the ABGs. The venous blood gas values reveal what has happened as the arterial blood has passed through the body.

TABLE 3-11	Normal and Abnormal Mixed Venous Blood Gas Values			
NORMAL VALUES				
Average: $S\bar{v}o_2$, 75%; $P\bar{v}o_2$, 40 torr; $P\bar{v}co_2$, 46 torr; pH 7.35				
Range: $S\bar{v}o_2$, 76%-70%; $P\bar{v}o_2$, 43-37 torr; $P\bar{v}co_2$, 46-44 torr; pH 7.36-7.34				
CRITICALLY ILL PATIENT				
	$P\bar{v}o_2$ (torr)		$S\bar{v}o_2$ (%)	
	Average	Range	Average	Range
Excellent cardio-vascular reserves	>37	40-35	>70	75-68
Limited cardio-vascular reserves	>32	35-30	>60	68-56
Failure of cardio-vascular reserves	<30	<30	<56	<56

Modified from Shapiro BA, Peruzzi WT, Kozelowski-Templin R: *Clinical application of blood gases,* ed 5, St Louis, 1994, Mosby.

Oxygen has been extracted, and carbon dioxide has been added to the blood. The difference between the arterial and venous oxygen levels reflects oxygen consumption by the body as well as cardiac output.

Because of this, the most critical venous blood gas values to measure are the $S\bar{v}o_2$ and $P\bar{v}o_2$. It is generally accepted that a $P\bar{v}o_2$ value of less than 30 torr or $S\bar{v}o_2$ of less than 56% indicates that the patient has tissue hypoxia. Both values can be obtained by analyzing a mixed venous blood sample taken through a pulmonary artery catheter. If the patient has a fiberoptic catheter, the $S\bar{v}o_2$ value can be monitored continuously. This is extremely helpful if the patient is unstable or having frequent changes in inspired oxygen or ventilator settings. (Pulmonary artery catheters are discussed in more detail in Chapter 5.)

5. Arterialized capillary blood gases

a. Review the patient's chart for arterialized capillary blood gas results (WRE code: IA5) [Difficulty: Ap, An]

This method of obtaining a blood gas sample is limited to neonatal patients when an arterial sample cannot be obtained.

b. Interpret the results of capillary blood gas analysis to evaluate the patient's response to respiratory care (WRE code: IB8e and IIIE4) [Difficulty: An]

This sampling method was described earlier. If the neonate's sampling site is well perfused and the sample properly obtained, the blood can be analyzed. Because this is not a true ABG sample, the following limitations are placed on interpreting the results.

a. The capillary pH (c pH) has a good correlation with the arterial pH.

b. The capillary CO_2 ($Pcco_2$) correlates with the $Paco_2$ about 50% of the time.

c. The capillary O_2 (Pco_2) does not correlate well with the $Paco_2$.

Based on these limitations, an arterialized capillary blood pH value can be clinically useful. The capillary CO_2 value should be viewed with suspicion. It should not be the only parameter monitored to judge the infant's ability to ventilate; however, the combination of a low pH and elevated CO_2 indicates hypoventilation. Evaluate the infant's vital signs, breathing efforts, chest radiograph, and so on to determine respiratory status.

Unfortunately, the capillary O_2 value is practically useless for judging the infant's oxygenation. Some infants may have a fairly close correlation with the Pao_2, whereas others do not. No way is known to predetermine those that will match and those that will not. Many practitioners view a low capillary oxygen level as a sign of clinical hypoxemia. The American Association for Respiratory Care (AARC) Clinical Practice Guideline, "Oxygen Therapy in the Acute Care Hospital," notes that a Pco_2 of less than 40 torr documents neonatal hypoxemia. An ABG sample remains the best way to determine the patient's respiratory status.

MODULE E
Pulse oximetry with first-generation units

1. Check the patient's chart for previous pulse oximetry results (WRE code: IA7d) [Difficulty: An]

Pulse oximetry (Spo_2) spectroscopically analyzes arterial blood to noninvasively determine the percentage of hemoglobin that is saturated with oxygen. It generally is indicated whenever a patient's oxygenation must be monitored. An Spo_2 of 92% or greater indicates that the patient is adequately oxygenated. Past values should be compared with current readings to monitor the patient's progress or response to treatment.

2. Make a recommendation to perform pulse oximetry (WRE code: IC3) [Difficulty: An]

Pulse oximetry is indicated in the following situations: during anesthesia and intraoperative monitoring of oxygenation, postoperatively when the patient is still sedated, when the patient is receiving sedatives or analgesics that can blunt the airway protective reflexes, during bronchoscopy, during a sleep study, and to evaluate the effectiveness of oxygen therapy. An exception to the use of first-generation pulse oximetry is when there is known or suspected carbon monoxide poisoning.

3. Get an appropriate pulse oximeter and related equipment (WRE code: IIA18) [Difficulty: Ap]

Each pulse oximeter reports a percentage of hemoglobin saturation with oxygen on a light-emitting diode (LED) display. Many newer units also display the patient's pulse rate. More expensive units print out a copy of Spo_2 percentage and pulse rate to be placed into the patient's chart if it is required. A variety of sensors fit the feet or hands of infants, an adult's fingers, the bridge of the nose, the forehead, and the earlobe. Choose a sensor designed to fit the site that is selected.

4. Put the equipment together and make sure that it works properly (WRE code: IIA18) [Difficulty: Ap]

Follow the manufacturer's suggestions for setup. The newer pulse oximetry systems visually display the strength of the pulse so that the best place for the probe can be found (Fig. 3-13). Keep bright light out of the patient site and transducer. Fig. 3-14 shows how to apply the finger probe properly.

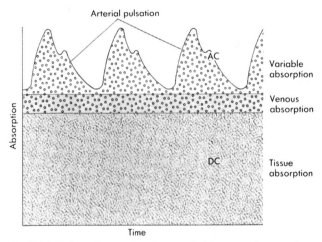

Fig. 3-13 Pulse oximetry signal strength. The strong surge of blood through the artery with each heartbeat results in variable absorption of the light emitted by the pulse oximeter. Venous and tissue absorption of light is stable when the heart is at rest. This absorption difference is used to find the patient's artery and measure the heart rate. (AC, variable absorption; DC, stable absorption.) *(From Ruppel G: Manual of pulmonary function testing, ed 6, St Louis, 1994, Mosby.)*

Fig. 3-14 Pulse oximetry transducer properly placed on a finger. Fold the OXISENSOR over the end of the digit. Align the other end of the OXISENSOR so that the two alignment marks are directly opposite each other. Press the OXISENSOR onto the skin. Wrap the adhesive flaps around the digit. *(Reprinted with permission of Nellcor Puritan Bennett Inc., Pleasanton, Calif.)*

5. Troubleshoot any problems with the equipment (WRE code: IIA18) [Difficulty: Ap]

The pulse signal will not be strong if the patient has poor circulation at the site of the oximeter probe. This can occur if the patient is hypothermic, hypotensive, or receiving a vasoconstricting medication. If the pulse signal is weak, the pulse-oximetry values may not be accurate. See Table 3-12 for common sources of error and their solutions.

6. Perform pulse oximetry on your patient (WRE code: IB7b and IIIE3a) [Difficulty: An]

First-generation pulse oximetry has gained wide acceptance because it offers a way to monitor continuously and noninvasively a patient's oxygenation by following the percentage of hemoglobin saturated with oxygen. The reported SpO_2% is the percentage of oxyhemoglobin.

Pulse oximetry makes practical use of two physical principles. The first is spectrophotometry, which is used to analyze the transmission of two wavelengths of light through the blood and body tissues. One wavelength is 660 nm, and the other is between 920 and 940 nm, depending on the manufacturer. The 660-nm wavelength can be seen as red and is preferentially absorbed by oxyhemoglobin (O_2Hb). The 920- to 940-nm wavelength is not visible, because it is in the infrared range. It is preferentially absorbed by reduced hemoglobin (RHb).

The second principle is plethysmography. It is used to find and then evaluate the amplitude of the arterial pulse waveform. See Fig. 3-13 for the plethysmographic arterial waveform. When the pulse-oximeter sensor is placed on a patient site, the fingertip for example, the two wavelengths of light shine through the blood, tissues, and bone within the finger. It is important that the sending LED and receiving (photodiode) sensors be opposite each other (see Fig. 3-14). Most units have a signal strength display that indicates when the photodiode is receiving a strong signal, and the patient's pulse has been detected. The microprocessor is designed to detect a baseline level of light absorption by the tissues and venous blood, containing more RHb, as well as the light absorption of arterial blood, containing more O_2Hb. It can then compare the absorptions of the two wavelengths to determine the level of saturated oxyhemoglobin. This is displayed as saturation by pulse oximetry, or SpO_2.

It must be realized that because first-generation pulse oximetry samples only two wavelengths of light, the technology is unable to recognize the presence or quantity of the nonfunctional hemoglobin species of COHb and MetHb. Instead, an ABG sample should be drawn and sent to the laboratory to be passed through a CO-oximeter for a complete fractional hemoglobin analysis. Even healthy persons have small amounts of COHb and MetHB. For this and other technical reasons, manufacturers report the following SpO_2 values for general accuracy at 1 standard deviation (SD) for a general population: ±2% from 100% to 70% saturation, and ±3% from 70% to 50% saturation. Because of these limitations, the following clinical guidelines have been created by a number of authors.

a. Do not use pulse oximetry on patients with significant levels of COHb or MetHB.

b. If in doubt about abnormal types of hemoglobin, analyze an ABG through a CO-oximeter and compare the true SaO_2 with the SpO_2 from pulse oximetry. Pulse oximetry can be used if the correlation of values is within 4%.

c. Question the SpO_2 value when the displayed heart rate is different from the actual heart rate.

d. Do not use pulse oximetry when the SpO_2 reading is less than 70%.

e. Pulse oximetry can be used on a term neonate or one that weighs 1500 g or more. Smaller neonates should have oxygenation measured by a transcutaneous oxygen monitor. This is because it is too easy to hyperoxygenate a small neonate when small

TABLE 3-12	Sources of Error in Pulse Oximetry
Sources of Error	**Remedy**
Light interference: xenon lamp, fluorescent light, infrared (bilirubin) light; probe fell off of patient	Cover the probe with an opaque wrap; put the probe back in place on the patient
Low perfusion: low blood pressure, hypothermia, vasoconstricting drugs	Use earlobe, bridge of nose, or forehead instead of finger or toe; discontinue use if still unreliable
Motion artifact	Secure the probe site; ensure that the SpO_2 reading is synchronized with the heart rate
Darkly pigmented patient	Use lightly pigmented site such as tip of finger or toe; SpO_2 value may overestimate PaO_2; discontinue use if still unreliable
Artificial or painted fingernails	Remove acrylic nails; remove black, blue, green, metallic, or frosted nail polish; use a different site
Venous pulsation being read as an arterial pulsation	Loosen a tight sensor; change the finger sensor site every 2-4 hr; loosen the cause of a tourniquet-like effect
The following vascular dyes will cause low SpO_2 readings: methylene blue, indigo carmine, indocyanine green	Do not use SpO_2

PaO_2, Partial pressure of O_2 in arterial blood; SpO_2, pulse oximeter.

changes in saturation can result in wide swings in Po_2. The risk of retinopathy of prematurity (formerly called retrolental fibroplasia) from hyperoxia is too great in the small neonate.

Table 3-13 lists common clinical ranges for Spo_2 values. For the aforementioned reasons, the minimum safe values are 2% higher than the corresponding Sao_2 value by CO-oximetry. It is important that the patient have good pulsatile blood flow to the measurement site to obtain an accurate reading.

7. Interpret a patient's pulse-oximetry value (WRE code: IB8b) [Difficulty: An]

The previously healthy patient who has cardiopulmonary failure should have the Spo_2 value kept at 92% or greater to ensure adequate oxygenation. The patient with COPD can probably tolerate an Spo_2 value of as low as 87%. The neonate should have the Spo_2 kept between 92% to 96%. Saturations below these values indicate hypoxemia in most patients.

Note the site at which the saturation was measured. This is especially important in neonates who may have congenital heart defects. A higher saturation in the right fingers or right earlobe compared with the rest of the body is seen with a patent ductus arteriosus (PDA). A higher saturation in the fingers and earlobes as compared with the toes is seen with a coarctation of the aorta.

Exam Hint

The patient with carbon monoxide poisoning should not be evaluated with a first-generation pulse oximeter because the units are unable to distinguish functional oxyhemoglobin from nonfunctional carboxyhemoglobin. These pulse oximeters show the level of only functional O_2Hb. Use only a CO-oximeter blood gas analyzer on a patient with known or suspected CO poisoning. Clinical examples include a patient removed from an enclosed house fire or a patient removed from a car with the engine running.

Second-generation pulse oximeters can measure and display both functional hemoglobin (Spo_2) and nonfunctional hemoglobin ($SpCO$ and $SpMet$). They *can* be used to monitor patients with carbon monoxide poisoning.

Exam Hint

Usually a question is related to an inaccurately low pulse oximeter reading due to poor local perfusion. See Table 3-12 for this and other examples of causes of inaccurate readings.

TABLE 3-13	Recommended Clinical Ranges for True Values in Saturation of O_2 in the Hemoglobin (Sao_2), Values in Pulse Oximetry (Spo_2),* and Their Correlation with Values in Partial Pressure of O_2 in Arterial Blood (Pao_2)		
	Sao_2	Spo_2	Approximate Pao_2 (torr)
ADULT			
Acute hypoxemia	90%-95%	92%-95%†	60-95
Chronic hypoxemia	85%-90%	87%-92%	50-60
NEONATE			
<1500 g or in the first week of life	About 97%	92%-96%	60-70
>1500 g or after the first week of life	90%-96%	90%-96%	50-70
>1 month of age with chronic lung disease	85%-90%	87%-92%	50-60

Note: The clinical goal with most neonates is to prevent both hypoxemia, defined as a Pao_2 < 45 torr, and hyperoxemia, defined as a Pao_2 > 90 torr.
*Based on the patient having normal carboxyhemoglobin and methemoglobin levels. Elevated level(s) result in an erroneously high Spo_2 reading and unsuspected hypoxemia.
†Black patients should have an Spo_2 of 95% maintained to ensure adequate oxygenation.

MODULE F
Transcutaneous oxygen monitoring

NOTE: Transcutaneous monitoring (TCM) involves the continuous monitoring of oxygen, carbon dioxide, or both as they diffuse through the skin. Each gas has its own individual electrode, and a combined electrode exists for both gases.

1. Review the patient's chart for a transcutaneous oxygen ($Ptco_2$) value (WRE code: IA7d) [Difficulty: An]

Transcutaneous oxygen monitoring ($Ptco_2$, $tcPo_2$, or Tco_2) enables any patient's oxygenation status to be followed on a continuous basis. In practice, neonates are monitored much more often than adults. Check the chart for a record of the patient's transcutaneous oxygen values. It is particularly important to compare the Pao_2 with the $Ptco_2$. In addition, note what the $Ptco_2$ values are when the inspired oxygen is changed, the patient is suctioned, or changes are made in continuous positive airway pressure (CPAP) or mechanical ventilation. Avoid clinical situations that have previously resulted in hypoxemia.

2. Recommend transcutaneous oxygen monitoring for additional data (WRE code: IC3) [Difficulty: An]

$PtcO_2$ monitoring has been used for the following purposes:

   a. To monitor oxygenation during transportation of an unstable neonate within the hospital or between two hospitals.

   b. To monitor intraoperative and postoperative oxygenation.

   c. To monitor oxygenation during changes in the inspired oxygen, during changes in mechanical ventilation, and to detect hypoxemia during an equipment failure.

   d. To help detect a right-to-left shunt. When a neonate has a PDA, the $PtcO_2$ is higher in the right upper chest than in the left upper chest, abdomen, or thighs.

   e. To help detect a coarctation of the aorta. When this defect is present, the $PtcO_2$ is higher in the right and left upper chest than in the abdomen or thighs.

   f. To determine the congenital heart disease patient's response to an oxygen challenge test.

3. Get the necessary equipment to perform transcutaneous oxygen monitoring (WRE code: IIA18) [Difficulty: An]

The electrode used for monitoring the patient's transcutaneous oxygen level is a miniaturized and modified Clark-type polarographic electrode similar to that used in the blood gas analyzer (Fig. 3-15). Some authors describe it as a *Huch* or *Hellige* electrode after two researchers who modified the original Clark electrode for their work with pediatric patients.

Fig. 3-15 Schematic drawing of the modified Clark electrode used to monitor transcutaneous oxygen tension. *1,* O-ring to hold the membrane to the electrode; *2,* polypropylene membrane permeable to oxygen; *3,* silver anode that surrounds the platinum cathode; *4,* electrolyte chamber with solution held in place by the polypropylene membrane; *5,* heating element; *6,* platinum cathode; *7,* electrolyte solution of sodium bicarbonate and sodium chloride held between the membrane and electrode; and *8,* negative temperature coefficient (NTC) resistor that serves to regulate the temperature of the sensor. *(From Shapiro BA, Peruzzi WT, Templin R: Clinical application of blood gases, ed 5, St Louis, 1994, Mosby.)*

4. Put the transcutaneous oxygen monitor together and make sure that it works properly (WRE code: IIA18) [Difficulty: An]

Always follow the manufacturer's recommendations for the assembly and care of the equipment. Select the proper electrode for the monitor based on the physician's order for evaluating transcutaneous oxygen, carbon dioxide, or both together.

5. Perform quality control procedures on a transcutaneous oxygen monitor (WRE code: IIC5) [Difficulty: Ap, An]

Always follow the manufacturer's recommendations for the assembly and care of the equipment. Select the proper electrode for the monitor based on the physician's order for evaluating transcutaneous oxygen, carbon dioxide, or both together.

Site selection. Care must be taken to select the best site for the electrode. A bad site will give incorrect information that can lead to mistakes in patient care. See Box 3-2 for a listing of site-selection guidelines.

Skin and electrode preparation and application of the skin electrode. An airtight seal between the skin and electrode is necessary for accurate readings. An air leak will result in

---

BOX 3-2 Optimal Sites and Sites to Avoid with Transcutaneous Gas Monitoring

OPTIMAL NEONATAL SITES
Upper part of the chest
Right upper chest if a preductal $PtcO_2$ value is desired
Abdomen
Inner aspect of either thigh

OPTIMAL ADULT SITES
Upper part of the chest
Inner aspect of the upper arm

SITES TO AVOID
Large fat deposit
Bony prominence
Pressure point
Thick skin
Skin edema
Hands and feet

CONDITIONS IN WHICH TRANSCUTANEOUS MONITORING SHOULD NOT BE USED
Locally cold skin or general, deep hypothermia
Locally decreased peripheral perfusion or general hypotension
Patient receiving vasoconstricting drugs such as tolazoline or dopamine
Cardiac index less than $1.9 \, L/min/m^2$ of body surface area
Halothane anesthesia will give erroneously high transcutaneous O_2 values unless a Teflon membrane is used

$PtcO_2$, Pressure of transcutaneous oxygen.

an increase in the PtcO$_2$ reading (and a decrease in the PtcCO$_2$ reading). The following steps should be taken to ensure that the skin site and electrode are prepared and an airtight seal is ensured:

1. Clean the skin. Usually, cleaning with an alcohol swab is enough to remove perspiration. Oily skin should be cleaned with soap and water.
2. Adults may need to have hair shaved from the site.
3. Adults may have dead skin cells removed by placing sticky adhesive tape against the site and pulling it off.
4. Prepare the electrode according to the manufacturer's guidelines. This usually includes placing a drop of the electrolyte solution on the electrode surface and placing a gas-permeable membrane with a double adhesive ring over the electrode.
5. The other side of the adhesive ring is pressed against the monitoring site to form an airtight seal.
6. As the electrode warms the skin, the patient values will fluctuate. Stabilization usually requires several minutes, after which the patient values should be clinically useful.

Limitations and patient precautions. Because the electrode is heated, it must be rotated to a different skin site on a routine basis. The general manufacturer's guidelines for site rotation are every 4 to 6 hours for neonates weighing between 1000 and 2500 g; every 3 to 5 hours for neonates weighing between 2500 and 3500 g; and 2 to 4 hours for neonates weighing more than 3500 g, pediatric patients, and adult patients. As a safety precaution, change the electrode on all patients at least every 4 hours, or at least every 3 hours if the patient is hypothermic. The manufacturer's range in times is based on the relative thickness of the patient's skin and the different electrode temperatures. It is important to adjust the site-rotation times on an individual patient basis. Some may tolerate longer times, and others will need more frequent rotations.

Care must be taken when removing the adhesive ring and electrode. It is possible to tear the thin, delicate skin of a premature neonate. Loosen the adhesive by running the edge of an alcohol wipe along the side that is being gently pulled up. After the electrode is removed, it is important to examine the skin; it is normal to see a red circle. This warmed, vasodilated area will stay red for some time and will gradually fade away, with no scarring or permanent injury. Rarely, the skin will have overheated and a blister is seen; this is a second-degree burn. Obviously, future site rotations must be made more frequently. Do not use this site again. Treat it as a burn, and avoid any further injury that might break the skin and lead to an infection.

Calibration. Two-point calibration must be performed with oxygen percentages that will cause Po$_2$ values beyond the clinical range that can be expected. Usually the first calibration point is a "zero" point because the electrode is exposed to no oxygen in a nitrogen-filled chamber. This point is usually quite stable. The second calibration point

is found when the electrode is exposed to room air (20.95% or 0.2095 oxygen). Always follow the manufacturer's written procedures during the calibration process. Generally, when environmental conditions include a fairly stable room temperature of 25° C and 50% relative humidity, the following equation can be used to predict the room air calibration point:

$$\text{Calibration Ptco}_2 = P_B \times 0.2095$$

in which P_B is the local barometric pressure, and 0.2095 is the oxygen fraction found in room air. Expose the electrode to room air to determine whether it matches the calculated calibration value. Adjust the instrument to match the calibration PtcO$_2$ if necessary. It is recommended that the room-air calibration point be rechecked every 24 hours when in continuous use, after changing the membrane, or after changing the electrolyte solution. A variation of up to ±5 torr is acceptable and can be corrected by adjusting the reading on the instrument. If the variation is greater than ±5 torr, the zero-point and room-air calibration procedures should be repeated.

6. Troubleshoot any problems with the equipment (WRE code: IIA18) [Difficulty: Ap]

Problems usually associated with too much electrode drift include electrode or membrane surfaces contaminated by debris such as blood or sweat, an improperly applied membrane, a worn-out membrane, an air bubble beneath the membrane, improper gas exposed to the membrane during the calibration, exhausted electrolyte solution in the electrode, or inaccurate calibration values. After correcting a problem, the calibration procedure should be repeated.

7. Interpret transcutaneous oxygen monitoring values to evaluate the patient's response to respiratory care (WRE code: IB8a) [Difficulty: R, Ap, An]

It has been found that heating the electrode speeds the diffusion of oxygen through the skin. Heating also provides a closer correlation with the patient's Pao$_2$ value. However, it must be remembered that the PtcO$_2$ value is not the same as the Pao$_2$ value. Current recommendations are that any unit should give PtcO$_2$ values that are within ±15% of the Pao$_2$ over the operating range of the instrument. The values should then correlate within ±15% as the patient's condition changes. This should always be confirmed.

An arterial blood gas sample should be drawn for Pao$_2$ every time transcutaneous oxygen monitoring is started. The Pao$_2$–Ptco$_2$ gradient can then be calculated as the difference between the two. For example, if the patient's Pao$_2$ is 100 torr, the PtcO$_2$ should be no less than 85 torr. If the PtcO$_2$ decreases to 70 torr, the Pao$_2$ should have decreased to no lower than 85 torr. Because of this close correlation, the patient's trend can be monitored with some assurance of accuracy. In addition, ABG samples do not need to be drawn as frequently for the Pao_2. This trending relation holds true for changes in the patient's pulmonary condition. It does not, however, hold true when the patient has cardiovascular problems such as hypotension, hypothermia, peripheral vascular disease, or cardiogenic shock with decreased tissue perfusion.

Always follow the manufacturer's recommendations for the proper electrode temperature. In general, the temperature ranges from 42.5°C for a 1000-g infant to 44°C for a 3500-g infant. A pediatric patient can tolerate a temperature of 44°C, whereas an adult can have an electrode temperature of 45°C. The higher temperatures are needed in older patients because their skin is thicker. Studies have shown that when the neonate's Pao_2 is greater than 100 torr, the $Ptco_2$ value underestimates it. This can lead to dangerous hyperoxemia. For this reason, it is recommended that the $Ptco_2$ be kept at less than 90 torr. In the adult, less correlation is found between the Pao_2 and $Ptco_2$ because of the thicker skin. $Ptco_2$ can still be used in the adult to follow trends in oxygenation, but the practitioner must realize that a decrease in the $Ptco_2$ value can be a result of hypoxemia, a decreased cardiac output, or cutaneous vasoconstriction. An arterial blood gas sample must be drawn to further evaluate the patient's status.

Correlation of $Ptco_2$ and local power consumption. As mentioned earlier, the electrode is heated to above body temperature. The amount of electrical current needed to keep the electrode at a constant temperature depends on the temperature of the blood and the speed at which the blood passes beneath the electrode. This is known as local power consumption or simply local power (LP). A change in the LP value and $Ptco_2$ can be used to indicate what is happening to the patient. For example:

   a. A normal LP seen with a decreased $Ptco_2$ indicates that the patient's pulmonary problem has worsened.
   b. A normal LP seen with an increased $Ptco_2$ indicates that the patient's pulmonary problem has improved.
   c. A decreased LP seen with a decreased $Ptco_2$ indicates that the patient's cardiac output has worsened.
   d. An increased LP seen with an increased $Ptco_2$ indicates that the patient's cardiac output has improved.

Exam Hint

If a sick neonate has normal cardiovascular status, the Pao_2 and $Ptco_2$ should correlate with each other (but not be identical) as the patient's pulmonary condition changes. For example, the neonate has infant respiratory distress syndrome. The Pao_2 and $Ptco_2$ values probably will not correlate when the patient has cardiovascular problems. For example, the neonate is hypotensive with low cardiac output.

MODULE G
Transcutaneous carbon dioxide monitoring

1. Review the patient's chart for a transcutaneous carbon dioxide value (WRE code: IA7d) [Difficulty: An]

Transcutaneous carbon dioxide monitoring ($Ptcco_2$, $tcPco_2$, or $Tcco_2$) enables any patient's ventilation status to be monitored on a continuous basis. In practice, neonates are monitored much more often than adults. Check the chart for a record of the patient's transcutaneous carbon dioxide values. It is particularly important to correlate these values with any ABG values, which allows comparison between the $Paco_2$ and the $Ptcco_2$. In addition, note the $Ptcco_2$ values when changes are made in CPAP or mechanical ventilation. Avoid clinical situations that have previously resulted in hypoventilation.

2. Recommend transcutaneous carbon dioxide monitoring for additional data (WRE code: IC3) [Difficulty: An]

$Ptcco_2$ monitoring has been used for the following purposes:
   a. To monitor ventilation during transportation of an unstable infant within the hospital or between two hospitals.
   b. To monitor intraoperative and postoperative ventilation.
   c. To monitor ventilation during changes in mechanical ventilation such as tidal volume, rate, minute ventilation, mechanical dead space, or a combination of these.
   d. To detect hypoventilation during an accidental disconnection from the ventilator.

3. Get the necessary equipment to perform transcutaneous carbon dioxide monitoring (WRE code: IIA18) [Difficulty: Ap]

The electrode used for monitoring the patient's transcutaneous carbon dioxide level is a miniaturized and modified Stow-Severinghaus–type electrode similar to the ABG electrode (Fig. 3-16).

4. Put the transcutaneous carbon dioxide monitor together, and make sure that it works properly (WRE code: IIA18) [Difficulty: Ap]

Always follow the manufacturer's recommendations for the assembly and care of the equipment. Select the proper electrode for the monitor based on the physician's order for evaluating transcutaneous carbon dioxide.

5. Perform quality control procedures on a transcutaneous carbon dioxide monitor (WRE code: IIC5) [Difficulty: Ap, An]

Much of the information on skin-site selection and so forth presented in the preceding discussion of transcutaneous

Fig. 3-16 Schematic drawing of the modified Stow-Severinghaus electrode used to monitor transcutaneous carbon dioxide tension. *1,* Epoxy resin; *2,* glass electrode with a chlorinated silver wire, a buffer solution (the inner liquid), and a pH-sensitive glass membrane; *3,* negative temperature coefficient (NTC) resistor that serves to regulate the temperature of the sensor; *4,* O-ring to hold the membrane to the electrode; *5,* electrolyte chamber with solution held in place by the polypropylene membrane; *6,* electrolyte solution of sodium bicarbonate and sodium chloride held between the membrane and electrode; *7,* polypropylene membrane permeable to carbon dioxide; *8,* heating element; and *9,* silver/silver chloride reference electrode. *(From Shapiro BA, Peruzzi WT, Templin R: Clinical application of blood gases, ed 5, St Louis, 1994, Mosby.)*

oxygen monitors applies here, as well. As with the transcutaneous oxygen electrode, it has been found that heating the Ptc_{CO_2} electrode speeds the diffusion of carbon dioxide through the skin. Always follow the manufacturer's recommendations for the proper electrode temperature. In general, the temperature is 44°C in both neonates and adults. It must be remembered that Ptc_{CO_2} value is not the same as the Pa_{CO_2} value. An arterial blood gas sample should be analyzed for Pa_{CO_2} every time transcutaneous carbon dioxide monitoring is started. Unlike transcutaneous oxygen monitoring, the correlation between Pa_{CO_2} and Ptc_{CO_2} is as good in adult as in neonatal patients. In addition, it is not as easily influenced by changes in the patient's skin blood flow.

Two-point calibration must be performed with carbon dioxide percentages that cause P_{CO_2} values beyond the expected clinical range. Usually the electrode is exposed to 5% and 10% carbon dioxide from prepared cylinders. Always follow the manufacturer's written procedures during the calibration process. Generally, when environmental conditions include a fairly stable room temperature of 25°C and 50% relative humidity, the following equation can be used to predict the two calibration points:

$$\text{Calibration } Ptc_{CO_2} = (P_B \times CO_2\% \text{ used}) - (X\ CO_2 \times \text{electrode temperature factor})$$

in which P_B is the local barometric pressure; $CO_2\%$ is the carbon dioxide fraction exposed to the electrode, either 10% (0.10) or 5% (0.05); and $X\ CO_2$ is the correction factor to equilibrate the Ptc_{CO_2} to Pa_{CO_2}. (This is discussed later.)

Electrode temperature factor. This is a factor determined by the manufacturer based on the electrode temperature. It is usually heated to 44°C.

Expose the electrode to 10% carbon dioxide in a sealed chamber to determine whether it matches the calculated calibration value. Adjust the instrument to match the calibration Ptc_{CO_2} if necessary. Next, expose the electrode to 5% carbon dioxide in the sealed chamber. Again, adjust the instrument to match the calibration Ptc_{CO_2} if necessary. It is recommended that the two-point calibration points be rechecked every 24 hours when in continuous use, after changing the membrane, or after changing the electrolyte solution. A variation of up to ±4 torr is acceptable and can be corrected by adjusting the reading on the instrument. If the variation is greater than ±4 torr, the two-point calibration procedures should be repeated.

6. Troubleshoot any problems with the equipment (WRE code: IIA18) [Difficulty: Ap]

Problems usually associated with too much electrode drift include electrode or membrane surfaces contaminated by debris such as blood or sweat, an improperly applied membrane, a worn-out membrane, an air bubble beneath the membrane, improper gas sample exposed to the membrane during the calibration, exhausted electrolyte solution in the electrode, or inaccurate calibration values. After correcting a problem, the calibration procedure should be repeated.

7. Interpret transcutaneous carbon dioxide monitoring values to evaluate the patient's response to respiratory care (WRE code: IB8a) [Difficulty: R, Ap, An]

The net effect of heating the carbon dioxide electrode and skin results in the Ptc_{CO_2} readings being 1.2 to 2 times (120% to 200%) greater than the Pa_{CO_2} values. Commonly, an average multiplier of 1.6 is found. The actual value varies among patients and can be found by dividing the Ptc_{CO_2} by the Pa_{CO_2}.

For example, a patient has a Pa_{CO_2} of 40 torr and a Ptc_{CO_2} of 64 torr. Calculate the gradient between the arterial and transcutaneous values.

$$\text{Gradient} = \frac{Ptc_{CO_2}}{Pa_{CO_2}} = \frac{64}{40} = 1.6$$

As long as the patient's cardiovascular status is fairly stable, the Pa_{CO_2} can be calculated by dividing the Ptc_{CO_2} by 1.6. For example, if the patient's Ptc_{CO_2} increases to 80 torr, calculate the Pa_{CO_2}.

$$Pa_{CO_2} = \frac{Ptc_{CO_2}}{1.6} = \frac{80}{1.6} = 50 \text{ torr}$$

Rather than perform these calculations every time a change occurs in the patient's status, some practitioners divide the CO_2 values found during the calibration procedure by 1.6. This results in "real" $PaCO_2$ values being given continuously on the monitor. This change must be clearly communicated to all staff members to avoid confusion between the original $PtcCO_2$ values and values that have been reduced to "arterialize" them.

MODULE H
Respiratory care plan

1. Analyze available information to determine the patient's pathophysiologic state (CSE code: IIIH1)

Many patients with pneumonia or other pulmonary conditions will have significant hypoxemia despite receiving supplemental oxygen. This gap between the alveolar oxygen level and the arterial oxygen level is called the alveolar-arterial oxygen pressure difference [$P(A-a)O_2$]. Measurement of this gap or difference gives an important indication of the seriousness of the patient's condition.

Perform the following to determine the alveolar-arterial O_2 pressure difference [$P(A-a)O_2$]:

a. Note the patient's inspired oxygen percentage.
b. Draw and analyze an ABG sample. Note the patient's PaO_2 and $PaCO_2$.
c. Note the patient's temperature. This is needed to determine the patient's pulmonary water vapor pressure (PH_2O). The value of 47 torr (mm Hg) is used if the patient's temperature is normal. Check published tables for the pulmonary water vapor pressure if the patient's temperature is higher or lower than normal.
d. Measure the local barometric pressure (P_B) in torr (mm Hg).
e. If possible, calculate the patient's respiratory exchange ratio. If this cannot be done, use the standard value of 0.8.
f. Calculate the patient's PAO_2. The formula presented here is the most commonly used of several versions:

$$PAO_2 = [(P_B - PH_2O) \, FIO_2] - \frac{PaCO_2}{0.8}$$

In which:

PAO_2 = Pressure of alveolar oxygen.

P_B = Barometric pressure of air. This is 760 torr (mm Hg) at sea level; it decreases as the altitude increases.

PH_2O = Pressure of water vapor in the lungs. This is 47 torr (mm Hg) at the normal temperature of 98.6°F/37°C. Remember that water vapor pressure increases if the patient has a fever and decreases if the patient is hypothermic.

FIO_2 = Fractional concentration (percentage) of inspired oxygen. Use whatever percentage of oxygen your patient is breathing in.

$\frac{PaCO_2}{8}$ = Effect of carbon dioxide and the patient's metabolism. The factor of 0.8 is based on how much oxygen a normal person uses and how much carbon dioxide is produced in 1 minute. The symbols for this metabolic value are R for respiratory exchange ratio and RQ for respiratory quotient. The following calculation is based on a normal person's metabolism:

$$R \text{ or } RQ = \frac{VCO_2}{VO_2} = \frac{200 \text{ mL/min}}{250 \text{ mL/min}} = 0.8$$

Because many sick patients do not react as expected, the factor has a range of 0.6 to 1.1, depending on oxygen consumption and carbon dioxide production. Assume that the factor is 0.8 unless you are told otherwise or measure otherwise.

g. Subtract the patient's PaO_2 from the PAO_2 to determine the $P(A-a)O_2$.

When you are interpreting the patient's value, remember that the $P(A-a)O_2$ in a normal young person should be no greater than 15 torr. The difference slowly increases as a normal person ages. Lung disease causes the value to increase significantly. The following are examples of some conditions in which the measurement of the $P(A-a)O_2$ aids in diagnosis or treatment:

1. Patients who are hypoxemic because they are hypoventilating (increased CO_2) have a normal $P(A-a)O_2$ when breathing room air. The hypoxemia can be corrected by increasing ventilation. Supplemental oxygen results in an expected increase in PaO_2.
2. Any condition in which a low ventilation-to-perfusion ratio is found reveals an elevated $P(A-a)O_2$ when the patient is breathing room air. Supplemental oxygen results in an increase in PaO_2; however, the increase is not as dramatic as that seen in the hypoventilating patient. Examples include asthma, bronchitis, emphysema, or any other condition in which unequal distribution of air into and out of the lungs but relatively normal perfusion is found.
3. Any shunt-producing disease or condition. Examples include ARDS and right-to-left anatomic shunt, such as could be seen in a ventricular septal defect. The $P(A-a)O_2$ becomes greater as the oxygen percentage is increased. It is commonly accepted that a $P(A-a)O_2$ of more than 350 torr, when 80% to 100% oxygen is administered, indicates that the patient is experiencing refractory hypoxemia. The patient probably needs to be supported by a mechanical ventilator. Commonly, positive end-expiratory pressure (PEEP) is administered so that the oxygen percentage can be reduced to a safer level.
4. Any disease producing a diffusion defect. Pulmonary fibrosis from any cause results in a wider than normal $P(A-a)O_2$. Supplemental oxygen results in an increase in the PaO_2, but not as great an increase as desired.

The following examples are offered to aid in the calculation of $P(A-a)O_2$ and the interpretation of the results.

EXAMPLE 1

You are working in a major teaching hospital in Miami. The patient's physician asks you to calculate the $P(A-a)O_2$ on a 30-year-old patient. The following conditions exist:

P_B = 760 torr
PH_2O = 47 torr because your patient's temperature is 98.6°F/37°C
FIO_2 = 0.21 because the patient is breathing room air
$PaCO_2$ = 40 torr from ABGs
PaO_2 = 90 torr from ABGs
R = 0.8

1. $PAO_2 = ([P_B - PH_2O]\, FIO_2) - PaCO_2/0.8$
2. $PAO_2 = ([760 - 47]\, 0.21) - 40/0.8$
3. $PAO_2 = ([713]\, 0.21) - 50$
4. $PAO_2 = (150) - 50$
5. $PAO_2 = 100$ torr
6. $P(A-a)O_2 = 100 - 90 = 10$ torr

Interpretation: A $P(A-a)O_2$ of 10 torr is normal for a patient of this age. It is normal to see a difference between the alveolar and arterial oxygen levels that starts in the range of 4 to 12 torr and slowly increases with age (Fig. 3-17).

EXAMPLE 2

You are working in a major teaching hospital in Denver. You are asked to calculate the alveolar-arterial difference in oxygen on a 40-year-old patient. The following conditions exist:

P_B = 710 torr

PH_2O = 50 torr because your patient's temperature is 100°F/38°C
FIO_2 = 0.35 because the patient is breathing 35% oxygen by mask
$PaCO_2$ = 55 torr from ABGs
PaO_2 = 65 torr from ABGs
R = 0.85

1. $PAO_2 = ([P_B - PH_2O]FIO_2) - PaCO_2/0.8$
2. $PAO_2 = ([710 - 50]\, 0.35) - 55/0.85$
3. $PAO_2 = ([660]\, 0.35) - 65$
4. $PAO_2 = (231) - 65$
5. $PAO_2 = 166$ torr
6. $P(A-a)O_2 = 166 - 65 = 101$ torr

Interpretation: The difference of 101 torr is elevated even though this patient is older than the patient in Example 1.

Exam Hint

The above calculation has been tested on the Written Registry Exam. Know that a widened alveolar-arterial (A–a) gradient indicates pulmonary disease. Diseases that result in true shunt or venous admixture result in a ventilation/perfusion mismatch. Giving supplemental oxygen may have little beneficial affect on the patient's oxygenation.

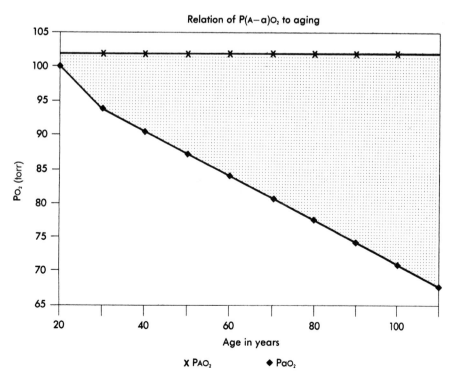

Relation of P(A–a)O₂ to aging

Fig. 3-17 The relation of $P(A-a)O_2$ to aging. As the PaO_2 naturally decreases with age, the $P(A-a)O_2$ increases at the rate of approximately 3 torr per decade beyond 20 years. *(From Lane EE, Walker JF: Clinical arterial blood gas analysis, St Louis, 1987, Mosby.)*

2. Determine the appropriateness of the prescribed therapy and goals for the identified pathophysiologic state (CSE code: IIIH3)

As part of the patient care team, you may need to evaluate the patient's blood gas values and other parameters to make a recommendation. For example, a patient with carbon monoxide poisoning is best treated by administering 100% oxygen through a nonrebreather mask. Pure oxygen reduces the half-life of COHb to 60 to 90 minutes. A first-generation pulse oximeter should not be used to measure this patient's saturation of oxyhemoglobin. These units are unable to identify COHb and will give misleadingly high saturation values for O_2Hb.

ABG analysis remains the "gold standard" by which all other values are judged. Typically, the arterial sample is analyzed through a standard blood gas analyzer. A CO-oximeter is needed if the patient has carbon monoxide poisoning. Mixed venous and capillary blood-sample analysis is limited in clinical application, but very helpful in the right patient situation. However, these offer only momentary insight into the patient's condition.

Pulse oximetry and transcutaneous oxygen monitoring offer continuous information on the patient's oxygenation. Transcutaneous carbon dioxide monitoring allows continuous monitoring of the patient's ventilation. As with all technology, these units have advantages, disadvantages, and limitations. It is up to the practitioner to make the correct choices. Some unstable patients can best be monitored through the combination of periodic evaluation of ABGs and these noninvasive continuous monitoring systems.

Exam Hint

Be prepared to make a recommendation regarding adjustment of the patient's inspired oxygen based on the PaO_2 (or related) value. Also be prepared to make a recommendation regarding adjustment of the patient's mechanical ventilation settings for tidal volume, rate, minute volume, mechanical dead space, or a combination of these based on the $PaCO_2$ (or related) value.

---

3. Stop the treatment or procedure if the patient has an adverse reaction to it (CSE code: IIIF1)

The hazards associated with drawing a sample of arterial blood were presented earlier. If a puncture site is not suitable, a different site must be selected.

4. Maintain records and communication on the patient's pulse-oximetry values (WRE code: IIIA1c) [Difficulty: An]

Pulse-oximetry values and their interpretation were covered earlier.

BIBLIOGRAPHY

Aloan CA, Hill TV, editors: *Respiratory care of the newborn and child,* ed 2, Philadelphia, 1997, Lippincott-Raven.

American Academy of Pediatrics: Task force on transcutaneous oxygen monitors, *Pediatrics* 83(1):122, 1989.

American Association for Respiratory Care: Clinical practice guideline: blood gas analysis and hemoximetry: 2001 revision and update, *Respir Care* 46:498-505, 2001.

American Association for Respiratory Care: Clinical practice guideline: transcutaneous blood gas monitoring for neonatal and pediatric patients: 2004 revision and update, *Respir Care* 49(9):1069–1072, 2004.

American Association for Respiratory Care: Clinical practice guideline: transcutaneous blood gas monitoring for neonatal and pediatric patients, *Respir Care* 39(12):1176, 1994.

American Association for Respiratory Care: Clinical practice guideline: capillary blood gas sampling for neonatal and pediatric patients, *Respir Care* 39(12):1180, 1994.

American Association for Respiratory Care: Clinical practice guideline: oxygen therapy in the acute care hospital, *Respir Care* 36(12):1410, 1991.

American Association for Respiratory Care: Clinical practice guideline: pulse oximetry, *Respir Care* 36(12):1406, 1991.

American Association for Respiratory Care: Clinical practice guideline: sampling for arterial blood gas analysis, *Respir Care* 37(8):913, 1991.

American Association for Respiratory Care: Clinical practice guideline: in-vitro pH and blood gas analysis and hemoximetry, *Respir Care* 38(5):505, 1993.

Barnes TA, editor: *Textbook of respiratory care practice,* ed 2, St Louis, 1994, Mosby.

Barnhart SL, Czervinske MP: *Perinatal and pediatric respiratory care,* Philadelphia, 1995, WB Saunders.

Blanchette T, Dziodzio J, Harris K: Pulse oximetry and normoximetry in neonatal intensive care, *Respir Care* 36(1):25, 1991.

Bohn DJ: Ask the expert, *Respiratory Tract,* 9, Feb 1988.

Branson RD, Hess DR, Chatburn RL, editors: *Respiratory care equipment,* ed 2, Philadelphia, 1999, Lippincott Williams & Wilkins.

Burton GC, Hodgkin JE, Ward JJ, editors: *Respiratory care: a guide to clinical practice,* ed 4, Philadelphia, 1997, Lippincott-Raven.

Cairo JM, Pilbeam SP: *Mosby's respiratory care equipment,* ed 7, St Louis, 2004, Mosby.

Czervinske MP: Arterial blood gas analysis and other cardiopulmonary monitoring. In Koff PB, Daily KE, Schroeder JS, editors: *Techniques in bedside hemodynamic monitoring,* ed 4, St Louis, 1989, Mosby.

Eitzman D, Neu J: *Neonatal and pediatric respiratory care,* ed 2, St Louis, 1993, Mosby.

Elser RC: Quality control of blood gas analysis: a review, *Respir Care* 31(9):807, 1986.

Federal government releases CLIA '88 final regulations, *AARC Times* 16(4):76, 1992.

Fell WL: Sampling and measurement of blood gases. In Lane EE, Walker JF, editors: *Clinical arterial blood gas analysis,* St Louis, 1987, Mosby.

Fink JB, Hunt GE, editors: *Clinical practice in respiratory care*, Philadelphia, 1999, Lippincott-Raven.

Garza D, Becan-McBride K: *Phlebotomy handbook*, ed 4, Stamford, Conn, 1996, Appleton & Lange.

Instrumentation Laboratories: *Operator's manual for the IL282 CO-oximeter*, Lexington, Mass.

Jubran A, Tobin MJ: Reliability of pulse oximetry in titrating supplemental oxygen therapy in ventilator-dependent patients, *Chest* 97:1420, 1990.

Lane EE, Walker JF: *Clinical arterial blood gas analysis*, St Louis, 1987, Mosby.

Levitzky MG, Cairo JM, Hall SM: *Introduction to respiratory care*, Philadelphia, 1990, WB Saunders.

Madama VC: *Pulmonary function testing and cardiopulmonary stress testing*, ed 2, Albany, NY, 1998, Delmar.

Mahoney JJ, Hodgkin JE, Van Kessel AL: Arterial blood gas analysis. In Burton GG, Hodgkin JE, Ward JJ, editors: *Respiratory care: a guide to clinical practice*, ed 4, Philadelphia, 1997, Lippincott-Raven.

Martin RJ: Transcutaneous monitoring: instrumentation and clinical applications, *Respir Care* 35(6):577, 1990.

Mathews P, Conway L: Arterial blood gases and noninvasive monitoring of oxygen and carbon dioxide. In Wyka KA, Mathews PJ, Clark WF, editors: *Foundations of respiratory care*, Albany, NY, 2002, Delmar.

Mohler JG, Collier CR, Brandt W: Blood gases. In Clausen JL, editor: *Pulmonary function testing guidelines and controversies*, Orlando, 1984, Grune & Stratton.

Moran RF: Assessment of quality control of blood gas/pH analyzer performance, *Respir Care* 26(6):538, 1981.

Moran RF: CLIA regulations. I. The cure might be worse than the disease, *AARC Times* 14(11):41, 1990.

Moran RF: CLIA regulations. II. An analysis of some technical requirements, *AARC Times* 14(12):25, 1990.

Nelson CM, Murphy EM, Bradley JK, et al: Clinical use of pulse oximetry to determine oxygen prescriptions for patients with hypoxemia, *Respir Care* 31(8):673, 1986.

Novametrics Medical Systems: product literature on transcutaneous monitoring, Wallingford, Conn.

Peters JA, Hodgkin JE, Collier CA: Blood gas analysis and acid-base physiology. In Burton GG, Hodgkin JE, Ward JJ, editors: *Respiratory care: a guide to clinical practice*, ed 3, Philadelphia, 1991, JB Lippincott.

Ruppel G: *Manual of pulmonary function testing*, ed 8, St Louis, 2003, Mosby.

Salyer JW: Pulse oximetry in the neonatal intensive care unit, *Respir Care* 36(1):17, 1991.

Scanlan CL, Wilkins RL: Analysis and monitoring of gas exchange. In Wilkins RL, Stoller JK, Scanlan CL, editors: *Egan's fundamentals of respiratory care*, ed 8, St Louis, 2003, Mosby.

Shapiro BA, Kacmarek RM, Cane RD, et al, editors: *Clinical application of respiratory care*, ed 4, St Louis, 1991, Mosby.

Shapiro BA, Peruzzi WT, Templin R: *Clinical application of blood gases*, ed 5, St Louis, 1994, Mosby.

Sonnesso G: Are you ready to use pulse oximetry? *Nursing* 21(8):60, 1991.

Walton JR, Shapiro BA: Value and application of temperature-compensated blood gas data, *Respir Care* 25(2), 1980.

Welch JP, DeCesare R, Hess D: Pulse oximetry: instrumentation and clinical applications, *Respir Care* 35(6):584, 1990.

Whitaker K: *Comprehensive perinatal and pediatric respiratory care*, ed 2, Albany, NY, 1997, Delmar.

White GC: *Equipment theory for respiratory care*, ed 3, Albany, NY, 1999, Delmar.

SELF-STUDY QUESTIONS

1. A 35-year-old patient with pneumonia is receiving mechanical ventilation with positive end-expiratory pressure (PEEP). You are ordered to calculate and interpret the patient's $P(A-a)O_2$. The following conditions exist:

    P_B = 750 torr. Normal is 760 torr for sea level.

    P_{H_2O} = 54 torr because your patient's temperature is 104°F/40°C. Normal is 47 torr for a normal temperature.

    FIO_2 = 0.5 for 50% inspired oxygen. Normal is 0.21 for room air.

    $PaCO_2$ = 36 torr

    PaO_2 = 60 torr

    Respiratory Exchange Ratio = 0.8

    $$PAO_2 = [(P_B - P_{H_2O})\, FIO_2] - \frac{PaCO_2}{0.8}$$

    Based on the listed conditions, what is the patient's PAO_2?
    A. 312 torr
    B. 303 torr
    C. 101 torr
    D. 95 torr

2. Based on the listed conditions, what is the patient's $P(A-a)O_2$?
    A. 248 torr
    B. 243 torr
    C. 232 torr
    D. 41 torr

3. How should the patient's $P(A-a)O_2$ results be interpreted?
    A. There is an error; check the blood gas analyzer.
    B. Normal oxygenation for 50% oxygen being inspired.
    C. Normal for a patient of this age.
    D. Larger than normal difference.

4. After performing a modified Allen's test on a patient's right wrist, it is found to take 25 seconds for the patient's hand to regain its color. What should be done now?
    A. Perform an Allen's test on the right wrist.

B. Draw an arterial blood sample on the right wrist.

C. Draw an arterial blood sample on the left wrist.

D. Perform a modified Allen's test on the patient's left wrist.

5. A 45-year-old patient is brought by ambulance into the Emergency Department from a business where there is a carbon monoxide leak. The patient is obtunded and has an irregular pulse. Which of the following is the *least* important to evaluate at this time?

A. Pulse oximeter value from a first-generation unit

B. 12-lead electrocardiogram

C. ABGs analyzed through a CO-oximeter

D. Glasgow coma analysis

6. For which of the following conditions should an arterial line be inserted?

I. Septic shock with vasopressor therapy

II. Suspected carbon monoxide poisoning

III. ARDS requiring mechanical ventilation with PEEP

IV. Anxiety-induced hyperventilation

A. I and II

B. I and III

C. II, III, and IV

D. All of the above

7. A 45-year-old patient has been admitted to the Emergency Department after having smoke inhalation from a house fire. He is wearing a nonrebreather mask set at 10 L/min of oxygen. The most appropriate way to evaluate his oxygenation status is by:

A. Pulse oximetry with a first-generation unit

B. Transcutaneous oxygen probe

C. Running an ABG sample through the blood gas analyzer

D. Running an ABG sample through the CO-oximeter

8. You are working with a postanesthesia patient who has a transcutaneous carbon dioxide monitor. The correlation factor between the $PaCO_2$ and $PtcCO_2$ is 1.4. The patient's previous $PtcCO_2$ was 63 torr. The nurse has called you because it is now 76 torr. The patient's approximate $PaCO_2$ would be calculated as:

A. 63 torr

B. 75 torr

C. 54 torr

D. 105 torr

9. Interpret the following blood gas drawn when the patient was breathing in 45% oxygen: PaO_2, 64 torr; SaO_2, 91%; pH, 7.38; $PaCO_2$, 59 torr; HCO_3^-, 39 mEq/L; and BE, +12 mEq/L.

I. Corrected hypoxemia

II. Uncorrected hypoxemia

III. Metabolic alkalosis

IV. Compensated respiratory acidosis

V. Metabolic acidosis

A. I, IV

B. I, III

C. II, V

D. II, IV

10. Interpret the following blood gas drawn when the patient was breathing in 30% oxygen: PaO_2, 82 torr; SaO_2, 94%; pH, 7.32; $PaCO_2$, 39 torr; HCO_3^-, 16 mEq/L; and BE, −6 mEq/L.

I. Corrected hypoxemia

II. Uncorrected hypoxemia

III. Compensated metabolic acidosis

IV. Uncompensated metabolic acidosis

V. Compensated respiratory acidosis

A. II, IV

B. I, IV

C. II, V

D. I, III

11. Interpret the following blood gas drawn when the patient was breathing in 24% oxygen: PaO_2, 125 torr; SaO_2, 99%; pH, 7.52; $PaCO_2$, 25 torr; HCO_3^-, 25 mEq/L; and BE, +1 mEq/L.

I. Normal oxygenation

II. Excessively corrected hypoxemia

III. Uncompensated respiratory alkalosis

IV. Uncompensated metabolic acidosis

V. Combined respiratory and metabolic alkalosis

A. II, III

B. II, V

C. I, III

D. I, IV

12. Interpret the following blood gas drawn when the patient was breathing in 40% oxygen: PaO_2, 75 torr; SaO_2, 93%; pH, 7.15; $PaCO_2$, 55 torr; HCO_3^-, 20 mEq/L; and BE, −8 mEq/L.

I. Uncorrected hypoxemia

II. Corrected hypoxemia

III. Uncorrected respiratory acidosis

IV. Uncorrected metabolic acidosis

V. Combined metabolic and respiratory acidosis

A. I, V

B. II, V

C. II, III

D. II, IV

13. Interpret the following blood gas drawn when the patient was breathing in 30% oxygen: PaO_2, 65 mm Hg; SaO_2, 91%; pH, 7.44; $PaCO_2$, 25 mm Hg; HCO_3^-, 17 mEq/L; and BE, −7 mEq/L.

I. Corrected hypoxemia

II. Uncorrected hypoxemia

III. Compensated respiratory alkalosis

IV. Uncompensated respiratory alkalosis

V. Combined metabolic and respiratory acidosis

A. I, III

B. I, IV

C. II, III

D. II, V

14. Which of the following clinical values indicates that a patient's tissues are hypoxemic?

    A. Pa_{O_2}, 55 torr

    B. $P\bar{v}_{O_2}$, 25 torr

    C. $S\bar{v}_{O_2}$, 80%

    D. Sa_{O_2}, 88%

15. You are working with a neonate in an incubator. She is being monitored with a transcutaneous oxygen electrode on her right upper chest. An hour ago, the patient's oxygen value was 52 torr, and now it is 115 torr. The nurse tells you that no change has occurred in the neonate's condition. What is the most likely explanation of this difference?

    A. The patient has a patent ductus arteriosus.

    B. Air has leaked under the electrode.

    C. The temperature inside the incubator has been increased.

    D. The patient's cardiac output and lung condition have improved.

16. A 17-year-old patient is receiving mechanical ventilation because of apnea resulting from a drug overdose. While the patient is breathing 25% oxygen, the following ABG values are analyzed:

    Pa_{O_2}, 155 torr

    Sa_{O_2}, 100%

    pH, 7.42

    Pa_{CO_2}, 41 torr

    HCO_3^-, 26 mEq/L

    BE, +2 mEq/L.

    What action should now be taken?

    A. Reduce the patient to 21% oxygen.

    B. Maintain the patient on present settings.

    C. Recheck the blood gas analyzer.

    D. Increase the tidal volume to hyperventilate the patient.

ANSWER KEY

1. **B.** Rationale: The patient's PA_{O_2} (pressure of alveolar oxygen) can be calculated as follows:

$$PA_{O_2} = ([P_B - PH_2O]\ FI_{O_2}) - \frac{Pa_{CO_2}}{0.8}$$
$$= ([750 - 54]\ 0.5) - \frac{36}{0.8}$$
$$= ([696]\ 0.5) - 45$$
$$= (348) - 45$$
$$= 303\ torr$$

2. **B.** Rationale: The patient's $P(A-a)_{O_2}$ (difference between alveolar and arterial pressure of oxygen) can be calculated as follows:

The patient's PA_{O_2} = 303 torr

The patient's Pa_{O_2} = −60 torr

243 torr

3. **D.** Rationale: The normal $P(A-a)_{O_2}$ difference should be no more than 25 torr for a healthy person of this age. The patient's difference of 243 torr is far greater than normal. No indication is found that the blood gas analyzer needs recalibration. If a normal person were breathing 50% oxygen, the Pa_{O_2} would be much higher (about 275 torr) than this patient's Pa_{O_2}. The difference is much larger than normal for a patient of this age (see Fig. 3-17).

4. **D.** Rationale: The modified Allen's test on the patient's right wrist is abnormal. It took 25 seconds for the return of adequate circulation through the ulnar artery. No arterial blood sample should be taken from the right radial artery because of poor collateral circulation through the ulnar artery (see Fig. 3-2). Check the circulation on the patient's left wrist by doing a modified Allen's test on it. Draw from the left radial artery if the test result is normal (less than 15 seconds for the return

of circulation). The Allen's test is a test of circulation through the radial artery, whereas the modified Allen's test is a test of circulation through the ulnar artery.

5. **A.** Rationale: A first-generation pulse oximeter value is of no use in evaluating a patient with carbon monoxide poisoning. This pulse oximeter technology is unable to distinguish carboxyhemoglobin from oxyhemoglobin; therefore the pulse-oximeter value will show a higher oxygen saturation than is actually present in the patient. A 12-lead electrocardiogram is needed to help determine the cause of the patient's irregular pulse. The patient may have had a heart attack as the result of profound hypoxemia. To evaluate the patient's oxygenation accurately, an arterial blood sample should be drawn and analyzed with a CO-oximeter. A CO-oximeter can distinguish between carboxyhemoglobin and oxyhemoglobin, so that the patient's actual Sa_{O_2} can be determined. A Glasgow Coma Scale analysis should be done to evaluate the patient's neurologic status. The patient may have had a stroke as the result of profound hypoxemia.

6. **B.** Rationale: A patient with septic shock who is receiving vasopressor therapy needs an arterial line to monitor blood pressure continuously. This is because the disease condition and the drugs result in considerable variation in blood pressure. A patient with ARDS who requires mechanical ventilation with PEEP needs frequent arterial blood sampling for gas analysis. Rather than puncture the patient's arteries for each sample, it is more humane and efficient to place an arterial line. In addition, the patient's blood pressure can be continuously monitored for the effects of PEEP. A patient

with suspected (or actual) carbon monoxide poisoning does not usually need more than one or two arterial blood samples taken for the diagnosis and the evaluation of treatment effectiveness. An arterial line is not justified. A patient with anxiety-induced hyperventilation is not hypoxic and does not need an ABG sample analyzed.

7. **D.** Rationale: The best way to assess the oxygenation status of a patient with carbon monoxide poisoning is to run an ABG sample through the CO-oximeter. The CO-oximeter is the only device that can accurately differentiate between carboxyhemoglobin and oxyhemoglobin (as well as other types of hemoglobin) and measure the amounts of each. Therefore it gives an accurate SaO_2 value. The first-generation pulse oximeter device is unable to distinguish between carboxyhemoglobin and oxyhemoglobin. This provides a false high value for SaO_2. The transcutaneous oxygen probe can be used to give an approximate tissue oxygen value. However, it is not the clinically accepted way to evaluate a patient with CO poisoning. Running an ABG sample through a standard blood gas analyzer results in measurements of oxygen, carbon dioxide, and pH. However, the SaO_2 value is calculated from the PaO_2. This can result in a falsely high value for the calculated SaO_2 if the patient is receiving supplemental oxygen and has an elevated PaO_2 (measured from the blood plasma).

8. **C.** Rationale: Because the correlation factor between the $PaCO_2$ and $PtcCO_2$ is 1.4, the solution to the problem requires that the patient's current $PtcCO_2$ of 76 torr be divided by 1.4, as follows:

$$\text{Approximate } PaCO_2 = PtcCO_2 \text{ of 76 torr} / 1.4$$
$$= 54 \text{ torr (actually 54.29 torr)}$$

9. **D.** Rationale: A PaO_2 of less than 80 torr is uncorrected hypoxemia. A compensated respiratory acidosis is indicated by the increased $PaCO_2$ coupled with an increased bicarbonate and increased base excess found with a normal pH. Review Tables 3-2 and 3-9 if needed.

10. **B.** Rationale: A PaO_2 of greater than 80 torr with supplemental oxygen is corrected hypoxemia. An uncompensated metabolic acidosis is indicated by the normal $PaCO_2$ coupled with a decreased bicarbonate and decreased base excess found with an acidotic pH. Review Tables 3-2 and 3-9 if needed.

11. **C.** Rationale: Normal oxygenation is indicated because the patient's PaO_2 is elevated secondary to hyperventilation ($PaCO_2$ of 25 torr). An uncompensated respiratory alkalosis is indicated by the low $PaCO_2$ coupled with a normal bicarbonate and normal base excess found with an alkalotic pH. Review Tables 3-2 and 3-9 if needed.

12. **A.** Rationale: A PaO_2 of less than 80 mm Hg is uncorrected hypoxemia. A combined metabolic and respiratory acidosis is indicated by the increased $PaCO_2$ coupled with a decreased bicarbonate and decreased base excess found with an acidotic pH. Review Tables 3-2 and 3-9 if needed.

13. **C.** Rationale: A PaO_2 of less than 80 mm Hg is uncorrected hypoxemia. A compensated respiratory alkalosis is indicated by the decreased $PaCO_2$ coupled with a decreased bicarbonate and decreased base excess found with a normal pH. Review Tables 3-2 and 3-9 if needed.

14. **B.** Rationale: A $P\bar{v}O_2$ value of 25 torr is quite low. A $P\bar{v}O_2$ value of 40 torr is normal, and a value below 30 torr usually indicates tissue hypoxia. An $S\bar{v}O_2$ of 80% is above the normal value of 75% and indicates above-normal tissue oxygenation. Review Table 3-11 if needed. Although a PaO_2 of 55 torr and SaO_2 of 88% are below normal, they do not necessarily indicate tissue hypoxia. Many patients with chronic lung disease live acceptable lives with values in this range.

15. **B.** Rationale: Because the PO_2 of room air is 150 torr, the only possible explanation for the dramatic increase in the patient's transcutaneous oxygen value has to be a leak of room air under the electrode. When the electrode is sealed to the patient's skin, the $PtcO_2$ value should decrease to the actual value. If the patient had a patent ductus arteriosus, a decrease in the $PtcO_2$ value would be found over the patient's left chest area and body. Usually a decrease in the $PtcO_2$ value over the right chest is not seen because this area receives preductal blood. An increased temperature inside the incubator would have no effect on the $PtcO_2$ value. However, a decrease in temperature inside the incubator could result in vasoconstriction and a resulting decrease in $PtcO_2$ value. Even if the patient's cardiac output and lung condition have improved, the $PtcO_2$ value is too high for a neonate breathing room air. (It is important also to realize that if a leak of room air occurs under the transcutaneous carbon dioxide electrode, a decrease in the $PtcCO_2$ value will be noted because room air contains virtually no carbon dioxide.)

16. **C.** Rationale: Recheck the blood gas analyzer for a problem with the PO_2 electrode. A calculation of the patient's PAO_2 shows that the maximum PaO_2 the patient can have is 127 torr. Until an accurate PaO_2 can be determined, no change should be seen in the patient's inspired oxygen percentage. Although no reason exists to doubt the pH and $PaCO_2$ values, no decision to maintain the patient on his or her present ventilator settings can be made until a correct PaO_2 value is obtained. No indication exists to hyperventilate this drug-overdose patient. Do not confuse this case with hyperventilation of a patient with a head injury and increased intracranial pressure.

4 Pulmonary Function Testing

Note 1: The National Board for Respiratory Care (NBRC) has released the *RRT Examination Matrix* (covering the testable items on the Written Registry Exam) and the *CSE Examination Matrix* (covering the testable items on the Clinical Simulation Exam). Turn to the appendices at the back of this book for both publications in their original format. This book is intended to cover all of the testable items in these two publications. This chapter (and all others) uses the abbreviation "WRE" for the coded items testable on the Written Registry Exam *and* Clinical Simulation Exam. The listed difficulty (R, Recall; Ap, Application; An, Analysis) relates to the question difficulty on the Written Registry Exam. The abbreviation "CSE" is used for the coded items testable on *only* the Clinical Simulation Exam. Because no question difficulty level is given for this exam, be prepared for anything.

Note 2: A review of the most recent Written Registry Examinations has shown an average of four questions (4% of the exam) that cover pulmonary function testing. The Clinical Simulation Exam is comprehensive and may include everything that should be known or performed by an advanced level respiratory therapist.

MODULE A

Review the patient's record for data on the following tests

1. Pulmonary function results (WRE code: IA4) [Difficulty: Ap, An]

Be prepared to review the results of all types of pulmonary function test (PFT) results. This chapter will cover the PFTs listed by the NBRC and other PFTs that have been tested by the NBRC.

2. Respiratory monitoring (WRE code: IA7b) [Difficulty: An]

Patients at risk of respiratory failure, such as those with neurologic disease, should have their breathing monitored regularly. Respiratory monitoring could include checking a patient's respiratory rate, tidal volume, minute volume, inspiratory/expiratory (I:E) ratio, maximum inspiratory pressure, maximum expiratory pressure, and airway graphics.

3. Lung compliance (WRE code: IA7c) [Difficulty: An]

Lung compliance is usually measured in patients with stiff lungs (as found with pulmonary fibrosis) or overly compliant lungs (as found with emphysema).

4. Airway resistance (WRE code: IA7c) [Difficulty: An]

Patients with asthma or chronic bronchitis may need to have airway resistance measured as part of their bronchodilator therapy management. Airway resistance will decrease if the proper type and amount of medication is taken.

MODULE B

Perform the following types of bedside spirometry tests

1. Lung mechanics tests

   a. Recommend lung mechanics tests to obtain additional data (WRE code: IC2) [Difficulty: Ap, An]

Different authors include various tests in the category of lung mechanics tests, including the following:
   a. Lung volumes and capacities except for those requiring the residual volume (RV).
   b. Spirometry for forced vital capacity (FVC) and flow values derived from the FVC. These values are needed to determine the degree of impairment in the obstructive diseases patient.
   c. Spirometry for flow-volume loop. This test is used to determine obstructive problems in the lungs or upper airway.
   d. Maximum inspiratory pressure (MIP) and maximum expiratory pressure (MEP). These values indicate the patient's overall respiratory muscle strength.

   b. Perform any of the lung mechanics (spirometry) tests (WRE Code: IIIE8) [Difficulty: An]

Discussion of the steps to perform and interpretation of the tests follow.

2. Tidal volume

a. Perform the procedure (WRE code: IB7c) [Difficulty: An]

The tidal volume (V_T) is the volume of gas breathed out in each respiratory cycle. Realize that individual tidal volumes are rarely identical. Fig. 4-1 shows several different tidal volumes before and after a nonforced (slow) vital capacity (VC). For that reason, it is recommended that the tidal volumes be accumulated for 1 minute (thus providing a minute volume [$\dot{V}_E$]) and the respiratory rate (f) counted. An average V_T is found by dividing the $\dot{V}_E$ by the respiratory f. If this cannot be done, find the average volume of at least six breaths. The average, predicted tidal volume for a resting, afebrile, alert adult should be about 3 to 4 mL/lb or 7 to 9 mL/kg of ideal body weight. For example, the predicted tidal volume range of a 154-lb (70-kg) patient is calculated as follows:

$$3 \text{ to } 4 \text{ mL/lb} \times 154 \text{ lb} = 462 \text{ to } 616 \text{ mL}$$
$$7 \text{ to } 9 \text{ mL/kg} \times 70 \text{ kg} = 490 \text{ to } 630 \text{ mL}$$

The patient should be allowed to relax before the test is performed so that the measured volume is accurate and not enlarged because of any undue stress or excitement. Keeping the instructions and demonstration simple and easy to follow help reduce the patient's anxiety. Some patients will not tolerate a full minute's tidal volume measurement. In that case, measure the accumulated tidal volumes for as long as possible, and divide by the number of respirations to obtain the average.

b. Interpret the results (WRE code: IB8c) [Difficulty: An]

A tidal volume that is larger or smaller than expected for the patient's size requires further evaluation. A small tidal volume may be seen in patients who have low metabolic rates, are asleep or in a coma, have neuromuscular diseases that make them unable to breathe deeply, or are alkalotic. A large tidal volume may be seen in patients with a high metabolic rate, fever, dead space–producing diseases, increased intracranial pressure, or acidotic conditions.

3. Monitor inspiratory/expiratory ratio (WRE code: IIIE9) [Difficulty: An]

The I:E ratio is the ratio of the patient's inspiratory time to the expiratory time. It can be simply measured at the bedside with a stopwatch. Again, make sure that the patient is relaxed and breathing in the normal pattern to get an accurate timing. Measure several of the patient's inspiratory times and expiratory times to figure an average for each. A spirometer that gives a printout is needed if a more complete analysis of the patient's breathing pattern is necessary.

The National Board of Respiratory Care (NBRC) is known to test the examinee's ability to calculate: (1) the inspiratory time (T_I) and expiratory time (T_E) from a given I:E ratio and respiratory rate; and (2) the I:E ratio from a given T_I and T_E. These examples should help.

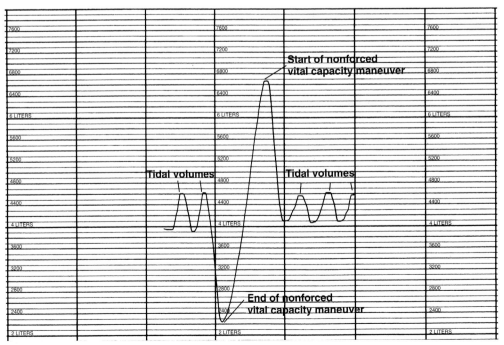

Fig. 4-1 Volume-time curve tracing of tidal volumes and nonforced vital capacity.

1. Calculate the patient's inspiratory time and expiratory time when the I:E ratio is 1:2 and the respiratory rate is 12/min.

    a. $\dfrac{60 \text{ sec/min}}{12 \text{ breaths/min}} = 5$ seconds/respiratory cycle

    b. $\dfrac{5 \text{ sec/respiratory cycle}}{3 \text{ parts of I and E}} = 1.66$ seconds for one part

    c. Inspiratory time = 1 part = 1.66 seconds

    d. Expiratory time = 2 parts = 3.32 seconds

2. Calculate the neonatal patient's I:E ratio when the inspiratory time is 0.3 seconds and expiratory time is 0.9 seconds.

    a. $I{:}E = \dfrac{I}{E} = \dfrac{0.3 \text{ seconds}}{0.9 \text{ seconds}}$

    b. $\dfrac{I}{E} = \dfrac{1}{3}$ (The I:E ratio is 1:3.)

A normal, spontaneously breathing patient has an I:E ratio of 1:2 to 1:4. A prolonged inspiratory time is often seen in patients with an upper airway obstruction. A prolonged expiratory time is often seen in patients with asthma or chronic obstructive pulmonary disease (COPD). Any abnormal I:E ratio should be investigated. For example, patients with Kussmaul's respiration, Cheyne-Stokes respiration, or Biot's respiration will have unusual I:E ratios.

4. Minute volume
a. Perform the procedure (WRE code: IB7c) [Difficulty: An]

The minute volume ($\dot{V}_E$) is the volume of gas exhaled in 1 minute. It is usually a more stable value than are individual tidal volumes. Minute volume is found by adding the accumulated tidal volumes for 1 minute. A simple handheld spirometer is often used to accumulate the tidal volume breaths. If the patient cannot perform the test for 1 minute, do it for 30 seconds, and double the value.

b. Interpret the results (WRE code: IB8c) [Difficulty: An]

The predicted range for a minute volume in a resting, afebrile, alert adult should be 5 to 10 L/min. The wide range is found in part because it is a product of two factors: tidal volume and respiratory rate. It is possible for either one or both of these factors to be normal, abnormally high, or abnormally low. For these reasons, the minute volume must be evaluated along with the tidal volume and respiratory rate to reach any conclusion about the patient's condition. The same factors that have an impact on the tidal volume affect the patient's minute ventilation.

5. Alveolar ventilation
a. Perform the procedure (WRE code: IB7c) [Difficulty: An]

Alveolar ventilation (V_A) is the amount of tidal volume that reaches the alveoli. It is calculated by subtracting the physiologic dead space (anatomic plus alveolar dead space) from the measured exhaled tidal volume. For a bedside test,

it is possible to subtract only the estimated anatomic dead space. It is estimated at 1 mL/lb or 2.2 mL/kg of ideal body weight. The alveolar dead-space measurement requires sophisticated equipment, which is usually available only in the pulmonary function testing laboratory. Clinically normal people have very little alveolar dead space.

EXAMPLE

A 154-lb/70-kg person has a measured tidal volume of 500 mL and an estimated anatomic dead space of about 154 mL. The calculated alveolar ventilation = 500 mL − 154 mL = 346 mL.

b. Interpret the results (WRE code: IB8c) [Difficulty: An]

The following examples show how the patient's alveolar ventilation can vary considerably because of changes in the respiratory rate and tidal volume even though the minute volume remains unchanged. These examples are included to show the importance of alveolar ventilation on the patient's Pa_{CO_2} values.

EXAMPLE 1

Normal patient: f = 12, tidal volume = 500 mL, anatomic dead space = 154 mL

$$\text{minute alveolar ventilation } (\dot{V}_A) = 12 \times (500 \text{ mL} - 154 \text{ mL})$$
$$= 12 \times 346 \text{ mL}$$
$$= 4152 \text{ mL}$$

This patient should have a normal carbon dioxide level.

EXAMPLE 2

Tachypneic patient: f = 24, tidal = volume 250 mL, anatomic dead space = 154 mL

$$\text{minute volume} = 24 \times \text{minute volume}$$
$$= 12 \times 500 \text{ mL} = 6000 \text{ mL}$$
$$\text{minute alveolar ventilation } (\dot{V}_A) = 24 \times (250 \text{ mL} - 154 \text{ mL})$$
$$= 24 \times 96 \text{ mL}$$
$$= 2304 \text{ mL}$$

This patient should have a high carbon dioxide level.

EXAMPLE 3

Bradypneic patient: f = 6, tidal volume = 1000 mL, anatomic dead space = 154 mL

$$\text{minute volume} = 6 \times 1000 \text{ mL} = 6000 \text{ mL}$$
$$\text{minute alveolar ventilation } (\dot{V}_A) = 6 \times (1000 \text{ mL} - 154 \text{ mL})$$
$$= 6 \times 846 \text{ mL}$$
$$= 5076 \text{ mL}$$

This patient should have a low carbon dioxide level.

6. Measure and interpret the patient's maximum inspiratory pressure at the bedside
a. Perform the procedure (WRE code: IB7g) [Difficulty: An]

The MIP is the greatest amount of negative pressure that the patient can create when inspiring against an occluded airway. It also is known as negative inspiratory force (NIF).

The following factors affect the test results: strength of the diaphragm and accessory muscles of inspiration, lung volume when the airway is occluded, ventilatory drive, and the length of time the airway is occluded. It is most commonly used to determine the weanability of mechanically ventilated patients. In addition, it is used to help monitor the strength of patients with a neuromuscular disease.

A study of the literature reveals that a number of measurement devices have been assembled and that different bedside techniques have been used to determine the effort of a patient breathing naturally, an intubated patient, and a patient breathing with assistance from a mechanical ventilator. Branson and colleagues and Kacmarek and colleagues make a strong case for the use of a double one-way valve to connect the intubated patient to the manometer (Fig. 4-2). Use of the one-way valve lets the patient exhale but prevents an inhalation when the practitioner occludes the opening. This forces the patient to inhale from closer to residual volume with each breathing effort. They also recommend that the patient make inspiratory efforts for 15 to 20 seconds.

Steps in the MIP procedure for a normally breathing patient include the following:

Fig. 4-2 Two systems for measuring maximal inspiratory pressure (MIP) on a patient with an artificial airway. System **A**, Simple occlusion. *A*, Pressure manometer; *B*, connecting tubing; *C*, port to be occluded during the MIP; *D*, connection of the adapter to the manometer; *E*, port to connect to the patient's airway. System **B**, One-way valve. *A*, Pressure manometer; *B*, connecting tubing; *C*, inspiratory port to be occluded during the MIP effort; *D*, expiratory port; *E*, port to be connected to the patient's artificial airway. *(From Kacmarek RM, Cycyk-Chapman MC, Young-Palazzo PJ, et al: Determination of maximal inspiratory pressure: a clinical study and literature review, Respir Care 34:868–878, 1989, with permission.)*

1. Obtain a pressure gauge capable of measuring at least −60 cm water pressure.
2. Have the patient sit upright. Place a note in the chart if the patient is lying down.
3. Describe the procedure to the patient.
4. Simulate a demonstration of the procedure.
5. Place nose clips over the patient's nose. Have the patient seal his or her lips and teeth around the mouthpiece and breathe through the open port.
6. Tell the patient to exhale completely. Seal the port when residual volume has been reached.
7. Tell the patient to breathe in as hard as possible and hold it for 1 to 3 seconds.
8. Reteach if necessary.
9. Repeat until at least three good efforts have been performed. Record the greatest stable value seen after the first second of effort. This eliminates any artifact created by the cheeks or by chest wall movement.

b. Interpret the results (WRE code: IB8f) [Difficulty: An]

Patients of either sex and of any age should be able to generate at least −60 cm H_2O. This is enough to offer assurance that the patient has enough strength and coordination to protect the airway, take a deep breath, and cough effectively. Patients with neuromuscular diseases, diseases of the respiratory muscles, thoracic injury or abnormality, and chronic obstructive lung diseases tend to have decreased strength. The patient who cannot generate at least −20 cm H_2O is at risk. This patient probably does not have the strength to cough effectively. Depending on the blood gas values and other physical parameters, the patient may need to be intubated and maintained on a mechanical ventilator.

Black and Hyatt published the following MIP prediction formulas for spontaneous breathing in nonintubated adult subjects between 20 and 86 years old who are breathing from residual volume. The values are in centimeters of water pressure (cm H_2O). As can be seen, the older the patient, the lower the predicted negative inspiratory force.

		Lower limits of normal
Males:	$143 - (0.55 \times age) =$	−75 cm H_2O
Females:	$104 - (0.51 \times age) =$	−50 cm H_2O

c. Monitor the patient (WRE code: IIIE9) [Difficulty: An]

A patient being weaned from mechanical ventilation or with a deteriorating neuromuscular condition should have the MIP measured on a regular, frequent basis. If the patient's pressure is only −20 cm H_2O, the physician should be notified. Mechanical ventilation is probably needed.

It is important to monitor any patient for signs of undue stress and hypoxemia such as tachycardia, bradycardia, ventricular dysrhythmias, hypertension, hypotension, and decreasing saturation on pulse oximetry. If any of these are seen, the procedure should be stopped and the patient reoxygenated and ventilated. Some patients achieve their best effort on the first or second inspiration and have decreasing effort as they continue trying. This is probably because of fatigue. Stop the procedure, and record the best effort.

7. Maximum expiratory pressure
a. Perform the procedure (WRE code: IB7g) [Difficulty: An]

The maximum expiratory pressure (MEP) is the greatest amount of positive pressure that the patient can create when expiring from total lung capacity (TLC) against an occluded airway. It also is known as a maximum expiratory force (MEF). The following factors affect the test results: patient cooperation and effort, strength of the expiratory muscles, lung volume when the airway is occluded, ventilatory drive, and the length of time the airway is occluded. It is used to determine the weanability of mechanically ventilated patients and to monitor the strength of patients with a neuromuscular disease.

As with the MIP test, a study of the literature reveals that a number of measurement devices have been assembled and that different bedside techniques have been used to determine the effort of a patient breathing naturally and the effort of one who is intubated and is breathing by way of a mechanical ventilator. A strong case can be made for the use of a double one-way valve to connect the intubated patient to the manometer (see Fig. 4-2). Use of the one-way valves lets the patient inhale but prevents an exhalation when the practitioner occludes the expiratory opening. This forces the patient to exhale from closer to TLC with each breathing effort. However, the expiratory efforts should not be held for more than 3 seconds. This test is similar to the Valsalva maneuver and can cause a reduction in the cardiac output because of the high intrathoracic pressure.

Steps in the MEP procedure for a normally breathing patient include the following:

1. Obtain a pressure gauge capable of measuring at least +60 cm water pressure.
2. Have the patient sit upright. Place a note in the chart if the patient is lying down.
3. Describe the procedure to the patient.
4. Simulate a demonstration of the procedure.
5. Place nose clips over the patient's nose. Have the patient seal his or her lips and teeth around the mouthpiece and breathe through the open port.
6. Tell the patient to inhale completely. Seal the port when TLC has been reached.
7. Tell the patient to breathe out as hard as possible. Hold it for 1 to 3 seconds.
8. Reteach if necessary.
9. Repeat until at least three good efforts have been performed. Record the greatest stable value seen after

the first second of effort. This eliminates any artifact created by the cheeks or chest wall movement.

It is important to monitor any patient for signs of undue stress and hypoxemia such as tachycardia, bradycardia, ventricular dysrhythmias, hypotension, and decreasing saturation on pulse oximetry. If any of these is seen, the procedure should be stopped, and the patient reoxygenated and ventilated.

b. Interpret the results (WRE code: IB8f) [Difficulty: An]

Clinically normal people of either sex and of any age should be able to generate at least +80 cm water pressure. Patients with neuromuscular diseases, thoracic injury or abnormality, and COPD tend to have decreased strength. A MEP value of +40 cm water is probably enough to offer assurance that the patient has enough strength and coordination to cough effectively to clear secretions. However, depending on the blood gas values and other physical parameters, the patient may need to be intubated and maintained on a mechanical ventilator.

Black and Hyatt published the following MEP prediction formulas for spontaneously breathing nonintubated adult subjects between 20 and 86 years old who are breathing from TLC. The values are in centimeters of water pressure. As can be seen, the older the patient, the lower the predicted maximum expiratory force.

	Lower limits of normal
Males: $268 - (1.03 \times age)$	$+ 140$ cm H_2O
Females: $170 - (0.53 \times age)$	$+ 95$ cm H_2O

8. Vital capacity
a. Perform the test (WRE code: IB7c) [Difficulty: An]

The nonforced (slow) vital capacity (VC or SVC) is the greatest volume of gas that the patient can exhale after the lungs have been completely filled. The therapist should demonstrate the procedure to the patient. He or she must understand that there is no need to blow out fast while emptying the lungs. The measurement device can be a simple, hand-held spirometer if a printout of the result is not needed. A portable, computer-based spirometer can be used, if needed, to generate a printout of the results or a graphic tracing. Normally at least *three* efforts are made, and the largest is recorded.

b. Interpret the results (WRE code: IB8c) [Difficulty: An]

See Fig. 4-1 for a graphic tracing of a nonforced VC. Compare it with the tracing on Fig. 4-3, which shows an FVC. In a patient without obstructive lung disease, the same volume should be found in a nonforced VC and FVC. The following discussion on the FVC includes predicted values for male and female patients and guidelines on the interpretation of the patient's results.

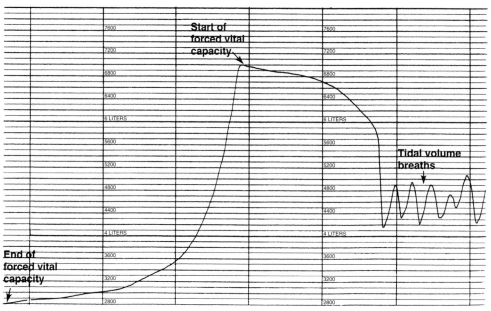

Fig. 4-3 Tracing of tidal volumes and forced vital capacity.

MODULE C

Advanced spirometry

1. Forced vital capacity

a. Perform the test (WRE code: IB7d and IIIE8) [Difficulty: An]

The FVC is the greatest volume of gas that the patient can exhale as rapidly as possible after the lungs have been completely filled. Normally, the FVC is the same volume as that found in a slow or nonforced VC. Careful instructions, demonstrations, and coaching are needed to ensure that the patient's efforts are the best possible. At least *three* proper efforts must be obtained.

If the measurement instrument does not give a printout, simply record the patient's efforts in the chart. If the measurement instrument does give a printout, include copies of the efforts. See Fig. 4-3 for the tracing of a properly performed FVC. The tracing enables us to compare the volumes exhaled in a series of 1-second intervals. Because of this, the tracing is often referred to as a *volume-time curve*. Notice that the start of the effort is smooth and without interruption. The initial fast flow of gas from the upper airway is seen as the nearly vertical part of the tracing. The rest of the tracing is smooth without any coughing or other interruptions in the patient's effort. The tracing becomes progressively more horizontal as the end of the effort is reached. Encourage the patient to try to push out as much air as possible as the end approaches. To be an acceptable FVC, the patient must show maximal effort without coughing or closing the glottis, and the expiratory effort must last at least 6 seconds. The patient's final 2 seconds of expiratory effort should show no appreciable airflow.

b. Interpret airway graphics (WRE code: IIIE8) [Difficulty: An]

Fig. 4-3 was made on a chain-compensated, water-seal spirometry system. Notice how the tracing progresses from the right to the left. The Stead-Wells system shows the same tracing "upside down" compared with the chain-compensated system. The tracing starts on the left and moves to the right (Figs. 4-4 and 4-5). Other tracings may show either the chain-compensated or Stead-Wells tracings in a mirror image or opposite shape.

> ### Exam Hint
>
> The NBRC can show a FVC tracing from any system and expect it to be interpreted. The start of the FVC effort can be determined by the near vertical portion of the tracing and the relatively small expiratory reserve volume (ERV) compared with the inspiratory reserve volume (IRV). You must be able to determine the various volumes and capacities from a spirometry tracing.

c. Interpret the results (WRE code: IB8d) [Difficulty: An]

Normal racial differences in the FVC must be taken into consideration. Most modern pulmonary function systems automatically adjust the measured values for racial differences when so programmed by the operator. If not, the predicted values should be mathematically adjusted by the therapist. The predicted white patient normal values in liters

Fig. 4-4 Forced vital capacity (FVC) tracings showing an obstructed flow pattern and a restrictive flow pattern. Note that the patient with the obstructive pattern has a slower than normal exhalation, whereas the patient with the restrictive pattern has a faster-than-normal exhalation. *(From Ruppel G: Manual of pulmonary function testing, ed 6, St Louis, 1994, Mosby.)*

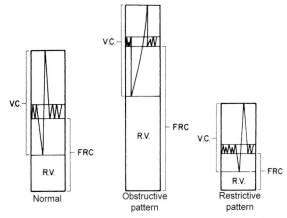

Fig. 4-5 Spirometry tracings of a normal, obstructed, and restricted patient. Note how the obstructed and restricted patients' volumes and capacities are out of proportion compared with those of the normal patient. VC, Vital capacity; RV, residual volume; FRC, functional residual capacity. *(From Cherniack RM: Pulmonary function testing, Philadelphia, 1977, WB Saunders.)*

for the FVC* were reported by Morris, Koski, and Johnson (1971) as

$$\text{Men: } [(0.148 \times \text{height in inches}) - (0.025 \times \text{age})]$$
$$- 4.24 \text{ [SD (1 standard deviation) 0.58]}$$

$$\text{Women: } [(0.115 \times \text{height in inches}) - (0.024 \times \text{age})]$$
$$- 2.85 \text{ (SD 0.52)}$$

EXAMPLE

Calculate the predicted FVC of a 50-year-old white man who is 6 feet (72 inches) tall.

$$\begin{aligned} \text{FVC} &= [(0.148 \times \text{height in inches}) - (0.025 \times \text{age})] - 4.24 \\ &= [(0.148 \times 72) - (0.025 \times 50)] - 4.24 \\ &= (10.656 - 1.25) - 4.24 \\ &= 9.406 - 4.24 \\ &= 5.166 \text{ L} \end{aligned}$$

It is known that blacks have a smaller lung capacity than whites of the same height. Because of this, a 10% to 15% adjustment should be made for the predicted FVC and TLC of a black patient. In other words, the predicted values for a black patient are 85% to 90% of those of a comparable white patient.

---

*The body, temperature, pressure, saturated (BTPS) correction has been calculated into these equations.
Note: These and some other researchers have already calculated a standard patient and room temperature and barometric pressure into their formulas.

Adjustments for Hispanic and Asian populations are not so well documented. It has been reported that the predicted FVC values should be adjusted down by 20% to 25% for Asians.

It has been commonly accepted that a measured FVC that is at least 80% of the predicted FVC is considered to be within normal limits for adults of all races. In addition, the forced expiratory volume in 1 second (FEV_1) and TLC measurements have been included in this 80% of predicted rule. More recent studies by Knudson, Kaltenborn, Knudson, and associates (1987) and Paoletti, Viegi, Pistelli, and associates (1985) suggest that normal values for most tests should be determined by finding the percentage of predicted value above which 95% of the population would be seen (the so-called "normal 95th percentile"). Even though this method finds 5% (1 in 20) of healthy nonsmokers to be abnormal, it offers more realistic predicted values. It is normal to see a decline in the FVC with age.

Restrictive problems such as advanced pregnancy, obesity, ascites, neuromuscular disease, sarcoidosis, and chest wall or spinal deformity can result in a small FVC. Patients with chronic obstructive lung diseases such as emphysema, bronchitis, asthma, cystic fibrosis, and bronchiectasis commonly have a small FVC. (Fig. 4-5 shows a comparison of the spirometry tracings of a normal, obstructed, and restricted patient.)

The limitations of this text prevent a discussion of back extrapolation to find the start of a less-than-perfect effort or the calculations for converting volumes and flows from atmospheric temperature, pressure, saturated (ATPS) to body temperature, pressure, saturated (BTPS). However, most PF textbooks discuss these topics.

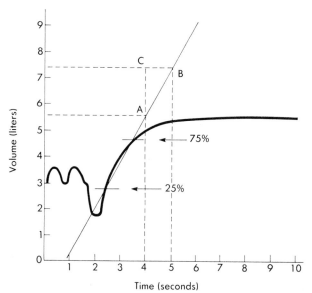

Fig. 4-6 One method of determining the 25% to 75% forced expiratory flow (FEF$_{25\%-75\%}$) value from a forced vital capacity (FVC) tracing. First, mark the 25% and 75% points from the start of the effort. These are found by multiplying the FVC value by 0.25 and 0.75, respectively, and measuring from the start of the effort. Second, draw a line through these two points to intersect the dashed time lines at points A and B. Horizontal dashed lines are added from A and B to cross the volume scale. The FEF$_{25\%-75\%}$ value is read as the distance between A and C or about 2 L/sec. BTPS correct this measurement. *(From Ruppel G: Manual of pulmonary function testing, ed 5, St Louis, 1991, Mosby.)*

Exam Hint

It may be necessary to calculate how close a patient's FVC or other breathing effort has come to his or her predicted value. This is known as the patient's percentage of predicted. It is found by this equation:

$$\frac{\text{Patient's actual test result}}{\text{Patient's predicted test value}} \times 100 = \text{Patient's \% of predicted}$$

For example, in the previous discussion on FVC, it was determined that a patient has a predicted FVC of 5.166 L. Calculate the percentage of predicted if the actual FVC result is 4.65 L.

$$\frac{4.65\ L}{5.116} \times 100 = \text{patient's \% of predicted}$$

$$= .90 \times 100 = 90\%$$

Therefore the patient exhaled 90% of predicted FVC and is within the normal range for that test result.

2. Peak flow

a. Perform the procedure (WRE code: IB7e and IIIE8) [Difficulty: An]

The peak flow (PF) is the greatest flow rate seen in a patient's forced expiratory effort. Some authors refer to the PF as the peak expiratory flow rate (PEFR). It is usually seen at the beginning of the FVC effort. The instructions for the test must emphasize that the patient must "blast" the air out as hard and fast as possible. It is not necessary to encourage the patient to empty the lungs completely to residual volume.

The patient's effort is easily directly measured with a handheld peak flowmeter. Usually at least three efforts are required to find two that are acceptably close. PF values that are consistent and low despite variable patient efforts probably indicate a malfunctioning unit that should not be used. It is reasonable to record the patient's effort in liters per second because the effort takes place in about that much time. However, do not be confused by some measurement instruments and other prediction equations giving the value in liters per minute. Simply multiply or divide by 60 to convert your patient's effort from one time frame to the other. For example, a young man's PF might be recorded as 10 L/sec or 600 L/min. Cherniack and Raber (1972) published the following formulas for predicting PF in liters per second[*]:

Men: [(0.144 × height in inches) − (0.024 × age)] + 2.225

Women: [(0.090 × height in inches) − (0.018 × age)] + 1.130

b. Interpret the results (WRE code: IB8c) [Difficulty: An]

The PF is directly related to height and indirectly related to age. Therefore the taller the patient, the greater the PF. The PF decreases with age. The PF is a rather nonspecific measurement of airway obstruction. It measures flow through the upper airways and is reduced in patients with an upper airway problem like a tumor, vocal cord paralysis, or laryngeal edema.

The PF test is most often given to patients having an asthma attack as a quick and easy measurement of small-airways obstruction. Current asthma guidelines state that if an asthma patient's peak flow is 80% to 100% of predicted or personal best, he or she is in the "green zone." This means that the patient's medications are adequately controlling the asthma. If the peak flow is 50% to 79% of predicted or personal best, he or she is in the "yellow zone." This means that the patient's medications are not adequately controlling the asthma. Increased doses are indicated if ordered by the physician. If the peak flow is less than 50% of predicted or personal best, he or she is in the "red zone." This means that the patient's medications

---

[*]The BTPS correction has been calculated into these equations.

are not adequately controlling the asthma. The patient should get medical help as soon as possible.

3. Timed, forced expiratory volumes

All of the timed, forced expiratory volume tests are derived from a properly performed FVC test. (see Fig. 4-3). When the FVC is done correctly, the following values can be properly calculated and evaluated to determine the patient's condition. As discussed earlier, an FVC that is within 80% of predicted is interpreted as within normal limits. Because of this, if the results of the following tests show patient values within 80% of predicted, the results are interpreted as being within normal limits.

a. Forced expiratory flow$_{25\%-75\%}$ (FEF$_{25\%-75\%}$)
1. Perform the procedure (WRE code: IB7m) [Difficulty: An]

The FEF$_{25\%-75\%}$ is the mean forced expiratory flow during the middle half of an acceptable FVC (see Fig. 4-6). The FVC effort to use for this test is the one that has the greatest combination of FVC volume and FEV$_1$. As mentioned earlier, the patient must give his or her best effort. The measurement is usually recorded in liters per second but may be recorded in liters per minute.

b. Interpret the results (WRE code: IB8i) [Difficulty: An]

The results are normally less than in the FEF$_{200-1200}$ and PF tests because the flow being measured comes from medium-size and small airways (smaller than 2 mm in diameter). The results should decline with age and be lower in women than in men. A patient with a restrictive lung disease may have a normal or increased value, whereas a low value is seen in a patient with obstructive lung disease. A small FEF$_{25\%-75\%}$ value when the FVC, FEV$_1$, and FEF$_{200-1200}$ values are normal is often taken to indicate early small airways disease. A normal 150-lb/68-kg young man should have values of 4 to 5 L/sec or 240 to 300 L/min. The following formulas[*] were developed by Morris, Koski, and Johnson (1971) and can be used to calculate the predicted values in liters per second:

Men: [(0.047 × height in inches) − (0.045 × age in years)] + 2.513 (SD 1.12)

Women: [(0.060 × height in inches) − (0.030 × age in years)] + 0.551 (SD 0.80)

c. Forced expiratory volume, timed (FEV$_T$)
1. Perform the procedure (WRE code: IB7d) [Difficulty: An]

The FEV$_T$ is the volume of air exhaled from an acceptable FVC in the specified time. The time increments are 0.5, 1, 2, and 3 seconds or more and are listed as FEV$_{0.5}$, FEV$_1$,

FEV$_2$, FEV$_3$, and so on. It is important that the FVC have a good start and a maximal effort to the end.

The FEV$_1$ is the most commonly used measurement, along with the FVC value, to judge the patient's response to inhaled bronchodilators, for bronchoprovocation testing to screen for asthmatic tendencies, to detect exercise-induced asthma, and for simple screening. BTPS correct all the measured values.

The timed forced expiratory volumes (FEV$_{.5}$, FEV$_1$, FEV$_2$, FEV$_3$) effectively "cut" the FVC into sections based on how much volume the patient forcibly exhales in 0.5, 1, 2, and 3 seconds. Some patients with severe obstructive lung disease require several more seconds to exhale completely. In these cases, simply keep measuring the volume exhaled in each additional second. See Fig. 4-7 for an FVC tracing that is subdivided at 0.5-, 1-, 2-, and 3-second intervals. Some bedside units give a numeric value for some or all the timed intervals; however, it is best to have a spirometer that produces a printed copy of the patient's FVC effort. The individual volumes can be determined by marking the vertical distance on the volume scale from the baseline (total lung capacity) to the respective arrow tips.

2. Interpret the results (WRE code: IB8d) [Difficulty: An]

The FEV$_T$ values are often reduced in both restrictive and obstructive lung diseases. Patients with a severe restrictive lung disease exhale almost all of their small FVC within the first second. Patients with severe obstructive lung disease

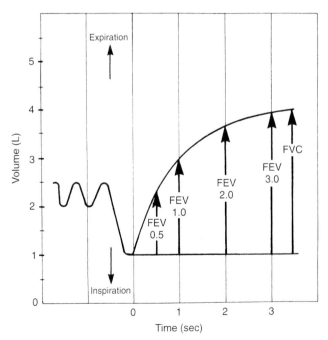

Fig. 4-7 Forced vital capacity divided into FEV$_{0.5}$, FEV$_{1.0}$, FEV$_{2.0}$, and FEV$_{3.0}$. *(From Ruppel G:* Manual of pulmonary function testing, *ed 4, St Louis, 1986, Mosby.)*

---

[*]The BTPS correction has been calculated into these equations.

show low values at all time intervals, with the volumes at $FEV_{2, 3, etc.}$ becoming progressively smaller. The most commonly evaluated values are the FEV_1 and the $FEV_{1\%}$. The following formulas[*] were developed by Morris, Koski, and Johnson (1971) and can be used to calculate the predicted values for FEV_1 in liters:

Men: $[(0.092 \times$ height in inches$) - (0.032 \times$ age in years$)]$
$- 1.260$ (SD .55)

Women: $[(0.089 \times$ height in inches$) - (0.024 \times$ age in years$)]$
$- 1.93$ (SD 0.47)

d. Forced expiratory volume/forced vital capacity ratio (FEV_T/FVC or $FEV_{T\%}$)
1. Perform the procedure (WRE code: IB7d) [Difficulty: An]

The FEV (timed)-to-FVC ratio compares by division the volume exhaled at 0.5, 1, 2, and 3 (or more) seconds (see Fig. 4-7) with the FVC. This results in a series of decimal fractions. These are multiplied by 100 to convert the answers to percentages.

It must be obvious that every person exhales different volumes for the FEV time intervals because each person's FVC is different. This procedure mathematically standardizes the results regardless of the patient's FVC. Therefore these percentage values can be standardized for all individuals despite different FVCs. The predicted values for normal patients are as follows:

$FEV_{0.5}$ = 50% to 60% of the FVC
FEV_1 = 75% to 85% of the FVC
FEV_2 = 94% of the FVC
FEV_3 = 97% of the FVC

2. Interpret the results (WRE code: IB8d) [Difficulty: An]

These values normally decrease slightly in the elderly patient. Most patients with normal lungs and airways are still able to completely exhale their FVC within 4 seconds.

Patients with restrictive lung diseases often exhale their FVC more quickly than expected. This abnormal finding is caused by these patients having a smaller-than-normal FVC and stiff lungs that recoil more quickly than expected to their resting volume. See Fig. 4-4 to compare the FVC curves of a patient with restrictive lung disease with the FVC curves of a patient with obstructive lung disease.

Patients with obstructive lung disease take longer than expected to exhale their FVC. As a result, the percentages of the FVC exhaled in the timed intervals listed are lower than normal. Obviously, the lower the percentage exhaled for any timed interval, the worse the obstruction to exhalation. A patient with restrictive lung disease exhales the

FVC too quickly, and all of the derived values are higher than expected.

Exam Hint

Of these tests, the FEV_1 is the most important to monitor. An FEV_1 of less than 70% of the FVC confirms obstructive lung disease.

MODULE D
Special purpose pulmonary function tests

1. Spirometry before and after an aerosolized bronchodilator has been inhaled
a. Perform the procedure (WRE code: IB7m) [Difficulty: An]

The following are common indications for the procedure:
1. Patient is known to have asthma or another type of chronic obstructive lung disease.
2. The patient has an $FEV_{1\%}$ of less than 70% (unless elderly).
3. The effectiveness of a new bronchodilator is being evaluated.

The most commonly administered tests are the PF and $FEV_{1\%}$ from an FVC. Before starting the test, make sure that the patient has not taken a bronchodilating drug in the previous 4 to 6 hours. If no bronchodilating drugs have been administered, the test can be performed. A PF or $FEV_{1\%}$ test should be performed, and the value(s) should be measured, and then a fast-onset sympathomimetic-type drug is given. The medication can be given by intermittent positive pressure breathing (IPPB), handheld nebulizer, or metered dose inhaler, as long as the method is done properly. Wait about 10 to 15 minutes for the medication to take effect and the patient's blood gas values to return to normal. Then repeat the PF or $FEV_{1\%}$ test. The percentage of improvement is calculated by using this formula:

$$\text{Percentage of change} = \frac{\text{after drug airflow} - \text{before drug airflow}}{\text{before drug airflow}} \times 100$$

b. Interpret the results (WRE code: IB8i) [Difficulty: An]

To prove that the medication is effective, the current standard requires the patient to have at least a 12% improvement in PF or $FEV_{1\%}$ or both and a 200-mL increase in exhaled volume. (The old standard required a 15% to 20% improvement in flow.) It is not uncommon to see patients with asthma improve much more than this. Other patients may not have this much improvement but do show increases in airflow and FVC and say that they feel better. In these cases, the physician may decide to continue the medication.

---

[*]The BTPS correction has been calculated into these equations.

2. Flow-volume loops

a. Perform the procedure (WRE code: IB7m) [Difficulty: An]

The flow-volume loop is a graphic display of the flow and volume generated during a forced expiratory vital capacity (FEVC) that is immediately followed by a forced inspiratory vital capacity (FIVC). It is used to identify inspiratory or expiratory flow at any lung volume.

As with the FVC test, the patient should be coached to inhale completely and blast the air out until he or she is completely empty. When you are sure that the patient has exhaled to residual volume, coach him or her to inhale as quickly as possible until the lungs are completely full. No hesitation at the start, leaks, glottis closing, or coughing should occur throughout the entire procedure.

The expiratory half of the curve is called the maximum expiratory flow-volume (MEFV) curve. It begins at TLC and ends at residual volume. The inspiratory half of the curve is called the maximum inspiratory flow-volume (MIFV) curve. It begins at residual volume and ends at TLC. Ideally, the two halves of the loop meet at the TLC. Flow is recorded in liters per second and graphed on the vertical (ordinate or Y) axis. Volume is recorded in liters and graphed on the horizontal (abscissa or X) axis. Both flow and volume should be BTPS adjusted.

b. Interpret the results (WRE code: IB8i) [Difficulty: An]

Flow-volume loops have gained great popularity because the shape of the curve is diagnostic of the patient's condition. In addition, peak inspiratory and peak expiratory flows can be determined. If the effort can be timed, all the parameters found on the previously discussed volume-time curves can be found on the flow-volume loop. The following examples show a normal flow-volume loop and representative abnormal loops.

Normal. A normal flow-volume loop is shown in Figs. 4-8 and 4-9. First look at Fig. 4-8, in which the various volumes are measured on the horizontal scale. The tidal volume (VT) of 500 mL is the small loop within the larger VC loop. The ERV and IRV are shown on both sides of the tidal volume. The FVC is shown as the total of all three volumes. Finally, TLC and residual volume (RV) are marked.

Fig. 4-9 shows the same normal flow-volume loop in which the various flows are measured on the vertical scale.

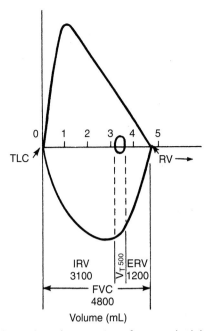

Fig. 4-8 Flow-volume loop tracing of a normal adult showing the positions and values of the lung volumes. *ERV*, Expiratory reserve volume; *FVC*, forced vital capacity; *IRV*, inspiratory reserve volume; *RV*, residual volume; *TLC*, total lung capacity.

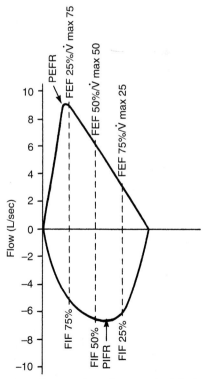

Fig. 4-9 Flow-volume loop tracing of a normal adult showing the positions and values of the various inspiratory and expiratory flows. *FEF*, Forced expiratory flow; *FIF*, forced inspiratory flow; *PEFR*, peak expiratory flow rate; *PIFR*, peak inspiratory flow rate.

Starting from TLC with the FEVC, the peak expiratory flow rate (PEFR) is seen as the greatest flow that is generated; it is about 9 L/sec. Starting from RV with the FIVC, the peak inspiratory flow rate (PIFR) is seen as the greatest flow that is generated; it is about 7 L/sec. It is normal for the PEFR to be greater than the PIFR.

To find the instantaneous flow at any FVC lung volume, the FVC must be divided by 4 to find the 25th, 50th, and 75th percentile points. In Fig. 4-8, the FVC is 4800 mL. Dividing by 4 gives 1200 mL per quarter of the FVC. These points are marked on the horizontal volume scale. If a vertical (dashed) line is drawn through these three points to the flow-volume tracing, the instantaneous flows at these volumes can be found. *Expiratory flows* are reported as

1. Flow at 75% of the FEVC = $\dot{V}_{max75}$ (maximum flow with 75% of the FVC remaining) or $FEF_{25\%}$ (forced expiratory flow with 25% of the FVC exhaled)
2. Flow at 50% of the FEVC = $\dot{V}_{max50}$ (maximum flow with 50% of the FVC remaining) or $FEF_{50\%}$ (forced expiratory flow with 50% of the FVC exhaled)
3. Flow at 25% of the FEVC = $\dot{V}_{max25}$ (maximum flow with 25% of the FVC remaining) or $FEF_{75\%}$ (forced expiratory flow with 75% of the FVC exhaled)

Inspiratory flows are reported as

1. Flow at 25% of the FIVC = $FIF_{25\%}$ (forced inspiratory flow with 25% of the FVC inhaled)
2. Flow at 50% of the FIVC = $FIF_{50\%}$ (forced inspiratory flow with 50% of the FVC inhaled)
3. Flow at 75% of the FIVC = $FIF_{75\%}$ (forced inspiratory flow with 75% of the FVC inhaled)

The PEFR and FEF_{25} or $\dot{V}_{max75\%}$ values should be about the same because they all measure flow through the large upper airways. Either test is a good gauge of the patient's effort because it will be low if the patient is not trying hard. The FEF_{50} or $\dot{V}_{max50\%}$ values should approximate the $FEF_{25\%-75\%}$ values because they both show flow through the medium to small airways in the middle half of the FVC effort. It is normal for the FIF_{50} to be greater than the FEF_{50}. The FEF_{75} or $\dot{V}_{max25\%}$ values are the best indicator of early small-airways disease because both show flow through the small airways as the patient approaches the residual volume. Note that the tracing from the FEF_{25} or $\dot{V}_{max75\%}$ point to the residual volume is close to a straight line. In normal people, the flow decreases in proportion to the decreasing lung volume, resulting in the straight-line tracing. Cherniack and Raber (1972) published formulas for predicting adult MEFV flows in liters per second; see the bibliography.

Small airways disease. Examples of conditions resulting in small-airways disease (less than 2 mm in diameter) include asthma, chronic bronchitis, bronchiectasis, cystic fibrosis, and emphysema. The obstruction can be from bronchospasm, mucus plugging, or damage to the alveoli and small airways, leading to their collapse on expiration.

Fig. 4-10 shows representative flow-volume loops of asthma and emphysema superimposed over a normal

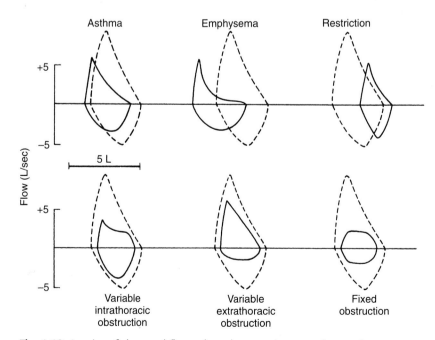

Fig. 4-10 A series of abnormal flow-volume loop tracings superimposed over a dashed-line tracing of a normal loop. *(From Ruppel G: Manual of pulmonary function testing, ed 6, St Louis, 1994, Mosby.)*

flow-volume loop. Notice that both loops are shifted to the left toward the TLC because the residual volumes are increased. Also notice that the flows are decreased more than normal as the patient exhales closer to the residual volume. This "scooped out" appearance is very characteristic of small airways disease. Having the patient inhale a bronchodilator and repeating the flow-volume loop shows the degree of reversibility. Some computer-based systems allow the before and after bronchodilator loops to be superimposed to show further the amount of improvement.

Restriction. A restriction can be caused by a pulmonary condition such as fibrosis; a thoracic condition such as pleural effusion, pneumothorax or hemothorax, or kyphoscoliosis; or obesity, advanced pregnancy, or ascites pushing up on the diaphragm. Only fibrosis and kyphoscoliosis are permanent. Fig. 4-10 shows a representative flow-volume loop for a patient with restrictive lung disease. Notice that the volume is small and shifted to the right toward the small residual volume.

Variable intrathoracic obstruction. A variable intrathoracic obstruction can be caused by a tumor or foreign body partially blocking a bronchus. Figure 4-10 shows a representative flow-volume curve. Note that the FVC volume is almost normal, with a greatly decreased peak expiratory flow rate.

Variable extrathoracic obstruction. A variable extrathoracic obstruction can be caused by vocal cord paralysis, laryngeal tumor, or a foreign body partially obstructing the upper airway. Fig. 4-10 shows a representative flow-volume curve. Note that the FVC volume is almost normal, with a greatly reduced inspiratory flow. This same pattern is commonly seen in patients with obstructive sleep apnea. The $FEF_{50\%}$ will be greater than the $FIF_{50\%}$.

Fixed large airway obstruction. A fixed large airway obstruction is usually caused by a tumor in the trachea or a main-stem bronchus. Fig. 4-10 shows a representative flow-volume loop. Again, the FVC volume is close to normal. Note the abnormally reduced inspiratory and expiratory flow rates. The tracing looks almost "squared off," with the $FEF_{50\%}$ and $FIF_{50\%}$ values being about the same.

3. Maximum voluntary ventilation

a. Perform the procedure (WRE code: IB7m) [Difficulty: An]

The maximum voluntary ventilation (MVV) is the volume of air exhaled in a specified period during a repetitive maximum respiratory effort. It is most commonly performed to evaluate a patient's ability to perform a stress test. It also may be used as a preoperative screening test to help determine the patient's chance of pulmonary complications.

The patient should breathe at a volume that is greater than the tidal volume but less than the VC, with a rate between 70 and 120 per minute. The minimal time for the test is 5 seconds, with a recommended time of 12 seconds. See Fig. 4-11 for two different tracings of the MVV effort.

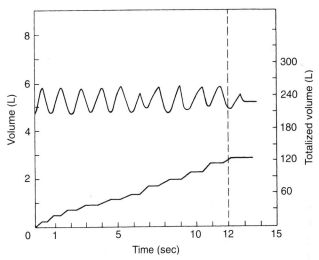

Fig. 4-11 Two tracings of the same maximum voluntary ventilation (MVV) effort. The saw-toothed tracing shows each individual volume effort and the respiratory rate. The stair-stepped tracing shows the cumulative volume during the effort. *(From Ruppel G:* Manual of pulmonary function testing, *ed 6, St Louis, 1994, Mosby.)*

The total volume exhaled in the given time period is mathematically adjusted for 1 minute so that the derived value is in liters per minute. This is done by multiplying a 5-second effort by 12 or a 12-second effort by 5. The derived value is then BTPS corrected to give the final value.

b. Interpret the results (WRE code: IB8i) [Difficulty: An]

The results of the MVV test are among the most difficult to evaluate. This is because the patient's effort, the condition of the respiratory muscles, lung/thoracic compliance, neurologic control over the drive to breathe, and airway and tissue resistance all have an influence. Abnormalities in any of these can cause the MVV value to decrease. Because more than one problem can exist, a decreased MVV does not point out the exact difficulty. A healthy young man can have an MVV of 150 to 200 L/min. Women tend to have smaller values, and the values of both sexes decrease with age. Because of the many factors involved in the MVV, normal predicted values may vary by as much as ±30%. Therefore unless a patient has an MVV value that is less than 70% of predicted, he or she cannot really be considered abnormal.

Cherniack and Raber (1972) published the following equations[*] for predicting the MVV in liters per minute:

Males: $[(3.03 \times \text{height in inches}) - (0.816 \times \text{age in years})] - 37.9$

Females: $[(2.14 \times \text{height in inches}) - [0.685 \times \text{age in years}]] - 4.87$

---

[*]The BTPS correction has been calculated into these equations.

When evaluating an abnormally low MVV result, the following considerations must be made:

1. Did the patient try his or her best? The respiratory therapist must make a professional judgment that the patient made his or her best effort. An objective way of judging this is to multiply the patient's FEV_1 × 35 to estimate the MVV. They should be close to the same volume. For example, if the patient's FEV_1 is 3 L, the estimated MVV is 105 L/min (3 L × 35). An MVV value that is much less than this indicates that the patient did not try very hard. Conversely, an MVV value that is much greater than this indicates that the FEV_1 value is too low and should be repeated.

2. What is the condition of the patient's respiratory muscles? Patients with neuromuscular abnormalities probably will not be able to breathe much more deeply than the normal tidal volume or keep up the great effort required for the duration of the test. Because of this, their results will be low.

3. What is the patient's lung/thoracic compliance? Patients with low compliance probably will not be able to sustain the greater than normal workload required by the MVV test. However, some patients are able to compensate for a small tidal volume by increasing their respiratory rate enough to generate an MVV value within normal limits. A printout of the MVV test would show a smaller than expected volume moved at a higher-than-expected respiratory rate.

4. What is the patient's neurologic control over the drive to breathe? Patients who have had an injury to the brain may have an abnormal drive to breathe. Because of this, they produce a low MVV result.

5. What is the patient's airway and tissue resistance? Patients with increased airway resistance usually have a low MVV result. This problem also may cause air trapping and force the patient to stop the effort. Increased tissue resistance, such as seen in pulmonary edema, obesity, and ascites, also results in a low MVV value.

Despite these difficulties in determining the cause of a decreased MVV value, doing so has proven helpful in preoperative evaluation and cardiopulmonary stress testing. Any patient with a lower-than-normal MVV value is at an increased risk of postoperative atelectasis and pneumonia. The risks of pulmonary complications related to MVV are low when the patient reaches 75% to 50% of predicted, moderate when the patient reaches 50% to 33% of predicted, and high when the patient reaches less than 33% of predicted. Patients with known moderate to severe COPD usually have to stop exercise testing because of their inability to breathe. An MVV value of less than 50 L/min is a good predictor of this.

4. Single-breath nitrogen washout test and closing volume

Note: This test is not listed on the NBRC's detailed content outlines. However, a question related to it was asked on a recent Written Registry Exam.

a. Perform the procedure

The single-breath nitrogen washout (SBN_2) is used to measure two things: (1) the evenness of the distribution of ventilation into the lungs during inspiration and (2) the emptying rates of the lungs during exhalation. It is a helpful diagnostic test in any adult patient who is known to have or suspected of having obstructive airways disease. The NBRC uses the phrase *nitrogen washout distribution test* for its examinations.

The closing volume is one part of the SBN_2 test. It marks the lung volume when small-airway closure begins and is used as an early indicator of small-airways disease.

The SBN_2 test is done by analyzing the nitrogen (N_2) percentage that is exhaled after an inspiratory vital capacity (IVC) of 100% oxygen. It is beyond the scope of this book to go into detail on all the steps of the procedure; however, the general steps include instructing the patient to perform an IVC test while inhaling oxygen. Tell the patient to exhale slowly and evenly until his or her lungs are empty again without any breath holding. The exhaled gases are sent through a rapid N_2 analyzer to measure the percentage, a spirometer to measure the volume, and a graphing device.

b. Interpret the results

Refer to Fig. 4-12 for a normal tracing showing these phases:

Fig. 4-12 Tracing of a normal single-breath nitrogen washout (SBN_2) test showing the four phases and other features. CC, Closing capacity; CV, closing volume; $\Delta N_{2\,750-1250}$, nitrogen percentage found in the 500 mL of gas exhaled between 750 and 1250 mL of the vital capacity; RV, residual volume; TLC, total lung capacity; VC, vital capacity. *(From Ruppel G: Manual of pulmonary function testing, ed 6, St Louis, 1994, Mosby.)*

Phase I shows gas exhaled from the anatomic dead space of the upper airway. Because it is made up of 100% oxygen, the nitrogen percentage shows a zero reading.

Phase II shows a mix of dead space gas and alveolar gas. The nitrogen percentage increases rapidly as the pure oxygen is exhaled and nitrogen-rich gas from the alveoli is brought out. The first 750 mL of gas that includes these first two phases is not used in the evaluation of the distribution of ventilation.

Phase III shows a fairly level plateau as alveolar gas from the lower lobes with a stable mix of oxygen and nitrogen is exhaled. Phase III is further evaluated in the following two ways:

1. $\Delta N_{2\ 750-1250}$ looks at the increase in the nitrogen percentage found in the 500 mL of gas exhaled between 750 mL and 1250 mL of the VC. It is normally no more than 1.5% in healthy young adults. It increases to between 3% and 4.5% in healthy older adults. Patients with severe airways and lung disease, such as emphysema, may have a finding of 6% to 10% or more.

2. Slope of phase III is found by drawing a straight line from the point where 30% of the VC is exhaled to the point where phase IV begins. It is normally no more than 0.5% to 1% N_2 per liter of exhaled volume in healthy young adults, but may vary widely.

Phase IV is seen as a sharp increase in the nitrogen percentage and continues to residual volume. This is seen when the nitrogen-rich gas from the upper airways continues to be exhaled as the basilar airways became compressed and close off near the end of the VC effort.

The start of phase IV is called the *closing volume* (CV). It marks the lung volume when small airway closure begins and is an early indicator of small airways disease. CV does not occur in healthy young adults until after about 80% to 90% of the VC has been exhaled. The closing capacity (CC) is found by adding the closing volume to the residual volume (found by another test). Healthy young adults have a CC that is about 30% of their TLC.

Problems can be indicated through the following: increases in the $\Delta N_{2\ 750-1250}$, the slope of phase III, and especially early onset of phase IV; increased closing volume; and increased closing capacity. The following diseases or conditions can cause these abnormal test results: small-airways disease, congestive heart failure with pulmonary edema, or obesity.

5. Functional residual capacity by the helium dilution method

NOTE: This test is not listed on the NBRC's detailed content outlines. However, questions related to interpreting the results of lung volume tests have been asked on recent Written Registry Exams.

a. Perform the procedure

The functional residual capacity (FRC) is the volume of gas left in the lungs at the end of a normal expiration. It cannot be measured through spirometry. An FRC is needed to calculate a patient's residual volume (RV) and TLC. It is necessary to know a patient's RV, FRC, and TLC to diagnose and determine the severity of obstructive lung disease and restrictive lung disease.

The helium (He) dilution method basically involves diluting the resident gases in the lungs (mainly nitrogen and oxygen) with helium to mathematically determine the FRC. This also is called the closed-circuit method because the patient and circuit are sealed off. Fig. 4-13 shows a schematic drawing of the components that make up the circuit. These include a two-way valve to switch the patient from breathing room air to the helium mix, soda lime to absorb the patient's exhaled carbon dioxide from the circuit, a combined CO_2 and water vapor absorber to prevent these gases from entering the helium analyzer, the helium analyzer, a variable speed blower to move the gases through the circuit, a spirometer for monitoring tidal volumes, attached kymograph to trace out the patient's breathing pattern, and an oxygen supply to meet the patient's needs. The helium supply is not shown.

It is beyond the scope of this text to cover all the steps in the helium dilution test; however, the following features of the procedure are important to know. Add enough helium to the room air in the circuit to create a 10% to 15% He mix. At the end of a normal elation, the patient is switched to breathing the mix so that the FRC can be determined. The patient breathes the gas mix until the helium is evenly distributed throughout the lungs and the helium percentage is stable. Typically, the test is performed for up to 7 minutes if needed to reach an equilibrium point. Extending the test longer may help to reach a stable equilibrium point in abnormal patients. The calculation of RV is rather complex and is usually done through the computer built into the pulmonary function system. Spirometry also must be performed because the ERV is subtracted from the FRC to find the RV. Commonly the test is repeated. The patient should be allowed to breathe room air for 5 minutes between tests to clear the helium from the lungs. Patients with severe obstructive lung disease may need more time. Bates, Macklem, and Christie (1971) published the following equations[*] for calculating the normal FRC in liters:

$$\text{Males} = (0.130 \times \text{height in inches}) - 5.16$$

$$\text{Females} = (0.119 \times \text{height in inches}) - 4.85$$

---

[*]The BTPS correction has been calculated into these equations.

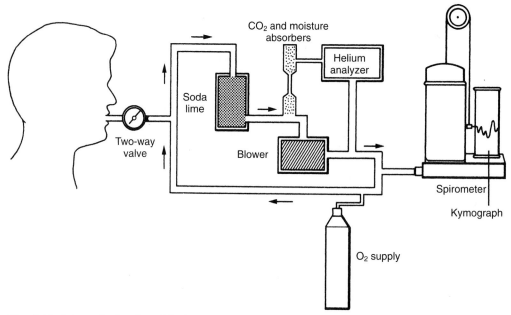

Fig. 4-13 Schematic drawing of the key components of a helium dilution system for measuring functional residual capacity. *(From Beauchamp RK: Pulmonary function testing procedures. In Barnes TA, editor:* Respiratory care practice, *St Louis, 1988, Mosby.)*

Goldman and Becklake (1959) published the following equations[*] for calculating the normal RV in liters:

$$\text{Males} = [(0.069 \times \text{height in inches}) + (0.017 \times \text{age in years})] - 3.45$$

$$\text{Females} = [(0.081 \times \text{height in inches}) + (0.009 \times \text{age in years})] - 3.90$$

b. Interpret the results

A normal young man has an FRC volume of about 2400 mL. As shown in Fig. 4-14, it is composed of the ERV and the RV. The FRC and RV values are invaluable in diagnosing obstructive and restrictive lung diseases. See Figure 4-6 for the relative volumes and capacities for a normal patient, a patient with an obstructive pattern, and a patient with a restrictive pattern. Note that the obstructive patient has a disproportionate increase in the RV, with a resulting decrease in the FVC. The TLC may be normal, as shown, or, more commonly, increased lung capacity. The patient with restrictive disease has a proportionate decrease in all the lung volumes and capacities. It is commonly accepted that the normal limits of TLC are about ±20% of the predicted value. This ±20% of the normal limit applies to the FRC and RV values as well. In other words, obstructive lung disease can be diagnosed by an RV, FRC, or TLC that is more than 120% of the predicted value. Common examples of obstructive diseases include asthma, bronchitis, and emphysema.

Restrictive lung disease can be diagnosed by an RV, FRC, or TLC that is less than 80% of the predicted value. Examples of restrictive diseases include fibrotic lung disease, air or fluid in the pleural space, obesity, kyphoscoliosis, pectus excavatum, and neuromuscular weakness or paralysis.

The following considerations should be accounted for to ensure that the measured values are accurate:

1. There should be no leaks in the system. A leak can result in an overestimation of the FRC because the lost helium results in a lower final helium percentage. A leak also can result in failure of the final helium percentage to stabilize as expected.

2. The patient must be breathing on the system long enough for the helium to reach all of the lung units and reach equilibrium. Usually this takes about 7 minutes; however, patients with severe obstructive lung disease will need more time and may never reach an equilibrium state. This results in an underestimation of the FRC.

6. Functional residual capacity by the nitrogen washout method

NOTE: This test is not listed on the NBRC's detailed content outlines. However, questions related to interpreting the results of lung volume tests have been asked on recent Written Registry Exams.

a. Perform the procedure

As discussed in the helium dilution method, the nitrogen (N_2) washout method is used to find the FRC so that the

---

[*]The BTPS correction has been calculated into these equations.

TLC 6000 mL	VC 4800 mL	IC 3600 mL	IRV 3100 mL	
			V_T500 mL	
		FRC 2400 mL	ERV 1200 mL	
	RV 1200 mL		RV 1200 mL	

<u>Volumes:</u> Four primary

A. Tidal volume (V_T). The volume of gas inspired *or* expired during normal respiration.
B. Inspiratory reserve volume (IRV): The maximum volume of gas that can be inspired beyond a normal inspiration.
C. Expiratory reserve volume (ERV): The maximum volume of gas that can be exhaled after a normal expiration.
D. Residual volume (RV): The volume of gas remaining in the lungs after a maximum expiration.

<u>Capacities:</u> Four, which include two or more primary volumes

A. Total lung capacity (TLC): The total amount of gas contained in the lungs after maximum inspiration. Includes all four primary volumes (TLC = V_T + IRV + ERV + RV).
B. Vital capacity (VC): The maximum amount of gas that can be exhaled after a maximum inspiration. Includes three primary volumes (VC = V_T + IRV + ERV).
C. Inspiratory capacity (IC): The maximum amount of gas that can be inspired after a normal expiration. Includes two primary volumes (IC = V_T + IRV).
D. Functional residual capacity (FRC): The total amount of gas remaining in the lungs after normal expiration. Includes two primary volumes (FRC = ERV + RV).

Fig. 4-14 Lung volumes and capacities for a clinically normal young man.

RV can be derived from it and TLC calculated. It is necessary to know a patient's RV, FRC, and TLC to diagnose and determine the severity of obstructive lung disease and restrictive lung disease.

The nitrogen washout method basically involves having the patient breathe in 100% oxygen until all the resident nitrogen is removed from the lungs. It also is called the open-circuit method because the patient inspires as much oxygen as needed to displace the nitrogen to a reservoir for measurement.

Fig. 4-15 shows a schematic drawing of the components that make up the automated nitrogen washout system and circuit. These include a solenoid valve to switch the patient from breathing room air to breathing pure oxygen, an oxygen source with demand valve, a nitrogen analyzer with recorder, a pneumotachometer, and a microprocessor that directs all the necessary activities for the test. It is beyond the scope of this text to go into the complete procedure for the test; however, the following features should be known. The circuit is filled with pure oxygen. The patient is switched from room air to oxygen at the end of a normal exhalation so that the nitrogen in the FRC can be determined. Typically, the test is performed for up to 7 minutes or until the nitrogen percentage falls below a target level. This target percentage has been reported by various authors as 1% (best results) up to 3%. Extending the test longer may help to reach a target level in patients with increased airway resistance or an increased lung volume. As before, the calculation of RV is rather complex and is usually done through the computer built into the pulmonary function system. Spirometry also must be performed because the ERV is subtracted from the FRC to find the RV. Commonly the test is repeated. The patient should be allowed to breathe room air for at least 15 minutes between tests to clear the oxygen from the lungs. Patients with severe obstructive lung disease may need more time.

Predicted patient values for FRC and RV can be determined with the same equations listed in the previous discussion of the helium dilution method of determining FRC.

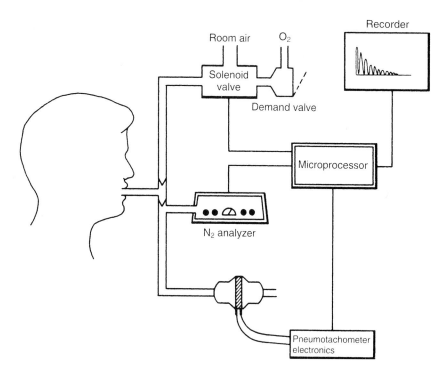

Fig. 4-15 Schematic drawing of the key components of the automated nitrogen washout system for measuring functional residual capacity. *(From Beauchamp RK: Pulmonary function testing procedures. In Barnes TA, editor:* Respiratory care practice, *St Louis, 1988, Mosby.)*

b. Interpret the results

As discussed earlier in the helium dilution test, the FRC and RV values are invaluable in diagnosing obstructive and restrictive lung diseases. When done properly, the helium dilution and nitrogen washout tests reveal similar patient values. If the nitrogen percentage is graphed over time, the shape of the washout curve also can be helpful in evaluating the degree of airway obstruction. Both the normal and abnormal tracings show rapid nitrogen washout from the upper-airway dead space. However, as the test continues, the patient with obstructive lung disease shows a progressive slowing of the nitrogen washout rate.

The following considerations should be accounted for to ensure that the measured values are accurate:

1. There should be no leaks in the system. A leak would be noticed as a sudden increase in the nitrogen percentage after a steady decrease. This results in an overestimation in the FRC value.
2. The patient must be breathing on the system long enough for the nitrogen to be washed out of all the lung units. Usually this takes less than 7 minutes; however, patients with severe obstructive lung disease need more time and may never reach the targeted percentage. This results in an underestimation of the FRC.

7. Total lung capacity

NOTE: This test is not listed on the NBRC's detailed content outlines. However, questions related to interpreting the results of lung volume tests have been asked on recent Written Registry Exams.

a. Perform the procedure

TLC is the volume of air in the lungs after inhaling a VC. As discussed earlier, it is necessary to determine a patient's TLC to diagnose obstructive or restrictive lung disease.

Refer to Fig. 4-14 for the relations of the lung volumes and capacities to each other. As can be seen, TLC can be found by adding several combinations of volumes and capacities. Most commonly, it is calculated by adding the FRC to the inspiratory capacity (IC) found through spirometry. However, be prepared to add or subtract various combinations of volumes and capacities to find the TLC.

b. Interpret the results

The TLC results cannot be interpreted without looking at the volumes and capacities that compose it. Fig. 4-5 shows representative TLC patterns for a normal patient and a patient with an obstructive pattern and a restrictive pattern. Note that with the abnormal patterns, the FRC and its components, the ERV and RV, are out of proportion. Patients with emphysema, bronchitis, or asthma often show the obstructive pattern with its large FRC of trapped gas. Patients with fibrotic lung disease, thoracic deformities, or obesity often show the restrictive pattern with its decreased FRC and other lung volumes.

Some practitioners use the general rule that a TLC that is more than 120% of predicted indicates an obstructive pattern, and a TLC that is less than 80% of predicted indicates a restrictive pattern. However, this may be an oversimplification. It is more reliable to calculate the RV-to-TLC (RV:TLC) ratio. This takes into account the interrelation of the two. Normal healthy adults have an RV:TLC ratio that is 0.20 (20%) to 0.35 (35%). An increased RV:TLC ratio is commonly seen in patients with emphysema and an increased RV. However, if the patient's TLC is increased in proportion to the RV, the ratio may be within normal limits. A decreased RV:TLC ratio is commonly seen in patients with fibrotic lung disease. The ratio will be normal, however, if the patient's TLC is decreased in proportion to the RV. Table 4-1 shows the relations of the lung volumes and capacities, TLC, and the RV:TLC ratio found in a number of conditions.

Exam Hint

Most examinations have at least one table that must be interpreted to determine if the patient has obstructive lung disease or has restrictive lung disease. The "20% rule" can help with this determination. Obstructive lung disease is identified by lung volumes (TLC, FRC, RV) that are 20% or more *greater* than predicted (more than 120% of predicted). Restrictive lung disease is identified by lung volumes (TLC, FRC, RV) that are 20% or more *smaller* than predicted (less than 80% of predicted).

---

8. Body plethysmography

The body plethysmography unit (sometimes called the *body bubble*) is a sealable chamber large enough for an adult to sit inside. Auxiliary equipment includes a differential pressure pneumotachometer, a monitor/storage oscilloscope, a computer, and a recording device (Fig. 4-16). The plethysmograph can be used to measure (1) the FRC and, from that, the RV and TLC; (2) lung compliance; and (3) airway resistance. Each of these tests is discussed later.

a. Thoracic gas volume

NOTE: This test is not listed on the NBRC's detailed content outlines. However, questions related to interpreting the results of lung volume tests have been asked on recent Written Registry Exams.

1. Perform the procedure

The volume of gas measured in the lungs at the end of exhalation by a plethysmograph is termed *thoracic gas volume* (TGV or VTG). When the unit is accurately calibrated and the test properly performed, the plethysmograph provides a more accurate FRC volume measurement than either the helium dilution or nitrogen washout methods. Once TGV is determined, the RV can be derived from it, and TLC calculated. It is necessary to know a patient's RV, FRC, and TLC to diagnose and determine the severity of obstructive lung disease and restrictive lung disease.

It is not possible to go into a complete discussion of the procedure; however, the following steps are important. The unit must be sealed so that it is airtight during the patient's breathing. The patient is instructed to breathe a normal tidal volume through the pneumotachometer. At the end of exhalation (FRC), a shutter is closed on the pneumotachometer so that no air leaks. The patient is instructed to continue to make tidal volume breathing efforts. The computer integrates the following two pressure changes: (1) a

---

TABLE 4-1 Lung Volumes and Capacities Seen in Various Disorders							
Disorder	**VC**	**IC**	**ERV**	**FRC**	**RV**	**TLC**	**RV:TLC**
Asthma or airway disease	D	N	D	N,I	I	N,I*	I
Emphysema	N	N	N	I	I	I	N,I
Diffuse parenchymal disease							
Early	N	N	N	D	N	N	N
Advanced (all volumes and							
capacities are equally reduced)							
Space-occupying lesions	N	N	N	N	D	N	D
Obesity	N	N	D	N,I†	N	N	I
Thoracic/skeletal disease	D	D	D	D	N	D	I

D, Decreased; ERV, expiratory reserve volume; FRC, functional residual capacity; I, increased; IC, inspiratory capacity; N, normal; RV, residual volume; TLC, total lung capacity; VC, vital capacity.
*When airway resistance is greater than about 3.5 cm H_2O/L/sec.
†When the weight:height (pounds:inches) ratio is greater than 5:1.
Modified from Snow MG: Determination of functional residual capacity, *Respir Care* 34(7):586, 1989.

Fig. 4-16 Schematic drawing of the layout of a body plethysmograph with its components. The patient sits within the sealed plethysmograph chamber for the tests. *(From Ruppel G: Manual of pulmonary function testing, ed 6, St Louis, 1994, Mosby.)*

decrease in mouth pressure as the patient attempts to inhale, and (2) an increase in plethysmograph chamber pressure as the patient's chest expands. The patient's TGV is then determined at FRC. Fig. 4-17, *A,* shows a normal TGV loop on the oscilloscope. Through spirometry, the patient's ERV, RV, and TLC can be calculated.

2. Interpret the results

The interpretation of the TGV and TLC results from a body plethysmograph are about the same as the interpretation of the FRC and TLC results from the helium dilution or nitrogen washout methods. (Review these earlier discussions if needed.) The only difference would be if the TGV were significantly larger than the FRC. This would indicate that the patient has trapped gas that was measured only in the plethysmograph. The TGV is commonly larger than the FRC measured by the preceding two methods when the patient has chronic obstructive pulmonary disease (COPD). This is because it includes *all* the gas found in the thorax. That gas may be found in normal alveoli connected by a patent airway to the atmosphere, but the TGV may also include gas trapped in emphysematous blebs and bullae, pneumothorax, pneumomediastinum, and so forth.

b. Lung compliance
1. Recommend the procedure (WRE code: IC2) [Difficulty: Ap, An]

Lung compliance (C_L) is the volume change per unit of pressure change in the lungs. It is recorded in liters or milliliters per centimeter of water pressure (L[mL]/cm H_2O). A lung compliance test is indicated in a patient with a known or suspected condition that caused the lungs to be either overly compliant (as in emphysema) or noncompliant (as in pulmonary fibrosis).

2. Perform the procedure (WRE code: IB7g and IIIE8) [Difficulty: An]

The patient must swallow a 10-cm-long balloon to the midthoracic level. A catheter connects the proximal end of the balloon to a pressure transducer outside of the patient. Air is injected into the balloon, and the transducer is calibrated accurately to measure changes in intrathoracic pressure as the patient breathes. The patient is then placed into a body plethysmograph that is sealed. He or she is told to breathe through the differential pressure pneumotachometer to measure lung volumes. The patient is then instructed to inhale slowly from the resting level (FRC) to TLC. As this is done, the pneumotachometer shutter is periodically closed to measure the intrathoracic pressure decrease at the increasing volumes (Fig. 4-18). As the patient slowly exhales from TLC, the shutter is again periodically closed to measure the increasing intrathoracic pressure as the patient returns to FRC volume. Lung compliance is usually calculated from the pressure and volume points of FRC and FRC + 500 mL (for a tidal volume).

3. Interpret the results (WRE code: IB8f) [Difficulty: An]

Normal lung compliance (C_L) in an adult is 0.2 L/cm water. Through other methods, the normal adult's thoracic compliance (C_T) has been determined also to be 0.2 L/cm water. However, because the lungs tend to collapse smaller and the thorax cage tends to expand out, the two opposing forces offset each other somewhat. Because of this, the lung/thoracic compliance (C_{LT}) is calculated as 0.1 L (or 100 mL)/cm water.

A number of diseases and conditions can affect lung, thoracic, and lung/thoracic compliance. Patients with emphysema are known to have a higher than normal lung compliance. Their lungs are overly distended. Decreased lung compliance is seen in pulmonary fibrosis (from sarcoidosis, silicosis, or asbestosis), lung tumor, pulmonary edema, atelectasis, pneumonia, or decreased surfactant. Decreased thoracic compliance is seen in patients with kyphoscoliosis, pectus excavatum, obesity, enlarged liver, or advanced pregnancy. All these conditions result in small, stiff lungs.

c. Airway resistance
1. Recommend the procedure (WRE code: IC2) [Difficulty: Ap, An]

Airway resistance (Raw) is the difference in pressure between the alveoli and the mouth that develops as air flows into and out of the lungs. It is recorded in centimeters of water pressure per liter of gas moved per second (cm water/L/sec). The test is performed on patients with a known or suspected condition of increased airway resistance. These include asthma, emphysema, and

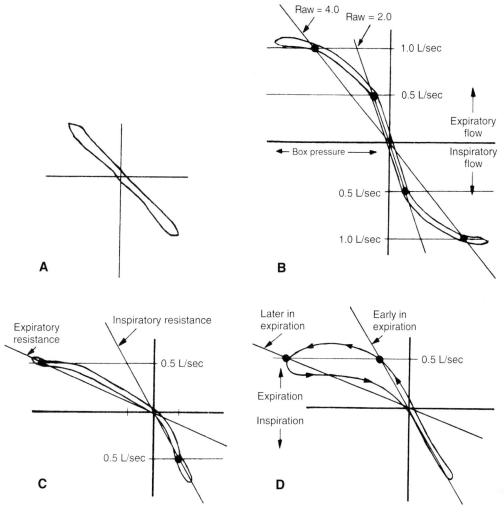

Fig. 4-17 Examples of body plethysmography tracings. Tracing **A** shows a normal thoracic gas volume loop. Tracing **B** shows a normal inspiratory and expiratory loop for airway resistance (Raw). Note that it is symmetrical. This patient has an Raw of 2 cm H_2O/L/sec at the standard flow of 0.5 L/sec. As the flow increases, the Raw increases as a result of the increased turbulence. The Raw of 4 cm H_2O/L/sec seen at the flow of 1 L/sec should not be recorded as the patient's value. Tracing **C** shows a patient who has an expiratory resistance that is greater than inspiratory resistance. In this case, either both resistances should be recorded in the chart or just the expiratory resistance if only one can be recorded. Tracing **D** shows a significant difference between early and late expiratory resistance. This is commonly seen in patients with obstructive airways disease such as emphysema. Record the late resistance because it better represents the patient's disease condition. *(From Zarins LP, Clausen JL: Body plethysmography. In Clausen JL, editor:* Pulmonary function testing guidelines and controversies, *Orlando, 1984, Grune & Stratton.)*

chronic bronchitis (COPD). The test confirms the patient's condition. Then it is used to help determine the proper dose of bronchodilator medications to help manage the problem.

2. Perform the procedure (WRE code: IB7g and IIIE8) [Difficulty: An]

The patient is placed into a plethysmograph that is sealed. He or she is instructed to breathe through a differential pressure pneumotachometer. With the pneumotachometer shutter open, the patient is told to pant several tidal volumes of about 500 mL at a rate of 1 breath per second. Data on flow rate, tidal volume, mouth pressure changes, and chamber pressure changes are recorded and graphed (Fig. 4-19). Then the shutter is closed at the patient's resting FRC volume. The patient is told to continue panting at the same volume and rate. Again, flow rate, tidal volume, mouth pressure changes, and chamber pressures are recorded and graphed. The computer integrates the data to calculate the patient's airway resistance during tidal volume breathing.

Fig. 4-18 Measurement of lung compliance (C_L) with the esophageal balloon technique. A balloon is swallowed to the midthoracic level, filled with air, and connected to a pressure transducer to measure intrapleural pressure. The patient sits within a body plethysmograph to measure inspiratory and expiratory volumes. *(From Ruppel G: Manual of pulmonary function testing, ed 6, St Louis, 1994, Mosby.)*

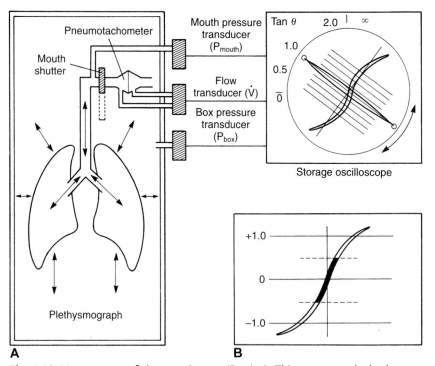

Fig. 4-19 Measurement of airway resistance (Raw). **A,** This represents the body plethysmograph that the patient sits within during the test. Tidal volume panting against an open and then closed pneumotachometer shutter is displayed on the storage oscilloscope. **B,** This represents a printout of the pressure changes as the patient pants a tidal volume of 500 mL/sec. *(From Ruppel G: Manual of pulmonary function testing, ed 6, St Louis, 1994, Mosby.)*

3. Interpret the results (WRE code: IB8f) [Difficulty: An]

Airway resistance is the pressure difference developed per unit of flow. This pressure is required to overcome the friction of moving the tidal volume through the airways to the lungs. It can be thought of as the ratio of alveolar pressure to airflow. It is calculated by this formula:

$$Raw = \frac{atmospheric\ pressure - alveolar\ pressure}{flow}$$

Ruppel (2003) reports the normal adult's airway resistance to range from 0.6 to 2.4 cm $H_2O/L/sec$. The standard inspiratory and expiratory flow rate during the test is 0.5 L/sec (500 mL/sec). This is to standardize air turbulence during the test. The usual components of airway resistance found in an adult are as follows:

1. Upper airway including the nose and mouth, 50%
2. Trachea and bronchi larger than 2 mm in diameter, 30%
3. Airways less than 2 mm in diameter, 20%

Increased airway resistance is abnormal. It is most readily noticed if the problem is in the upper airway, trachea, or major bronchi, because most resistance is normally found there. Patients with asthma, bronchitis, and emphysema have most of their resistance in the airways that are 2 mm or less in diameter. Because of this, significant disease must be present before a large enough airway resistance is noticed to alert the therapist or physician to the problem. Fig. 4-17, *B* through *D*, shows normal and increased expiratory resistance curves. Madama (1998) lists the following airway resistance values and their severity

Raw [cm $H_2O/L/sec$]	Severity
2.8–4.5	mild
4.5–8	moderate
>8	severe

9. Diffusing capacity
a. Perform the procedure (WRE code: IB7m) [Difficulty: An]

The diffusing capacity (D_L or $D_{L\ CO}$) tests look at the capacity for carbon monoxide to diffuse through the lungs into the blood. Carbon monoxide is used because its high affinity for hemoglobin virtually eliminates blood as a barrier to diffusion. The measured value can then be correlated to the ability of oxygen to diffuse through the lungs. This test is indicated when it is important to know the extent of lung disability causing hypoxemia. This is most common with patients having emphysema, but it also is important in patients with fibrotic lung disease.

At the time of this writing, the single-breath carbon monoxide diffusing capacity test ($D_{L\ CO}$ SB) is the only version that has a widely adopted standard technique for administration. It is recorded in milliliters of carbon monoxide (CO) per minute per millimeter of mercury at 0° C, 760 mm Hg, and dry standard temperature and pressure (STPD).

The following are key steps in the procedure. A reservoir or spirometer is filled with a mix of .3% CO, 10% He, 21% O_2, and the balance of N_2 (Fig. 4-20). The patient is connected to the apparatus and breathes room air while being instructed in the test. After the patient is told to exhale completely (to RV), the practitioner switches the patient to the gas mix. The patient is instructed to rapidly inhale an IVC. A shutter automatically closes so that the patient cannot exhale for 10 seconds. This allows time for some of the carbon monoxide to diffuse into the patient's bloodstream.

After the breath hold, the shutter opens, and the patient is told to exhale to resting volume. The equipment is designed to automatically let 750 to 1000 mL of exhaled gas pass through to the spirometer. The next 500 mL of gas is diverted into the end-tidal gas sampler. This sample is then analyzed for He% and CO%. The remainder of the patient's exhaled volume is passed through into the spirometer. The various measured parameters are integrated into the equations in the computer to give the patient's $D_{L\ CO}$ SB value.

This test is done only after the patient has been measured for both RV and TLC. That is because the patient's lung volume directly affects the diffusibility of carbon monoxide.

b. Interpret the results (WRE code: IB8i) [Difficulty: An]

Interpretation is limited to the results of the $D_{L\ CO}$ SB test. Ruppel (2003) reports the average resting normal adult $D_{L\ CO}$ SB as 25 mL CO/min/mm Hg STPD (standard temperature, pressure, dry, conditions). Gaensler and Wright (1966) report the following $D_{L\ CO}$ SB prediction equations with values in mL CO/min/mm Hg STPD:

Males: [(0.250 × height in inches) − (0.177 × age in years)] + 19.93

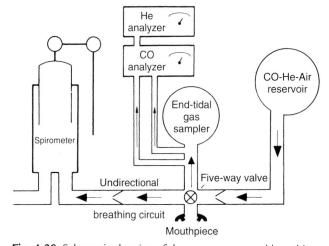

Fig. 4-20 Schematic drawing of the components and breathing circuit used when performing a single-breath lung-diffusion test ($D_{L\ CO}$SB). Analysis of the patient's exhaled helium (He) and carbon monoxide (CO) percentages is critical to the test. *(From Ruppel G: Manual of pulmonary function testing, ed 6, St Louis, 1994, Mosby.)*

Females: $[(0.284 \times$ height in inches$) - (0.177 \times$ age in years$)]$
$+ 7.72$

It should be noted that a number of other authors have developed their own prediction equations. In general, patients who show $D_{L\,CO}$ SB results within ±20% of the predicted values (80% to 120% of predicted) are considered to be within normal limits. A patient who has actual results that are significantly below the predicted values (<80% of predicted) has a problem with lung diffusion. Fig. 4-21 shows a number of common conditions that can lead to poor lung diffusion. The following factors also should be taken into consideration when interpreting the measured values:

1. Increased hematocrit and hemoglobin values result in an increased $D_{L\,CO}$, whereas decreased values result in a decreased $D_{L\,CO}$. An actual value should be used to calculate a patient's D_L CO.
2. An increased carboxyhemoglobin level results in a decreased $D_{L\,CO}$ value. Patients who smoke should be instructed not to smoke the night before the test so that the COHb level will decrease to normal.
3. An increased alveolar carbon dioxide level results in a lowered alveolar oxygen level. This, in turn, results in an increased $D_{L\,CO}$ value. A decreased alveolar carbon dioxide level results in a decreased $D_{L\,CO}$ value.

4. Increased altitude results in an increased $D_{L\,CO}$. This is probably a concern only if the patient is tested in a mountainous area.
5. An increased pulmonary capillary blood volume results in an increased D_L CO.
6. The patient should breathe room air for at least 4 minutes before the test is repeated.

It is well known that diffusibility is directly related to lung volume. This is the reason that blacks have lower diffusion rates than whites. To eliminate this as a factor in interpreting the D_L value, it is necessary to divide the diffusion value by the TLC. Blacks have the same normal values as whites when this calculation is performed.

MODULE E
Pulmonary function equipment

1. Water, mercury, and aneroid-type manometers (pressure gauges)
a. Get the necessary equipment for the procedure (CSE code: IIA19)

Mercury or water-type manometers have a vertical column of the liquid, as in a sphygmomanometer, for measuring blood pressure. An aneroid (spring-loaded) unit is most commonly used. This is because it does not have to be kept

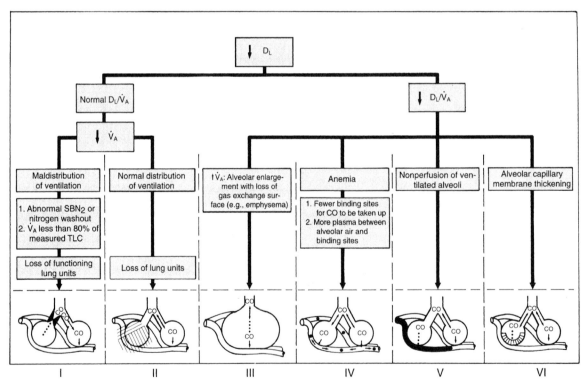

Fig. 4-21 Six factors that can cause decreased lung diffusion (D_L). Factors I and II result in a decrease in D_L that is in proportion to the decrease in alveolar volume. Factors III, IV, V, and VI result in a decrease in D_L that is greater than the decrease in alveolar volume. Therefore these later conditions are more harmful to the patient's pulmonary function and well-being. SBN$_2$, Single-breath nitrogen washout; TLC, total lung capacity; V$_A$, alveolar ventilation. *(From Ayers LN, Whipp BJ, Ziment I: A guide to the interpretation of pulmonary function tests, ed 2, New York, 1978, Roerig.)*

upright to measure accurately. Aneroid manometers can be calibrated in either millimeters of mercury (mm Hg) or centimeters of water (cm H_2O) pressure and look like a Bourdon gauge.

b. Put the equipment together and make sure that it works properly (CSE code: IIA19)

These pressure gauges come preassembled by the manufacturer. It is necessary to attach the pressure source only to the inlet port on the unit to measure a pressure change. This connection must be airtight or a leak will occur and the measured pressure will be less than actually exists. Accuracy of the unit can be checked by opening the inlet port to room air and reading the pressure. A reading of zero should be seen (indicating no pressure change from atmospheric). Next, a known pressure is applied to the gauge. Often this is done by attaching it to a sphygmomanometer and pumping up the pressure to a known level, such as 50 mm Hg. The pressure gauge should show the same.

c. Troubleshoot any problems with the equipment (CSE code: IIA19)

If, during the calibration procedure, the set pressure does not match the pressure in the gauge, a leak may be present in the system or the pressure gauge is miscalibrated. Tighten all connections and attempt to calibrate again. Do not use a pressure gauge that cannot be calibrated.

2. Inspiratory or expiratory force meters (pressure gauges)
a. Get the necessary equipment for the procedure (CSE code: IIA19)

The maximum inspiratory pressure and maximum expiratory pressure tests are usually recorded in centimeters of water pressure. However, millimeters of mercury can be used. If a centimeters of water pressure gauge is used, it should be able to record a negative and positive pressure of at least 100 cm H_2O. However, a unit that can record ±60 cm H_2O is probably adequate.

b. Put the equipment together and make sure that it works properly (CSE code: IIA19)

No standard setup exists for these devices. See Fig. 4-2 for a possible assembly. The system can be sealed and pressure checked with a known force to make sure that the pressure manometer is accurate and all the connections are airtight.

c. Troubleshoot any problems with the equipment (CSE code: IIA19)

If, during the calibration procedure, the set pressure does not match the pressure in the gauge, a leak may be present in the system, or the pressure gauge is miscalibrated. Tighten all connections, and attempt to calibrate again. Do not use a pressure gauge that cannot be calibrated. The one-way valves must function so that the patient can exhale or inhale only as needed for the test.

3. Pressure transducer
a. Get the necessary equipment for the procedure (CSE code: IIA19)

Pressure transducers are used in the body plethysmograph for measuring mouth pressure and chamber pressure. They come with the unit and are supplied by the manufacturer. Another type of transducer is used with an esophageal balloon when performing a lung compliance measurement. Follow the balloon manufacturer's recommendations for the proper transducer.

b. Put the equipment together and make sure that it works properly (CSE code: IIA19)
c. Troubleshoot any problems with the equipment (CSE Code: IIA19)

Each type of pressure transducer should be assembled as described by the manufacturer. As seen in Fig. 4-22, the differential pressure transducer has small bore tubing connecting it before and after a resistive element. These small tubes transmit the pressures before and after the resistance

Fig. 4-22 Cutaway view of a differential pressure pneumotachometer. Flow is measured as the pressure decreases between *A* and *B*, which are ports leading to a differential pressure transducer. The resistive element may consist of a mesh screen, a network of parallel capillary tubes, or other devices. *(From Beauchamp RK: Pulmonary function testing procedures. In Barnes TA, editor:* Respiratory care practice, *St Louis, 1988, Mosby.)*

element to the transducer as gas flows through the large, main tube. Make sure that the tubing is properly connected to the main tube and transducer. If a tube were to disconnect, the transducer would give a reading of zero.

4. Pneumotachometer respirometers

a. Get the necessary equipment for the procedure (CSE code: IIA20)

b. Put the equipment together and make sure that it works properly (CSE code: IIA20)

c. Troubleshoot any problems with the equipment (CSE code: IIA20)

All pneumotachometers convert one type of physical information or signal to another (for example, converting an *airflow* or pressure signal to an electrical signal). Two common types are discussed next. Either type should be acceptable for performing bedside spirometry. Make sure that the unit you select is capable of performing the ordered test. Be sure that you select a unit capable of printing out a hard copy of the patient's test results and spirometry tracings if they are required for the chart.

Differential-pressure (flow sensing) pneumotachometer. Some articles refer to a differential pressure pneumotachometer as a *Fleisch-type* device. These units have a resistive element (tubes or mesh screen) in the flow tube. The faster the flow of gas through the flow tube, the greater the pressure difference before and after the resistance. Hoses connect the flow tubes before and after the resistive element to the differential pressure transducer. The transducer converts this pressure difference into an electrical signal. A microprocessor calculates the various patient values from this information (see Fig. 4-22).

Assembly requires the addition of the patient's mouthpiece to the inspiratory port so that no air leak occurs. The expiratory port should be kept completely open so that the only obstruction to the patient's airflow is from the resistive element. A volume calibration check is performed by forcing a known amount of air from a supersyringe (certified volume standard syringe) through the pneumotachometer. Minimally, several repetitions of a known 3-L volume should reveal identical measured volumes. As long as the measured volumes are within ±3% or 50 mL (whichever is less), the unit is acceptably accurate.

Common problems with accuracy include an air leak around the mouthpiece; cracked, disconnected, or obstructed pressure-relaying hoses; water condensation or mucus on the resistive element; or obstructed upstream or downstream port. The resistive element is usually heated to minimize any condensation.

Heat-transfer pneumotachometer. Some articles refer to a heat-transfer pneumotachometer as a *thermistor-type device* or *hot-wire anemometer*. These units have a heated thermistor that is cooled as the gas flows past it. The temperature transducer automatically increases and measures the flow of electricity to the thermistor to keep

Fig. 4-23 Cutaway view of a heat-transfer pneumotachometer. *(From Ruppel G: Manual of pulmonary function testing, ed 6, St Louis, 1994, Mosby.)*

it at the required temperature. A microprocessor calculates the various patient values from this information. The earlier discussion on assembly, calibration, and troubleshooting applies to the heat-transfer–type pneumotachometers, except that no pressure-relaying hoses are present (Fig. 4-23).

5. Bedside pulmonary function screening equipment

a. Get the necessary equipment for the procedure (CSE code: IIA27)

b. Put the equipment together and make sure that it works properly (CSE code: IIA27)

c. Troubleshoot any problems with the equipment (CSE code: IIA27)

Volume displacement (also called *positive displacement*) respirometers are mechanical devices. They are called *volume displacement respirometers* because the patient's exhaled gas fills and moves a sealed bell or accordion-like bellows. These systems are self-contained and sealed rather than being open to room air, as are the other devices. They can have residual volume and lung diffusion test hardware added on. The three general categories are discussed here: water-seal spirometers, dry rolling-seal spirometers, and wedge-type spirometers.

Water-seal spirometers. Water-seal spirometers are the commonly found chain-compensated and Stead-Wells units made by Collins Medical, Inc. (see Fig. 4-24 for the cutaway appearance of the chain-compensated type). The bell falls and rises as the patient breathes in and out. A pulley system attached to the bell and the marking pens record the patient's efforts on the rotating kymograph paper. Note that the tracing is inverted from the patient's actual breathing effort. The Stead-Wells units have the marking pen attached directly to the bell; therefore the tracing directly shows the patient's breathing efforts (Fig. 4-25). The newer chain-compensated and Stead-Wells units also have microprocessors for calculating patient information.

Gas analyzers for helium, nitrogen, carbon monoxide, and other extra equipment can be added for RV and lung

Fig. 4-24 Cutaway view of a chain-compensated water-seal spirometer. CO, carbon monoxide; CO_2, carbon dioxide, He, helium; N_2, nitrogen. *(From Ruppel G: Manual of pulmonary function testing, ed 6, St Louis, 1994, Mosby.)*

diffusion measurements. The carbon dioxide absorber should be left out of the breathing circuit for FVC tests because it interferes with the fast flow of gas; however, it must be put in line for any testing that will last more than 15 seconds and involves breathing repeatedly into the closed system. Supplemental oxygen must be added to the circuit for any tests that require the patient to breathe repeatedly from the closed system. The following is a checklist for setup and where to look when problem solving:

1. Make sure the water level is correct (not too high or too low).
2. Use a 7-L bell for children and a 14-L bell for adults.
3. Make sure all circuit tubing and one-way valve connections are tight.
4. Check the following kymograph features: paper on correctly; pens contain ink; kymograph speeds are adjustable to 32, 160, and 1920 mm/sec.

Fig. 4-25 Cutaway view of a Stead-Wells water-seal spirometer. CO, carbon monoxide; CO_2, carbon dioxide, He, helium; N_2, nitrogen. *(Courtesy Warren E. Collins, Inc, Braintree, Mass.)*

5. The carbon dioxide absorber should be out of the circuit for FVC tests; it should be in the circuit for RV and lung-diffusion tests.
6. Oxygen should be added to the system for RV and lung-diffusion tests.
7. Make sure the various gas analyzers are calibrated properly.
8. As discussed earlier, do not be confused by the various ways the tracing is presented. Always find the start of the FVC by the near-vertical slope of the tracing.

Dry rolling-seal spirometers. Dry rolling-seal spirometers are sometimes called *piston spirometers.* As can be seen in Fig. 4-26, these units use a flexible silicone rubber (Silastic) or Teflon-coated rubber seal instead of water. The large volume piston moves in and out as the patient breathes. The patient's efforts can be directly recorded by pen on paper. Newer units also have microprocessors for calculating the information.

They are still rather large and are best suited for the pulmonary function laboratory. These units also can be outfitted with a carbon dioxide absorber and various gas analyzers, so they too can be used for the full range of lung function tests. The previous checklist for setup and problem-solving ideas apply in this case except for those items that are specific to the chain-compensated and Stead-Wells systems.

Wedge-type spirometers. Wedge-type spirometers are sometimes called *bellows spirometers* (Fig. 4-27). Note that these units have plastic or rubber bellows that are fixed on one side and are flexible like an accordion on other sides. The bellows move in and out as the patient breathes. The patient's efforts can be directly recorded by pen on paper. Newer units also have microprocessors for calculating the information.

All the earlier information on the dry rolling-seal spirometers applies here except what is specific to those units. The same setup and problem-solving ideas apply here also.

6. CO, He, O$_2$, and specialty gas analyzers
a. Get the necessary equipment for the procedure (WRE code: IIA21) [Difficulty: R, Ap, An]

These analyzers are needed for a variety of special purpose tests as described earlier:

A Piston spirometer   **B** Piston spirometer (schematic)

Fig. 4-26 Outside **(A)** and cutaway **(B)** views of a dry rolling-seal or piston spirometer. *(From Beauchamp RK: Pulmonary function testing procedures. In Barnes TA, editor: Respiratory care practice, St Louis, 1988, Mosby.)*

A Wedge spirometer **B** Wedge spirometer (schematic)

Fig. 4-27 Outside **(A)** and cutaway **(B)** views of a wedge-type spirometer. *(From Beauchamp RK: Pulmonary function testing procedures. In Barnes TA, editor:* Respiratory care practice, *St Louis, 1988, Mosby.)*

1. Carbon monoxide is analyzed in single-breath carbon monoxide diffusing capacity test.
2. Helium (He) is analyzed in the single-breath carbon monoxide diffusing capacity test and the helium dilution test to find FRC.
3. Oxygen (O_2) is analyzed in the single-breath carbon monoxide diffusing capacity test and the helium dilution test to find FRC.
4. Nitrogen (N_2) is analyzed in the single-breath nitrogen washout test and the nitrogen washout method of finding FRC.

b. Put the equipment together and make sure that it works properly (WRE code: IIA21) [Difficulty: R, Ap, An]

Check the label on the tank to be sure it is the correct gas at the correct percentage. Review Table 6-1 for color codings for tanks, if needed. Each specialty gas has its own diameter index safety system (DISS) reduction valve to connect to the tank. A high-pressure hose connects the reduction valve outlet to the pulmonary function testing machine inlet.

c. Troubleshoot any problems with the equipment (WRE code: IIA21) [Difficulty: R, Ap, An]

The problems that can occur with specialty gas cylinders, pressure reducing valves, and connecting high-pressure hoses are the same as can occur with oxygen cylinders. Review the discussion in Chapter 6 if needed.

MODULE F
Respiratory care plan

1. Analyze available information to determine the patient's pathophysiologic state (CSE code: IIIH1)

Even though a physician must legally determine the patient's diagnosis, a therapist must be able to understand the cause, pathophysiology, diagnosis, treatment, and prognosis for patients with cardiopulmonary disorders. Interpretation of patient data that is tested by the NBRC was discussed earlier. The following is a brief categorization of the conditions that may be diagnosed by pulmonary function testing.

Obstructive airways disease. The patient with severe obstructive lung disease shows low gas flow at all time intervals. However, a decreased FEV_3 and the $FEF_{25\%-75\%}$ are early markers of small-airways disease. Quite commonly, the RV is increased as a result of air trapping. This increases the FRC and often the TLC. Despite the increased lung volume, the patient's diffusing ability is decreased. Examples of conditions that cause obstructive lung disease include asthma, emphysema, bronchitis, and bronchiolitis. Excessive mucus, foreign bodies, and airway tumors also cause bronchospasm and air trapping.

> **Exam Hint**
>
> **M**ost examinations have tested the understanding and interpretation of data to determine whether a patient has obstructive or restrictive lung disease. This usually involves the assessment of patient data on a table. A key finding in patients with *obstructive lung disease* is air trapping resulting in the RV, FRC, and TLC being greater than 120% of predicted. A key finding in patients with *restrictive lung disease* is the RV, FRC, and TLC being less than 80% of predicted.

Restrictive lung disease. In restrictive lung disease, all lung volumes and capacities are reduced, and lung diffusion is reduced. Expiratory flows such as FEV_1 are increased. Examples of conditions that cause restrictive lung disease include fibrosis, pulmonary edema, hemothorax or pneumothorax, acute or infant respiratory distress syndrome, chest wall deformities, obesity, and various neuromuscular disorders.

> **Exam Hint**
>
> **C**ommonly, examinations have at least one question that deals with recommending tests for assessing a patient with airway obstruction or evaluating the results of PFTs on a patient with airway obstruction. This can include interpreting a table of data, a volume-time tracing, a flow-volume loop, or calculating the results of a before and after bronchodilator study.

2. Determine the appropriateness of the prescribed therapy and goals for the identified pathophysiologic state (CSE code: IIIH3)

The care plan depends on the patient's diagnosis and the degree of limitation. If the patient has reversible small-airways disease, he or she should be counseled to stop smoking and avoid all airborne irritants. Inhaled or systemic bronchodilators or both should be prescribed to relax the airways as much as possible. If the patient has restrictive lung disease, he or she should also be counseled to avoid any airborne irritants. Whether any medications or other procedures can be performed to offer some relief depends on the specific cause of the patient's disorder.

MODULE G

Quality assurance and quality control

1. Develop outcomes of quality improvement programs (WRE code: IIIH4a) [Difficulty: An]

2. Perform respiratory care quality assurance (WRE code: IIIH3) [Difficulty: Ap]

3. Record and monitor the outcomes of quality assurance programs by using accepted statistical methods (WRE code: IIC6) [Difficulty: Ap]

4. Perform quality control procedures for pulmonary function equipment (WRE code: IIC3) [Difficulty: Ap, An]

Every pulmonary function testing laboratory must have a quality control/quality improvement program. Regular maintenance of equipment and calibration must be performed and documented.

Spirometry equipment. The volume-displacement respirometers should have the following quality control procedures performed on a regular basis:

a. A supersyringe with at least a 3-L capacity should be pumped repeatedly into and out of the unit. A reading that is accurate to within ±3% or ±50 mL must be measured. The flow rates should be varied to ensure that they do not have any influence on the measured volumes. It is recommended that 1- and 2-L volumes also be pumped into the unit to check for linearity.

b. To check for leaks in the circuit, perform the following steps:
   1. Pump a 3-L volume into the bellows.
   2. Close the mouthpiece to the atmosphere to seal the circuit.
   3. Add a weight to the bell to speed up any small leaks.
   4. Turn on the kymograph at a slow speed, and put the pen on the paper to record any decrease in volume.
   5. If a leak is noted, it must be located and sealed.

c. Turn on the kymograph to its various speeds, and check its accuracy with a stopwatch. The manufac-

turer's literature should tell how far the kymograph will travel at its set speeds.

d. The thermometer reading should be compared with that of a laboratory quality unit.

e. Replace or repair any component that fails to meet the manufacturer's or established American Thoracic Society–American College of Chest Physicians (ATS-ACCP) standards.

Nitrogen washout equipment for measuring functional residual capacity. See Fig. 4-15 for the basic setup and breathing circuit of a nitrogen washout system. Review the troubleshooting of volume displacement and pneumotachometer spirometers; they are used with the nitrogen washout procedure to find the FRC. The nitrogen washout type RV test uses an emission spectroscopy ionization chamber analyzer for nitrogen. It is more commonly called a *Giesler tube ionizer*. It uses a vacuum pump to draw a gas sample into the ionization chamber. The intensity of the light spectrum given off by the ionized nitrogen directly relates to its percentage in the sample. A two-point calibration check should be performed at least every 6 months to check for linearity. It involves the following steps:

1. Draw a room-air sample into the unit and check the nitrogen meter reading. It should read about 78% nitrogen.
2. Adjust the meter reading, if necessary, to the manufacturer's specified value.
3. Turn off the needle valve so that no air can be drawn into the unit.
4. Check to see that the nitrogen meter reading decreases to zero nitrogen as the vacuum pump removes all gas from the ionization chamber.

Linearity (three-point calibration) can be checked by introducing from 5% to 10% nitrogen into the unit to see if the nitrogen meter measures that value. Do not use an analyzer that is inaccurate.

Helium dilution equipment for measuring functional residual capacity. See Fig. 4-13 for the basic setup of the helium dilution equipment and breathing circuit. Again, review the troubleshooting of volume displacement and pneumotachometer spirometers; they are used with the helium dilution procedure to find the FRC. Both the helium dilution FRC test and the lung diffusion tests require the analysis of helium in the gas mixture. A thermal conductivity analyzer is typically used. It operates under the principle of a Wheatstone bridge, in which differences in gas density lead to different cooling rates of heated thermistor beads. The different rates of cooling change electrical resistances and cause different electrical currents to flow. In a helium analyzer, the greater the helium concentration, the faster the thermistor bead cools, and the more electricity flows through the circuit. This is then read off a meter as the helium percentage.

The thermal conductivity helium analyzer should be linear over the clinically used range of helium to an accuracy of ±0.2% He. Minimally, a two-point calibration should be performed. A room-air sample can be drawn into the analyzer and should read zero helium. A known helium concentration may then be added and analyzed (for example, heliox, which contains 80% helium and 20% oxygen). A third point can be checked if needed by analyzing another known helium percentage.

Body plethysmography. See Fig. 4-16 for the basic components of the system. The plethysmograph chamber must be airtight when the door and all vents are closed. This can be confirmed by attaching a pressure manometer to a chamber port and applying a known volume or pressure into the sealed chamber. The pressures should be identical between the chamber pressure gauges and outside pressure manometer. The differential-pressure pneumotachometer must also read accurately when a known volume is pumped through it. Most manufacturers have a series of calibration check procedures listed in the equipment literature.

BIBLIOGRAPHY

American Association for Respiratory Care: Clinical practice guideline: spirometry, 1996 update. *Respir Care* 41(7):629-636, 1996.

American Association for Respiratory Care: Clinical practice guideline: spirometry, *Respir Care* 36(12):1414, 1991.

American Association for Respiratory Care: Clinical practice guideline: single-breath carbon monoxide diffusing capacity, *Respir Care* 38(5):511, 1993.

American Association for Respiratory Care: Clinical practice guideline: single-breath carbon monoxide diffusing capacity, 1999 update, *Respir Care* 44(1):91, 1999.

American Association for Respiratory Care: Clinical practice guideline: static lung volumes, 2001 revision and update, *Respir Care* 46(5):531-539, 2001.

American Association for Respiratory Care: Clinical practice guideline: static lung volumes, *Respir Care* 39(8):830, 1994.

American Association for Respiratory Care: Clinical practice guideline: infant/toddler pulmonary function tests, *Respir Care* 40(7):761, 1995.

American Association for Respiratory Care: Clinical practice guideline: bronchial provocation, *Respir Care* 37(8):902, 1992.

American Association for Respiratory Care: Clinical practice guideline: body plethysmography, 2001 revision and update, *Respir Care* 46(5):506-513, 2001.

American Association for Respiratory Care: Clinical practice guideline: assessing response to bronchodilator therapy at point of care, *Respir Care* 40(12):1300, 1995.

American Thoracic Society: Standardization of spirometry: 1987 update, *Am Rev Respir Dis* 136:1285, 1987.

Ayers LN, Whipp BJ, Ziment I: *A guide to the interpretation of pulmonary function tests,* ed 2, New York, 1978, Roerig.

Bates DV, Macklem PT, Christie RV: *Respiratory function in disease,* ed 2, Philadelphia, 1971, WB Saunders.

Beauchamp RK: Pulmonary function testing procedures. In Barnes TA, editor: *Respiratory care practice,* Chicago, 1988, Mosby.

Black LF, Hyatt RE: Maximal respiratory pressures: normal values and relationship to age and sex, *Am Rev Respir Dis* 99:696, 1969.

Branson RD, Hurst JM, Davis K Jr, et al: Measurement of maximal inspiratory pressure: a comparison of three methods, *Respir Care* 34(9):789, 1989.

Buist SA, Ross BB: Predicted values for closing volumes using a modified single-breath nitrogen test, *Am Rev Respir Dis* 111:405, 1975.

Cairo JM: Assessment of pulmonary function. In Cairo JM, Pilbeam SP, editors: *Mosby's respiratory care equipment,* ed 7, St Louis, Mosby, 2004.

Cherniack RM: *Pulmonary function testing,* ed 2, Philadelphia, 1992, WB Saunders.

Cherniack RM, Raber MD: Normal standards for ventilatory function using an automated wedge spirometer, *Am Rev Respir Dis* 106:38, 1972.

Clausen JL, editor: *Pulmonary function testing guidelines and controversies,* Orlando, 1984, Grune & Stratton.

Clausen JL: Clinical interpretation of pulmonary function test, *Respir Care* 34(7):638, 1989.

Crapo RO: Reference values for lung function tests, *Respir Care* 34(7):626, 1989.

Douce FH: Pulmonary function testing. In Wilkins RL, Stoller JK, Scanlan CL, editors: *Egan's fundamentals of respiratory care,* ed 8, St Louis, 2003, Mosby.

Enright PL, Hodgkin JE: Pulmonary function tests. In Burton GG, Hodgkin JE, Ward JJ, editors: *Respiratory care: a guide to clinical practice,* ed 4, Philadelphia, 1997, Lippincott-Raven.

Gaensler EA, Wright GW: Evaluation of respiratory impairment, *Arch Environ Health* 12:146, 1966.

Gardner RM: Pulmonary function laboratory standards, *Respir Care* 34(7):651, 1989.

Goldman HI, Becklake MR: Respiratory function tests: normal values at median altitudes and the prediction of normal results, *Am Rev Tuberculosis* 79:457, 1959.

Gursel G, Adams AB: Pulmonary function testing. In Hess DR, MacIntyre NR, Mishoe SC, et al, editors: *Respiratory care principles and practice,* Philadelphia, 2002, WB Saunders.

Hess D: Measurement of maximal inspiratory pressure: a call for standardization, *Respir Care* 34:857, 1989.

Holland SA: Pulmonary function testing. In Wyka KA, Mathews PJ, Clark WF, editors, *Foundations of respiratory care,* Albany, NY, 2002, Delmar.

Hunt GE: Diagnostic procedures at the bedside. In Fink JB, Hunt GE: *Clinical practice in respiratory care,* Philadelphia, 1999, Lippincott Williams & Wilkins.

Kacmarek RM, Cycyk-Chapman MC, Young-Palazzo PJ, et al: Determination of maximal inspiratory pressure: a clinical study and literature review, *Respir Care* 34:868, 1989.

Knudson RJ, Kaltenborn WT, Knudson DE, et al: The single-breath carbon monoxide diffusing capacity, *Am Rev Respir Dis* 135:805, 1987.

Knudson RJ, Lebowitz MD, Holberg CJ, et al: Changes in the normal maximal expiratory flow-volume curve with growth and aging, *Am Rev Respir Dis* 127:725, 1983.

Kory RC, Callahan R, Syner JC: The Veterans Administration-Army cooperative study of pulmonary function, I: clinical spirometry in normal men, *Am J Med* 30:243, 1961.

MacIntyre NR: Diffusing capacity of the lung for carbon monoxide, *Respir Care* 34(6):489, 1989.

Madama VC: *Pulmonary function testing and cardiopulmonary stress testing*, ed 2, Albany, NY, 1998, Delmar.

Morris JF, Koski A, Johnson LC: Spirometric standards for healthy nonsmoking adults, *Am Rev Respir Dis* 103:57, 1971.

National Institutes of Health: Practical guide for the diagnosis and management of asthma, Pub No 97-4053, Atlanta, 1997, U.S. Department of Health and Human Services.

Paoletti P, Viegi G, Pistelli G, et al: Reference equations for the single-breath diffusing capacity, *Am Rev Respir Dis* 132:806, 1985.

Ruppel G: *Manual of pulmonary function testing*, ed 8, St Louis, 2003, Mosby.

Single breath carbon monoxide diffusing capacity (transfer factor): recommendations for a standard technique, *Am Rev Respir Dis* 136:1299, 1987.

Snow MG: Determination of functional residual capacity, *Respir Care* 34(7):586, 1989.

Sue D: Exercise testing and the patient with cardiopulmonary disease. In Goldman AL, editor: *Problems in pulmonary disease* 2(1):1, Spring 1986.

Wanger J: *Pulmonary function testing*, ed 2, Baltimore, 1996, Williams & Wilkins.

Zamel N, Altose MD, Speir WA Jr: Statement on spirometry, *Chest* 3:547, 1983.

SELF-STUDY QUESTIONS

1. After performing complete spirometry on a 50-year-old patient, the following data are found:

	Predicted	Actual	% Predicted
TLC (L)	5.9	8.1	137
RV (L)	1.1	1.8	164
FVC (L)	5.0	2.6	52
$FEF_{25\%-75\%}$ (L/sec)	4.2	1.5	36
FEV_1/FVC	75%	20%	27

How should the data be interpreted?
   A. Mild restrictive lung disease
   B. Severe restrictive lung disease
   C. Mild obstructive lung disease
   D. Severe obstructive lung disease

2. A nitrogen washout test for residual volume has been performed on a patient for 7 minutes and has not reached the desired nitrogen percentage. What could explain this situation?
   A. There is an oxygen leak into the system.
   B. The patient has an abnormally high respiratory exchange ratio.
   C. The patient has severe air trapping.
   D. Nitrogen has been absorbed into the patient's tissues.

3. An order is received to perform the following bedside spirometry tests on a patient: tidal volume, FVC, and peak flow. Which device would you take with you to perform the tests?
   A. Stead-Wells water-seal spirometer
   B. Maximum inspiratory pressure manometer
   C. Differential pressure pneumotachometer
   D. Body plethysmograph

4. Which section of the following spirometry tracing represents the inspiratory reserve volume?

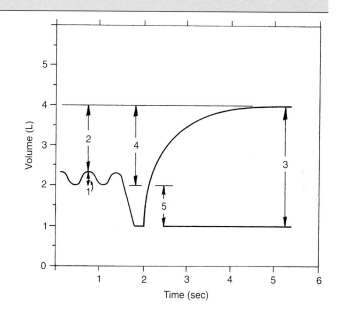

   A. 2
   B. 3
   C. 4
   D. 5

5. Which section of the spirometry tracing in question 4 represents the expiratory reserve volume?
   A. 1
   B. 2
   C. 3
   D. 4

6. After performing spirometry, it is important that patient flow rates be reported at:
   A. ATPS
   B. BTPS
   C. STPD
   D. ATPD

7. Your patient is performing a residual volume test on a water-seal spirometer in the pulmonary function laboratory. After breathing on the system for 1 minute, he takes out the mouthpiece and complains of being short of breath. What is the most likely problem in the pulmonary function system?
   A. The carbon dioxide absorber was accidentally left in the circuit.
   B. There is too much water around the spirometer bell.
   C. The carbon dioxide absorber has been left out of the circuit.
   D. Nose clips were left off of the patient.

8. Which of the following studies produces the most accurate determination of the TLC in a patient with severe emphysema?
   A. Single-breath nitrogen washout test
   B. Seven-minute nitrogen washout test
   C. Helium dilution test
   D. Body plethysmography test

9. In which type of patient is a carbon dioxide response curve test indicated?
   A. History of COPD
   B. History of asthma attacks
   C. History of ARDS
   D. History of asbestos exposure

10. Before having a patient perform a forced vital capacity test, the water-sealed spirometer should have all the following done *except*:
    A. Make sure that the circuit is airtight.
    B. Place a carbon dioxide–absorbing material in line with the circuit.
    C. Pump a 3-L volume into and out of the circuit to check for leaks.
    D. Check the kymograph speeds.

11. A properly performed FVC test will not have:
    I. Any coughing or leaks
    II. A weak patient effort
    III. An unsatisfactory start to the test
    IV. Excessive variability among test results
       A. I, II
       B. II, III
       C. I, II, IV
       D. I, II, III, IV

12. A patient has a suspected diagnosis of asthma. Which of the following tests would be the *least* helpful in assessing the patient for this condition?
    A. Before and after bronchodilator study
    B. Flow-volume loop
    C. Diffusion study
    D. Bronchoprovocation

13. A patient with a history of COPD has been admitted. To help clarify her diagnosis between emphysema and asthma, which of the following should the respiratory therapist recommend?
    A. Flow-volume loop
    B. Maximum voluntary ventilation
    C. Spirometry before and after an inhaled bronchodilator
    D. Peak flow test

14. Based on the flow-volume loops that are shown in the following figure, which one represents the most severe small airways obstruction?

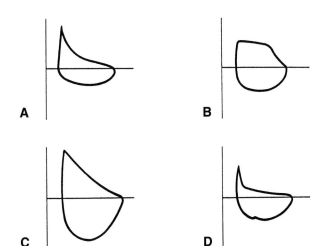

    A. Tracing *A*
    B. Tracing *B*
    C. Tracing *C*
    D. Tracing *D*

15. Based on the flow-volume loops that are shown in question 14, which one represents the fixed extrathoracic obstruction?
    A. Tracing *A*
    B. Tracing *B*
    C. Tracing *C*
    D. Tracing *D*

16. Based on the flow-volume loops that are shown in question 14, tracing *A* represents a patient with asthmatic bronchitis, and tracing *C* represents the same patient 1 hour after receiving an inhaled bronchodilator medication. What conclusion can be reached?
    A. The patient's condition is treatable.
    B. The patient is not giving his or her best effort.
    C. The patient's condition has worsened.
    D. The patient needs another bronchodilator treatment.

ANSWER KEY

1. **D.** Rationale: All of the data on the table indicate severe obstructive lung disease. The TLC and RV are both greater than 120% of predicted, indicating significant air trapping. All three flow measurements are far lower than predicted. If the patient had restrictive lung disease, the TLC and RV values would be smaller than predicted.

2. **C.** Rationale: Patients with severe air trapping, as found with emphysema, take much longer than normal to "wash" the nitrogen out of their lungs. Often the test must be prolonged for several minutes past the usual 7-minute duration to eliminate enough nitrogen to complete the test. The nitrogen washout test requires the patient breathe in 100% oxygen to displace the resident nitrogen found in the lungs. The respiratory exchange ratio has to do with oxygen consumption and carbon dioxide production; it has nothing to do with nitrogen elimination. Nitrogen is not active in metabolism. The normal amount of nitrogen found in the body is not significantly affected by the nitrogen washout test.

3. **C.** Rationale: A differential-pressure pneumotachometer is portable enough to be taken to a patient's bedside. It can be used to determine a patient's tidal volume, FVC, and peak flow. A Stead-Wells water-seal spirometer is not typically moved because it is large and the water will be splashed about while moving it. The device can be used for all three listed tests when done in the pulmonary function laboratory. A maximum inspiratory pressure manometer is used for the maximum inspiratory pressure (MIP) test. It may be reconfigured for a maximal expiratory pressure (MEP) test but cannot measure any gas flows. A body plethysmograph is far too large to move to a patient's bedside. However, it can be used for all three listed tests when done in the pulmonary function laboratory.

4. **D.** Rationale: The inspiratory reserve volume (IRV) is found from the end of a tidal volume inspiration to the TLC. It represents the additional volume that can be inhaled after a normal tidal volume. Review Fig. 4-14 if needed. Do not be confused by vital capacity efforts that look "upside down" compared with others. Review the various volume-time curve tracings in the chapter for extra practice determining volumes. Volume number 2 is the ERV. Volume number 3 is the vital capacity. Volume number 4 is the ERV and tidal volume combined. Volume number 1 is the tidal volume.

5. **B.** Rationale: The expiratory reserve volume (ERV) represents the volume of air that can be exhaled after a normal tidal volume is exhaled. Review Fig. 4-14 if needed. Do not be confused by vital capacity efforts that look "upside down" compared with others. Review the various volume-time curve tracings in the

chapter for extra practice determining volumes. Volume number 1 is the tidal volume. Volume number 3 is the vital capacity. Volume number 4 is the ERV and tidal volume combined.

6. **B.** Rationale: All patient flows, volumes, and capacities must be mathematically converted from ATPS (atmospheric temperature, pressure, saturated) to BTPS (body temperature, pressure, saturated) conditions. This results in the exhaled flows or volumes measured at room temperature being adjusted for the expansion of gas found at the patient's body temperature. STPD (standard temperature, pressure, dry) conditions are used only with diffusing-capacity tests. ATPD (atmospheric temperature, pressure, dry) is not used for reporting any pulmonary function results.

7. **C.** Rationale: It is necessary to place a carbon dioxide absorber in the PFT system when the patient has to breathe on a closed system for an extended period. Without one, the patient will rebreathe his or her own exhaled carbon dioxide. If too much water is around the spirometer bell, some splashing may occur. However, too much water will not cause the patient to feel short of breath. If nose clips were left off the patient, he or she may breathe through the nose instead of the mouth. This will not cause a feeling of shortness of breath.

8. **D.** Rationale: A body plethysmography test for total lung capacity (TLC) will be the most accurate for a patient with severe emphysema because it can measure the volume of *all* gas within the chest. This includes gas in damaged parts of the lungs that do not ultimately connect to larger airways and the outside atmosphere. The 7-minute nitrogen washout test and helium dilution test measure only the gas in areas of the lungs that connect to the larger airways and outside atmosphere. This may result in an undermeasurement of the patient's true lung volumes. The single-breath nitrogen washout test is not used to measure the TLC. It is used to assess the evenness of inspiratory and expiratory gas flow.

9. **A.** Rationale: A patient with a history of COPD can have a carbon dioxide response curve test performed to determine if his or her central chemoreceptors are responding normally to the stimulation of carbon dioxide. Some COPD patients do not increase their breathing as much as expected when exposed to higher than normal levels of carbon dioxide. Patients with a history of asthma, acute respiratory distress syndrome (ARDS), and asbestos exposure do not have their central chemoreceptors affected adversely.

10. **B.** Rationale: Because the FVC test lasts for only a few seconds, the patient will not rebreathe significant amounts of carbon dioxide; therefore a carbon dioxide

absorber is not needed. In addition, in some pulmonary function systems, a carbon dioxide absorber slows the flow of exhaled gas and results in lower reported FVC values than are actually present. The PFT circuit must be airtight to prevent any leakage and resulting lower volumes and flows. Volume calibration is done by pumping a known volume (3 L) into and out of the spirometer. Any leak will result in a lower-than-expected volume being found. The kymograph should have its speed settings checked to make sure that the timing of the test is accurate.

11. **D.** Rationale: All listed items must be avoided to ensure an accurate FVC test. Coughing causes variable flows and cuts off the full FVC volume. A leak results in a loss of volume. A weak patient effort results in a slower expiratory flow than the patient can optimally provide. When tests are done properly, they show consistent results. Excessive variability shows inconsistent patient effort.

12. **C.** Rationale: A diffusion study measures carbon monoxide diffusion to evaluate oxygen diffusion across the alveolar-capillary membrane. It is not helpful in the diagnosis of asthma. The other three listed tests can be very useful in diagnosing asthma. With a before and after bronchodilator study, an asthmatic who is responsive to inhaled bronchodilator medications shows improved flows after inhaling the medication. A patient with an asthma problem often reveals a distinctive flow-volume loop tracing (see Fig. 4-8). A bronchoprovocation test often produces decreased expiratory flows in a patient with asthma.

13. **C.** Rationale: Spirometry before and after an inhaled bronchodilator is the best test to differentiate between asthma and emphysema. Most asthmatic patients have some reversibility to their bronchospasm. Their spirometry should show improved expiratory flows after inhaling a bronchodilating medication. Patients with emphysema have very little if any improvement in expiratory flows after inhaling a bronchodilating medication. This is because it is the alveoli, and not the airways, that are damaged. The other three listed tests may not show significant differences between patients with asthma and those with emphysema.

14. **D.** Rationale: Tracing D shows a severe "scoop" during the expiratory part of the patient effort after the peak flow. This dramatic decrease in expiratory flow is characteristic of severe small-airways obstruction. Tracing A shows a less-severe decrease in expiratory flow after the peak flow. Tracing B shows a severely reduced peak flow that is characteristic of a fixed extrathoracic obstruction. Tracing C shows a normal flow-volume loop. Review Fig. 4-8 if needed for a comparison of different flow-volume loops.

15. **B.** Rationale: Tracing B shows a severely reduced peak flow that is characteristic of a fixed extrathoracic obstruction. This might be caused by a laryngeal tumor, paralyzed vocal cord, or other upper airway problem. Tracing D shows a severe "scoop" during the expiratory part of the patient effort after the peak flow. This dramatic decrease in expiratory flow is characteristic of severe small-airways obstruction. Tracing A shows a less severe decrease in expiratory flow after the peak flow. Tracing C shows a normal flow-volume loop. Review Fig. 4-10 if needed for a comparison of different flow-volume loops.

16. **A.** Rationale: Tracing C shows an increased peak flow compared with tracing A and correction of the expiratory "scoop" seen in tracing A. In addition, the inspiratory flow on tracing C is greater than that on tracing A. All of these changes show significant improvement, indicating that the patient's condition is treatable. The patient's effort or lack of effort cannot be determined by looking at the two tracings. Tracing C is normal and does not justify the patient receiving another bronchodilator treatment.

5

Advanced Cardiopulmonary Monitoring

Note 1: The National Board for Respiratory Care (NBRC) has released the *RRT Examination Matrix* (covering the testable items on the Written Registry Exam) and the *CSE Examination Matrix* (covering the testable items on the Clinical Simulation Exam). Turn to the appendices at the back of this book for both publications in their original format. This book is intended to cover all of the testable items in these two publications. This chapter (and all others) uses the abbreviation "WRE" for the coded items testable on the Written Registry Exam *and* Clinical Simulation Exam. The listed difficulty (R, Recall; Ap, Application; An, Analysis) relates to the question difficulty on the Written Registry Exam. The abbreviation "CSE" is used for the coded items testable on *only* the Clinical Simulation Exam. Because no question difficulty level is given for this exam, be prepared for anything.

Note 2: A review of the most recent Written Registry Examinations has shown an average of three questions (3% of the exam) that cover advanced cardiopulmonary monitoring. The Clinical Simulation Exam is comprehensive and may include everything that should be known or performed by an advanced level respiratory therapist.

MODULE A

Cardiopulmonary monitoring procedures

1. Capnography (exhaled CO₂ monitoring)

a. Review capnography data in the patient's chart (WRE code: IA7d) [Difficulty: An]

Capnography is the analysis of graphic and numeric data showing the pattern and amount of exhaled carbon dioxide (CO_2). It is wise to look for previous capnography data before measuring the patient's exhaled CO_2 level again. Look for numeric values as well as a printout of the tracing of exhaled CO_2. Be prepared to compare the previous information with the new data to help evaluate the patient's condition. It also is useful to compare the patient's pressure of CO_2 in arterial blood ($PaCO_2$) with the capnography information, even though they should not be expected to be the same.

b. Perform the bedside procedure (WRE code: IB7b and IIIE3c) [Difficulty: An]

The capnometer is a device that measures the concentration of CO_2 in a gas sample from a patient. The

principle of operation of most bedside units is based on the absorption by carbon dioxide of infrared light in a narrow wavelength band (4.3 mm). Infrared light at this wavelength is passed through the gas sample to a receiving unit. The difference between what is sent out and what is received is directly related to how much carbon dioxide is in the gas sample. In other words, the greater the difference between the sent and the received infrared light, the greater the concentration of carbon dioxide in the gas sample.

The capnometer is calibrated by comparing a gas sample without carbon dioxide (possibly room air) with a second gas sample containing a known amount of carbon dioxide. The first gas sample without CO_2 should give a "zero" reading. Adjust the calibration control to zero if needed. The second sample usually contains 5% to 10% carbon dioxide. The capnometer should read out a CO_2 level that matches the amount in the known gas sample. Adjust the calibration control as necessary. The carbon dioxide level can be read as a percentage or fraction ($FACO_2$) or as partial pressure ($PACO_2$).

The capnograph is a strip-chart recorder that provides a copy of the patient's exhaled carbon dioxide curve. At least two paper speeds are useful for different purposes. The fast speed is most useful for evaluating sudden changes in the patient's condition. Each individual breath is easily seen (Fig. 5-1). The slow speed is most useful for trend monitoring (Fig. 5-2).

Two different gas sampling methods exist: mainstream and sidestream. The mainstream method involves having the infrared sensing unit at the airway; usually it is attached directly to the endotracheal/tracheostomy tube. If the patient is on a ventilator, the sampling adapter must be placed between the endotracheal tube and the ventilator circuit (with or without mechanical dead space). All inspired and expired gas passes through the sensor (Fig. 5-3).

The sidestream method uses a capillary tube placed so that a small sampling of the patient's exhaled gas can be drawn into the capnometer for analysis. It is not necessary for the patient's entire breath to pass through the sampling adapter; therefore it can be used in an unintubated patient by taping the sampling catheter a short

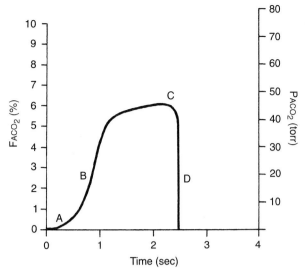

Fig. 5-1 Normal capnograph tracing taken at a fast speed. The percentage of exhaled alveolar CO_2 is shown on the left vertical scale as $FACO_2$. The partial pressure of exhaled alveolar CO_2 is shown on the right vertical scale as $PACO_2$. The tracing of exhaled gas can be divided into these four components: *A,* the beginning of exhalation, which shows no carbon dioxide in the upper airway anatomic dead space; *B,* the addition of alveolar gas, rich in carbon dioxide, to the anatomic dead space gas causes a rapid increase in measured CO_2; *C,* pure alveolar gas with a stable amount of CO_2 causes a plateau. The end-tidal CO_2 point is shown at *C* just before inspiration; and *D,* inspiration with a rapid decrease in carbon dioxide to zero. A fast-speed tracing is more useful for determining the cause of a patient's changing condition than a slow-speed tracing.

Fig. 5-3 Schematic drawing of a mainstream exhaled carbon dioxide analyzer sensor. The infrared sensor is attached to the patient's airway so that all of the exhaled and inhaled gas passes through it. *(From Szaflarski NL, Cohen NH: Use of capnography in critically ill adults.* Heart Lung *20:363–374, 1991.)*

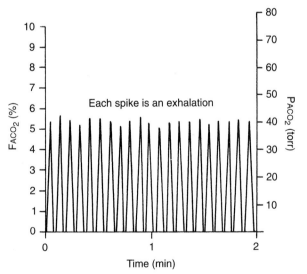

Fig. 5-2 Normal capnograph tracing taken at a slow speed. The percentage of exhaled alveolar CO_2 is shown on the left vertical scale as $FACO_2$. The partial pressure of exhaled alveolar CO_2 is shown on the right vertical scale as $PACO_2$. The slow speed results in a blending of parts *A, B,* and *C* of the fast-speed tracing (see Fig. 5-1). Each spike is part *C* of the curve and marks an exhalation. A slow-speed tracing is more useful in trend monitoring of a patient than a fast-speed tracing.

distance into a nostril. If the patient is on a ventilator, the sampling adapter must be placed between the endotracheal tube and the ventilator circuit (with or without mechanical dead space). Remember that the patient's exhaled tidal volume (V_T) and minute volume (V_E) is reduced by the amount that is drawn into the capnometer (Fig. 5-4).

c. Interpret the results from the procedure (WRE code: IB8b) [Difficulty: An]

It is known that carbon dioxide diffuses from a higher concentration in the tissues to the venous blood and to the lungs to be exhaled. Fig. 5-5 shows the normal physiology behind capnography. This diffusion or "flow" of CO_2 results in a measurable gradient or difference. In a normal, upright sitting person, a close relation exists between the carbon dioxide levels in the venous blood, exhaled carbon dioxide gas, and arterial blood. The carbon dioxide level at the end of exhalation is the most commonly monitored for patient care. This is called the *end-tidal carbon dioxide pressure* ($PetCO_2$). When ventilation and perfusion match well, as in a normal upright person, the gradient between the arterial carbon dioxide level ($PaCO_2$) and the $PetCO_2$ is between 1 and 5 torr. The gradient will show the $PetCO_2$ to be less than the $PaCO_2$. This is because the $PetCO_2$ is an average of exhaled carbon dioxide from all lung areas.

Box 5-1 lists normal values of capnography. Three factors influence the use of capnography and the interpretation of the results. First is the patient's metabolism. The average resting adult produces about 200 mL of CO_2 per minute, and fever and exercise increase this value.

Fig. 5-4 Representation of a sidestream capnometry system. A capillary tube is placed into the ventilator circuit to sample the exhaled and inhaled gases.

Hypothermia, sleep, and sedation decrease CO_2 production. Exhaled CO_2 is monitored during a cardiopulmonary resuscitation (CPR) attempt to determine the effectiveness of circulation and ventilation attempts and to determine whether the efforts should be continued or stopped. If no carbon dioxide is being exhaled, a patient's metabolism has stopped altogether, and death has occurred. Nothing is to be gained by continuing CPR efforts.

Second, although not a major factor, is the patient's cardiac output. Sepsis, which might double a patient's cardiac output, reduces the Pco_2 only a few torr (millimeters of mercury [mm Hg]). Cardiogenic shock, which reduces the cardiac output, increases the partial pressure of CO_2 (Pco_2) only a few torr.

Third, and most important, is alveolar ventilation. A doubling of alveolar ventilation, under steady-state conditions for carbon dioxide production, results in a halving of the Pco_2 in arterial blood and alveolar gas. However, a reduction of alveolar ventilation to half of its previous level will result in the $Paco_2$ and $Petco_2$ being doubled (Fig. 5-6).

V_T and respiratory rate are directly related to alveolar ventilation. Of the two, tidal volume is more important because it relates to the patient's dead space (V_D) to V_T

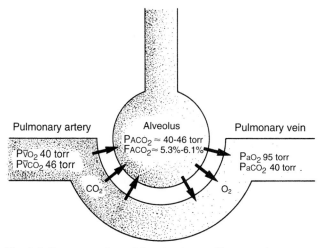

Fig. 5-5 Representation of the alveolar-capillary membrane showing the diffusion of oxygen and carbon dioxide and the arterialization of venous blood. Also shown are alveolar CO_2 values measured by capnography.

BOX 5-1 Normal Blood Gas and Capnography Values (Based on a Sea-Level Barometric Pressure of 760 torr)[*]

$Paco_2$ is approximately 40 torr.
$P\bar{v}co_2$ is approximately 46 torr.
The pressure of exhaled alveolar CO_2 ($PAco_2$) ranges from approximately 35 to 43 torr with the breathing cycle.
The pressure of exhaled end-tidal CO_2 ($Petco_2$) ranges from 35 to 43 torr. This shows the CO_2 level varying between the arterial and mixed venous blood levels. This value is often correlated with the $Paco_2$.
The percentage of exhaled CO_2 ($FAco_2$) ranges from 5% to approximately 6% with the breathing cycle.
The percentage of end-tidal CO_2 ($FAco_2$) is approximately 5% to 6% and correlates with the $Paco_2$.

---

[*]Both $PAco_2$ and $FAco_2$ may be seen listed as end-tidal CO_2. End-tidal CO_2 may be abbreviated as $ETco_2$, $Etco_2$, $etco_2$, or $Petco_2$.
$FAco_2$, Fraction (percentage) of CO_2 level; $Paco_2$, partial pressure of CO_2 in arterial blood; $PAco_2$, partial pressure of alveolar CO_2 level; $P\bar{v}co_2$, partial pressure of carbon dioxide in mixed venous blood.

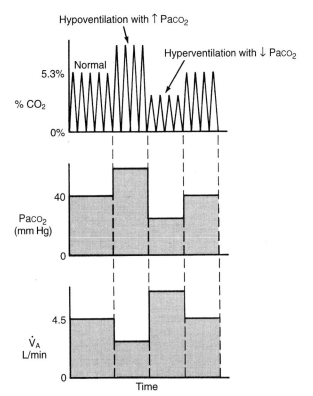

Fig. 5-6 Relation between alveolar ventilation, Pa_{CO_2}, and exhaled CO_2 percentage. *(From Pilbeam SP: Mechanical ventilation: physiological and clinical applications, ed 3, St Louis, 1998, Mosby.)*

ratio (V_D/V_T). A decrease in the patient's V_T results in less alveolar ventilation and an increase in Pet_{CO_2}. Conversely, an increase in the V_T results in more alveolar ventilation and a decrease in the Pet_{CO_2}.

Capnography is most accurate and correlates best with the Pa_{CO_2} if the patient's ventilation and perfusion match. The more ventilation and perfusion mismatching or the more unstable the pulmonary perfusion, the wider or less reliable the gradient between the patient's arterial carbon dioxide and alveolar carbon dioxide levels will be. The following procedures should be performed to help understand the patient's condition and interpret the capnography results.

> ### Exam Hint
>
> **R**emember that millimeters of mercury (mm Hg) and torr (Torricelli) are equivalent units of pressure. The National Board of Respiratory Care (NBRC) uses these two units for different items in its questions. It uses millimeters of mercury for blood pressure measurements and torr for blood gas values (such as Pa_{CO_2} and $P\bar{v}_{O_2}$). However, in questions dealing with capnography, the NBRC has used both units in its questions that relate to exhaled CO_2 (such as PA_{CO_2} and Pet_{CO_2}).

1. Calculate and interpret the arterial–end-tidal carbon dioxide gradient

The arterial–end-tidal carbon dioxide gradient [$P(a–et)_{CO_2}$] is useful, because once it is reliably determined, the patient's ventilatory condition can be monitored by capnography alone. Drawing an arterial blood sample to measure the Pa_{CO_2} level is less necessary if the patient is stable.

The normal gradient is 1 to 5 torr or less. However, most patients using capnography are not normal. The possible gradient ranges from –6 to + 20 torr in unstable patients with cardiopulmonary abnormalities. For example, the patient who is breathing shallowly may have an end-tidal CO_2 that is greater than the arterial CO_2. This is because the patient is not exhaling completely to empty alveolar gas. Therefore determining each patient's own gradient is important.

Follow these steps:

a. Simultaneously draw an arterial blood gas (ABG) sample for Pa_{CO_2} measurement and take an end-tidal gas sample for Pet_{CO_2} measurement.

b. The difference is the $P(a–et)_{CO_2}$ gradient. The alveolar sample commonly shows a lower CO_2 level than the arterial sample.

EXAMPLE 1

A patient is seen in the recovery room after surgery and has the following P_{CO_2} levels:

$$\begin{array}{rl} Pa_{CO_2} = & 40 \text{ torr} \\ Pet_{CO_2} = & -36 \text{ torr} \\ \hline P(a–et)_{CO_2} = & 4 \text{ torr} \end{array}$$

The usefulness of this gradient is demonstrated when monitoring a patient's spontaneous breathing during weaning or making ventilator changes in the tidal volume or minute volume. It may be possible to avoid drawing as many ABG samples.

EXAMPLE 2

The patient in Example 1 is seen later and has the following capnography reading: Pet_{CO_2} = 54 torr. The patient's Pa_{CO_2} can be easily calculated by subtraction:

$$\begin{array}{rl} Pet_{CO_2} = & 54 \text{ torr} \\ P(a–et)_{CO_2} \text{ gradient} = & +4 \text{ torr} \\ \hline \text{Estimated } Pa_{CO_2} = & 58 \text{ torr} \end{array}$$

It can be concluded that the patient is not breathing as deeply as before. Appropriate action should be taken to awaken the patient, further reverse the anesthesia, or begin artificial ventilation.

Review the components of a fast-speed capnography tracing in Fig. 5-1 to understand a normal person's expiratory pattern. Fig. 5-7 shows eight different abnormal fast-speed capnography tracings. See the figure legend for

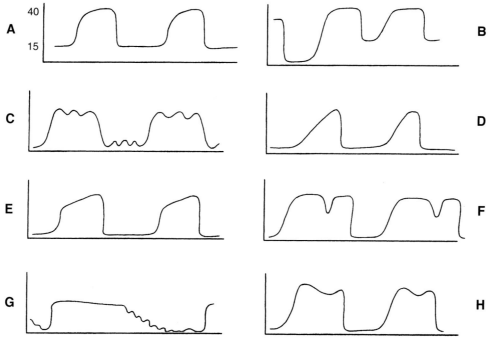

Fig. 5-7 A series of abnormal fast-speed capnography tracings. **A,** A mechanically ventilated patient with a malfunctioning exhalation valve. Note that the baseline CO_2 level is elevated because the patient's exhaled breath is measured during an inspiration. Correction of the exhalation valve should result in normal inhalation and exhalation. **B,** This rapidly rising baseline gas pressure and failure to return to baseline are usually seen when moisture or secretions block the capillary tube. Clearing the obstruction enables the patient's gas to again reach the analyzer. **C,** Distortions in the tracing from incomplete exhalation. These may be caused by hiccups, chest compressions during cardiopulmonary resuscitation, or inconsistent tidal volume efforts during an asthma attack. **D,** An obstructive lung disease patient with ventilation and perfusion mismatching. No alveolar plateau with a stable CO_2 level is seen. Inhaling a bronchodilator should result in the tracing returning closer to normal. **E,** A patient with restrictive lung disease showing no plateau of alveolar gas emptying. This is because the alveoli do not empty evenly. **F,** A sudden decrease in carbon dioxide level in the middle of an exhalation indicates that the patient attempted inspiration. This "cleft" is usually seen when a patient who has been pharmacologically paralyzed begins to regain movement. **G,** Uneven carbon dioxide levels seen at the end of exhalation can be caused by (1) The patient's heartbeat pumping fresh blood and CO_2 to the emptying lungs. The cardiogenic oscillations should match the heart rate; (2) The ventilator's exhalation valve is fluttering open and closed. **H,** The alveolar plateau is biphasic. This has been seen in patients with lungs that are different in compliance and ventilation/perfusion matching (e.g., single-lung transplantation). *(From Shapiro BA, Peruzzi WT, Templin R: Clinical application of blood gases, ed 5, St Louis, 1994, Mosby.)*

an explanation of each problem. As the patient returns to normal, the tracing should approach that shown in Fig. 5-1.

2. Calculate and interpret the arterial–residual volume alveolar carbon dioxide gradient

If the patient is cooperative and will exhale maximally to residual volume (RV), this measurement provides more clinically useful information. The usual $P(a-RV)CO_2$ gradient in a normal person is less than 7 torr. The wider the gradient, the more ventilation-to-perfusion ($\dot{V}/\dot{Q}$) mismatching there is. A gradient of more than 13 torr is

considered to be markedly abnormal. This may be the case in patients with chronic obstructive pulmonary disease (COPD), pulmonary emboli, left heart failure (LHF), or hypotension.

When comparing the normal (solid line) tracing in Fig. 5-8 with the $\dot{V}/\dot{Q}$ mismatching (dashed line) tracing, note the increased gradient at end-tidal CO_2. With continued exhalation to RV, the LHF and COPD patients have a narrowing of the gradient. This can be used clinically to monitor these patients' progress and response to treatment. The patient with large pulmonary emboli will not have such a narrowing of the gradient as he or she exhales to RV. This patient's gradient will narrow to

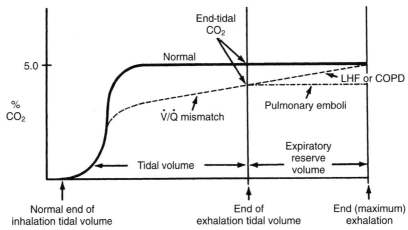

Fig. 5-8 Comparison of several fast-speed capnograph tracings showing how the exhaled carbon dioxide level changes as the patient exhales to residual volume. A normal tracing is matched against abnormal tracings of pulmonary emboli, left heart failure (LHF), and chronic obstructive pulmonary disease (COPD). The normal patient has the same end-tidal CO_2 as residual volume CO_2, showing good matching of ventilation and perfusion. LHF and COPD patients have a narrowing of the gradient as residual volume is approached. The patient with a pulmonary embolism keeps the same gradient at the residual volume as that found at the end of the tidal volume. *(From Pilbeam SP: Mechanical ventilation: physiological and clinical applications, ed 3, St Louis, 1998, Mosby.)*

normal as the emboli are resolved and the physiologic dead space returns to normal.

2. Review dead space to tidal volume ratio data in the patient's chart (WRE code: IA7d) [Difficulty: An]

The dead space to tidal volume test (V_D/V_T) is most commonly performed to document the amount of dead space (wasted ventilation) in a patient with a pulmonary embolism. A number of other clinical situations, discussed later, can justify the procedure. Review previous data before repeating the test to understand whether the patient's condition has changed or is abnormal. Be prepared to compare the previous information with the new data to help evaluate the patient's current condition.

The normal adult's V_D/V_T ratio ranges from 0.2 (20%) to 0.4 (40%). Anatomic dead space is normally greater in men than in women. The normal 3-kg neonate's dead space to tidal volume ratio is 0.3 (30%). Physiologic dead space (also known as respiratory dead space) is gas that is

ventilated into the lungs but does not take part in gas exchange. This is because the alveoli are not perfused or are underperfused for the amount of gas that they receive.

Physiologic dead space is made up of the following:

1. Anatomic dead space, or the gas in the connecting airways from the nose and mouth to the terminal bronchioles. Generally it is assumed to be about 1 mL/lb of ideal body weight, or 2.2 mL/kg of ideal body weight.
2. Alveolar dead space that is made up of nonfunctioning alveoli that are ventilated but not perfused is minimal in a normal person. The previous "normal" adult example has the expected amount of dead space for his or her weight.

The following conditions or pulmonary disorders can cause the ratio to vary from the normal range:

1. Decreased V_D/V_T ratio
   a. Lung resection or pneumonectomy because the airways are removed; the patient will maintain his or her tidal volume in the other lung segments.
   b. Asthma attack because the airways are narrowed.
   c. Insertion of an endotracheal or tracheostomy tube because the upper airway is bypassed.
   d. Exercise in the normal person because the increased blood pressure increases perfusion of the apices (zone 1).
2. Increased V_D/V_T ratio
   a. Vascular tumor because of decreased perfusion to ventilated alveoli.
   b. Pulmonary embolism because of lack of blood flow to ventilated alveoli. Consider this if the patient is a

candidate for a pulmonary embolism and suddenly deteriorates.

3. Increased dead space effect with ventilation greater than perfusion ($\dot{V} > \dot{Q}$)
   a. Rapid, shallow ventilations because the upper-airway dead space is overventilated compared with the alveoli.
   b. Mechanical dead space added to the ventilator circuit. This is an intentional effort to have the patient retain some of his or her exhaled carbon dioxide to correct for a respiratory alkalosis.
   c. COPD (bronchitis, bronchiectasis, cystic fibrosis, emphysema) because varying degrees of bronchospasm, mucous plugging, and tissue destruction lead to increased ventilation and perfusion mismatching.

Many clinicians believe that a dead space/tidal volume ratio of 0.6 (60%) or more is an indication for mechanically ventilating the patient. A person who is wasting 60% or more of his or her ventilation will soon tire from the work of breathing and go into ventilatory failure.

> ### Exam Hint
>
> **R**emember that a pulmonary embolism is the most likely cause of a sudden increase in dead space. This concept is often tested. In addition, a question usually relates to identifying that a COPD patient will have an increased V_D/V_T value.

MATH REVIEW

Calculate the dead space to tidal volume ratio. NOTE: The NBRC does not list this calculation as testable on the current advanced practitioner exams. However, it was tested on the previous generation of Written Registry Exams. The calculation is included here as an aid to the exam taker. The procedure is the mathematical comparison of a person's dead-space volume with his or her tidal volume. Steps in the procedure follow and are shown in Fig. 5-9:

1. Determine the *average* exhaled CO_2 ($P\bar{E}CO_2$) value by either of these methods:
   a. Collect the patient's entire exhaled gas sample over several minutes in a large airtight bag. Count

Fig. 5-9 A schematic presentation of the procedure for gathering patient samples for calculating the dead space–to–tidal volume ratio (V_D/V_T). An anesthesia or other airtight bag is used to gather all exhaled gas to determine the average exhaled carbon dioxide pressure. An arterial sample is collected for $PaCO_2$. *(From Pilbeam SP: Mechanical ventilation: physiological and clinical applications, ed 2, St Louis, 1992, Mosby.)*

the number of breaths that occurred. Calculate the average tidal volume breath by dividing the total exhaled volume by the total rate. Put all or part of this gas sample through the blood gas analyzer for the P_{CO_2} value.

    b. Have the patient's exhaled gas pass through a capnometer that can give you an average value (not end-tidal CO_2). A number of breaths should be averaged for greater P_{CO_2} accuracy. Measure or calculate the patient's average tidal volume over the time of the test.

2. Draw an arterial sample at the same time that you are performing either step 1a or 1b. Have the blood sample analyzed for Pa_{CO_2}.

3. Calculate the results by using either of two methods.

Determine the decimal fraction or percentage of dead space. Place both carbon dioxide values into this formula, which is derived from the original Bohr formula:

$$V_D/V_T \text{ (or } V_D) = \frac{(Pa_{CO_2} - P\overline{E}_{CO_2})}{Pa_{CO_2}}$$

In which:

V_D/V_T or V_D = The patient's physiologic dead space
Pa_{CO_2} = The patient's arterial carbon dioxide pressure
$P\overline{E}_{CO_2}$ = The patient's average exhaled carbon dioxide pressure

The following example is based on an abnormal adult:
Pa_{CO_2} = 45 torr
$P\overline{E}_{CO_2}$ = 18 torr

$$V_D = \frac{(45 - 18)}{45}$$

$$= \frac{27}{45} = .6$$

The patient's V_D fraction can be recorded as 0.6 or 60%. (Note that this equation must be used when the patient's tidal volume is not known.)

Determine the dead space volume. Place both carbon dioxide values into this formula, which is derived from the original Bohr formula:

$$V_D/V_T \text{ (or } V_D) = \frac{(Pa_{CO_2} - P\overline{E}_{CO_2})}{Pa_{CO_2}} \times V_T$$

In which:

V_D/V_T or V_D = The patient's physiologic dead space
V_T = Average exhaled tidal volume
Pa_{CO_2} = The patient's arterial carbon dioxide pressure
$P\overline{E}_{CO_2}$ = The patient's average exhaled carbon dioxide pressure

The following example is based on a normal adult:
V_T = 500 mL
Pa_{CO_2} = 40 torr
$P\overline{E}_{CO_2}$ = 28 torr

$$V_D = \frac{(40 - 28)}{40}$$

$$= \frac{12}{40} \times 500 = 0.3 \times 500 \text{ mL} = 150 \text{ mL}$$

The patient's physiologic V_D volume = 150 mL (Note that this equation must be used when the patient's tidal volume is known.) In addition, the preceding equation allows for calculation of the patient's V_D/V_T ratio. In this example, it is 150/500, 0.3, or 30%, depending on how it is written.

Note: The recent advent of *volumetric capnography* technology allows the patient's dead space to be rapidly determined. These units can simultaneously measure the patient's exhaled tidal volume and the variable percentage of carbon dioxide found during the exhalation (Fig. 5-10). The computer that is integrated with the volumetric capnography unit then calculates the volume of dead space as a fraction of the exhaled tidal volume.

3. Mixed venous blood sampling
a. Review the patient's chart for data on mixed venous oxygen values (WRE code: IA5) [Difficulty: Ap, An]

A patient with a functioning pulmonary artery catheter can have a sample of blood withdrawn through it and analyzed for the mixed venous oxygen ($P\overline{v}_{O_2}$) value (and the other blood gas values as well). As always, the $P\overline{v}_{O_2}$ value(s) should be reviewed before measuring it again. (See Chapter 3 for information on mixed venous blood gas values.)

b. Perform mixed venous oxygen sampling at the bedside (WRE code: IIIE2b) [Difficulty: An]

Currently three methods are used to perform the bedside procedure. All methods require that a pulmonary

Fig. 5-10 A graphic representation of the factors involved in the calculation of a patient's dead space volume, or dead space to tidal volume (V_D/V_T) ratio, through volumetric capnography. These units can measure exhaled carbon dioxide (by pressure or percentage) at time intervals as the patient's tidal volume is exhaled. Review Fig. 5-1, as needed, for a normal capnograph tracing.

artery catheter (PAC) be placed into the patient. NOTE: The NBRC refers to PACs as "flow-directed balloon-tipped catheters." The catheter also is commonly called a Swan-Ganz catheter after the inventors who lent their names to a particular brand. They come in different lengths and diameters and have variable features for pediatric or adult patients. See Fig. 5-11 for a typical adult catheter.

Perform the procedure through the distal lumen of a PAC as it is being inserted. This method is used when trying to determine whether a ventricular septal defect is present. The procedure is commonly done on neonates with suspected congenital heart defects, but it may be used in adults as well. With sterile technique, blood samples are withdrawn serially from the right atrium, right ventricle, and sometimes from the pulmonary artery. See Fig. 5-12 for the blood sampling sites as the catheter is advanced through the heart.

Normally, the $P\bar{v}O_2$ and $S\bar{v}O_2$ values are the same in all blood samples. The patient with a ventricular septal defect shows an increase in $P\bar{v}O_2$ and $S\bar{v}O_2$ values going from the right atrium to the right ventricle and pulmonary artery. This is because the oxygenated blood from the left ventricle is forced though the ventricular septal defect to increase the oxygen value of the right ventricular blood.

Use a pulmonary artery catheter with reflectance oximetry capability. These catheters have fiberoptic bundles built into them and use technology similar to that used in pulse oximeters (Fig. 5-13). The processing unit sends a narrow waveband of light down the transmitting fiberoptic bundle to be shined on the passing blood in the pulmonary artery. Oxyhemoglobin in the red blood cells absorbs some of the light. The rest is reflected. The receiving fiberoptic bundle picks up some of this light and transmits it back to the monitoring unit.

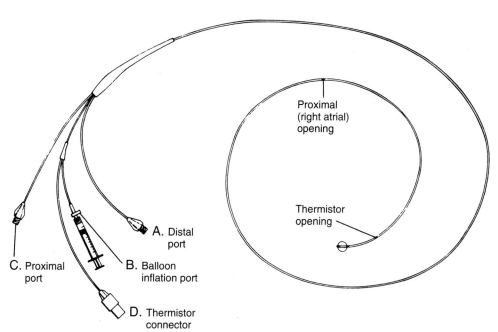

Fig. 5-11 A 7F quadruple-lumen thermodilution pulmonary artery catheter. *A,* Distal port goes to the tip of the catheter. It is used for measuring pulmonary artery pressure, pulmonary capillary wedge pressure (PCWP), and sampling blood for $P\bar{v}O_2$. *B,* Balloon inflation port is used to inflate the balloon for inserting the catheter and for obtaining a PCWP reading. *C,* Proximal port is used for measuring central venous pressure and for injecting iced saline for a thermodilution cardiac output study. The iced saline exits from the right atrial opening. *D,* Thermistor connector attaches to the cardiac output computer. A bimetallic wire runs through the catheter to the thermistor opening, where it is exposed to temperature changes of the blood and cold injectate. (Note: Not all catheters are capable of measuring cardiac output. Some catheters have other special features such as continuously measuring venous saturation or cardiac pacemaker leads.) *(From Oblouk Darovic G:* Hemodynamic monitoring, *Philadelphia, 1987, WB Saunders.)*

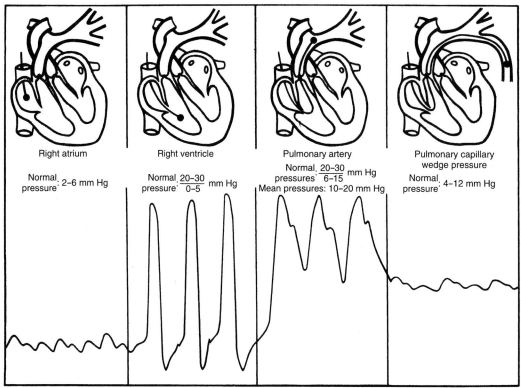

Fig. 5-12 Sequence of pressures and pressure waveforms seen as the pulmonary artery catheter advances through the *right atrium, right ventricle,* and *pulmonary artery* until it wedges. Be observant of premature ventricular contractions (PVCs) as the catheter is advanced through the right ventricle. *(From Wilkins RL, Sheldon RL, Krider SJ:* Clinical assessment in respiratory care, *ed 4, St Louis, 2000, Mosby.)*

$S\bar{v}o_2$ is determined by the monitoring unit based on the light waves that were transmitted and what was received. Care must be taken when using this catheter in patients with elevated carboxyhemoglobin or methemoglobin levels. As with pulse oximetry, COHb and MetHb will be interpreted as oxyhemoglobin; thus inaccurately high readings will be seen.

An actual mixed venous blood sample can be taken with this catheter through the distal lumen, as described next. The advantage of the reflectance oximetry system is that it gives continuous monitoring of the patient's venous oxygen level. In addition, high and low saturation alarms can be set. If the tip should become lodged in the wall of the artery or if a clot should form at the tip, the $S\bar{v}o_2$ will decrease or fluctuate dramatically. The alarms should warn the clinician of a problem with the equipment.

Use the distal lumen of a "standard" pulmonary artery catheter. A true mixed venous blood sample is obtained by withdrawing blood from the distal lumen of the catheter. This is the same lumen that is used for the pulmonary artery pressure (PAP) and pulmonary capillary wedge pressure (PCWP) readings. With sterile technique, a 5- to 10-mL syringe is used to pull out the heparinized

solution in the lumen until about 1 to 2 mL of blood is removed. A second preheparinized syringe is then used to withdraw about 2 mL of mixed venous blood. It is important to withdraw the intravenous (IV) solution and blood at a rate of no faster than 0.5 mL per second. Drawing any faster can pull preoxygenated blood back through the capillary bed and give falsely elevated oxygen values. After the blood is sampled, the lumen must be fast-flushed with the heparinized solution to prevent the blood from clotting (Fig. 5-14). Flush for several seconds until the solution flows freely. This blood sample may be reliably analyzed for $S\bar{v}o_2$, $P\bar{v}o_2$, and $P\bar{v}co_2$.

c. Interpret the mixed venous blood sample results (WRE code: IB8e and IIIE4) [Difficulty: An]

This topic is discussed in some detail in Chapter 3. The normal values follow:

$P\bar{v}o_2$ of 40 torr (range of 37 to 43 torr)

$S\bar{v}o_2$ of 75% (range of 70% to 76%)

Mixed venous blood oxygen values are useful for monitoring the patient's oxygen consumption. The most

A

B

Fig. 5-13 Mixed venous oxygen saturation ($S\bar{v}O_2$) can be monitored continuously by reflection spectroscopy in the appropriate pulmonary artery catheter. **A,** Detail of the fiberoptic bundles in the catheter. Specific wavelengths of light are directed at passing blood. Some of the light is absorbed by the passing red blood cells, and some is reflected back to the photodetector. The microprocessor calculates the $S\bar{v}O_2$%. **B,** Components of the system include (1) microprocessor that connects to the catheter, displays $S\bar{v}O_2$% values, and has high and low saturation alarms; (2) strip-chart recorder to copy the saturation values over time; and (3) reflective spectroscopy-type pulmonary artery catheter. The catheter also can be used for measuring pulmonary artery pressure, pulmonary capillary wedge pressure, and cardiac output; and taking a mixed venous blood gas sample.*(A, From Ruppel GL: Manual of pulmonary function testing, ed 8, St. Louis, 2003, Mosby. B, Courtesy Hospira, Inc., Lake Forest, Ill.)*

accurate methods of calculating percentage shunt and cardiac output (Fick method) use mixed venous blood oxygen values with arterial blood oxygen values. A $P\bar{v}O_2$ value of less than 30 torr or $S\bar{v}O_2$ of less than 56% is considered to show tissue hypoxemia. Quick steps must be taken to reverse this. Increase the inspired oxygen percentage as needed. Low stroke volume and cardiac output can be increased by giving digoxin (Lanoxin) or other inotropic agents. Low blood pressure can be increased by giving vasopressors such as dopamine HCl (Intropin).

Fig. 5-14 The various components of the pulmonary artery monitoring system. It includes a fluid source such as normal saline that is pressurized to 300 mm Hg to maintain a flow of fluid through the tubing system. The continuous flush device (made by Sorenson) is designed to allow three drips of fluid per minute through the tubing system; pulling on the fast-flush valve gives a continuous flow of fluid to clear air or blood from the system. The transducer converts a pressure signal to an electrical signal that is sent to the monitor for display as numeric data and a pressure waveform. The high-pressure tubing transfers the patient's pressure accurately to the transducer. The double stopcocks are used to close off the tubing system or sample blood from the patient. This then connects to the distal port of the pulmonary artery catheter. This same monitoring system can be used with an arterial catheter for continuous pressure monitoring and blood sampling. *(From Oblouk Darovic G:* Hemodynamic monitoring, *Philadelphia, 1987, WB Saunders.)*

MODULE B
Cardiopulmonary monitoring equipment

1. Perform quality control procedures on capnography equipment (WRE code: IIC5) [Difficulty: Ap, An]

As discussed earlier, a capnograph is used to measure a patient's exhaled carbon dioxide level and expiratory pattern. Two different types of capnography systems are found. Their main difference is in how the gas is sampled from the patient. Fig. 5-3 shows the patient connection for a mainstream capnograph. Fig. 5-4 shows a sidestream capnograph. Both work equally well if the patient is intubated. The capnography connector is attached between the endotracheal tube and the ventilator circuit or T-piece (Brigg's adapter). The sidestream unit also may be used with a spontaneously breathing patient because the capillary tube may be taped into a patient's nostril for gas sampling.

The following are components of a capnography system:
1. Airway attachment: The mainstream and sidestream units must have both inhaled and exhaled gas pass through the sensor or connector, respectively. Connections must be airtight and free of obstructions.
2. The gas sampling capillary tube of the sidestream unit must be kept clear of water or secretions.

3. Capnometer: Periodically calibrate the unit with two gases of different CO_2 content. Room air is used for the "zero" value, and either 5% or 10% CO_2 in a preanalyzed cylinder is used for the "high" value. Both values should calibrate within the manufacturer's specifications.
4. Capnograph: Check that the paper speeds and marker work properly.

Relatively few things can go wrong with capnography systems. The sidestream capnometer units must be kept dry. An external water trap is located between the capillary tube and the capnometer itself. Make sure that the water is drained periodically. Either capnography system can be disconnected from the patient. This is seen as a decrease in exhaled carbon dioxide to zero. The alarm should activate if it has been set.

As presented earlier, both capnography units are calibrated by using two points. Room air is used to set the zero point, and either 5% or 10% carbon dioxide from a cylinder is used to set the high point. Follow the manufacturer's guidelines regarding how much adjustment for low or high point can be tolerated. Do not use a machine that cannot be properly calibrated.

2. Pressure transducer
a. Get the necessary equipment for the procedure (CSE code: IIA19)

Hemodynamic monitoring requires a transducer that converts a blood pressure signal into an electrical signal. Select a strain gauge–type transducer to do this. The strain-gauge transducer uses a fine wire screen that bends proportionately to the pressure put against it.

b. Put the strain gauge transducer equipment together and make sure that it works properly (CSE code: IIA19)

Check to see that the wire screen of the transducer is not bent, damaged, or fouled with old blood or other debris. The transducer's wire cable and monitor-connecting prongs should not be bent or damaged. Carefully insert the prongs into the receiving jack on the monitor.

A disposable, sterile, clear plastic dome should be firmly screwed onto the transducer. Noncompliant pressure tubing should connect the transducer with the patient's arterial or pulmonary artery catheter. The automatic fluid drip system (Sorenson) should be pressurized to 300 mm Hg. Heparin must be added to the fluid (usually normal saline) to prevent clotting in the patient's catheter. Because this is a continuous fluid "plumbing" system, all connections must be tightly screwed together to be watertight (Fig. 5-15).

The transducer must be kept at the patient's midchest (midheart) level during calibration and measurement. Calibrate the electronics in the monitor by putting

Fig. 5-15 Schematic diagram of a strain-gauge pressure transducer. The wire mesh resistance wires are arranged like a Wheatstone bridge so that a pressure change results in a proportional change in the electrical resistance. *(From Armstrong PW, Baigrie RS: Hemodynamic monitoring in the critically ill, Philadelphia, 1980, Harper & Row.)*

known pressures against the fluid system. The electronics should first be adjusted to "zero" pressure by opening the transducer to room air (atmospheric pressure). Adjust the electronic controls as needed. A sphygmomanometer is then used to pressurize the fluid system. A PAC system is pressurized to relatively low pressures, such as 30 and 50 mm Hg. An arterial system is adjusted to higher pressures, such as 100 and 150 mm Hg. The monitored pressure should match the sphygmomanometer pressure. If not, adjust the electronic controls on the monitor to match.

c. Troubleshoot any problems with the equipment (CSE code: IIA19)

As mentioned earlier, all connections must be watertight. If not, the IV solution will drip out when it is pressurized. This also can result in the patient's measured pressures being less than true. Stopcocks must be opened or closed properly to allow the patient's pressure to be measured by the transducer. Electronics that will not calibrate to match the known pressures should not be used.

3. In-dwelling arterial catheters

a. Get the necessary equipment for arterial catheterization (WRE code: IIA17) [Difficulty: R, Ap, An]

As discussed earlier, a neonate can have its umbilical artery catheterized. An adult usually has the radial artery catheterized. Following are the general supplies necessary for catheterizing either of these arteries for drawing blood gases and continuously monitoring blood pressure:

1. Sterile 20-gauge or 21-gauge needle with a flexible plastic sheath. After placement into the artery, the needle is withdrawn, and the sheath is left in place (Fig. 5-16). A neonate needs a long catheter of the correct gauge based on its body weight.
2. Sterile surgical drape for covering the area surrounding the insertion site.
3. Disinfectant such as 70% isopropyl alcohol or povidine-iodine (Betadine) solution.
4. Local anesthetic such as 4% lidocaine in a syringe and needle for injection into the insertion site.
5. One or two sterile 3-mL or 5-mL syringes for blood sampling.
6. Equipment for setting up a pressurized intravenous drip system so that the catheter does not clot.

b. Put the equipment together and make sure that it works properly (WRE code: IIA17) [Difficulty: R, Ap, An]

See Fig. 5-17 for an illustration of how the pressure transducer, connecting tubing, stopcocks, infusion system, and monitoring electronics are assembled. See Fig. 5-18 for a completed radial artery system. Clinical experience is needed with these types of systems.

The process of calibrating the monitor for systemic artery pressures was briefly discussed earlier. Regardless of whether the catheter is placed into a systemic artery, pulmonary artery, umbilical artery, or superior vena cava, the equipment must be properly calibrated to ensure accurate data. When performing two-point calibration, all pressures should read "zero" when exposed to atmospheric pressure. This is the low point. The high point pressure for arterial pressure monitoring is commonly 100 mm Hg.

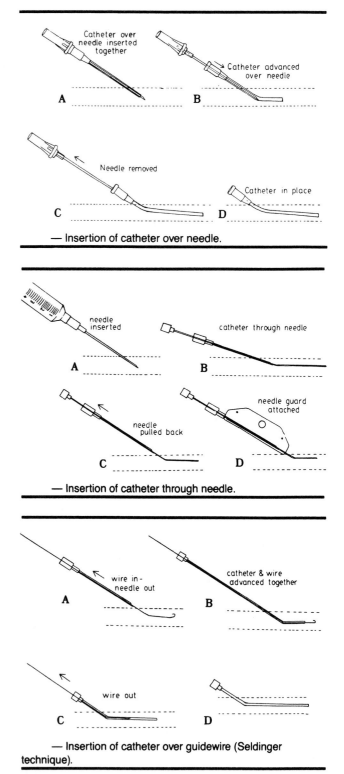

— Insertion of catheter over needle.

— Insertion of catheter through needle.

— Insertion of catheter over guidewire (Seldinger technique).

Fig. 5-16 Steps in the procedure for the percutaneous insertion of an arterial catheter for the continuous measurement of arterial pressure. Once inserted into the artery, the proximal end of the catheter is connected to a tubing circuit and pressure transducer, as shown in Figs. 5-17 and 5-18. *(From Oblouk Darovic G:* Hemodynamic monitoring, *Philadelphia, 1987, WB Saunders.)*

Fig. 5-17 Common steps in the assembly of the tubing circuit and pressure transducer to attach to an arterial or pulmonary artery catheter. Sterile technique must be maintained at all times. (Note: Individual institutions will vary these steps. Clinical practice is very important in this assembly.) **A,** Obtain a 250- to 500-mL bag of sterile, normal saline. Add 1 to 2 units of heparin per milliliter of solution. Attach an IV line with a macrodrip chamber. **B,** Insert the solution bag into a pressure bag. Inflate the pressure to about 100 mm Hg to force the fluid through the IV tubing. The pressure bag will be pumped up to 300 mm Hg at the end of this procedure to ensure that 3 drops of fluid flow through the tubing per minute to keep it patent. **C,** Attach the strain-gauge pressure transducer to an IV pole. Let it and the monitor warm up. **D,** Attach the IV tubing to the continuous-flush device (Sorenson Intraflow). **E,** Screw the continuous-flush device into the transducer stopcock. **F,** Backflush the continuous-flush device and transducer, with open stopcocks, so that all air is removed and replaced with the saline solution. **G,** Zero and calibrate the pressure transducer and monitor. **H,** Attach high-pressure tubing to the continuous-flush device. Flush the air out of it. **I,** Attach the high-pressure tubing to the patient's arterial line or pulmonary artery catheter. Ensure that no air bubbles are present and that a continuous saline-to-blood connection is present. Accurate patient pressures should now be seen on the monitor. *(From Oblouk Darovic G:* Hemodynamic monitoring, *Philadelphia, 1987, WB Saunders.)*

Fig. 5-18 Example of a complete setup for monitoring the arterial pressure. *(From Daily EK, Schroeder JS: Techniques in bedside hemodynamic monitoring, ed 5, St Louis, 1994, Mosby.)*

c. Troubleshoot any problems with the equipment (WRE code: IIA17) [Difficulty: R, Ap, An]

Table 5-1 lists problems, causes, prevention, and treatment for inaccurate pressure measurements with arterial or pulmonary artery catheters. Table 5-2 specifically lists problems with arterial lines. Fig. 5-19 shows common problem areas with arterial lines. Pulmonary artery catheters can have problems in the same areas.

MODULE C
Respiratory care plan

1. Analyze available information to determine the patient's pathophysiologic state (CSE code: IIIH1)

Exam Hint

Memorize the values listed in Box 5-2. Expect to see questions in which these values are used as patient data or as options to answer a question. Question areas include hemodynamic monitoring, oxygen and nitric oxide therapy, and mechanical ventilation. The normal values must be understood to identify abnormal values and know why they are abnormal.

The NBRC does not currently specifically list the following areas as testable on the advanced practitioner exams. However, in the previous generation of Written Registry Exams, information on these patient values was incorporated into questions about hemodynamic monitoring and mechanical ventilation. If the exam taker has the time, it is recommended that this material be reviewed.

a. Central venous pressure monitoring

A central venous catheter (also called a central venous pressure [CVP] line) is inserted into many patients for one or more reasons: (1) to monitor the patient's right-side heart pressure, (2) to administer a large volume of intravenous fluids rapidly, and (3) to give cardiac medications during a CPR attempt (preferred route). The catheter is usually inserted into the right jugular vein or right subclavian vein and advanced to just above the superior vena cava. When set up for monitoring pressure, it measures the right atrial pressure. It is important that the patient breathe spontaneously if at all possible. Peak pressures during inspiration on a mechanical ventilator may artificially increase the CVP reading. Positive end-expiratory pressure (PEEP) also may increase the CVP reading. If the patient cannot be removed from the ventilator, take the reading during exhalation. Make a note of the settings and that the reading

TABLE 5-1	Inaccurate Pressure Measurements		
Problem	**Cause**	**Prevention**	**Treatment**
Damped waveforms and inaccurate pressures	Partial clotting at catheter tip	Use continuous drip with 1 unit heparin/1 mL IV fluid. Hand flush occasionally. Flush with large volume after blood sampling. Use heparin-coated catheters.	Aspirate, then flush catheter with heparinized fluid (*not* in PAW position).
	Tip moving against wall	Obtain more stable catheter position.	Reposition catheter.
	Kinking of catheter	Restrict catheter movement at insertion site.	Reposition to straighten catheter. Replace catheter.
Abnormally low or negative pressures	Incorrect air-reference level (above midchest level)	Maintain transducer air-reference port at midchest level; rezero after patient position changes.	Remeasure level of transducer air reference and reposition at midchest level; rezero.
	Incorrect zeroing and calibration of monitor	Zero and calibrate monitor properly.	Recheck zero and calibration of monitor.
	Loose connection	Use Luer-Lok stopcocks.	Check all connections.
Abnormally high pressure reading	Pressure trapped by improper sequence of stopcock operation	Turn stopcocks in proper sequence when two pressures are measured on one transducer.	Thoroughly flush transducers with IV solution; rezero and turn stopcocks in proper sequence.
	Incorrect air-reference level (below midchest level)	Maintain transducer air-reference port at midchest level; recheck and rezero after patient position changes.	Check air-reference level; reset at midchest and rezero.
Inappropriate pressure waveform	Migration of catheter tip (e.g., in RV or PAW instead of in PA)	Establish optimal position carefully when introducing catheter initially.	Review waveform; if RV, inflate balloon; if PAW, deflate balloon and withdraw catheter slightly.
		Suture catheter at insertion site and tape catheter to patient's skin.	Check position under fluoroscope and/or radiograph after reposition.
No pressure available	Transducer not open to catheter	Follow routine, systematic steps for pressure measurement.	Check system, stopcocks.
	Amplifiers still on *cal, zero,* or *off*		
Noise or fling in pressure waveform	Excessive catheter movement, particularly in PA	Avoid excessive catheter length in ventricle.	Try different catheter tip position.
	Excessive tubing length	Use shortest tubing possible (<3 to 4 feet).	Eliminate excess tubing.
	Excessive stopcocks	Minimize number of stopcocks.	Eliminate excess stopcocks.

PAW, Pulmonary artery wedge; RV, right ventricle; PA, pulmonary artery.
From Daily and Schroeder: *Techniques in bedside hemodynamic monitoring,* ed 5, St Louis 1995, Mosby.

was taken with the patient on the ventilator. Record the data in the patient's chart or flow sheet.

As noted earlier, the CVP is a measure of the pressure in the right atrium. The two main factors that influence the right atrial pressure are the blood volume returning to it and the functioning of the right ventricle (see Box 5-2 for the normal CVP readings). A decreased CVP reading usually means that the patient is hypovolemic. Hypotension confirms this. An increased CVP may suggest one of the following possibilities:

TABLE 5-2   Problems Encountered with Arterial Catheters

Problem	Cause	Prevention	Treatment
Hematoma after withdrawal of needle	Bleeding or oozing at puncture site	Maintain firm pressure on site during withdrawal of catheter and for 5–15 min (as necessary) after withdrawal. Apply elastic tape (Elastoplast) firmly over puncture site. For femoral arterial puncture sites, leave a sandbag on site for 1–2 hr to prevent oozing. If patient is receiving heparin, discontinue 2 hr before catheter removal.	Continue to hold pressure to puncture site until oozing stops. Apply sandbag to femoral puncture site for 1–2 hr after removal of catheter.
Decreased or absent pulse distal to puncture site	Spasm of artery	Introduce arterial needle cleanly, nontraumatically.	Inject lidocaine locally at insertion site and 10 mg into arterial catheter.
	Thrombosis of artery	Use 1 unit heparin/1 mL IV fluid	Arteriotomy and Fogarty catheterization both distally and proximally from the puncture site result in return of pulse in more than 90% of cases if brachial or femoral artery is used.
Bleedback into tubing, dome, or transducer	Insufficient pressure on IV bag	Maintain 300 mm Hg pressure on IV bag.	Replace transducer. "Fast flush" through system.
Hemorrhage	Loose connections Loose connections	Use Luer-Lok stopcocks; tighten periodically. Keep all connecting sites visible. Observe connecting sites frequently. Use built-in alarm system. Use Luer-Lok stopcocks.	Tighten all connections. Tighten all connections.
Emboli	Clot from catheter tip into bloodstream	Always aspirate and discard before flushing. Use continuous flush device. Use 1 unit heparin/1 mL IV fluid. Gently flush < 2–4 mL.	Remove catheter.
Local infection	Forward movement of contaminated catheter	Carefully suture catheter at insertion site. Always use aseptic technique. Remove catheter after 72–96 hr.	Remove catheter. Prescribe antibiotic.
	Break in sterile technique Prolonged catheter use	Inspect and care for insertion site daily, including dressing change and antibiotic or iodophor ointment.	
Sepsis	Break in sterile technique Prolonged catheter use	Use percutaneous insertion. Always use aseptic technique. Remove catheter after 72–96 hr.	Remove catheter. Prescribe antibiotic.
	Bacterial growth in IV fluid	Change IV fluid bag, stopcocks, dome, and tubing every 24–48 hr. Do not use IV fluid containing glucose. Use sterile dead-ender caps on all ports of stopcocks. Carefully flush remaining blood from stopcocks after blood sampling.	

From Daily and Schroeder: *Techniques in bedside hemodynamic monitoring,* ed 5, St Louis 1995, Mosby.

Fig. 5-19 Common problem areas with arterial and pulmonary artery catheters. *(From Oblouk Darovic G:* Hemodynamic monitoring, *Philadelphia, 1987, WB Saunders.)*

a. Fluid overload. Check for an elevated blood pressure and crackles in the bases of the lungs. Unfortunately, an elevated CVP is a late finding with this problem.

b. Tricuspid valve or pulmonic valve insufficiency or stenosis. Abnormal electrocardiogram or echocardiogram findings or abnormal heart sounds (heart murmur) help to specify the problem.

c. Right ventricular failure. A right ventricular heart attack can be identified on an electrocardiogram.

If a COPD patient with pulmonary hypertension has right ventricular failure, the condition is called *cor pulmonale.*

d. Cardiac tamponade (blood filling the pericardium). Watch for a decrease in the blood pressure, tachycardia, and distended jugular veins. This problem can be rapidly fatal if not quickly corrected.

e. Atrial septal defect or ventricular septal defect with a left-to-right intracardiac shunt. These congenital conditions are usually detected in a young child by

---

BOX 5-2 Normal Cardiopulmonary Values

CENTRAL VENOUS PRESSURE (CVP)
Range for a normal adult is 2–8 cm water or 1–6 mm Hg
Range for a normal infant is 1–5 mm Hg
Range for a normal neonate is 0–3 mm Hg

PULMONARY ARTERY PRESSURE (PAP)
Range for a normal adult is 15–28/5–16 mm Hg
 (about 25/10 mm Hg)
Range for a normal adult mean PAP is 10–22 mm Hg
Range for a normal child is 15–30/5–10 mm Hg
Range for a normal neonate is 30–60/2–10 mm Hg

PULMONARY CAPILLARY WEDGE PRESSURE (PCWP)
Range for a normal PCWP (mean) is 6–15 mm Hg
 (about 8 mm Hg)

CARDIAC OUTPUT
Range for a normal adult is 4–8 L/min
Range for a normal neonate is 0.6–0.8 L/min

STROKE VOLUME
Adults: 50–120 mL/beat
School-age children: 35 mL/beat
Preschoolers: 15 mL/beat
Neonates: 5 mL/beat

CARDIAC INDEX
2.5–4.0 L/min/sm^2 of body surface area

ARTERIAL-VENOUS OXYGEN CONTENT DIFFERENCE
$[C(a–\bar{v})O_2]$
Range of normal is 3.0–5.5 vol % of O_2

SHUNT
5% or less of cardiac output

PULMONARY VASCULAR RESISTANCE
80–240 dynes • sec • cm^{-5}

SYSTEMIC VASCULAR RESISTANCE
900–1400 dynes • sec • cm^{-5}

an abnormal electrocardiogram or echocardiogram finding or an abnormal heart sound (heart murmur).

f. Pulmonary embolism. This condition should be suspected when a patient who is prone to the problem experiences sudden onset of hypoxemia and clinical deterioration. A pulmonary angiogram showing blocked blood flow through the lung(s) confirms the problem.

Exam Hint

During hemodynamic monitoring for blood pressure, the pressure transducer must be kept at the midchest level. Usually a mark is placed on the patient's chest for a consistent measurement point. Raising the transducer above the mark (or lowering the patient below the transducer) results in an incorrectly low reading. Lowering the stopcock below the mark (or raising the patient above the transducer) results in an incorrectly high reading.

---

b. Pulmonary artery pressure monitoring

The PAP is the systolic and diastolic pressure found in either pulmonary artery. It can be measured only through a pulmonary artery catheter (PAC). (The NBRC often refers to this as a flow-directed balloon-tipped pulmonary artery catheter.) Review the patient's previous values before taking another to make a comparison. Box 5-2 shows normal cardiopulmonary values. PAP is important to measure in patients with severe pulmonary or cardiovascular problems, pulmonary hypertension, myocardial infarction, congestive heart failure, hypertension, and hypotension.

To read the PAP, a PAC must be inserted through a vein and passed through the right atrium and right ventricle into the pulmonary artery. The common insertion sites, in descending order of preference, are the basilic vein in either the right or left arm, the right internal jugular or subclavian vein, or the right or left femoral vein. The PAC also is commonly called a Swan-Ganz catheter after the inventors who lent their names to a particular brand. The catheters come in different lengths and diameters for pediatric and adult patients. See Fig. 5-11 for an illustration of a 7F quadruple-lumen thermodilution PAC. Besides PAP, it is capable of being used to measure cardiac output. Fig. 5-14 shows how a PAC could be arranged with a pressure transducer and pressure monitor. Fig. 5-12 shows a representation of the series of pressure waveforms seen as the catheter is advanced through the heart and into the wedged position in a branch of the pulmonary

artery. To read the PAP accurately, the equipment must be set up and calibrated properly, the distal lumen of the catheter must be patent and connected to the transducer, and the catheter's balloon must be deflated.

See Box 5-2 for normal values. Elevated PAP values are usually seen with the following conditions:

1. Left ventricular failure/congestive heart failure, acute myocardial infarction, or fluid overload. To better determine the pathophysiologic problem, it is necessary to evaluate the following kinds of clinical information:
   a. Known history of heart disease or of sudden illness suggesting a heart attack
   b. Crackles heard in the bases of the lungs
   c. Decreased static lung compliance
   d. Elevated PCWP
   e. Decreased cardiac output or low blood pressure or both
   f. The normal gradient (difference) between the pulmonary artery diastolic pressure (PAd) and the PCWP is 5 mm Hg or less.

EXAMPLE

An adult patient has the following PAC values: PAP is 35/25 mm Hg, and PCWP is 22 mm Hg. Calculate the patient's PAd pressure minus PCWP (PAd − PCWP) gradient as follows:

Pulmonary artery diastolic is:	25 mm Hg
Pulmonary capillary wedge pressure is:	−22 mm Hg
The PAd − PCWP gradient is:	3 mm Hg

It can be concluded that this person's PAd − PCWP gradient is normal.

2. Pulmonary hypertension from COPD (usually emphysema). To better determine the pathophysiologic problem, it is necessary to evaluate the following kinds of clinical information:
   a. The patient usually has a known history of COPD.
   b. Systolic PAP may exceed 40 mm Hg if the problem is of long standing.
   c. The gradient (difference) between the PAd pressure and the PCWP (PAd − PCWP) is greater than 5 mm Hg.

EXAMPLE

An adult patient has the following PAC values: PAP is 35/25 mm Hg, and PCWP is 8 mm Hg. Calculate the patient's PAd pressure minus PCWP (PAd − PCWP) gradient as follows:

Pulmonary artery diastolic is:	25 mm Hg
Pulmonary capillary wedge pressure is:	−8 mm Hg
The PAd − PCWP gradient is:	17 mm Hg

It can be concluded that this person's PAd − PCWP gradient is elevated.

3. Pulmonary hypertension from a pulmonary embolism. The better to determine the pathophysiologic problem, it is necessary to evaluate the following kinds of clinical information:
   a. The patient's history matches that of a sudden onset of shortness of breath and other pulmonary problems.
   b. The systolic PAP is less than 40 mm Hg. This is because the relatively thin-walled right ventricle cannot rapidly increase its muscle mass to increase the driving pressure.
   c. The gradient (difference) between the PAd pressure and the PCWP (PAd − PCWP) is greater than 5 mm Hg if the embolism is large.
4. Pulmonary hypertension in the neonate with persistent pulmonary hypertension of the newborn (PPHN). This condition is often seen in the premature neonate with the infant respiratory distress syndrome (RDS). When these neonates become hypoxic, the pulmonary vascular bed constricts. This causes the infant to revert to fetal circulation. Giving 100% oxygen and hyperventilating the infant usually reverses the processes. The PAP then returns to normal.
5. Decreased PAP values are not frequently seen. Patients with hypovolemic shock, anaphylaxis (allergic shock), or excessive use of vasodilating drugs may have a decreased PAP. The most obvious clinical sign in these patients is a low systemic blood pressure.

c. Pulmonary capillary wedge pressure monitoring

The PCWP refers to the pressure measured in the pulmonary capillary bed under no-flow conditions. It is important to review previous patient data before measuring another pressure. Normal values are listed in Box 5-2. A PAC must be placed into a patient's pulmonary artery for the PCWP to be measured. Measuring the PCWP is important in patients with severe pulmonary or cardiovascular problems, including pulmonary hypertension, myocardial infarction, congestive heart failure, hypertension, and hypotension.

The PCWP is obtained by inflating the balloon at the tip of the catheter. This blocks off that branch of the pulmonary artery so that the downstream pressure from the left ventricle is seen on the monitor (see Fig. 5-12). The balloon volume varies with the diameter of the catheter. The needed volume is printed on the catheter near where the air is injected into the balloon. For example, the 5F catheter balloon holds 0.8 mL of air, and the 7F catheter balloon holds 1.5 mL of air. It is important to put in only the required amount. Overinflating may burst the balloon or rupture the pulmonary artery. If the balloon wedges at less than the required volume, the catheter is probably too far down in the artery and may need to be

withdrawn a short distance. The balloon is inflated only long enough to obtain the PCWP, and then the balloon is deflated. Pulmonary infarction will occur if the balloon is left inflated and the blood in the pulmonary artery is stagnant and allowed to clot. Record the PCWP value in the patient's chart or flow sheet.

As noted earlier, the PCWP refers to the pressure measured in the pulmonary capillary bed under no-flow conditions. This pressure reflects downstream pressure from the left side of the heart. At diastole, in the patient without pulmonary hypertension or mitral valve disease, the PCWP parallels left atrial pressure (LAP) and left ventricular end-diastolic pressure (LVEDP). The literature reveals that a variety of terms and initials are used to describe the same physiologic value. Do not be confused by reading about the pulmonary capillary pressure (PCP), pulmonary wedge pressure (PWP), pulmonary artery wedge pressure (PAWP), or wedge pressure.

Elevated PCWP is generally held to be greater than 10 mm Hg and can indicate:
1. Intravascular fluid overload: Look at the patient's history to see whether the patient is in renal failure or has recently had a large amount of oral or intravenous fluids. Perform a physical examination to see whether the patient has edema in the ankles or back if he or she has been lying down. Look for jugular vein distention when the patient lies down. Listen for crackles in the bases of the lungs.
2. Left ventricular dysfunction with congestive heart failure: Perform the same steps listed in point 1. In addition, look for a history of chronic heart failure or acute myocardial infarction.
3. Mitral valve insufficiency: Blood regurgitating back into the left atrium is shown as an elevated PCWP.

These conditions result in serious problems for the patient's lung function. When the PCWP reaches 20 to 25 mm Hg, fluid begins to leak into the pulmonary interstitium. This makes the lungs less compliant and increases the patient's work of breathing. A PCWP of 25 to 30 mm Hg results in frank pulmonary edema and dramatically decreases the patient's PaO_2.

Decreased PCWP is commonly held to be less than 4 mm Hg and can indicate:
1. Low intravascular volume: Look in the patient's history for an illness resulting in dehydration (vomiting and diarrhea). A physical examination will show tachycardia; low blood pressure; low urine output with a high specific gravity; tenting of the skin when pinched, showing poor turgor; and flat jugular veins when the patient is lying down.
2. Sepsis: The patient's history will reveal infection, usually a septicemia. The physical examination will reveal tachycardia, hypotension, and oliguria, as noted in point 1. A major difference is that the

patient will appear to be fluid overloaded because of the peripheral edema. This finding is produced when an infectious organism (often *Staphylococcus aureus*) causes a dilation of the peripheral vascular bed and leakage of fluids out of the vascular bed into the tissues. The patient will have weak peripheral pulses and feel warm.

d. Cardiac output

Cardiac output (CO) is defined as the product of heart rate for 1 minute and stroke volume (CO = HR × SV). It is a measurement of the heart's pumping ability to meet the body's needs. As always, review previous data before repeating the test. Box 5-2 lists normal values. A CO measurement is performed on patients with serious cardiovascular disease to assess the patient's condition. A major change in vital signs or a new treatment justifies a measurement. The patient must have a PAC in place that is capable of measuring CO.

The bedside procedure involves the use of a special four-lumen PAC designed for thermodilution CO studies. Both catheter types require additional hardware and supplies, including a computer designed to calculate the CO. The first type of thermodilution catheter that was developed is used to inject a cool solution into the heart. This cool solution is diluted with the patient's blood. As the blood and cool solution mix passes a thermistor at the catheter tip, the computer calculates the patient's CO based on the time required to pump the cooler blood past the thermistor (see Fig. 5-11). A newer CO catheter makes use of a thermal filament (a heated wire) that wraps around the catheter. With this catheter, the computer periodically directs electricity to the filament. This results in periodic warming of the blood from the heated wire. The computer calculates the patient's CO by determining the time needed to pump the heated blood past the thermistor at the tip of the catheter. The advantages of the "heated wire" CO catheter are that it gives an updated CO value every 30 seconds, requires no additional time from the nurse or respiratory therapist after the initial setup, and does not add any additional fluid to the patient's intake.

As listed in Box 5-2, the normal, resting adult has a CO in the range of 4 to 8 L/min and a normal, resting neonate has a CO in the range of 0.6 to 0.8 L/min. CO can increase markedly in a person with a normal heart who is stressed, exercising, has a fever, or has any other reason for an increased metabolism. All these conditions increase the person's demand for oxygen, which is primarily met by increasing CO. (To a lesser extent, the tissues extract more oxygen from the blood.) Sepsis is the one serious condition that results in a high CO.

The most common causes of decreased CO are hypovolemia, increased peripheral resistance, and heart failure. A patient with low CO often has a low blood pressure. If the CO and blood pressure are too low, metabolic acidosis will develop from peripheral hypoxemia. Death can result if this is not corrected.

e. Stroke volume

Stroke volume (SV) is defined as the volume of blood ejected with each heartbeat. It is the difference between the volume of blood in each ventricle at the end of diastole and the volume left in the ventricles at the end of systole (after ejection). The normal SV is based on a person's age. See Box 5-2 for normal values. SV can be determined through a cardiac ultrasound procedure or calculated from the patient's heart rate and CO.

For example, calculate an adult patient's stroke volume when the heart rate is 100 beats/min and CO is 8 L/min (8000 mL/min):

$$SV = \frac{CO}{HR} = \frac{8000 \text{ mL}}{100} = 80 \text{ mL}$$

The SV is the same for both ventricles except under pathologic conditions. Usually, however, only the left ventricle is of concern. The Frank-Starling curve shows us that as the heart muscle is stretched with greater volume, it contracts and pumps more completely, resulting in a larger SV. A left ventricle that has been damaged by a myocardial infarction does not pump as effectively, and the SV decreases. A decrease in SV results in a decrease in CO unless the heart rate can increase to make up the difference. This is seen in many patients with heart disease. In addition, when a normal right ventricle continues to pump more blood than the damaged left ventricle, the unpumped blood backs up into the pulmonary circulation and results in pulmonary edema (congestive heart failure).

f. Cardiac index

The cardiac index (CI) is the CO per square meter of body surface area (BSA). CO is usually measured by one of the CO PACs, as discussed earlier. The BSA can be determined from the DuBois Body Surface Chart.

A normal, resting CI is 2.5 to 4 L/min/m² of BSA. The CI is a much more accurate way of determining whether the patient's oxygen demands are being met than by simply looking at the CO. For example, a resting CO of 4 L/min is considered normal. This CO might be fine for a small adult but not for a large one. The CI takes into account the difference in body sizes. A normal CI indicates that the patient is receiving enough oxygen to meet the body's needs. A low CI should be a cause for concern; it usually indicates that the patient is not getting enough blood and oxygen to his or her tissues. Check to see whether the patient's CO and blood pressure also are low and whether he or she has hypoxemia or acidemia. If these exist, they must be corrected as quickly as possible to prevent dire consequences. A high CI indicates that the patient is pumping more blood than appears necessary. Investigate why this is so. See the earlier discussion on CO and the factors that affect it to understand the factors that affect CI as well.

g. Arterial-venous oxygen content difference

The arterial-venous oxygen content difference $[C(a-\bar{v})O_2]$ is a calculation of oxygen consumption by the body. It is the difference between the oxygen content of arterial blood and the oxygen content of mixed venous blood. Box 5-2 lists the normal values. As always, check for previous values to compare with present values to understand whether the patient's condition has changed.

The normal range for the $C(a-\bar{v})O_2$ difference is 3 to 5.5 vol %. Figures in this range show normal oxygen consumption by the tissues, CO, and cardiopulmonary function. A $C(a-\bar{v})O_2$ difference of greater than 5.5 to 6 vol % is seen in patients with a low CO. As the blood flows more slowly than normal through the tissues, more oxygen is consumed per milliliter of blood. The $S\bar{v}O_2$ and $P\bar{v}O_2$ values decrease, and the $C(a-\bar{v})O_2$ difference widens.

A $C(a-\bar{v})O_2$ difference of less than 4 vol % in the healthy patient commonly indicates good cardiovascular reserve with an increased CO. As the blood flows more quickly than normal through the tissues, less oxygen is consumed per milliliter of blood. The $S\bar{v}O_2$ and $P\bar{v}O_2$ values increase, and the $C(a-\bar{v})O_2$ difference narrows. The septic patient may have a narrowed $C(a-\bar{v})O_2$ difference because of peripheral shunting and decreased oxygen consumption by the tissues caused by the infection. The $C(a-\bar{v})O_2$ difference is necessary to accurately calculate the percent of pulmonary shunting as discussed next.

h. Shunt study

Shunt ($\dot{Q}s/\dot{Q}t$) is the amount of blood pumped by the heart that passes through the lungs but does not participate in gas exchange. A PAC must be inserted into the patient for a shunt study to be performed. Review previous $\dot{Q}s/\dot{Q}t$ study results and compare with current information to see if a change has occurred in the patient's status. See Box 5-2 for normal values. A shunt study is very useful to find out how much ventilation-to-perfusion mismatch a patient has. Most patients with refractory hypoxemia and requiring mechanical ventilation have an increased amount of pulmonary shunting. When an optimal PEEP study is performed, a shunt study should be performed with each change in the PEEP level.

As noted earlier, shunt is the amount of blood pumped by the heart that does not participate in gas exchange through the lungs. It is wasted CO and wasted effort by the heart. The normal person has a shunt of no more than 5% of CO. This shunted blood has a low oxygen content and dilutes the oxygen content of all the blood. The larger the percentage of shunted blood, the more the heart and body are stressed. Many clinicians believe that an indication for mechanical ventilation is a shunt of 15% to 20%. Most agree that 30% or more shunt can be life threatening.

The ventilator is used to reduce the patient's work of breathing and oxygen consumption. Supplemental oxygen can be more carefully controlled, and PEEP may be added to increase the patient's functional residual capacity (FRC) as needed.

i. Pulmonary vascular resistance

Pulmonary vascular resistance (PVR) is the total resistance of the pulmonary vascular bed to the blood being pumped through it by the right ventricle. CO and pulmonary blood pressure determine the PVR. To gather the necessary hemodynamic information, the patient must have a CO pulmonary artery catheter inserted.

The normal range for PVR in the adult is 1 to 3 mm Hg/L/min. Multiplying this value by 80 gives the units of dynes/sec/cm^{-5}. PVR is listed this way in some cardiology studies. The normal range of PVR in an adult is between 80 and 240 dynes $\cdot$ sec $\cdot$ cm^{-5}. (see Box 5-2). With a normal PVR, the difference between the pulmonary artery diastolic pressure and the PCWP is 5 mm Hg or less. Any of the following can cause an elevated PVR:

1. Decreased oxygen in the lungs
2. COPD
3. Acute respiratory distress syndrome (ARDS)
4. Persistent pulmonary hypertension of the newborn (PPHN/persistent fetal circulation)
5. Primary pulmonary hypertension
6. Pulmonary embolism
7. Excessive PEEP
8. Increased pulmonary blood flow from a left-to-right intracardiac shunt such as an atrial septal defect or ventricular septal defect

Additional clinical data must be gathered to confirm the diagnosis. An increased PVR is a serious problem because it can lead to right ventricular hypertrophy. The COPD patient is at risk for developing cor pulmonale. This is right ventricular failure secondary to lung disease and increased PVR.

j. Systemic vascular resistance

Systemic vascular resistance (SVR) is the total resistance of the systemic vascular bed to the blood being pumped through it by the left ventricle. CO and systemic blood pressure determine the SVR. To gather the necessary hemodynamic information, the patient must have a CO pulmonary artery catheter, arterial line, and CVP line (if this cannot be measured from the PAC).

The normal range of SVR in the adult is 15 to 20 mm Hg/L/min. Multiplying this value by 80 gives us the units of dynes/sec/cm^{-5}. SVR is listed this way in some cardiology studies. When multiplied by 80, an adult's SVR has a range of between 900 and 1400 dynes $\cdot$ sec $\cdot$ cm^{-5} (see Box 5-2). Note that the normal range may vary with different references.

> ### Exam Hint
>
> **K**now both sets of normal values for PVR and SVR. The cardiology version of the PVR or SVR values can be written in several ways. The preferred versions have units listed in "dynes/sec/cm^{-5}" or "dyne sec/cm^{-5}." However, the NBRC has listed these values in units of "dynes • seconds • cm^{-5}" and "dynes • s • cm^{-5}"

> ### Exam Hint
>
> **C**losely review the following concepts because they have been tested on previous examinations.

A patient with hypertension will have an elevated SVR. It also will increase if the patient is given a vasoconstricting drug and decrease if the patient is given a vasodilating drug. Some allergic reactions result in anaphylaxis with a dramatic decrease in the SVR and blood pressure despite an increase in the CO.

2. Determine the appropriateness of the prescribed therapy and goals for the identified pathophysiologic state (CSE code: IIIH3)

Each clinical problem presented in this section requires its own individualized treatment. Be prepared to make recommendations to change the inspired oxygen percentage, give fluids if the patient is dehydrated, give diuretic medications to increase urine output if the patient is fluid overloaded, give vasodilator medications if the patient is hypertensive, or give vasoconstrictor medications if the patient is hypotensive.

See Fig. 5-20 for examples of diagnostic pathways. These can be used to help the clinician evaluate all the patient data. The diagnosis or pathophysiologic state can be determined by following the data down a given pathway. Normal values and common conditions associated

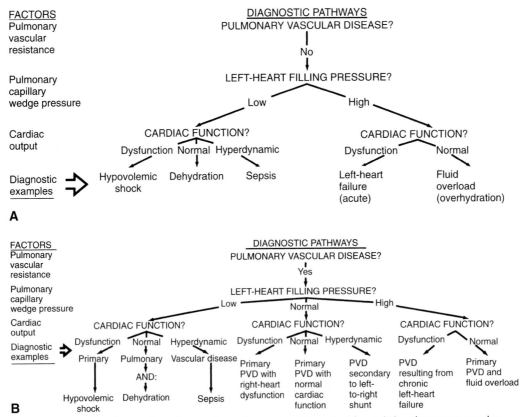

Fig. 5-20 Possible diagnostic pathways for patients with **(A)** and without **(B)** pulmonary vascular disease (PVD). In both cases, the pulmonary vascular resistance, pulmonary capillary wedge pressure, and cardiac output are measured. High, normal, or low values lead down different pathways. Previous discussions and clinical experience are needed to determine the final diagnosis. Sepsis may be associated with normal left-heart filling pressures. Primary PVD may be caused by pulmonary emboli, pulmonary artery disease (vasculitis, "primary" pulmonary hypertension), respiratory distress syndromes, hypoxic vasoconstriction, or drugs. *(From Osgood CF, Watson MH, Slaughter MS, et al: Hemodynamic monitoring in respiratory care, Respir Care 29(1):25–34, 1984.)*

with abnormal values were discussed earlier in this chapter. Interpret the information given by the intravascular monitor.

1. Interpretation of PAP. An increased PAP is usually associated with one of the following: fluid overload, heart failure or pulmonary hypertension (increased pulmonary vascular resistance) from COPD (emphysema), pulmonary embolism, or PPHN.

2. Interpretation of PCWP. An increased PCWP is usually associated with one of the following: fluid overload, heart failure, mitral valve insufficiency, cardiac tamponade, or constrictive pericarditis. Treatment for fluid overload or heart failure or both usually includes fluid restriction and diuretics (furosemide [Lasix]) and digitalis-type drugs (Lanoxin). A decreased PCWP is usually associated with dehydration (treated with increased fluids) or vasodilation (treated with vasoconstricting drugs like dopamine [Intropin]). When interpreting the PAP and PCWP together, it is very important to calculate the difference between the PAP diastolic pressure and the PCWP. Normally, the difference, or gradient, is 5 mm Hg or less. In other words, if the PAP diastolic pressure minus the PCWP is 5 mm Hg or less, the patient does not have pulmonary hypertension. A gradient of more than 5 mm Hg indicates pulmonary hypertension.

3. Interpretation of PVR. As noted earlier, determine the difference between the PAP diastolic pressure and the PCWP. Also know the normal PVR value from Box 5-2. An increased PVR is associated with COPD, primary pulmonary hypertension in an adult, and PPHN. NBRC questions that ask about the treatment for these conditions require the use of supplemental oxygen or nitric oxide (NO) to cause pulmonary vasodilation. Review nitric oxide therapy in Chapter 6.

4. Interpretation of SVR. Know the normal SVR value from Box 5-2. A low SVR is associated with hypovolemia, shock, or sepsis. Treatment can include increased fluids or a vasoconstricting drug (dopamine [Intropin]). A high SVR is associated with fluid overload or hypertension. Treatment can include diuretics (furosemide [Lasix]) or a vasodilating drug.

5. Interpretation of CO. A decreased CO is usually caused by hypovolemia (treated with increased fluids) or heart failure (treated with digitalis-type drugs [Lanoxin]). CO also may be decreased on a ventilator-dependent patient with high peak pressures or PEEP level. These can cause an increased intrathoracic pressure. When this is the situation presented in an NBRC question, and a request for care is called for, the best response is to decrease the PEEP level.

3. Maintain records and communicate information related to capnography and the patient's response to therapy (WRE code: IIIA1c) [Difficulty: An]

Review the previous discussion about the use of capnography to monitor the patient's breathing pattern (see Fig. 5-7).

BIBLIOGRAPHY

American Association for Respiratory Care: Clinical practice guideline: capnography/capnometry during mechanical ventilation, 2003 revision & update, *Respir Care* 48(5):534, 2003.

Anton WR, Raghu G: Measuring end-tidal carbon dioxide tension at maximal exhalation to improve its utility during T-piece weaning trials, *Respir Care* 35(11):1082, 1990.

Bakow ED: A limitation of capnography, *Respir Care* 27(2):167, 1982.

Branson RD, Campbell RS: Cardiovascular monitoring. In Branson RD, Hess DR, Chatburn RL, editors: *Respiratory care equipment*, ed 2, Philadelphia, 1999, Lippincott Williams & Wilkins.

Cairo JM: Assessment of physiologic function. In Cairo JM, Pilbeam SP, editors: *Mosby's respiratory care equipment*, ed 7, St Louis, 2004, Mosby.

Carlon GC, Ray C Jr, Miodownik S, et al: Capnography in mechanically ventilated patients, *Crit Care Med* 16(5):550, 1988.

Clark DB, Marshall SG: Mixed venous oxygen saturation measurement, II: general and specific clinical applications, *Respir Ther* 16:39, 1986.

Daily EK, Schroeder JS: *Techniques in bedside hemodynamic monitoring*, ed 4, St Louis, 1989, Mosby.

Deshpande VM, Pilbeam SP, Dixon RJ: *A comprehensive review in respiratory care*, East Norwalk, Conn, 1988, Appleton & Lange.

Divertie MB, McMichan JC: Continuous monitoring of mixed venous oxygen saturation, *Chest* 85(3):423, 1984.

Fahey PJ, Harris K, Vanderwarf C: Clinical experience with continuous monitoring of mixed venous oxygen saturation in respiratory failure, *Chest* 86(5):748, 1984.

Fink JB, Hunt GE, editors: *Clinical practice in respiratory care*, Philadelphia, 1999, Lippincott-Raven.

Harris K: Noninvasive monitoring of gas exchange, *Respir Care* 32(7):544, 1987.

Hess D: Capnometry and capnography: technical aspects, physiologic aspects, and clinical applications, *Respir Care* 35(6):557, 1990.

Hess D: Respiratory care monitoring. In Burton GG, Hodgkin JE, Ward JJ, editors: *Respiratory care: a guide to clinical practice*, ed 4, Philadelphia, 1997, Lippincott.

Hess DR, Branson RD: Noninvasive respiratory monitoring equipment. In Branson RD, Hess DR, Chatburn RL, editors: *Respiratory care equipment*, ed 2, Philadelphia, 1999, Lippincott Williams & Wilkins.

Hunt GE: Diagnostic procedures at the bedside. In Fink JB, Hunt GE, editors: *Clinical practice in respiratory care*, Philadelphia, 1999, Lippincott-Raven.

Jaquith SM: The Oximetrix Opticath: what is it, and how can it facilitate nursing management of the critically ill patient? *Crit Care Nurse* 4(3):55, 1984.

Kandel G, Aberman A: Mixed venous oxygen saturation: its role in the assessment of the critically ill patient, *Arch Intern Med* 143:1400, 1983.

Kinasewitz GT: Use of end-tidal capnography during mechanical ventilation, *Respir Care* 25(2):169, 1982.

Krider SJ: Cardiac output assessment. In Wilkins RL, Sheldon RL, Krider SJ, editors: *Clinical assessment in respiratory care*, ed 3, St Louis, 1995, Mosby.

Krider SJ: Invasively monitored hemodynamic pressures. In Wilkins RL, Sheldon RL, Krider SJ, editors: *Clinical assessment in respiratory care*, ed 3, St Louis, 1995, Mosby.

Malinowski T: Respiratory monitoring in the intensive care unit. In Wilkins RL, Krider SJ, Sheldon RL, editors: *Clinical assessment in respiratory care*, ed 3, St Louis, 1990, Mosby.

Marini JJ: Obtaining meaningful data from the Swan-Ganz catheter, *Respir Care* 30(7):572, 1985.

Mathews PJ, Gregg BL: Monitoring and management of the patient in the ICU. In Scanlan CL, Wilkins RL, Stoller JK, editors: *Egan's fundamentals of respiratory care*, ed 7, St Louis, 1999, Mosby.

McMichan JC: Continuous monitoring of mixed venous oxygen saturation in clinical practice, *Mt Sinai J Med* 51(5):569, 1984.

Nuzzo PF, Anton WR: Practical applications of capnography, *Respir Ther* 12, Nov/Dec 1986.

Oblouk Darovic G: *Hemodynamic monitoring*, ed 2, Philadelphia, 2000, WB Saunders.

Paulus DA: Invasive monitoring of respiratory gas exchange: continuous measurement of mixed venous oxygen saturation, *Respir Care* 32(7):535, 1987.

Pilbeam SP: *Mechanical ventilation, physiological and clinical applications*, ed 3, St Louis, 1998, Mosby.

Ramage JE Jr: Hemodynamic and gas exchange monitoring. In Hess DR, MacIntyre NR, Mishoe SC, et al, editors: *Respiratory care principles and practice*, Philadelphia, 2002, WB Saunders.

Ruppel G: *Manual of pulmonary function testing*, ed 8, St Louis, 2003, Mosby.

Scanlan CL, Wilkins RL: Analysis and monitoring of gas exchange. In Wilkins RL, Stoller JK, Scanlan CL, editors: *Egan's fundamentals of respiratory care*, ed 8, St Louis, 2003, Mosby.

Shapiro BA, Peruzzi WT, Templin R, et al: *Clinical application of blood gases*, ed 5, Chicago, 1994, Mosby.

Shapiro BA, Kacmarek RM, Cane RD, et al, editors: *Clinical application of respiratory care*, ed 4, St Louis, 1991, Mosby.

Whitaker K: *Comprehensive perinatal and pediatric respiratory care*, ed 2, Albany, NY, 1997, Delmar.

White GC: *Equipment theory for respiratory care*, ed 3, Albany, NY, 1999, Delmar.

Wiedemann HP: Invasive monitoring techniques in the ventilated patient. In Kacmarek RM, Stoller JK, editors: *Current respiratory care*, Toronto, 1988, BC Decker.

SELF-STUDY QUESTIONS

1. A 3-day postoperative open-heart surgery patient has an arterial catheter in the right radial artery for continuous blood pressure measurements. Because of retained secretions, the respiratory therapist places him into a head-down position for postural drainage therapy. The nurse notices that the patient's blood pressure is less than before being placed into this new position. After the patient is returned to the original position, the blood pressure is the same as it was originally. How can the therapist explain the blood pressure changes?
   A. There was an air bubble in the arterial catheter.
   B. There was a clot in the arterial catheter.
   C. The patient's body was below the level of the pressure transducer.
   D. Postural drainage positions always cause the blood pressure to decrease.

2. A patient with advanced emphysema is admitted to the respiratory intensive care unit. He is placed on a 24% Venturi-type mask and has a pulmonary artery catheter inserted. His initial pulmonary vascular resistance (PVR) is 300 dynes • sec • cm^{-5}, and the PaO_2 is 57 torr. The physician orders him increased to 28% oxygen. The resulting PVR is 220 dynes • sec • cm^{-5}, and the PaO_2 is 63 torr. Based on this information, what would you recommend?
   A. Decrease the oxygen to 24%.
   B. Place the patient on a ventilator.
   C. Administer a bronchodilating agent such as albuterol.
   D. Keep the patient on 28% oxygen.

3. Capnography will be used to monitor a patient's recovery from anesthesia. What gas should be used for the "zero" calibration?
   A. Room air for 0% carbon dioxide
   B. Room air for 21% oxygen
   C. 5% carbon dioxide
   D. The same concentration of anesthetic gas as used with the patient

4. Your patient is in the intensive care unit and is being monitored with a pulmonary artery catheter. She has the following parameters: PAP of 35/20 mm Hg, PCWP of 9 mm Hg, central venous pressure of 9 cm water. You would interpret the data to indicate that she:
   A. Has right ventricular failure/cor pulmonale.
   B. Has left ventricular failure.
   C. Has increased pulmonary vascular resistance.
   D. Is hypovolemic.

5. A 40-year-old patient receiving mechanical ventilation has an arterial line in place. It is noticed that a significant difference exists between the blood pressure taken by cuff on the left arm and blood pressure taken by arterial line on the right arm. What could explain this difference?
   I. A clot is at the tip of the catheter.
   II. There is an air bubble in the arterial line.
   III. The ventilator's peak pressure is too high.
   IV. The patient has a ventricular septal defect.
   A. I and II
   B. II and III
   C. I, III, and IV
   D. I, II, III, and IV

6. An adult patient is receiving mechanical ventilation when the following data are gathered:

	9:00 AM	**11:00 AM**
Pa_{O_2}	75 torr	53 torr
PVR	120 dynes • sec • cm^{-5}	340 dynes • sec • cm^{-5}
PCWP	8 mm Hg	10 mm Hg
PAP	25/10 mm Hg	42/21 mm Hg

How should the results be interpreted?
A. Pulmonary edema
B. Pulmonary embolism
C. Pneumonia
D. Cardiac tamponade

7. A patient is receiving mechanical ventilation with the SIMV mode and a mandatory rate of 10/minute. End-tidal carbon dioxide monitoring is being done, and the following data are recorded:

	4:00 PM	**6:00 PM**
Set tidal volume	700 mL	700 mL
Set rate	10	10
Pet_{CO_2}	33 torr	41 torr
Pa_{CO_2}	42 torr	43 torr

How can these data be explained?
A. Ventilation better matches perfusion.
B. Pulmonary edema has developed.
C. The patient is hyperventilating.
D. The patient's cardiac output has increased.

8. A patient has had an arterial line inserted. What should be done to ensure that accurate blood pressure readings are obtained?
   I. Open the stopcock to room air to "zero" the transducer.
   II. Make sure that air fills the transducer dome.
   III. Have the patient lie flat to measure the blood pressure.
   IV. Fill the pressure tubing with saline solution.
   A. I and II
   B. II and IV
   C. I, II, and III
   D. I, III, and IV

9. A 35-year-old patient in the intensive care unit has the following hemodynamic data. Which of them indicates a problem with the patient?
   A. SVR of 600 dynes • sec • cm^{-5}
   B. CI of 3 L/min/m^2 of body surface area
   C. $P\bar{v}_{O_2}$ of 38 torr
   D. Shunt of 4%

10. A patient with a history of congestive heart failure is inadvertently given intravenous fluids of 2000 mL instead of the ordered amount of 200 mL. Which of the following is most likely to be seen?
    A. Decreased lung markings on chest radiograph
    B. Increased pulmonary capillary wedge pressure
    C. Increased Pa_{O_2}
    D. Decreased pulmonary artery pressure

11. A patient hospitalized with a deep-vein thrombosis in the leg experiences sudden shortness of breath. Which of the following should be recommended to evaluate the patient's situation?
    A. Lung compliance
    B. Electrocardiogram
    C. Chest radiograph
    D. V_D/V_T

12. An unconscious 25-year-old patient is admitted with viral pneumonia, vomiting, and diarrhea. Mechanical ventilation is initiated, and a flow-directed pulmonary artery (Swan-Ganz) catheter is inserted. The following data are gathered:
    Pulmonary artery pressure, 22/8 mm Hg
    Pulmonary capillary wedge pressure, 3 mm Hg
    Central venous pressure, 0 mm Hg
    Blood pressure, 90/60 mm Hg
    Pulse, 142/min
    What is the most likely cause of these findings?
    A. Hypovolemia
    B. High ventilating pressures
    C. Bronchospasm
    D. Rupture of the balloon on the catheter

ANSWER KEY

1. **C.** Rationale: A pressure transducer for blood pressure monitoring should be "zero" calibrated at the patient's midchest level. This will result in accurate blood pressure measurements. If the patient is below the level of the transducer, the measured blood pressure will be less than actual. Conversely, if the patient is above the level of the transducer, the measure blood pressure will be greater than actual. If an air bubble or clot were in the arterial catheter, the problem would not go away when the patient's position was changed. Although postural drainage positions can cause a decrease in blood pressure, this does not always happen or fit the circumstances in this situation.

2. **D.** Rationale: The patient should be kept on 28% oxygen because the pulmonary vascular resistance has decreased to the normal range (see Box 5-2) and PaO_2 has increased from 57 to 63 torr compared to when the patient was breathing 24% oxygen. The patient is not hypoxemic; no indication is seen to begin mechanical ventilation. A bronchodilating agent such as albuterol may help the patient's breathing somewhat, but it is not effective at reducing pulmonary vascular resistance.

3. **A.** Rationale: A capnograph is zero calibrated on room air because it contains only a trace of carbon dioxide. A capnograph cannot measure oxygen percentage or anesthetic gases. Either 5% or 10% carbon dioxide is often used for the second point (high point) in two-point calibration of the capnograph.

4. **C.** Rationale: The patient's pulmonary vascular resistance can be found by calculating the pulmonary artery diastolic pressure minus the pulmonary capillary wedge pressure (PAd – PCWP) as follows:

   PAd   20 mm Hg
   PCWP   −9 mm Hg
               11 mm Hg

   Because a normal PAd – PCWP gradient is no more than 5 mm Hg, this patient's value of 11 mm Hg indicates increased pulmonary vascular resistance. Even though the patient's PAP is elevated at 35/20 mm Hg, that pressure alone does not give enough information to determine that the patient has right ventricular failure/cor pulmonale. An increased right ventricular pressure in a patient with COPD indicates right ventricular failure/cor pulmonale. Because the patient has a normal PCWP of 9 mm Hg, she does not have left ventricular failure. This problem is identified by an increased PCWP. This same normal PCWP of 9 mm Hg indicates normal blood volume. Hypovolemia is identified by a PCWP that is less than 4 mm Hg.

5. **A.** Rationale: If a clot is at the tip of the catheter, it will prevent the patient's blood pressure from being transmitted back to the transducer to be measured. If the clot is withdrawn, the lumen of the catheter will be open, and the blood pressure can be measured. If an air bubble is in the arterial line, the measured blood pressure will be less than actual. This is because the patient's blood pressure will partially collapse the gas bubble (Boyle's law) and transmit a lower pressure to the transducer. Withdrawing the air bubble allows the patient's blood pressure to be accurately sent to the transducer. If the ventilator's peak pressure is too high, the patient's cardiac output will be reduced. This will result in a decrease in blood pressure that will be measured equally on both arms. No evidence exists that the patient has a ventricular septal defect. Even if a septal defect were present, the blood pressure would be the same in both arms.

6. **B.** Rationale: The two significant changes in the patient's parameters indicate that the patient has a pulmonary embolism. First, the patient's pulmonary vascular resistance has almost tripled in 2 hours. Second, the patient's pulmonary artery diastolic pressure minus the pulmonary capillary wedge pressure (PAd – PCWP) difference has increased significantly.

	9:00 AM	**11:00 AM**
PAd	10 mm Hg	21 mm Hg
PCWP	− 8 mm Hg	−10 mm Hg
	2 mm Hg	11 mm Hg
	(Normal)	(Increased)

   The fact that both of these parameters have quickly increased significantly, combined with the sudden decrease in the patient's oxygen level, indicates a cause that can be only a pulmonary embolism. Because the patient's pulmonary capillary wedge pressure (PCWP) remains normal at 8 mm Hg and 10 mm Hg, pulmonary edema is not supported as a diagnosis. Pulmonary edema results in an increased PCWP. Pneumonia will result in hypoxemia. However, the other parameters do not match this diagnosis. Cardiac tamponade will decrease the patient's cardiac output but will not increase pulmonary vascular resistance or PCWP.

7. **A.** Rationale: The narrowing of the difference between arterial and exhaled $CO_2 [P(a-et)CO_2]$ from 9 torr to 2 torr correlates with better matching of ventilation to perfusion No data correlate with pulmonary edema (such as an increased pulmonary capillary wedge pressure). If the patient were hyperventilating, the $PetCO_2$ would have decreased instead of increased, and the $PaCO_2$ would have decreased. No data correlate with an increased cardiac output (such as a decreased difference between the oxygen content of arterial blood and the oxygen content of venous blood).

8. **D.** Rationale: It is necessary to "zero" the transducer by exposing it to local barometric pressure. Adjust the transducer so that it reads zero when exposed to room barometric pressure. The patient must lie flat in bed with the transducer at midchest level to give accurate blood pressure readings. If the patient sits up, the blood pressure will read low. If the patient's head is lower than his or her body, the blood pressure will read too high. Saline must fill the pressure tubing, transducer dome, and arterial catheter so that the patient's blood pressure is measured accurately. If air fills the transducer dome, it will be variably compressed, based on the patient's systolic and diastolic blood pressure changes. This is the result of Boyle's law and results in a lower-than-actual blood pressure being measured.

9. **A.** Rationale: A normal adult's systemic vascular resistance (SVR) has a range of 900 to 1400 dyne • sec • cm^{-5}. This patient's SVR value of 600 dyne • sec • cm^{-5} is well below normal. This may result from vasodilation or hypovolemia. All of the other values are within the normal range. See Box 5-2, Table 3-11, and discussion earlier in the chapter.

10. **B.** Rationale: If excessive fluid is given to a patient with congestive heart failure, the fluid is likely to back up into the pulmonary vessels because the left ventricle cannot pump effectively. This backup of fluid into the lungs will increase the pulmonary capillary wedge pressure. The patient should be watched for pulmonary edema. If pulmonary edema develops, a chest radiograph will show increased rather than decreased lung markings and fluid in the lungs. The patient's Pao$_2$ can be expected to decrease rather than increase if pulmonary edema develops. If fluid backs up from the left ventricle into the pulmonary vessels, the pulmonary artery pressure will increase along with the pulmonary capillary wedge pressure.

11. **D.** Rationale: The patient's history and current situation suggest that a pulmonary embolism has occurred. The VD/V$_T$ test should be performed to determine whether the patient's dead space has increased. If it has, this will match the clinical suspicion of a pulmonary embolism. It is doubtful that the patient's lung compliance will change if a pulmonary embolism has occurred. No specific change in the electrocardiogram corresponds with a pulmonary embolism or other sudden cause of shortness of breath. Chest radiograph changes are unlikely soon after a pulmonary embolism has occurred.

12. **A.** Rationale: The patient's history of vomiting and diarrhea would lead to a loss of body fluids. Hypovolemia correlates with tachycardia and all of the patient's low blood pressure values. High ventilating pressures can result in a decrease in the cardiac output. This can cause the systemic blood pressure to decrease, but is unlikely to result in all of the hemodynamic values being low. In addition, no information given relates to the patient's ventilating pressures, with no mention of the patient's breath sounds revealing bronchospasm. Even if bronchospasm were present, it would not cause all of the low hemodynamic values. If the balloon on the catheter were to rupture, a small volume of gas would be released into the pulmonary circulation. This would act as a small gas embolism. Although not good for the patient, this small gas embolism is unlikely to cause a decrease in all of the hemodynamic pressures.

6

Oxygen and Medical Gas Therapy

Note 1: The National Board for Respiratory Care (NBRC) has released the *RRT Examination Matrix* (covering the testable items on the Written Registry Exam) and the *CSE Examination Matrix* (covering the testable items on the Clinical Simulation Exam). Turn to the appendices at the back of this book for both publications in their original format. This book is intended to cover all of the testable items in these two publications. This chapter (and all others) uses the abbreviation "WRE" for the coded items testable on the Written Registry Exam *and* Clinical Simulation Exam. The listed difficulty (R, Recall; Ap, Application; An, Analysis) relates to the question difficulty on the Written Registry Exam. The abbreviation "CSE" is used for the coded items testable on *only* the Clinical Simulation Exam. Because no question difficulty level is given for this exam, be prepared for anything.

Note 2: A review of the most recent Written Registry Examinations has shown an average of seven questions (7% of the exam) that cover oxygen and medical gas therapy. The Clinical Simulation Exam is comprehensive and may include everything that should be known or performed by an advanced level respiratory therapist.

MODULE A

Ensure that the patient is adequately oxygenated

1. Oxygen administration

a. Recommend changes in the patient's position to minimize hypoxemia (WRE code: IIG2a) [Difficulty: An]

b. Minimize hypoxemia by positioning the patient properly (WRE Code: IID5) [Difficulty: Ap, An]

Usually a patient who is short of breath when lying supine should be repositioned to sit more upright in a Fowler's or semi-Fowler's position. This seems to work best in patients with bilateral pulmonary problems such as congestive heart failure or pneumonia. If the patient cannot sit up and the lung problem is one sided, roll the patient so that the more functional lung is down. The good lung should be positioned up in the following exceptions:

1. Undrained pulmonary abscess that should not be drained into the good lung.
2. Neonatal congenital diaphragmatic hernia in which the good lung should not be compressed by the bowel in the chest cavity.
3. Pulmonary interstitial emphysema in which, by lying on the bad lung, the air leak and functional residual capacity can be reduced.

In either case, always ask the patient whether the new position helps to make breathing easier. If not, reposition the patient until breathing is more comfortable with less shortness of breath.

c. Administer oxygen as needed and make a recommendation to change the fractional inspired oxygen concentration or oxygen flow to spontaneously breathing patients (WRE code: IIIG2c and IIID4a) [Difficulty: An]

Oxygen (O_2) must be administered in doses (up to 100%) that are adequate to treat hypoxemia, decrease the patient's work of breathing, or decrease the work of the heart. Because the Food and Drug Administration has declared supplemental oxygen to be a drug, a physician's order must exist to give it to a patient or to make a change in the percentage. The only exceptions are when recognized protocols exist in your institution to give oxygen under certain limited conditions. For example, all patients with a diagnosed heart attack are given a nasal cannula at 2 L/min, or all patients undergoing cardiopulmonary resuscitation (CPR) receive 100% oxygen.

See Chapter 3 (Module A) for a listing of indications for drawing blood for an arterial blood gas (ABG) measurement. This list should be fairly complete for conditions that justify the need for supplemental oxygen. In general, the goal of giving supplemental oxygen is to keep the patient's Pao_2 level between 60 and 100 torr. Exceptions include carbon monoxide poisoning, severe anemia, and CPR, when the hope is to fully saturate the hemoglobin and increase the plasma oxygen content as much as possible. Oxygen should not be given without proof of hypoxemia or another clinical justification. When those conditions have been corrected, the oxygen percentage should be adjusted accordingly.

Giving supplemental oxygen is not without risk. The following are oxygen-related problems that may be clinically seen:

O$_2$-induced hypoventilation. This is something to watch for in patients who have an elevated carbon dioxide level because of severe emphysema, chronic bronchitis, or both (known as chronic obstructive pulmonary disease [COPD]). A common clinical goal is to keep the Pao$_2$ level between 50 and 60 torr. Check the blood gases frequently for the oxygen and carbon dioxide levels.

Retinopathy of prematurity (formerly called retrolental fibroplasia). This type of blindness is found in some premature neonates who were given high levels of supplemental oxygen. The exact cause is not completely understood but is related primarily to the degree of prematurity. Keeping the Pao$_2$ in the range of 50 to 60 torr for the first week and 50 to 70 torr after that should help to prevent the problem.

Denitrogenation absorption atelectasis. Giving more than 80% oxygen can result in atelectasis of underventilated alveoli after the oxygen has been taken up by the blood.

Central nervous system abnormalities. A patient who is breathing 100% oxygen in a hyperbaric chamber can have muscle tremors and seizures.

Pulmonary O$_2$ toxicity. In general, it appears that patients can breathe up to 50% oxygen for prolonged periods without significant damage. If clinically possible, many practitioners try to limit their patients to no more than 48 to 72 hours of breathing more than 50% oxygen.

Exam Hint

The National Board of Respiratory Care (NBRC) is known to ask questions that relate to the proper use of oxygen and the hazards associated with its use. Expect to see at least one question that deals with the need to decrease the oxygen percentage for a COPD patient who has shown an increased Paco$_2$ when given too much supplemental oxygen.

---

d. Measure the patient's oxygen percentage, oxygen liter flow, or both (WRE code: IIIE10) [Difficulty: Ap, An]

Always measure the patient's inspired O$_2$ percentage (Fio$_2$) if possible. The gas sample should be taken as close as possible to the patient to minimize the chance of dilution from room air. Record the oxygen percentage on the ABG order slip, in the department records, and in the patient's chart if needed. As discussed in Chapter 3,

the oxygen percentage must be known to interpret the patient's Pao$_2$ level.

The oxygen liter flow is all that can be recorded with the following devices: nasal cannula, nasal catheter, simple mask, partial-rebreather mask, nonrebreather mask, and transtracheal oxygen catheter. A direct relation is found between the liter flow and the oxygen percentage, but it is not predictably accurate.

e. Prevent the patient from becoming hypoxemic by using proper technique (WRE code: IIID6) [Difficulty: An]

Use caution and plan ahead to minimize any time that the oxygen supply to the patient is cut off or reduced. When changing equipment of any kind, have the replacement set up and tested for proper function before replacing the current setup.

It is well known that suctioning the airway reduces the patient's oxygen level. This can result in dangerous dysrhythmias. Remember to increase the patient's inspired oxygen percentage about 1 minute before, during, and for at least 1 minute after suctioning. It is acceptable and safe to give 100% oxygen for short periods like this. Remember to reduce the oxygen percentage or liter flow to the previous level once the patient is stable after the procedure. Reanalyze the percentage if possible.

2. Oxygen and specialty gas analyzers
   a. Get the necessary equipment for the procedure (WRE code: IIA21) [Difficulty: R, Ap, An]
   b. Put the equipment together, and make sure that it works properly (WRE code: IIA21) [Difficulty: R, Ap, An]
   c. Troubleshoot any problems with the equipment (WRE code: IIA21) [Difficulty: R, Ap, An]

Because so many different models are available, consult an equipment book or the manufacturer's literature for details of the various analyzers. All portable, hand-held analyzers fall into one of the following categories: electric, physical/paramagnetic, and electrochemical.

Electric analyzers. These analyzers basically operate by comparing the cooling effects of an oxygen-enriched gas sample on a heated wire with the cooling effects of a room air gas sample on a heated wire. The oxygen-enriched gas cools faster than the room air gas. This is known as the principle of thermal conductivity. Each sample must be drawn into the analyzer through a capillary line. These analyzers are designed to work only in oxygen and nitrogen gas mixes. Do *not* use them around flammable gases such as those found in anesthesia. Failure to calibrate can be caused by a weak battery, a plugged capillary line, or a defect in an electrical component.

Physical/paramagnetic analyzers. These analyzers make use of the fact that oxygen is attracted toward a magnetic field (paramagnetic property). The more oxygen is in a sample gas, the more the magnetic field is altered. These units can be used with all types of gases and are safe in the operating room with flammable and explosive anesthetics. A silica gel–filled container is in line with the capillary tube to dry out the sample gas before it gets to the analyzing chamber. Failure to calibrate can be caused by water or a defect in the analyzing chamber, a weak battery, or a plugged capillary line.

Electrochemical analyzers: polarographic and galvanic fuel cell. Both the polarographic and galvanic fuel cells make use of the fact that each oxygen molecule accepts up to two electrons and becomes chemically reduced. The more oxygen in the gas sample, the more electrons are released from an oxidizing electrolyte solution. This is measured as an electrical current that is proportional to the oxygen percentage. These analyzers can continuously monitor and display the oxygen percentage. Both types are safe by themselves in the presence of flammable gases, but the added alarm systems are electrically powered and may make the units unsafe. Polarographic analyzers use a battery to polarize the gas sampling probe. Because of this, they have a faster response time than do the galvanic fuel cell types. Galvanic fuel cell analyzers do not need a battery for power. However, they usually include alarms that are battery powered.

Failure to calibrate either type can be caused by a weak battery, an exhausted supply of chemical reactant in the gas sampling probe, or an electronic failure. The galvanic units must have their probes kept dry to read accurately. Both types are pressure sensitive. High altitude causes them to display a lower-than-true oxygen percentage, and high pressure as seen in a ventilator circuit with positive end-expiratory pressure (PEEP) causes the units to display a higher-than-true oxygen percentage.

Specialty gas analyzers. The specialty gas analyzers (helium, nitrogen, and carbon monoxide) are used mainly with pulmonary function testing procedures and are discussed in Chapter 4. It may be necessary to use a helium analyzer if a helium and oxygen mix is given to a patient.

Nitric oxide (NO) is delivered through the INOvent delivery system. It is able to deliver set amounts of therapeutic NO and to continuously monitor the amount of NO given to the patient along with nitrogen dioxide (NO_2) and oxygen.

3. Perform quality control procedures for oxygen analyzers (WRE code: IIC2) [Difficulty: Ap]

A two-point calibration procedure is done on all oxygen analyzers by sampling room air, adjusting a calibration control if necessary to have the unit show 21% oxygen (first point or low oxygen check), sampling 100% oxygen, and adjusting a calibration control if necessary to have the unit show 100% oxygen (second point or high oxygen check). When room air is sampled again, the analyzer should read 21% oxygen. In general, always follow the manufacturer's guidelines for setup and calibration. If an analyzer does not pass the two-point calibration check, it should not be used.

MODULE B
Storage, hardware, and distribution of medical gases

1. **Oxygen and other gas cylinders, bulk storage systems, and manifolds**
   a. **Get the necessary equipment for the procedure (WRE code: IIA9b) [Difficulty: Ap, An]**
   b. **Put the equipment together and make sure that it works properly (WRE code: IIA9b) [Difficulty: Ap, An]**
   c. **Troubleshoot any problems with the equipment (WRE code: IIA9b) [Difficulty: Ap, An]**

Oxygen and other gas cylinders. The different types of gases in cylinders are identified by the color code of the cylinder and the cylinder label. Note that only E cylinders have mandatory color coding. The color codings on the other cylinders are voluntary but are usually followed by the manufacturers. However, always read the label to be sure of the contents of the cylinder. The most important cylinder colors to remember are those of oxygen and air, but all are included in Table 6-1 for the sake of completeness.

TABLE 6-1	Color Codes for Gas Cylinders
Gas	**Color**
Oxygen	Green (white for international)
Air	Yellow
Helium	Brown
Helium and oxygen	Brown and green (check the label for the percentage of each gas)
Carbon dioxide	Gray
Carbon dioxide and oxygen	Gray and green (check the label for the percentage of each gas)
Nitrous oxide	Light blue
Cyclopropane	Orange
Ethylene	Red

The NBRC is known to ask the examinee to calculate how long a certain cylinder lasts at a given gas flow. To date, only the durations of E-, H-, and K-sized oxygen cylinders have had to be calculated.

To review how to calculate the duration of flow of a type of cylinder, see Table 6-2 for the cylinder duration factors, the following equation, and the following examples.

Minutes of flow (divide by 60 to calculate hours) =
$$\frac{\text{Gauge pressure in psig} \times \text{Cylinder factor}}{\text{liter flow}}$$

1. Calculate the duration of flow of an E cylinder with 1500 pounds per square inch gauge (psig) that is running at 6 L/min.

Minutes of flow (divide by 60 to calculate hours) $= \dfrac{1500 \text{ psig} \times 0.28}{6 \text{ L}}$

$= \dfrac{420}{6}$

Minutes of flow $= 70 \left(\begin{array}{c}1.16 \text{ hr, or } 1 \text{ hr} \\ \text{and } 10 \text{ min}\end{array}\right)$

2. Calculate the duration of flow of an H cylinder with 1950 psig that is running at 9 L/min.

Minutes of flow (divide by 60 to calculate hours) $= \dfrac{1950 \text{ psig} \times 3.14}{9 \text{ L}}$

$= \dfrac{6123}{9}$

Minutes of flow $= 680.33 \left(\begin{array}{c}11.34 \text{ hr, or } 11 \text{ hr} \\ \text{and } 20 \text{ min}\end{array}\right)$

Bulk storage systems. The bulk liquid oxygen (LOX)-storage system is the main source of a hospital's oxygen. A reducing valve is used to decrease the gas pressure to 50 pounds per square inch gauge (psig) before it is piped throughout the hospital for easy access. Alarms will sound

TABLE 6-2	Oxygen Cylinder Duration of Flow Factors	
Cylinder Size	**Factor (L/psig)**	
E	0.28	
H	3.14	
K	3.14	
D	0.16	
M	1.36	
G	2.41	

psig, Pounds per square inch gauge.

if the pressure is low or too high. Pressure relief valves will open if the pressure is greater than 75 psig. Zone valves are located throughout the hospital to turn off the gas if a leak develops or if a fire occurs.

Manifolds. A manifold is a piping system that connects the bulk storage system and hospital gas piping system with a bank of H- or K-sized cylinders. These freestanding cylinders are a backup source of oxygen in case the bulk system fails. A 24-hour supply of gas must be available.

The manifold system includes a reducing valve to decrease the gas pressure to 50 psig. Check valves are built into the manifold so that a leak in one cylinder connection cannot result in all of the gas cylinders leaking out.

2. **Adjunct hardware: reducing valves, flowmeters, regulators, pulse-dose systems, and high-pressure hose connectors**
   a. **Get the necessary equipment for the procedure (WRE code: IIA9a) [Difficulty: Ap, An]**
   b. **Put the equipment together and make sure that it works properly (WRE code: IIA9a) [Difficulty: Ap, An]**
   c. **Troubleshoot any problems with the equipment (WRE code: IIA9a) [Difficulty: Ap, An]**

Reducing valves. Reducing valves are used to reduce the high pressure seen in a bulk oxygen storage system, manifold, or gas cylinder. One or more stages (pressure reducing steps) can be used to reach the working pressure of 50 psig. Single-stage reducing valves reach the pressure in a single step. Multiple-stage reducing valves give finer control over pressure and flow by decreasing pressure in the first stage to about 200 psig and to 50 psig in the second stage. Occasionally, three stages are seen. All reducing valves (and regulators [combined reducing valve and flowmeter]) have the following built-in safety features:
   a. A frangible disk that breaks to release gas pressure in the event of a mechanical failure or breakage
   b. A fusible plug that melts to release gas pressure in the event of a fire
   c. American Standard Compressed Gas Cylinder Valve Outlet and Index Connections (usually called the American Standard system), which prevent the accidental connection of the wrong reducing valve (or regulator) to a large gas cylinder
   d. The Pin Index Safety System (PISS) is a special section of the American Standard system that applies to gas cylinders that are E-sized and smaller. It is designed to prevent an accidental connection of the wrong gas to a reducing valve or regulator. These reducing valves and regulators are designed with a

Fig. 6-1 Locations of the Pin Index Safety System holes in the cylinder valve face. *(From Branson RD, Hess DR, Chatburn RL: Respiratory care equipment, ed 2, Philadelphia, 1999, Lippincott Williams & Wilkins.)*

specifically pinned yoke to wrap around the valve stem of a gas cylinder. A soft plastic O-ring washer is included to help ensure a tight seal. Fig. 6-1 shows the location of the pinholes in the cylinder valve face. Table 6-3 shows the gases and pinhole positions. It is important to know the positions for oxygen and air; the others are included for the sake of completeness.

It is necessary to "crack" or blow some gas out of a cylinder before putting any reducing valve or regulator onto it to prevent any dust or debris from being forced into the reducing valve or regulator, which might cause a fire.

Flowmeters. Flowmeters are designed to regulate and indicate flow. They also come with the following safety features so that they cannot be attached to the wrong reducing valve, regulator, high-pressure hose, or appliance:

a. Diameter Index Safety System (DISS) inlets and outlets that are specific to the various gases so that a mix-up cannot be made with the wrong appliance or connector. The DISS system applies to flowmeters that attach to all American Standard and DISS reduction valves.

b. Flowmeters with quick-connect inlet adapters instead of DISS inlets. These quick-connects are designed specifically for the hospital's piped-in oxygen and air outlets. They are not interchangeable between gases or between manufacturers. Occasionally a piped oxygen outlet will jam open and let gas rapidly escape. Insert the proper flowmeter into the outlet, and turn the flowmeter off. This stops the leak until the defective wall outlet can be repaired.

Flowmeters are usually categorized by how they react to backpressure. To complicate matters further, we must remember that the three different manufactured types of flowmeters may or may not be backpressure compensated.

a. Non–backpressure-compensated (pressure-uncompensated) flowmeters will *inaccurately* indicate the flow through them in the face of backpressure. Figs. 6-2 and 6-3 show non–backpressure-compensated kinetic and Thorpe types of flowmeters, respectively. Note that the Thorpe and kinetic flowmeters have

TABLE 6-3	Pin Index Safety System Gases and Pinhole Locations
Gas	**Pinhole Locations**
Oxygen	2-5
Air	1-5
Oxygen/carbon dioxide (≤7%)	2-6
Oxygen/carbon dioxide (>7%)	1-6
Oxygen/helium (not >80% helium)	2-4
Oxygen/helium (helium >80%)	4-6
Nitrous oxide	3-5
Ethylene	1-3
Cyclopropane	3-6

Fig. 6-2 Kinetic-type non–backpressure-compensated (pressure-uncompensated) flowmeter. *(Modified from McPherson SP: Respiratory care equipment, ed 4, St Louis, 1990, Mosby.)*

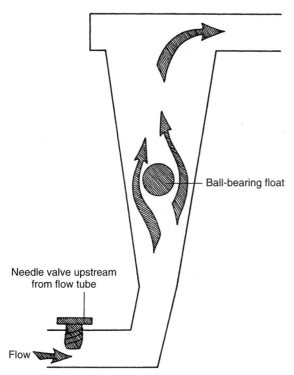

Fig. 6-3 Thorpe-type non–backpressure-compensated (pressure-uncompensated) flowmeter. *(Modified from McPherson SP: Respiratory care equipment, ed 4, St Louis, 1990, Mosby.)*

the flow-control valve upstream from the meter. They read accurately if they are kept upright and do not have to "push" against any backpressure. If laid on their sides, the plunger and ball bearing do not indicate the set flow. They both read a *lower* flow than that actually delivered when faced with a backpressure.

b. The Bourdon flowmeter is designed like the Bourdon gauge in the reducing valve (Fig. 6-4). The face piece is marked in liters of flow rather than pressure. It is the flowmeter of choice in a transport

Fig. 6-4 Bourdon-type non–backpressure-compensated (pressure-uncompensated) flowmeter. *(From McPherson SP: Respiratory care equipment, ed 4, St Louis, 1990, Mosby.)*

situation because it may be laid flat without affecting its flow if no backpressure is present. These flowmeters will display a *higher* flow than that actually delivered when faced with a backpressure.

c. Backpressure-compensated (pressure-compensated) flowmeters *accurately* indicate the flow through them in the face of backpressure. For this reason, they should be used whenever possible. Figs. 6-5 and 6-6 show backpressure-compensated kinetic and Thorpe types of flowmeters, respectively. Note that both of these flowmeters have the flow-control valve downstream from the meter. Because of this, they read accurately in the face of backpressure as long as they are kept upright. Besides reading the label, this simple test enables the practitioner to tell whether a flowmeter is backpressure compensated:

1. Make sure the flowmeter is turned off.
2. Plug the flowmeter into a gas outlet.
3. If the float or ball bearing bounces, the flowmeter is backpressure compensated.

d. Perform quality control procedures for flowmeters (CSE code: IIC5)

When performing a quality control procedure for a flowmeter, it is critical that a known flow be sent through it so that the flowmeter can be checked for accuracy. This

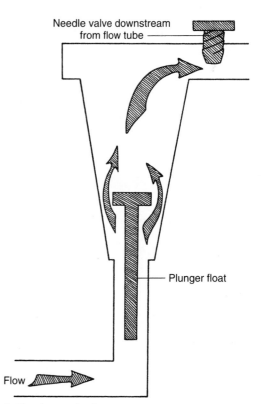

Fig. 6-5 Kinetic-type backpressure-compensated (pressure-compensated) flowmeter. *(Modified from McPherson SP: Respiratory care equipment, ed 4, St Louis, 1990, Mosby.)*

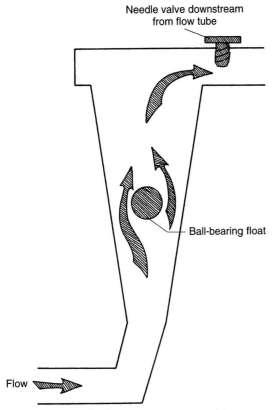

Needle valve downstream
from flow tube

Ball-bearing float

Flow

Fig. 6-6 Thorpe-type backpressure-compensated (pressure-compensated) flowmeter. *(Modified from McPherson SP: Respiratory care equipment, ed 4, St Louis, 1990, Mosby.)*

should be done without any backpressure against the flowmeter. Review the previous discussion on troubleshooting flowmeters for the effects of backpressure on non–backpressure-compensated flowmeters and Bourdon flowmeters. Do not use any flowmeter that does not give an accurate reading.

Exam Hint

Choose a backpressure-compensated flowmeter in all situations except during patient transport when the oxygen tank and flowmeter might be laid flat. Then a Bourdon flowmeter should be used.

Regulators. Regulators combine a reducing valve and a flowmeter. Everything that has been discussed so far relates to regulators. Bourdon gauge reducing valves are usually seen and can have either a second Bourdon gauge added as a flowmeter or a Thorpe or kinetic flowmeter. As mentioned earlier, use a backpressure-compensated flowmeter in all situations except for patient transport.

Pulse-dose systems. A pulse-dose oxygen delivery system (the NBRC calls it a *demand oxygen conserver*) is used in the home care setting to reduce the patient's oxygen use and to save money. The unit takes the place of a regulator and flowmeter on the oxygen source. Some units are designed for a low-pressure LOX system. Others are designed for a high-pressure E tank of oxygen. Be careful not to place a low-pressure unit on a high-pressure gas source, because it will be damaged. In all units, the distal end of a regular nasal cannula is attached to a pressure sensor on the pulse-dose system. It senses a decrease in pressure as the patient inspires. The sensor then triggers a solenoid valve that delivers a burst of oxygen to the cannula. A pulse-dose unit can be adjusted to change several factors such as how long the oxygen is delivered, how much is delivered, and whether the patient receives oxygen every breath or every second or third breath.

Make sure that the patient can feel a flow of gas from the cannula after he or she starts to inhale. The gas should stop during exhalation. Check the patient's pulse oximetry value at rest and during exercise to ensure that desaturation does not occur. Adjust the pressure sensor or solenoid if needed to meet the patient's oxygen needs.

If the patient cannot feel any oxygen flowing, the following should be considered: (1) the source of oxygen might be empty, (2) the tubing might be disconnected or kinked, or (3) the sensor is not detecting the patient's effort. The patient or therapist can switch to a second oxygen source and look for disconnections or kinks in the tubing. The therapist must adjust the nasal cannula or pulse-dose unit to correct for a sensitivity problem. Do not use a system that is malfunctioning and cannot be adjusted.

High-pressure hose connectors. These connectors and other adapters connect high-pressure hoses, flowmeters, and oxygen appliances. They have DISS inlets and outlets so that the gases cannot be cross-fitted to the wrong equipment.

3. Air compressors
   a. Get the necessary equipment for the procedure (WRE code: IIA9b) [Difficulty: R, Ap]
   b. Put the equipment together and make sure that it works properly (WRE code: IIA9b) [Difficulty: R, Ap]
   c. Troubleshoot any problems with the equipment (WRE code: IIA9b) [Difficulty: R, Ap]

Air compressors are used whenever a high-pressure gas source other than oxygen is needed. All three systems are alike in that they use an electrically powered motor, filter the room air as it enters and exits the compressor, and have a condenser to remove water vapor as it leaves the compressor.

Rotary-type compressors. Rotary-type compressors generate pressure with a rotating fan. They are commonly used in volume ventilators and in the home to power handheld medication nebulizers and intermittent positive-pressure breathing (IPPB) units.

Diaphragm-type compressors. Diaphragm-type compressors generate pressure with a diaphragm that moves up and down within a cylinder-like piston. They also are commonly used in the home to power hand-held medication nebulizers and IPPB units.

Piston-type compressors. Piston-type compressors generate pressure by piston action within a cylinder. They are much more powerful than the previous two types of compressors. Because they are designed to generate pressures of 50 psig or greater, they are used in the hospital with its piped air system. They also are used in the home setting in oxygen concentrators.

Make sure that all of these units are operational by checking that the inlet and outlet filters are cleaned. Dirty filters prevent proper airflow. Check the unit's pressure gauge to make sure that it is able to meet its manufacturer's specified pressure. Empty the water trap on the condensing unit as needed.

4. Air/oxygen proportioners (blenders)
a. **Get the necessary equipment for the procedure (WRE code: IIA9a and IIIF4b) [Difficulty: Ap, An]**
b. **Put the equipment together and make sure that it works properly (WRE code: IIA9a and IIIF4b) [Difficulty: Ap, An]**
c. **Troubleshoot any problems with the equipment (WRE code: IIA9a) [Difficulty: Ap, An]**

These units are designed to change the ratio of oxygen and air to blend the specific percentage of oxygen from 21% to 100% (Fig. 6-7). To do that, both source gases must be pressurized to 50 psi. The oxygen percentage will remain close to that desired even if a small decrease in either one or both line pressures occurs. Always analyze the oxygen percentage to confirm that it is correct. The blended gas can be sent directly to a ventilator or other device that uses 50 psi or through an added flowmeter.

Keep the gas inlets and outlets clear of any debris. All current units give an audible whistle if either one or both of the line pressures decrease to an unsafe level (often about 30 psig). If the unit has a water trap at the compressed air inlet, keep it emptied of any condensate.

Fig. 6-7 Example of an oxygen blender. Note the high-pressure air and oxygen hoses entering the bottom of the unit, the dial to set the oxygen percentage (75%), and the blended oxygen outlet to the right. In this case, a Wye connector has been attached with two oxygen flowmeters. *(From Cairo JM, Pilbeam SP: Mosby's respiratory care equipment, ed 7, St. Louis, 2004, Mosby.)*

5. Oxygen concentrators (enrichers)
a. **Get the necessary equipment for the procedure (WRE code: IIA9b) [Difficulty: R, Ap]**

Two different types of oxygen concentrators are available for the delivery of continuous low-flow oxygen in the home: molecular sieve and permeable plastic membrane.

Molecular sieve. Molecular sieve–type oxygen concentrators use an air compressor to push room air through two canisters of zeolite pellets (inorganic sodium-aluminum silicate) to remove nitrogen and water vapor. The remaining oxygen is delivered to the patient through a flowmeter (Fig. 6-8). Be aware that with this unit, the oxygen percentage varies inversely with the flow that is delivered (Table 6-4).

Permeable plastic membrane. Permeable plastic membrane oxygen concentrators make use of a 1-μm-thick plastic membrane as a filter. Room air is pulled through it by a vacuum pump. Molecular oxygen and water vapor can pass through the membrane faster than nitrogen. Any excess water vapor is removed by a simple condenser system. No need exists to add an external humidification system to the flowmeter (Fig. 6-9). The

Fig. 6-8 Drawing of the components of a molecular-sieve oxygen concentrator. The molecular-sieve beds remove nitrogen and pass oxygen through to the patient. *(Courtesy Sunrise Medical, Inc., Somerset, Penn.)*

TABLE 6-4	Comparison of Flow Rates and Oxygen Percentages in Oxygen Concentrators
Flow (L/min)	**Approximate Oxygen Percentage**
MOLECULAR SIEVE CONCENTRATOR	
1–2	>90%
3–5	80%–90%
6	about 74%
8	about 60%
10	50%
PERMEABLE MEMBRANE CONCENTRATOR	
1–10	40%

oxygen percentage is fixed at 40% in these units; however, the flow can be varied from 1 to 10 L/min, as shown in Table 6-4.

When deciding which type of concentrator to use, it is important to know the patient's required oxygen percentage and flow. As can be seen from Table 6-4, the molecular-sieve types can deliver a higher oxygen percentage at any liter flow as compared with the permeable plastic membrane units.

It should be noted that a home oxygen concentrator combined with a compressor is available. This allows a small portable oxygen tank to be filled, in the home, from the oxygen concentrator. This unit, the Invacare Venture HomeFill II oxygen filling system, allows the home care patient great flexibility in home and portable oxygen delivery.

b. Put the equipment together, and make sure that it works properly (WRE code: IIA9b and IIIF4c) [Difficulty: R, Ap, An]

c. Troubleshoot any problems with the equipment (WRE code: IIA9b) [Difficulty: R, Ap]

The molecular sieve–type units deliver dry gas; therefore a humidification system is frequently added to the flowmeter. With the permeable plastic membrane–type units, the condensed water vapor must be emptied from the collection jar. In both types of oxygen concentrators, it is important to check the air-inlet filter on a monthly basis to keep it clean of dust and debris. Follow the manufacturer's requirements for when filters should be replaced. The delivered oxygen concentration also should be checked each month. Follow the manufacturer's guidelines for its

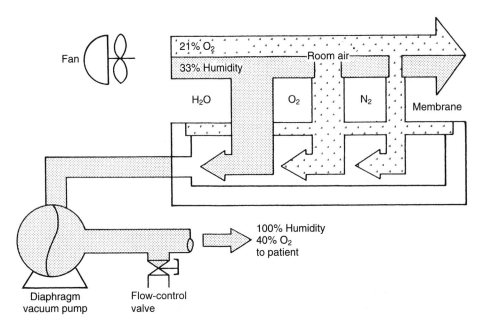

Fig. 6-9 Functional schematic of a semipermeable-membrane oxygen concentrator. The membrane permits more oxygen and water vapor than nitrogen to pass through. *(Courtesy of the Oxygen Enrichment Company, Schenectady, NY.)*

preventive maintenance needs. The molecular sieve-type units must have the zeolite pellet canisters replaced on a scheduled basis.

Some units have a visual or audio alarm that warns when a problem occurs, such as decreased flow. Because this is not a low-oxygen percentage alarm, some home care practitioners have recommended the addition of an external analyzer with an alarm system. This alerts the patient to call the home care company to repair the equipment. If a patient says that he or she cannot feel any gas coming out of the cannula, have the patient place the prongs into a glass of water. If no bubbling is seen, have the patient check the tubing for any disconnections. If the concentrator is malfunctioning, have the patient turn it off and switch to oxygen from the backup oxygen cylinder until repairs can be made.

Exam Hint

Most past examinations have included a question related to a malfunctioning oxygen concentrator used in the home. A patient may be expected to check for oxygen flowing through a cannula by placing the prongs under water to look for bubbling or switching from the concentrator to a backup source of oxygen such as an oxygen cylinder (tank). The patient should not be expected to troubleshoot problems with the concentrator or perform maintenance work on it. That is the home care respiratory therapist's job.

6. Portable liquid oxygen systems

a. Get the necessary equipment for the procedure (WRE code: IIA9b) [Difficulty: R, Ap]

An LOX system is used in the home when it is found to be more cost effective than an oxygen concentrator or battery of oxygen cylinders. An additional advantage is that the patient can carry a smaller portable unit in a shoulder bag for added mobility. It also is less conspicuous than wheeling an E cylinder about. An early widely known liquid oxygen system was the Linde (Union Carbide) Walker System. Fig. 6-10 shows the large liquid oxygen reservoir that is kept in the patient's home. Fig. 6-11 shows its smaller companion, the portable Linde Walker, which can be filled from the large reservoir.

b. Put the equipment together and make sure that it works properly (WRE code: IIA9b and IIIF4c) [Difficulty: R, Ap, An]

The Linde Walker reservoir tank weighs about 11 pounds and can be carried over the shoulder by a strap. It can be refilled from the larger reservoir tank kept in the home. The flow rate can be adjusted to meet most patients' needs. Humidification is provided by the patient's own

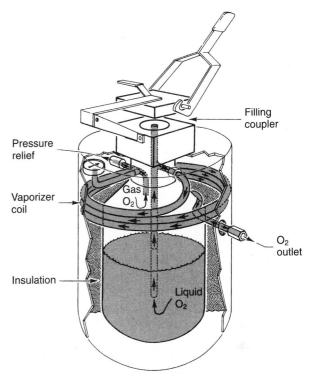

Fig. 6-10 Drawing of the components of a home liquid oxygen supply unit. *(From Lampton LM: Home and outpatient oxygen therapy. In Brashear RE, Rhodes ML, editors:* Chronic obstructive lung disease, *St Louis, 1978, Mosby.)*

airway. As with any pressurized system, all fittings must be kept tight to prevent leakage.

The National Fire Protection Agency (NFPA) has established a number of regulations to ensure that home LOX

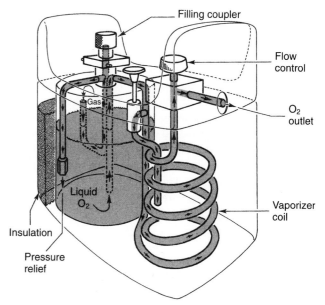

Fig. 6-11 Drawing of the components of a portable liquid oxygen unit. *(From Lampton LM: Home and outpatient oxygen therapy. In Brashear RE, Rhodes ML, editors:* Chronic obstructive lung disease, *St Louis, 1978, Mosby.)*

systems are safely installed. The key safety regulations include the following:

1. Stabilize the unit to prevent it from being tipped over.
2. The reservoir unit should not be set up near any radiators, steam pipes, or heat ducts to reduce the rate of oxygen loss.
3. No open flames or sources of ignition can be within 5 feet of the unit.
4. "No smoking" signs must be posted.
5. The patient and family must be instructed in how to use the equipment. This includes how to fill the Walker from the large reservoir tank. The person filling the Walker should wear safety goggles with side shields, loose-fitting insulated gloves, and high-top boots.
6. If liquid oxygen spills and contacts skin, it can cause frostbite. Medical attention should be sought immediately.
7. Avoid contact for at least 15 minutes with any equipment or the floor where liquid oxygen has spilled.

c. Troubleshoot any problems with the equipment (WRE code: IIA9b) [Difficulty: R, Ap]

Check that all connections are airtight to avoid spills and minimize the loss of oxygen. Make sure that the unit is functioning at its designed working pressure. The Linde unit operates at 90 psig. Make sure that the pressure relief valve operates properly and that the proper flow is delivered.

Exam Hint

Most past examinations have questioned either the need to set up a liquid oxygen supply unit and portable unit for a home care patient or troubleshooting problems with the system. A patient may be expected to check for oxygen flowing through a cannula by placing the prongs under water to look for bubbling or switching from the liquid oxygen system to a backup source of oxygen such as an oxygen cylinder (tank). The patient should not be expected to troubleshoot problems with the LOX system or perform maintenance work on it. That is the home care respiratory therapist's job.

---

7. Other therapeutic gases
a. Get the necessary equipment for the procedure (WRE code: IIA15) [Difficulty: R, Ap, An]

The NBRC specifically lists He/O_2 (heliox) as a testable item. In addition, O_2/CO_2 (carbogen) and inhaled NO (nitric oxide) are included in this discussion because they

may be administered to patients. The discussion of patient indications for each of these is presented in Module D.

All of these gases come in high-pressure cylinders and require the use of an American Standard system reducing valve (or regulator) designed specifically for the gas or gas mix. As shown in Table 6-3 and Fig. 6-1, a reducing valve or regulator for an E cylinder must match the appropriate pinholes on the cylinder valve face. Corresponding high-pressure hoses may also be needed. Table 6-1 shows the color codes for the various gas cylinders. Note that pure carbon dioxide comes in a gray cylinder, whereas a carbon dioxide and oxygen mix (carbogen) has a gray and green cylinder. Pure helium comes in a brown cylinder, whereas helium and oxygen mixes come in brown and green cylinders. Always check the cylinder label for the exact percentage of the gases within it. For example, heliox comes in mixes of 80% He/20% O_2, 70% He/30% O_2, and 60% He/40% O_2.

If carbogen is needed for a carbon dioxide response curve test the gas mix can be delivered from the cylinder flowmeter to the pulmonary function testing breathing circuit through small-bore tubing and a T-piece. The same simple assembly can deliver the carbogen to a patient's face mask or ventilator circuit. In both cases, the carbon dioxide level should be monitored by a capnometer added into the system (see Chapter 5).

A helium flowmeter can be used to set a flow of one of the heliox mixes to a patient's face mask. However, if a helium flowmeter is not available, an oxygen flowmeter can be added to the reducing valve on a heliox mix cylinder to set the flow of gas to the patient. (The calculation for determining the flow of a heliox mix through an oxygen flowmeter is shown in the following discussion.) If a patient requires helium through a mechanical ventilator, an air/oxygen proportioner (blender) is needed. Substitute 100% helium for the air side; oxygen will go through on its side of the unit, as usual. Simply dial the oxygen percentage as needed to adjust the mix of the two gases. For example, giving the patient 35% oxygen results in the patient also receiving 65% helium. Be aware that some ventilators do not accurately read the tidal volume when a helium/oxygen mix is delivered rather than the standard nitrogen/oxygen mix. The ventilator volume-measuring device (usually a flow-type pneumotachometer) may have to be recalibrated, or use a bellows-type spirometer to measure the exhaled tidal volume. Use a polarographic or galvanic fuel cell oxygen analyzer to monitor the patient's oxygen percentage.

The Food and Drug Administration (FDA) has granted approval of therapeutic inhaled nitric oxide (NO) and its delivery system to INO Therapeutics, Inc. The gaseous mixture is called INOmax and contains 0.8% nitric oxide and 99.2% nitrogen. The INOvent delivery system is needed to deliver inhaled nitric oxide to a mechanical ventilator or anesthesia machine. It is designed to deliver a precise dose of nitric oxide to either unit, as well as to monitor the NO level, nitrogen dioxide (NO_2) level, and oxygen level.

b. Put the equipment together and make sure that it works properly (WRE code: IIA15) [Difficulty: R, Ap, An]

When an oxygen flowmeter is used with a helium/oxygen regulator, the following adjustments must be made to the flow seen on the flowmeter. This is done because helium is less dense than oxygen. The heliox factor used to determine actual flow through an oxygen flowmeter varies with the ratio of helium to oxygen as follows:

Helium/oxygen ratio	Heliox factor
1. 80% helium/20% oxygen	1.8
2. 70% helium/30% oxygen	1.6
3. 60% helium/40% oxygen	1.4

The following examples show how actual flow can be calculated:

1. When using an 80% helium and 20% oxygen mix, multiply the observed flow by the heliox factor of 1.8. For example, an observed flow of 10 L/min × 1.8 = 18 L/min actual flow.
2. When using a 70% helium and 30% oxygen mix, multiply the observed flow by the heliox factor of 1.6. For example, an observed flow of 10 L/min × 1.6 = 16 L/min actual flow.
3. When using a 60% helium and 40% oxygen mix, multiply the observed flow by the heliox factor of 1.4. For example, an observed flow of 10 L/min × 1.4 = 14 L/min actual flow.
4. If a specific heliox flow is needed, the flow observed on the oxygen flowmeter must be divided by the heliox factor. For example, to get an actual flow of 7.5 L/min of 70/30 heliox, set the oxygen flowmeter at 12 L/min. Solution:

$$\frac{\text{Observed flow of 12 L/min}}{1.6 \text{ heliox factor}} = 7.5 \text{ L/min of actual flow}$$

Exam Hint

There is often one question that requires the calculation of actual flow of a heliox mixture through an oxygen flowmeter. The heliox factor must be known to do the calculation.

---

c. Troubleshoot any problems with the equipment (WRE code: IIA15) [Difficulty: R, Ap, An]

Each of the therapeutic gases discussed earlier needs its own particular hardware accessories as described. In addition, other types of respiratory care equipment such as face masks, pulmonary function testing equipment, or a mechanical ventilator are needed, based on the patient's situation.

A helium-oxygen mix is the most widely used of the therapeutic gases besides oxygen. With heliox therapy, the type of mask, delivery tubing, and humidifier chosen depend on whether the patient needs an aerosol delivered. If an aerosol is not needed, a nonrebreather mask with all of its one-way valves and small bore oxygen tubing is used. Attach a bubble humidifier with sterile water to the flowmeter. Connect the small bore tubing to the humidifier nipple and to the nonrebreather mask nipple. If aerosol is required, an aerosol mask with one-way exhalation valves and reservoir is needed. Screw the nebulizer filled with sterile water to the flowmeter. Make sure that the air entrainment control is set to deliver 100% source gas of heliox (no room air should be entrained). Connect the large bore, aerosol tubing to the nebulizer and the mask. Make sure the mask is adjusted to give as tight a fit to the face as is practical and comfortable. In either system, it is extremely important that all connections be tight because helium easily leaks out of any openings.

MODULE C
Administration of oxygen therapy

1. Oxygen hoods and oxygen tents

a. Get the necessary equipment for the procedure (WRE code: IIA1a) [Difficulty: Ap, An]

b. Put the equipment together and make sure that it works properly (WRE code: IIA1a) [Difficulty: Ap, An]

c. Troubleshoot any problems with the equipment (WRE code: IIA1a) [Difficulty: Ap, An]

Oxygen hoods. Oxygen hoods are used to provide a warmed aerosol, humidity, and a controlled oxygen percentage to pediatric patients who weigh no more than 18 lb (8.2 kg) (Fig. 6-12). When using an oxygen hood, the following procedures should be observed:

a. Use an air/oxygen proportioner with a flowmeter to control the oxygen percentage and flow to the hood. The flow should be at least 7 L/min to prevent the buildup of exhaled carbon dioxide. A flow of 10 to 15 L/min is needed to keep a stable oxygen percentage. Keeping the hood sealed as much as possible and minimizing the gap between the infant's neck and the opening to the hood also helps to stabilize the oxygen percentage.

b. A warmed humidifier is needed to provide a high humidity level and to warm the oxygen to the infant's body temperature. Care must be taken with infants to ensure that they are neither heated nor cooled by the gas blowing over their heads. A thermometer should be kept in the hood to note the temperature.

c. An oxygen analyzer should continuously monitor how much oxygen is inside the hood. The analyzer

Fig. 6-12 Infant in an oxygen hood. *(From Gaebler G, Blodgett D: Gas administration. In Blodgett D, editor:* Manual of pediatric respiratory care procedures, *Philadelphia, 1982, Lippincott.)*

Fig. 6-13 Child in an oxygen tent. *(From Gaebler G, Blodgett D: Gas administration. In Blodgett D, editor:* Manual of pediatric respiratory care procedures, *Philadelphia, 1982, Lippincott.)*

probe should be placed at the same level as the infant's nose. This is because oxygen is heavier than air and tends to settle toward the bottom of the hood. The advantages of the hood over the tent are that the patient's body is accessible, and the head can be reached by lifting the top off of the hood. Be aware of the noise level inside the hood to minimize damage to the infant's hearing. The sound level should be monitored and kept well below 65 dB.

Oxygen tents. Oxygen tents were formerly used for adults but are now used only for children who are too large and active for a hood. The tent is used to control the environment by providing a cooled aerosol, humidity, and controlled oxygen percentage (Fig. 6-13). In addition, the following procedures should be observed:

a. Set an oxygen flowmeter to deliver 8 to 10 L/min to small tents and 12 to 15 L/min to large tents. Flows of 30 L/min or greater are needed to keep the oxygen percentage close to the 50% maximum that can be reliably maintained. (Commonly, between 35% and 50% oxygen can be kept in a tent.)

b. The oxygen should flow through a nebulizer or ultrasonic unit to provide the needed humidity. Try to keep the relative humidity at 60% or greater to minimize any risk of a spark causing a fire inside the tent.

c. The tent must be cooled to prevent the patient from overheating the enclosed space. If the infant put into a tent has croup, the cooled air is therapeutic. Be careful not to chill the infant.

d. As with hoods, an oxygen analyzer should continuously monitor how much oxygen is inside the tent. The analyzer probe should be placed at the same

level as the infant's nose. Keep the tent sealed and the bottom edges tucked under the mattress to try to keep the oxygen percentage as high and stable as possible. The child should not be allowed to have any electrically powered toys inside the tent to minimize the risk of a spark and fire.

2. Air entrainment devices and masks

a. Get the necessary equipment for the procedure (WRE code: IIA1b) [Difficulty: An]

b. Put the equipment together and make sure that it works properly (WRE code: IIA1b) [Difficulty: An]

c. Troubleshoot any problems with the equipment (WRE code: IIA1b) [Difficulty: An]

Air entrainment masks are designed to provide the patient with a controlled oxygen percentage at a flow rate high enough to ensure that all of the patient's needs are met (Fig. 6-14). To be sure that this happens, the total flow through the mask must be equal to or greater than the patient's peak inspiratory flow. (The interested learner is encouraged to read about the Bernoulli principle, which regulates the mixing of fluids as a result of a decrease in pressure caused by a jet.) These masks are sometimes called Venturi masks, Venti masks, jet-mixing, and high airflow with oxygen enrichment (HAFOE) systems. See Table 6-5 for specific information on available air entrainment masks.

These masks are recommended in any clinical situation in which a known, certain oxygen percentage must be given to the patient who has a variable respiratory rate, inspiratory/expiratory (I:E) ratio, tidal volume, or minute volume. Common situations include a COPD patient and a patient in respiratory failure who needs increasing

Fig. 6-14 Adult wearing an air entrainment mask. **A,** High velocity jet; **B,** an area of reduced lateral pressure (Bernoulli's principle); **C,** room air entrainment. *(From White GC: Basic clinical lab competencies for respiratory care, an integrated approach, Albany, NY, 1988, Delmar.)*

oxygen percentages. Because it is difficult to ensure that the patient's peak inspiratory flow is matched by the gas flow through the mask, the following guidelines are recommended:

a. Make sure that the total flow through the mask is at least 40 L/min in a resting patient. More may be needed if the patient is breathing rapidly.

b. Provide the patient with a total flow that is 4 to 6 times his or her measured minute volume.

The total flow through the mask can be raised by increasing the oxygen flow. This should not significantly change the oxygen percentage because more room air is entrained to keep the same ratio. However, to be certain, analyze the oxygen percentage inside the mask to ensure that it is as prescribed. The total flow through the mask can be calculated by adding the total of the ratio parts and multiplying by the oxygen flow rate.

MATH REVIEW
Air entrainment mask calculations
EXAMPLE 1

Your patient has on a 28% air entrainment mask with an oxygen flow of 4 L/min. His condition worsens, and he increases his minute volume to 15 L/min. To ensure that he still receives his prescribed oxygen percentage, someone makes a recommendation to you to increase the oxygen liter flow to 6 L/min. The new total flow through the mask can be calculated as follows:

A 28% air entrainment mask has an air/oxygen ratio of 10:1.

a. The sum of the ratio parts is 10 + 1 = 11.

b. Total flow = 11 × 6 L/min oxygen flow = 66 L/min.

c. This flow is more than 4 times the patient's current minute volume. He should have all of his flow needs met.

d. Reanalyze the delivered oxygen percentage to make certain that it is as prescribed.

Exam Hint

It has been necessary on past exams to calculate the needed change in the oxygen flow to increase the total flow to meet or exceed a patient's peak inspiratory flow, which ensures that the proper oxygen percentage is delivered.

EXAMPLE 2

Your patient is wearing a 40% air entrainment mask that has the manufacturer's suggested 8 L/min of oxygen running into it. Her peak inspiratory flow is about 48 L/min (0.75 L/sec). To what should her oxygen flow be changed to ensure that the total gas flow is greater than her peak inspiratory flow? The new oxygen flow to the mask can be calculated as follows:

a. 40% air entrainment mask has an air/oxygen ratio of 3:1.

b. The sum of the ratio parts is 3 + 1 = 4.

c. Divide the sum of the ratio parts into the peak inspiratory flow: 48/4 = 12

d. Increase the oxygen flow from 8 to 12 L/min.

Some patients may complain that the gas coming through the mask is dry. To resolve this problem, some manufacturers have designed an aerosol adapter to add at

TABLE 6-5	Specifications for Air Entrainment Devices and Masks			
Oxygen (%)	Approximate Air/oxygen Ratio	Total Ratio Parts	Oxygen Flow Rate (L/min)*	Total Flow (L/min)
24	25:1	26	4	104
28	10:1	11	4	44
30	8:1	9	6	54
35	5:1	6	8	48
40	3:1	4	10	40
45	2:1	3	15	45
50	1.7:1	2.7	15	40.5

*These flow rates were selected to ensure that the minimum total flow through the system would be ≥ 40 L/min. The manufacturers may recommend other minimal O$_2$ flow rates.

the jet. A separate bland aerosol is then added to the room air that enters the jet stream. Make sure that the adapter fits properly and does not interfere with or block the jet or room air entrainment ports. Do *not* add a bubble-type humidifier to the jet on the mask because the high back-pressure through the jet will cause the pressure relief (pop-off) valve to open, and the oxygen will leak out.

The two different types of air entrainment devices are based on the physical principles seen in the Bernoulli effect. It is important to know about the two different types to understand what can go wrong with them and how they can be fixed. Make sure that the correct liter flow of oxygen, jet size, and air entrainment port setting are selected to get the desired total flow and oxygen percentage.

Variable jet diameter. Notice that the jets have different diameters, but the room air entrainment ports are the same size. You will see that the *smaller* the jet diameter is, the *lower* the oxygen percentage is. This is because as the jet becomes smaller, the lateral pressure is lower. This results in more room air being brought into the entrainment ports to dilute the oxygen and increase the total flow.

Make sure that the jets are not obstructed by mucus or anything else, or the oxygen percentage will be decreased. An obstruction downstream from the jet prevents the appropriate amount of room air from being brought into the mask. This results in the oxygen percentage increasing and the total flow decreasing.

Variable air entrainment ports. Notice that the jet size is fixed, but the room air entrainment ports have different sizes. The smaller the entrainment ports, the *higher* the oxygen percentage. This is because less room air can be entrained to dilute the oxygen. The total flow is also reduced when the entrainment ports are smaller.

Make sure that the entrainment ports are not obstructed by the patient's sheet or anything else, or the oxygen percentage will increase. An obstruction downstream from the jet prevents the appropriate amount of air as from being brought into the mask. This results in the oxygen percentage increasing and the total flow decreasing.

3. Nasal cannula
  a. Get the necessary equipment for the procedure (WRE code: IIA1a) [Difficulty: Ap, An]
  b. Put the equipment together and make sure that it works properly (WRE code: IIA1a) [Difficulty: Ap, An]
  c. Troubleshoot any problems with the equipment (WRE code: IIA1a) [Difficulty: Ap, An]

The nasal cannula is an oxygen delivery tube that has been modified with two short prongs to deliver oxygen to the nostrils (Fig. 6-15). They come in neonatal, pediatric, and

Fig. 6-15 Adult wearing a nasal cannula. *(From Thalken FR: Medical gas therapy. In Scanlan CL, Spearman CB, Sheldon RL, editors: Egan's fundamentals of respiratory care, ed 5, St Louis, 1990, Mosby.)*

adult sizes based on the diameter of the prongs. Care must be taken to make sure that the nares are patent and not plugged by a common cold, deviated septum, or other unseen problem. This low-flow oxygen delivery device is very widely used because it is more comfortable for many patients than an air entrainment or other types of face masks.

If a humidifier is used, make sure that it is properly filled with sterile water and that the oxygen bubbles through it. Check the high-pressure pop-off valve for pressure release and a whistling sound. Before placing the cannula on the patient, check to see that the oxygen is flowing through the tubing. If available, use a cannula with curved prongs. They direct the gas flow toward the back of the nasal passages for better natural humidification and are better for patient comfort. Take care not to pull the elastic restraining band too tightly around the head. Some brands loop the oxygen tubing over the ears to be drawn up snugly under the chin. Often this is more comfortable than the types that have an elastic band.

The problem with a nasal cannula is that the delivered oxygen percentage is unreliable. Variations in the patient's respiratory rate, I:E ratio, tidal volume, and minute volume result in different inhaled oxygen percentages. This is clearly unacceptable in an unstable patient in whom the PaO_2 values are being used to help judge the changing cardiopulmonary status. Because of this clinical limitation, this device and the other low-flow oxygen delivery systems in the discussions that follow should be used only with stable patients. In the adult, the delivered oxygen percentage can be *estimated* at approximately 4% for each liter of oxygen per minute (Table 6-6).

TABLE 6-6	Estimated Delivered Oxygen Percentage in Adults Based on the Oxygen Liter Flow through a Nasal Cannula	
Oxygen (L/min)	**Estimated Delivered Oxygen (%)**	
1	24	
2	28	
3	32	
4	36	
5	40	
6	44	

Flows are usually limited to 6 L/min to avoid excessive irritation to the nasal passages.

Flows are usually limited to no more than 1 to 2 L/min in infants and 4 L/min in older children. The pulse oximetry value or Pao$_2$ level should be checked in patients of any age whenever a flow change is made or the patient's condition changes significantly.

The traditional cannulas just described are common in hospitals for short-term patient use. However, in the home setting for long-term use, it is more economical to use one of the newer cannulas with a built-in oxygen reservoir because less oxygen is used.

Oxygen conserving nasal cannula. Oxygen conserving nasal cannulas are used for patients who need long-term oxygen therapy and wish to reduce their costs. When such a cannula is combined with a pulse-dose oxygen delivery system, the patient's oxygen delivery costs can be significantly cut. At least two different types of oxygen-conserving cannulas are found. Fig. 6-16 shows a reservoir nasal cannula and how it operates. It has an 18-mL reservoir that fills when the patient exhales and gives up its oxygen bolus during the next inspiration. Fig. 6-17 shows a pendant nasal cannula with its reservoir that hangs on the chest. Both types can have problems with tubing disconnections or kinks that can happen with any type of cannula. The only problem that is unique to both of these units is failure of the diaphragm that moves back and forth as the reservoir fills and empties. This membrane may wear out after about a week and prevent the reservoir from filling or emptying properly. Watch as the patient breathes to make sure that the diaphragm is moving properly. If not, replace the cannula.

4. **Oxygen masks: simple oxygen mask, partial-rebreathing mask, nonrebreathing mask, and face tent**
   a. **Get the necessary equipment for the procedure (WRE code: IIA1a) [Difficulty: Ap, An]**
   b. **Put the equipment together and make sure that it works properly (WRE code: IIA1a) [Difficulty: Ap, An]**

Fig. 6-16 Drawing of the Oximizer reservoir nasal cannula and its functions. *(Courtesy of CHAD Therapeutics, Chatsworth, Calif.)*

Fig. 6-17 Drawing of a patient wearing a pendant reservoir nasal cannula made by CHAD Therapeutics. *(From Wyka KA: Respiratory home care. In Scanlon CL, Spearman CB, Sheldon RL: Egan's fundamentals of respiratory care, ed 5, St Louis, 1990, Mosby.)*

c. Troubleshoot any problems with the equipment (WRE code: IIA1a) [Difficulty: Ap, An]

Simple oxygen mask. This mask, like all others, is designed to fit over the patient's nose and mouth and act as an oxygen reservoir for the next breath (Figs. 6-18 and 6-19). Various adult and pediatric sizes are available, and the patient should wear one that best fits the facial contours and size of the face. This is for comfort, as well as to try to increase the inspired oxygen percentage by decreasing the amount of room air that is inspired. Exhaled breath escapes through the exhalation ports. The patient's breathing pattern affects the amount of room air that is breathed in through the same exhalation ports. These ports also are important in case the oxygen flow to the mask is cut off.

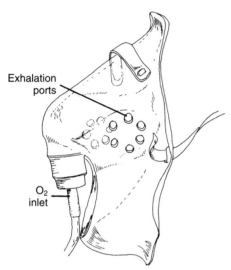

Fig. 6-18 Close-up view of a simple oxygen mask. *(From McPherson SP: Respiratory care equipment, ed 4, St Louis, 1990, Mosby.)*

Fig. 6-19 Child wearing a simple oxygen mask. *(From Gaebler G, Blodgett D: Gas administration. In Blodgett D, editor: Manual of pediatric respiratory care procedures, Philadelphia, 1982, Lippincott.)*

Because the oxygen reservoir in the mask is not large enough to meet the patient's tidal volume, the inspired oxygen percentage is unpredictable. Oxygen flows between 5 and 10 L/min should provide *approximately* 35% to 60% inspired oxygen. The pulse oximetry value or PaO_2 level should be checked whenever a flow change is made or the patient's condition changes significantly.

A bubble humidifier is often added so that the gas is not dry. Make sure that it works properly and that oxygen is flowing through the tubing before putting it on the patient. This and all other masks use an adjustable elastic strap that goes behind the head to hold it in place. Make sure that the mask fits snugly but not so tight as to cut off circulation.

Partial-rebreathing mask. The partial-rebreathing mask has a 500- to 1000-mL plastic bag added to the mask to act as an oxygen reservoir for the next breath (Figs. 6-20, 6-21, and 6-22). Child- and adult-size masks are commonly available. When properly applied, the first third of the patient's exhaled gas from the anatomic dead space is exhaled back into this bag. This gas is close to pure oxygen and has no carbon dioxide. Exhaled breath escapes through the exhalation ports. The patient's breathing pattern affects the amount of room air that is breathed in through the same exhalation ports. These ports also are important in case the oxygen flow to the mask is cut off. The added reservoir of oxygen results in a higher percentage being given to the patient than in a simple oxygen mask. An oxygen flow of between 6 and 10 L/min should provide *approximately* 35% to 80% inspired oxygen.

A bubble humidifier is often added so that the gas is not dry. Make sure that it works properly, that the oxygen is flowing through the tubing, and that the reservoir bag has been filled before putting it on the patient. Adjust the flow as needed to ensure that the reservoir does not collapse by more than one third on inspiration. This ensures that the mask and reservoir are filled with as much oxygen as possible. A pulse oximetry value or PaO_2 level should be checked whenever a flow change is made or the patient's condition changes significantly.

Nonrebreathing mask. The nonrebreathing mask looks initially like the partial-rebreathing mask with its plastic bag added as an oxygen reservoir for the next breath (Figs. 6-23 and 6-24). However, notice that a one-way valve has been added between the mask and the reservoir bag. This allows the bag to be filled with pure oxygen that is available for the next breath. No exhaled gas can enter the reservoir. Two (sometimes one) one-way valves are added to the exhalation ports on the mask. These ensure that the patient breathes in only oxygen and not room air. Exhaled breath escapes through the exhalation ports as with the partial-rebreathing mask. Not shown is an emergency pop-in valve that allows room air to be drawn into the mask if the oxygen supply is cut off. Adult and pediatric

Fig. 6-20 Outside view of a partial-rebreathing mask. *(From McPherson SP: Respiratory care equipment, ed 4, St Louis, 1990, Mosby.)*

sizes are available. The mask should be conformed to fit the patient's facial contours and size as much as possible. As mentioned earlier, this is for comfort and to try to increase the inspired oxygen percentage by decreasing the amount of room air that is inspired. It is, in theory, possible to deliver 100% oxygen with this mask if the oxygen flow is high enough and the mask is airtight over the face. However, experience has shown that the disposable masks that are usually available in the hospital do not prevent room air from being drawn in. Oxygen flows between 8 and 10 L/min should provide *approximately* 60% to 80% (or more) inspired oxygen.

A bubble humidifier is often added so that the gas is not dry. Make sure that it works properly, that the oxygen is flowing through the tubing, and that the reservoir bag has been filled before putting it on the patient. Adjust the flow as needed to ensure that the reservoir does not collapse by more than one third on inspiration. This ensures that the mask and reservoir are filled with oxygen and that the patient's tidal volume comes completely from the reservoir bag. The patient's pulse oximetry value or PaO_2 level should be checked whenever a flow change is made or the patient's condition changes significantly.

Open exhalation ports also allow emergency air intake

Exhaled air

O_2

Fig. 6-21 Cutaway view of a partial-rebreathing mask showing gas flow. *(From Thalken FR: Medical gas therapy. In Scanlan CL, Spearman CB, Sheldon RL, editors: Egan's fundamentals of respiratory care, ed 5, St Louis, 1990, Mosby.)*

Fig. 6-22 Child wearing a partial-rebreathing mask. *(From Gaebler G, Blodgett D: Gas administration. In Blodgett D, editor: Manual of pediatric respiratory care procedures, Philadelphia, 1982, Lippincott.)*

Valves

Fig. 6-23 Outside view of a nonrebreathing mask. *(From McPherson SP: Respiratory care equipment, ed 4, St Louis, 1990, Mosby.)*

Exam Hint

Expect to see one question that deals with the need to switch from a low oxygen percentage mask to a nonrebreather mask to give the seriously hypoxemic patient as much oxygen as possible. Also expect to see one question dealing with the reservoir bag collapsing on inspiration. Usually this involves the patient receiving a helium and oxygen (heliox) mix. Solve the problem by increasing the flow of therapeutic gas to the mask and bag.

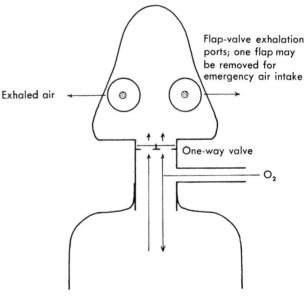

Fig. 6-24 Cutaway view of a nonrebreathing mask showing gas flow. *(From Thalken FR: Medical gas therapy. In Scanlan CL, Spearman CB, Sheldon RL, editors: Egan's fundamentals of respiratory care, ed 5, St Louis, 1990, Mosby.)*

Face tent. These masks are designed to fit around the patient's neck, under the jaw, and around the cheeks in front of the ears. The front edge should be higher than the level of the patient's nostrils (Fig. 6-25). These are sometimes used to provide oxygen to a patient who cannot wear a mask or cannula because of oral and nasal trauma, burns, or surgery. The patient using a face tent should be sitting as upright as possible. This is because oxygen is heavier than air and tends to settle in the mask around the patient's nose and mouth if the fit is tight. If the patient is lying flat or if the mask fits loosely, the oxygen will simply "pour" down out of it. This makes it difficult to know with any certainty what inspired oxygen percentage is available to the patient. Flows of 5 to 10 liters of oxygen per minute are commonly used with adults.

A face tent is usually ordered with the oxygen run through a humidifier or nebulizer so that the gas is not dry. Make sure that the humidifier or nebulizer is filled with sterile water, that the high-pressure pop-off works, and that gas is flowing through the tubing before the face tent is put on the patient. Try to analyze the oxygen percentage close to the patient's nose and mouth with as much accuracy as possible. A pulse oximetry value or PaO_2 level should be checked whenever a change in the oxygen percentage is made or the patient's condition changes significantly.

Fig. 6-25 Young adult wearing a face tent.

5. Transtracheal oxygen catheter

a. Get the necessary equipment for the procedure (WRE code: IIA1a) [Difficulty: Ap, An]

b. Put the equipment together and make sure that it works properly (WRE code: IIA1a) [Difficulty: Ap, An]

The transtracheal oxygen (TTO_2) catheter is a 20-cm long flexible, hollow plastic tube (Fig. 6-26, *A*). It is inserted into the trachea via a puncture procedure at the suprasternal notch. To date, only adults with COPD have had the procedure performed. Oxygen is delivered directly into the trachea. The patient's oxygenation can be maintained at lower oxygen flows than needed by a regular face mask or nasal cannula. The following equipment is needed:

1. Proper size transtracheal catheter (9F is the usual adult size)
2. Guide wire/stylet
3. Chain-link necklace to hold the catheter in place
4. Regular small-bore oxygen tubing to connect to the distal end of the catheter

Fig. 6-26 Transtracheal oxygen catheter. **A** *(top)*, Photograph of a flexible, plastic transtracheal oxygen catheter. The part to the left of the flange is inserted into the patient's trachea. The part to the right of the flange is attached to standard oxygen tubing. **A** *(bottom)*, The metal stylet may be used to help keep the catheter stiff during insertion and to clear the catheter of an obstruction. **B**, Drawing of a chain-link necklace keeping the external part of the catheter and flange secure. **C**, Cutaway drawing showing the catheter inserted into the trachea. *(From White GC: Equipment theory for respiratory care, Albany, NY, 1992, Delmar.)*

5. Flowmeter and oxygen source
6. Optional bubble humidifier with sterile water for patient comfort

Under normal working conditions, regular oxygen tubing is used to connect the oxygen source to the catheter. The oxygen flow to the catheter is set high enough to keep a satisfactory PaO_2 or SpO_2 level. Usually this is less than previously needed by nasal cannula. When combined with a portable LOX system or a pulse-dose oxygen delivery system, the patient has a real opportunity for increased mobility and decreased cost.

c. Troubleshoot any problems with the equipment (WRE code: IIAa1) [Difficulty: Ap, An]

The patient needs to be instructed to disconnect the oxygen tubing and flush the catheter with 3 mL of sterile saline twice a day. A cleaning rod also can be pushed through the catheter to make sure that no mucus accumulates. As with any tubing system, the components can become disconnected. Make sure that all connections are tight. If the saline or cleaning rod cannot be pushed through the catheter, an obstruction is likely. The patient should come into the hospital to have the catheter removed and replaced if necessary. It is possible that the proximal catheter tip has twisted into the tracheal mucosa. This can lead to subcutaneous emphysema. The patient should be instructed on how to identify the signs of this and to turn off the oxygen to the catheter. He or she should go back to using a nasal cannula for oxygen and call the physician for guidance.

6. Tracheostomy appliances: mask/collar and Brigg's adapter/T-piece

a. Get the necessary equipment for the procedure (WRE code: IIA1a) [Difficulty: Ap, An]

b. Put the equipment together and make sure that it works properly (WRE code: IIA1a) [Difficulty: Ap, An]

c. Troubleshoot any problems with the equipment (WRE code: IIA1a) [Difficulty: Ap, An]

Tracheostomy mask/collar. The adult or pediatric tracheostomy mask or collar is shaped to fit over a tracheostomy tube or stoma to provide oxygen and aerosol (Fig. 6-27). Because the patient's upper airway is bypassed, a nebulizer is used for humidity. It is usually an air entrainment type, so the oxygen percentage can be adjusted. Make sure that the nebulizer is filled with sterile water, that the high-pressure pop-off valve is working, and that adequate mist is flowing through to the mask before putting it on the patient.

Because the tracheostomy mask is an open system without reservoir, it is difficult to guarantee the patient's

Fig. 6-27 Adult wearing a tracheostomy mask/collar.

inspired oxygen percentage. Set the gas flow high enough to make a "cloud" of aerosol around the tracheostomy. If an excess of aerosol can be seen around the tracheostomy during inspiration, it is likely that the desired oxygen percentage is being delivered. Analyze the oxygen percentage from inside the mask to try for as much accuracy as possible. A pulse oximetry value or PaO_2 level should be checked whenever a flow change or oxygen percentage change is made or the patient's condition changes significantly.

Brigg's adapter/T-piece. The Brigg's adapter or T-piece is designed to provide air or supplemental oxygen and aerosol to an endotracheal or tracheostomy tube. It has one 15-mm inner-diameter (ID) opening that fits over any endotracheal or tracheostomy tube adapter. The other two openings are 22 mm outer diameter (OD) so that aerosol tubing can be added (Fig. 6-28). A nebulizer is commonly used for humidity because the patient's upper airway is bypassed. Make sure that the nebulizer is filled with sterile water, that the high-pressure pop-off valve is working, and that adequate mist is flowing through to the adapter before putting it on the patient. The nebulizer is usually an air entrainment type, so the oxygen percentage can be adjusted.

The addition of a length of aerosol tubing downstream from the adapter acts as a reservoir so that the inspired oxygen percentage is ensured. A reservoir of 50 to 100 mL of aerosol tubing is commonly needed for the adult. Care must be taken to adjust the gas flow so that it is high enough to meet the patient's peak inspiratory flow rate. This can be determined by watching the aerosol flow past the adapter and reservoir. Make sure that during inspiration the aerosol is still flowing past the tracheostomy/

Fig. 6-28 Child with intubated airway with a Brigg's adapter/
T-piece and aerosol tubing added to the endotracheal tube.
*(From Gaebler G, Blodgett D: Gas administration. In Blodgett D,
editor:* Manual of pediatric respiratory care procedures,
Philadelphia, 1982, Lippincott.)

endotracheal tube and into the reservoir. Inadequate flow
could result in the patient rebreathing gas from the reservoir. This gas has just been exhaled and is high in carbon
dioxide and low in oxygen.

> **Exam Hint**
>
> **K**now to increase the aerosol flow to either a
> tracheostomy mask or Brigg's adapter/T-piece if the
> aerosol cannot be seen during a patient's inspiration.
> The NBRC usually calls this a T-piece rather than a
> Brigg's adapter in its questions.

MODULE D

**Modify specialty gas therapy by changing the
mode of administration, adjusting the flow, and
adjusting the gas concentration (WRE code:
IIIF5) [Difficulty: R, Ap, An]**

The indications for all of the specialty gases are listed
in Box 6-1. Although none of these gases is widely
used in respiratory care, they can be very beneficial when
indicated.

O₂/CO₂ (carbogen) therapy. A child with hypoplastic
left-heart syndrome (HLHS) is usually being mechanically
ventilated. The infant with this congenital heart defect
must maintain an open foramen ovale and patent ductus
arteriosus (PDA) for adequate systemic circulation.
Carbogen is added by small-bore tubing connecting the
gas cylinder with a T-piece connected into the ventilator
circuit. Usually enough carbogen flow is added to result in
1% to 4% carbon dioxide being measured on a capnometer.

**BOX 6-1 Indications for the Special Therapeutic
Gases: O₂/CO₂ (Carbogen), He/O₂
(Heliox), and NO (Nitric Oxide)**

CARBOGEN USES
Hypoplastic left-heart syndrome (HLHS)
Carbon dioxide response curve test
Singultus (hiccup)

HELIOX USES
Upper airway obstruction
  Tracheal tumor
  Laryngotracheobronchitis (croup)
  Postextubation stridor
Lower airway obstruction
  Status asthmaticus
  May reduce work of breathing in other conditions such as
    COPD, bronchiolitis, or small endotracheal tube

NITRIC OXIDE USES
Treatment of term and near-term (>34 weeks) neonates with
  hypoxic respiratory failure associated with clinical, or
  echocardiographic evidence of pulmonary hypertension
Possible use in acute respiratory distress syndrome (ARDS)

Because increased carbon dioxide is a pulmonary vasoconstrictor, the PDA can be maintained. The infant's vital
signs and ABG values must be closely monitored to guide
the adjustment in carbogen.

The carbon dioxide response curve test is a measurement of the increase in minute volume caused by breathing different concentrations of carbon dioxide when the
patient's oxygen level is normal. The test is performed on
patients with COPD to determine whether their breathing
will increase when their carbon dioxide level is increased.
Depending on the method of test performed, the patient
inhales between 1% and 7% carbon dioxide. The flow and
concentration must be adjusted to maintain the desired
carbon dioxide level as measured on a capnometer. An
oxygen analyzer also should be included in the system to
make sure that the patient does not inhale less than 21%
oxygen.

The treatment of hiccups usually requires only that the
patient rebreathe from a paper bag. If necessary, a small
amount of carbon dioxide can be added to stop the
hiccups.

He/O₂ (heliox) therapy. Patients who benefit from
He/O₂ therapy can have an upper airway obstruction problem (tumor) or lower airway obstruction problem (asthma).
Because helium atoms are so much smaller than nitrogen
molecules, patients find that their work of breathing is
greatly reduced. Normoxic patients are usually given a mix
of 80% helium and 20% oxygen, whereas hypoxic patients
are given 70% helium and 30% oxygen or 60% helium and

40% oxygen. If more oxygen is needed, small-bore oxygen tubing can be used to add it into the mask or reservoir bag, or a special closed system will have to be assembled from components.

Ideally any helium/oxygen delivery system should have a reservoir bag. Usually the nonrebreathing mask and reservoir are used. The reservoir should be filled with the He/O_2 mix before the mask is placed on the patient's face. Again, the fit should be as tight as possible to minimize leaks. Adjust the flow so that the reservoir bag does not collapse by more than one third during an inspiration. If it does, increase the flow. The flow should be increased if the patient complains of shortness of breath. Signs of increased work of breathing include agitation, increased use of accessory muscles of respiration, sweating, and increased respiratory rate, heart rate, and blood pressure.

> **Exam Hint**
>
> There is usually one question about heliox therapy for the management of asthma to reduce the patient's work of breathing.

Nitric oxide therapy. Because nitric oxide is a pulmonary vasodilator, it has been shown to be effective in the treatment of newborns with pulmonary hypertension (persistent pulmonary hypertension of the newborn [PPHN]). The Food and Drug Administration has approved the use of INOmax (0.8% nitric oxide and 99.2% nitrogen) to deliver inhaled nitric oxide to these patients. The currently recommended dosing range of inhaled NO is 5 to 15 parts per million (ppm). To deliver this concentration of nitric oxide and supplemental oxygen, the INOvent delivery system is also needed. It is used to set the desired mix of INOmax to the newborn's ventilator and monitor the level of NO, nitrogen dioxide (NO_2), and oxygen delivered. Inhaled NO has not been approved for adult patients. However, some reports of nitric oxide being administered to patients with pulmonary hypertension and acute respiratory distress syndrome (ARDS) show promising results.

> **Exam Hint**
>
> Usually one question deals with treating a patient with pulmonary hypertension. Inhaled nitric oxide in the range of 5 to 15 parts per million (ppm) is indicated. The question often includes information that shows the patient has an increased pulmonary vascular resistance (PVR), indicating pulmonary hypertension. See Chapter 5 and Box 5-2 for more information on PVR.

MODULE E
Respiratory care plan

1. Analyze available information to determine the patient's pathophysiologic state (CSE code: IIIH1)

The goal of oxygen therapy is to correct the patient's hypoxemia. Obtain an ABG sample or perform pulse oximetry, as needed, to determine the patient's oxygenation. Review the complete discussion of these subjects in Chapter 3.

2. Determine the appropriateness of the prescribed therapy and goals for the identified pathophysiologic state (CSE code: IIIH3)
   a. Stop the treatment or procedure if the patient has an adverse reaction to it (CSE code: IIIF1)
   b. Discontinue treatment based on the patient's response (WRE code: IIIG1e) [Difficulty: An]

As discussed at the beginning of the chapter, several possible hazards occur with the use of oxygen therapy. The NBRC is most likely to ask questions related to the use of oxygen on a patient with COPD.

MODULE F
Respiratory care protocols

1. Develop the outcomes of respiratory care protocols (WRE code: IIIH4b) [Difficulty: An]
2. Apply respiratory care protocols to patient care situations (WRE code: IIIH6) [Difficulty: Ap]
3. Monitor the outcomes of respiratory care protocols (WRE code: IIIH5) [Difficulty: An]

Look for signs of hypoxemia and be prepared to recommend a change in the patient's oxygen delivery system or oxygen percentage to correct the problem. Tachycardia and tachypnea are common findings in hypoxemic patients. Proper oxygen therapy should relieve the problem so that the patient's vital signs return toward normal. An abnormal heart rhythm as a result of hypoxemia should return to normal with the relief of the problem. Check the patient's pulse oximetry or PaO_2 value whenever a change in the inspired oxygen percentage or a significant change in the patient's clinical condition occurs.

   a. Change the oxygen percentage (WRE code: IIIF4a) [Difficulty: An]
   b. Change the flow of oxygen (WRE code: IIIF4a) [Difficulty: An]

c. Change the method of administering the oxygen (WRE code: IIIF4a) [Difficulty: An]

Every patient's oxygen percentage or flow must be tailored to meet the patient's clinical goals. Usually this means keeping the patients who are acutely hypoxemic with a PaO_2 level between 60 and 100 torr and an SpO_2 value between 90% and 97%. Exceptions, when the blood oxygen level is kept as high as possible, include cardiopulmonary resuscitation and the treatment of carbon monoxide poisoning. Another exception is the COPD patient who is hypoxemic and hypercarbic. Usually these patients' conditions are maintained with a moderate hypoxemia. The PaO_2 level should be between 50 and 60 torr and the SpO_2 value between 85% and 90%. It is imperative to keep the oxygen in this relatively narrow range. Further hypoxemia will result in pulmonary hypertension and cor pulmonale. Cardiac dysrhythmias or arrest and death can occur if the hypoxemia is severe (<40 torr). Oxygen levels in the normal range (>60 torr) may result in blunting of the hypoxic drive. This can result in bradypnea and even greater carbon dioxide retention with corresponding acidemia. When the carbon dioxide pressure ($PaCO_2$) level exceeds 80 to 90 torr, many patients become drowsy or somnolent. The treatment is to decrease the FiO_2 to reduce the PaO_2 level to 50 to 60 torr. This, in turn, stimulates the hypoxic drive so that the patient increases his or her ventilation.

Exam Hint

Know the advantages, disadvantages, and possible oxygen ranges for the various oxygen appliances discussed earlier. Be prepared to make recommendations to change from one appliance to another or to change the oxygen percentage or flow. Expect to see one question that deals with the need to reduce the inspired oxygen percentage to a COPD patient with hypercarbia. In addition, usually one question deals with needing to increase the inspired oxygen percentage to a COPD patient who is too hypoxemic.

---

4. Communicate the outcomes of therapy and change the therapy based on the protocol (WRE code: IIIA5) [Difficulty: An]

The physician, respiratory therapist, nurse, patient, and the patient's family members must all understand the patient's oxygen therapy goal. This is especially important for the home care patient to ensure that the proper oxygen administration device and oxygen flowrate are used.

BIBLIOGRAPHY

AARC Clinical Practice Guideline: Oxygen therapy in the acute care hospital, *Respir Care* 36:1410-1413, 1991.

AARC Clinical Practice Guideline: Oxygen therapy in the home or extended care facility, *Respir Care* 37(8):918-922, 1992.

American Association for Respiratory Care: Clinical practice guideline: oxygen therapy for adults in the acute care facility: 2002 revision and update, *Respir Care* 47:717, 2002.

American Association for Respiratory Care: Clinical practice guideline: selection of an oxygen delivery device for neonatal and pediatric patients: 2002 revision and update, *Respir Care* 47:707, 2002.

Bageant RA: Oxygen analyzers, *Respir Care* 21:410-416, 1976.

Burton GG, Hodgkin JE, Ward JJ, editors: *Respiratory care, a guide to clinical practice,* ed 4, Philadelphia, 1997, Lippincott-Raven.

Cairo JM, Pilbeam SP: *Mosby's respiratory care equipment,* ed 7, St Louis, 2004, Mosby.

Dantzker DR, MacIntyre NR, Bakow ED, editors: *Comprehensive respiratory care,* Philadelphia, 1995, WB Saunders.

Datex-Ohmeda: INOvent delivery system. Available at: http://www.datex-ohmeda.com. Accessed January 1, 2001.

Eubanks DH, Bone RC: *Comprehensive respiratory care,* ed 2, St Louis, 1990, Mosby.

Fink JB, Hunt GE, editors: *Clinical practice in respiratory care,* Philadelphia, 1999, Lippincott-Raven.

Gaebler G, Blodgett D: Gas administration. In Blodgett D, editor: *Manual of pediatric respiratory care procedures,* Philadelphia, 1982, Lippincott.

Gluck EH, Onorato DJ, Castriotta R: Helium-oxygen mixtures in intubated patients with status asthmaticus and respiratory acidosis, *Chest* 98(3):693-698, 1990.

Heuer AJ, Scanlan CL: Medical gas therapy. In Wilkins RL, Stoller JK, Scanlan CL, editors: *Egan's fundamentals of respiratory care,* ed 8, St Louis, 2003, Mosby.

Hill KV: Oxygen therapy. In Aloan CA, Hill TV, editors: *Respiratory care of the newborn and child,* ed 2, Philadelphia, 1997, Lippincott-Raven.

Hollman GA, Shen G, Zeng L, et al: Helium-oxygen improves clinical asthma scores in children with acute bronchiolitis, *Crit Care Med* 26(10):1731-1736, 1998.

Hunt GE: Gas therapy. In Fink JB, Hunt GE, editors: *Clinical practice in respiratory care,* Philadelphia, 1999, Lippincott-Raven.

INOTherapeutics: Homepage, Available at: http://www.inotherapeutics.com. Accessed January 1, 2001.

Kass JE, Castriotta RJ: Heliox therapy in acute severe asthma, *Chest* 107(3):757-760, 1995.

Kemper KJ, Ritz RH, Benson MS, Bishop MS: Helium-oxygen mixture in the treatment of postextubation stridor in pediatric trauma patients, *Crit Care Med* 19(3):356-359, 1991.

Kudukis TM, et al: Inhaled helium-oxygen revisited: effect of inhaled helium-oxygen during the treatment of status asthmaticus in children, *J Pediatr* 131(2):333-334, 1997.

McPherson SP: *Respiratory care equipment,* ed 5, St Louis, 1995, Mosby.

Scanlan CL, Heuer A: Medical gas therapy. In Scanlan CL, Wilkins RL, Stoller JK, editors: *Egan's fundamentals of respiratory care,* ed 7, St, Louis, 1999, Mosby.

Schaffer EM, Pohlman A, Morgan S, Hall JB: Oxygenation in status asthmaticus improves during ventilation with helium-oxygen, *Crit Care Med* 27(12):2666–2670.

Shapiro BA, Kacmarek RM, Cane RD, et al, editors: *Clinical application of respiratory care*, ed 4, St Louis, 1991, Mosby.

Shapiro BA, Harrison RA, Cane RD, et al: *Clinical application of blood gases*, ed 4, St Louis, 1989, Mosby.

Tassaux D et al: Calibration of seven ICU ventilators for mechanical ventilation with helium-oxygen mixtures, *Am J Respir Crit Care Med* 160:22–32, 1999.

Vines DL, Scanlan CL: Storage and delivery of medical gases. In Wilkins RL, Stoller JK, Scanlan CL, editors: *Egan's fundamentals of respiratory care*, ed 8, St Louis, 2003, Mosby.

Ward JJ: Equipment for mixed gas and oxygen therapy. In Branson RD, Hess DR, Chatburn RL, editors: *Respiratory care equipment*, ed 2, Philadelphia, 1999, Lippincott Williams & Wilkins.

Ward JJ: Medical gas therapy. In Burton GC, Hodgkin JE, Ward JJ, editors: *Respiratory care: a guide to clinical practice*, ed 4, Philadelphia, 1997, Lippincott-Raven.

Whitaker K: *Comprehensive perinatal and pediatric respiratory care*, ed 2, Albany, NY, 1997, Delmar.

White GC: *Equipment theory for respiratory care*, ed 3, Albany, NY, 1999, Delmar.

Wojciechowski WV: *Respiratory care sciences: an integrated approach*, ed 3, Albany, NY, 2000, Delmar.

Youtsey JW: Oxygen and mixed gas therapy. In Barnes TA, editor: *Core textbook of respiratory care practice*, ed 2, St Louis, 1994, Mosby.

SELF-STUDY QUESTIONS

1. A COPD patient is going home. After doing a hospital exercise test, it has been determined that she will require 1 L/min of supplemental oxygen when exercising on her stationary bicycle or when she feels short of breath. Which of the following oxygen delivery systems should the respiratory therapist recommend?
   A. Molecular-sieve oxygen concentrator
   B. Linde Walker portable liquid oxygen system
   C. Semipermeable membrane oxygen concentrator
   D. Piston compressor

2. You are attempting to calibrate a polarographic oxygen analyzer but find that it cannot be done. Possible reasons for this include:
   I. The membrane is torn on the probe.
   II. The gas sampling capillary tube is plugged with debris.
   III. The electrode solution has evaporated.
   IV. The battery needs to be replaced.
   V. Water has condensed on the membrane.
      A. I and III
      B. II and III
      C. III, IV, and V
      D. I, III, IV, and V

3. A 3-year-old child with bronchitis is being kept in an oxygen tent. He is supposed to be in a 40% oxygen environment. When analyzing the percentage, you find the tent to contain 35% oxygen. To increase the oxygen percentage, you would do all the following *except:*
   A. Make sure that the bottom edge of the tent canopy is tucked under the mattress.
   B. Increase the flow of oxygen.
   C. Adjust the air entrainment nebulizer to give a more dense mist.
   D. Make sure that all patient access ports are closed.

4. An adult patient who was rescued from a house fire is being received in the Emergency Department. He is wearing a simple oxygen mask at 5 L/min. The SpO_2 value by pulse oximeter is 100%, and his SaO_2 value from an arterial blood gas sample analyzed on a CO-oximeter is 73%. What would you recommend be done at this time?
   A. Maintain the simple oxygen mask at the present flow.
   B. Change the patient to a nonrebreather mask.
   C. Decrease the oxygen flow to the simple oxygen mask to 4 L/min.
   D. Maintain present therapy and recalibrate the CO-oximeter.

5. Which of the following is the best device for giving 35% oxygen to an alert 2-year-old?
   A. Oxygen tent
   B. Nasal cannula at 3 L/min
   C. Simple mask at 3 L/min
   D. Incubator

6. You are called to evaluate a patient known to have advanced emphysema. She is wearing a nasal cannula at 6 L/min. The nurse says that she has become drowsy and less responsive since the oxygen was given to her an hour ago. Her arterial blood gas (ABG) results on the oxygen show:
   PaO_2, 84 torr
   $PaCO_2$, 65 torr
   pH, 7.32
   Which of the following would you would recommend?
   I. Leave her on the cannula.
   II. Change her to 24% O_2 on an air entrainment mask and repeat the ABGs in 20 minutes.
   III. Change her to a simple oxygen mask and repeat the ABGs in 20 minutes.
   IV. Let her rest undisturbed.

V. Monitor her closely for becoming more alert.
   A. I and IV
   B. III and IV
   C. II and V
   D. III and V

7. You are assisting with a bronchoscopy to obtain a biopsy of a suspicious laryngeal node on your patient. Afterward, the patient complains of shortness of breath and a "tight" throat. Which of the following recommendations could you give to the physician?
   A. Give the patient a 20% oxygen/80% helium mix to breathe.
   B. Put the head of the bed down 30 degrees.
   C. Give the patient a carbogen mix to breathe.
   D. Do a 7-minute helium dilution test.

8. You receive a call at the office from one of your home care patients. She reports that the high-pressure pop-off valve on the bubble humidifier to her transtracheal oxygen catheter is venting. In addition, she cannot flush out the catheter with saline or push the cleaning rod through it. What should you tell her to do?
   A. Remove the humidifier and double the oxygen flow rate to the catheter.
   B. Force the saline through the catheter until the obstruction is cleared.
   C. Force the cleaning rod through the catheter until the obstruction is cleared.
   D. Switch her oxygen from the transtracheal catheter to a nasal cannula.

9. You are working with a patient who has a tracheal tumor. He is wearing a nonrebreather mask with 20% oxygen and 80% helium. The patient says that it is harder to breathe and has increased his respiratory rate. You notice that the reservoir bag has collapsed. The most appropriate action is to:
   A. Decrease the flow of gas.
   B. Switch to an air entrainment mask and deliver 24% oxygen.
   C. Increase the flow of gas.
   D. Switch to a 30% oxygen/70% helium mix.

10. A 58-year-old patient with advanced emphysema is admitted with an acute exacerbation of his condition. While breathing 2 L/min of oxygen through a transtracheal oxygen catheter, he has the following arterial blood gas results:
    pH, 7.38
    $Paco_2$, 57 torr
    HCO_3^-, 31 mEq/L
    Pao_2, 47 torr
    Sao_2, 80%

Based on these findings, what do you think should be done?
    A. Change the patient to 24% oxygen by an air entrainment mask.
    B. Initiate bilevel mask ventilation.
    C. Change the patient to a nonrebreathing mask with 10 L/min of oxygen.
    D. Increase the oxygen flow to the current system to 3 L/min.

11. A 36-week gestational age neonate is hypoxic despite mechanical ventilation and has clinical evidence of persistent pulmonary hypertension of the newborn. What can be done to correct the hypoxemia?
    A. Instill intratracheal surfactant.
    B. Begin nitric oxide (NO) therapy.
    C. Begin 10 cm water PEEP.
    D. Begin carbogen therapy.

12. While you are working as the respiratory therapist assigned to the Emergency Department, a 24-year-old patient with status asthmaticus is transferred by ambulance from a small, rural hospital. The patient has been given continuous bronchodilator therapy and intravenous corticosteroids and aminophylline. She is becoming exhausted but refuses to allow intubation and mechanical ventilation. What should be recommended?
    A. Begin heliox therapy.
    B. Begin nitric oxide therapy.
    C. Intubate and ventilate the patient despite her protests.
    D. Allow the patient to die.

13. A 50-year-old male patient has primary pulmonary hypertension and is receiving mechanical ventilation. Before receiving 15 ppm of nitric oxide therapy, his PVR was 290 dynes • s • cm $^{-5}$. His current PVR is 180 dynes • s • cm^{-5}. What do you recommend be done at this time?
    A. Discontinue the nitric oxide therapy.
    B. Decrease the nitric oxide to 10 ppm.
    C. Maintain the current therapy.
    D. Increase the nitric oxide therapy to 20 ppm.

14. A 16-year-old patient with status asthmaticus is started on a 70% helium/30% oxygen (heliox) mix through a nonrebreather mask. It is noticed that the reservoir bag is not staying inflated despite the oxygen flowmeter showing a delivery of 8 L/min of gas. What is the actual heliox gas flow?
    A. 5 L/min
    B. 8 L/min
    C. 12.8 (13) L/min
    D. 14.4 (14) L/min

ANSWER KEY

1. **A.** Rationale: At a flow of 1 L/min, a molecular-sieve oxygen concentrator delivers at least 90% oxygen to the patient. A Linde Walker portable LOX system is not needed if the patient is not actively and frequently mobile. A semipermeable membrane oxygen concentrator delivers only about 40% oxygen to the patient. A piston compressor is useful to deliver pressurized air to power a small volume nebulizer. It does not deliver more than 21% oxygen (room air) to the patient.

2. **D.** Rationale: A polarographic oxygen analyzer does not have a gas sampling capillary tube; the paramagnetic type does. The other four listed problems can cause a polarographic analyzer to fail. The probe has a membrane through which oxygen diffuses. It must not be torn or have water, blood, or mucus covering it. An adequate amount of electrolyte solution must be within the probe for the oxygen-related chemical reaction to take place. A functional battery is needed to drive the chemical reaction within the electrolyte solution.

3. **C.** Rationale: Because an air entrainment nebulizer is powered by air and entrains air, it cannot affect the oxygen percentage. The three other items can affect the patient's oxygen percentage inside the tent. Because oxygen is more dense than air, it will leak out the bottom of the tent unless the plastic canopy is tightly tucked under the mattress. Increasing the flow of oxygen into the tent directly increases the oxygen percentage. All patient access ports must be closed to prevent oxygen from leaking out and reducing the oxygen percentage.

4. **B.** Rationale: The significant discrepancy between the pulse oximeter reading and the CO-oximeter can be explained only by the patient having carbon monoxide poisoning. In this situation, only the CO-oximeter reading will be accurate. A CO-oximeter reading of 73% indicates severe hypoxemia. Therefore the patient should be changed to a nonrebreather mask with enough flow to keep the reservoir bag inflated. This maximizes the inspired oxygen percentage to the patient. Maintaining the simple oxygen mask at the present flow or decreasing the oxygen flow to the simple oxygen mask to 4 L/min will worsen rather than improve the patient's condition. Nothing indicates that the CO-oximeter is malfunctioning and should be recalibrated.

5. **A.** Rationale: An oxygen tent will provide 35% oxygen to an alert 2-year-old patient without restricting normal movement. It is doubtful that an alert, active 2-year-old will keep either a nasal cannula or simple mask in place as needed. In addition, the actual oxygen percentage cannot be measured through these devices. This child is too large for an incubator.

6. **C.** Rationale: The patient's arterial blood gas results show her PaO_2 to be 84 torr. This is too high for many COPD patients. It is likely that her hypoxic drive to breathe has become blunted. This has resulted in her hypoventilating, with an increasing carbon dioxide level and secondary drowsiness. Although it is not possible to know the patient's inspired oxygen percentage with a 6 L/min nasal cannula, this flow has resulted in the PaO_2 being too high. It is best to switch her to an air entrainment mask so that a known low oxygen percentage (24%) can be administered. She should then be closely monitored for returning alertness, and another arterial blood gas sample should be obtained. This should be evaluated for a lower, but safe, PaO_2 and a lower $PaCO_2$. The patient should not be left on her present oxygen flow through the nasal cannula because of her unnecessarily high oxygen level, hypoventilation, increasing carbon dioxide level, and secondary drowsiness. Changing her from a cannula to a simple face mask at the same oxygen flow will not correct these problems. She needs to be awakened because her drowsiness is not the result of simple fatigue.

7. **A.** Rationale: It is likely that the biopsy site has developed some edema, which is causing the shortness of breath and "tight" throat feeling. Giving the patient 20% oxygen and 80% helium should help to ease the patient's shortness of breath because helium is less dense than nitrogen. Putting the patient's head down 30 degrees is commonly used when a patient's blood pressure is low; it is unlikely to ease a feeling of shortness of breathing. Carbogen (carbon dioxide and oxygen mix) stimulates the breathing center of the brain but will not relieve the patient's shortness of breath caused by laryngeal edema. The 7-minute helium dilution test is performed in the pulmonary function laboratory to measure the patient's residual volume. It is not intended to relieve the patient's feeling of shortness of breath from laryngeal edema.

8. **D.** Rationale: Because a major obstruction exists in the transtracheal oxygen catheter, it should be replaced, but first the patient must switch her oxygen delivery system to a nasal cannula. Attempts to force out the obstruction by doubling the oxygen flow or forcing the saline or cleaning rod through the catheter can result in injury to the trachea.

9. **C.** Rationale: Because the reservoir bag has collapsed, the flow of helium and oxygen must be increased. Ideally, the reservoir bag should not collapse by more than one third on inspiration. Decreasing the flow of gas to the patient will worsen the problem of shortness of breath, not improve it. When the flow of gas to the mask is inadequate, it does not matter if the patient is given 24% oxygen or changed to a 30% oxygen and 70%

helium mix. In addition, no indication is noted that the patient is hypoxemic.

10. **D.** Rationale: The patient's current blood gases show unacceptable hypoxemia with a Pao$_2$ of 47 torr and Sao$_2$ of 80%. Increasing the patient from 2 to 3 L/min through the transtracheal oxygen catheter should help to correct the situation. The patient should be monitored for a possible increasing carbon dioxide level as well as an improving oxygen level. Changing the patient to 24% oxygen by an air entrainment mask will probably not change his actual inspired oxygen percentage. In addition, no indication is reported that the transtracheal oxygen catheter has failed. The patient's ventilation is stable, with no indication that bilevel mask ventilation is needed. Changing the patient to a nonrebreathing mask with 10 L/min of oxygen is potentially dangerous. This much oxygen may blunt his hypoxic drive to breathe.

11. **B.** Rationale: Inhaled nitric oxide (INOmax) is indicated to dilate the pulmonary vascular bed of a newborn with persistent pulmonary hypertension of the newborn (PPHN). When the pulmonary vascular bed dilates, more blood flows through the lungs, and oxygenation should improve. The instillation of intratracheal surfactant is indicated only in a newborn with infant respiratory distress syndrome (RDS). Surfactant therapy is not indicated in PPHN. Although PEEP increases the functional residual capacity of an infant with RDS and improves oxygenation, PEEP must be used with great care, if at all, in a newborn with PPHN. Ten-centimeter water PEEP may overexpand the alveoli of a newborn with PPHN and prevent blood from flowing through the capillary bed. Oxygenation will worsen rather than improve.

Carbogen (carbon dioxide and oxygen mix) may be harmful to a newborn with PPHN. This is because an increased carbon dioxide level further constricts the newborn's pulmonary vascular bed. Carbogen is indicated in a newborn with hypoplastic left-heart syndrome.

12. **A.** Rationale: Heliox therapy should be helpful in reducing the patient's work of breathing. This should allow more time for the corticosteroid and aminophylline medications to begin working. Nitric oxide is a pulmonary vasodilator and not indicated for status asthmaticus. Review Box 6-1 if needed. It is not necessary at this time to go against a patient's wishes and begin mechanical ventilation without first trying heliox therapy. Absolutely no reason justifies allowing this patient to die of status asthmaticus! It should not be fatal if managed appropriately and aggressively.

13. **B.** Rationale: Because the patient's pulmonary vascular resistance (PVR) is now in the normal range, the concentration of nitric oxide can be reduced. The patient's PVR should then be reassessed. It is more prudent to wean off the nitric oxide level rather than discontinue the gas in one step. No need exists to increase the NO to 20 ppm because the patient's PVR is in the normal range. It also is possible that this level of NO could be toxic.

14. **C.** Rationale: The heliox factor for a 70% helium/30% oxygen mix is 1.6. To calculate the total flow of this heliox mix through an oxygen flowmeter, the following calculation is made:

8 L/min of gas observed on the flowmeter × 1.6 = 12.8 (13) L/min actual heliox gas flow

7

Hyperinflation Therapy

Note 1: The National Board for Respiratory Care (NBRC) has released the *RRT Examination Matrix* (covering the testable items on the Written Registry Exam) and the *CSE Examination Matrix* (covering the testable items on the Clinical Simulation Exam). Turn to the appendices at the back of this book for both publications in their original format. This book is intended to cover all of the testable items in these two publications. This chapter (and all others) uses the abbreviation "WRE" for the coded items testable on the Written Registry Exam *and* Clinical Simulation Exam. The listed difficulty (R, Recall; Ap, Application; An, Analysis) relates to the question difficulty on the Written Registry Exam. The abbreviation "CSE" is used for the coded items testable on *only* the Clinical Simulation Exam. Because no question difficulty level is given for this exam, be prepared for anything.

Note 2: A review of the most recent Written Registry Examinations has shown an average of two questions (2% of the exam) that cover hyperinflation therapy. The Clinical Simulation Exam is comprehensive and may include everything that should be known or performed by an advanced level respiratory therapist.

MODULE A

Perform coughing and deep-breathing procedures with the patient to help make breathing more effective

1. Teach the patient the best techniques for breathing efficiently (WRE code: IIID1a) [Difficulty: Ap]

Teach the following steps to patients with obstructive airways diseases:

  a. Have the patient lie in a comfortable supine position; knees can be flexed.
  b. Instruct the patient to relax physically as much as possible, especially the shoulders.
  c. Use soothing music, meditation, or other techniques for mental relaxation.
  d. Instruct the patient to concentrate on breathing more slowly.
  e. Emphasize pursed-lip breathing where the patient with relaxed abdominal muscles breathes in slowly through the nose and out slowly through pursed (slightly opened) lips. Breathing with pursed lips

keeps some backpressure on the airways so that they stay open longer. The technique helps to improve gas exchange so that the patient feels less dyspnea.

2. Teach the patient techniques for strengthening the inspiratory muscles (WRE code: IIID1b) [Difficulty: Ap]

In addition to the first three steps described earlier, teach the following steps to patients with obstructive airways diseases.

The practitioner places his or her hands and the patient's hands gently over the area(s) where the patient is to concentrate the breathing effort. Usually this is the abdominal area just below the sternum. This encourages the patient to use the diaphragm more effectively and to strengthen it. With diaphragmatic breathing, the hands move out during an inspiration.

The same hands-on technique can be used to aid in segmental breathing over an area that is underventilated or has atelectasis.

Breathing *in* against an obstruction can also increase strength and endurance of inspiratory muscles. A variety of devices exist. One type of device is a mouthpiece with selectable, variably sized openings at the other end (Fig. 7-1). The patient breathes in through the largest opening and progresses to smaller openings as tolerated.

Increasing strength and endurance of inspiratory muscles usually requires a training program similar to the following:

  a. Plug the nose with nose clips.
  b. Inspire a normal tidal volume (V_T) at a rate of 12 to 15 breaths/min through the largest opening.
  c. Continue for 10 to 15 min/day for a total of three to five times per week in the first week. If the patient notices shortness of breath, a noticeably increased pulse rate, or increased fatigue, the exercise should be stopped until the symptoms are gone. Resume the exercise when the patient is comfortable again.
  d. Gradually increase the duration to about 30 minutes per session or two 15-min sessions per day.
  e. When this schedule can be easily tolerated three times per week, switch to the next smallest hole.

Fig. 7-1 PFLEX inspiratory muscle trainer. The body of the device features a dial selector with inspiratory holes. The holes range from the 1 setting (largest opening) to the 6 (smallest opening). A one-way valve allows the patient to expire. The mouthpiece can be directly attached to the body or have a monitoring/oxygen adapter added between them. This adapter allows oxygen to be added to meet the patient's needs. An inspiratory-force meter also can be added to determine the amount of negative pressure the patient is generating at each of the inspiratory hole settings. *(Courtesy of Respironics HealthScan Asthma & Allergy Products, Inc., Cedar Grove, NJ.)*

    f. Repeat steps **a** to **e** as tolerated. The most beneficial exercise is tiring but not exhausting. The device may be adjusted to the next larger hole setting if the patient becomes too tired. The whole process usually takes 4 to 6 weeks to see positive results.

    g. A maintenance program necessitates that the exercise be done every other day.

3. Reinforce to the patient the need to breathe deeply (WRE code: IIID1a) [Difficulty: Ap]

Explain to the patient that taking in deep breaths keeps the lungs inflated and healthy and decreases the chance of pneumonia developing. Deep breathing and coughing are indicated in patients with atelectasis, pulmonary infiltrates, or pneumonia. These exercises should help to raise secretions. It is especially important to prevent or limit atelectasis and pneumonia by deep breathing and coughing in patients who have just had abdominal surgery, such as cholecystectomy or splenectomy. Ideally the patient is taught these techniques before surgery. If not, teach them postoperatively:

    a. Minimize traction or tension on the incision, to decrease the pain, by placing your or the patient's hands on both sides of the incision. A pillow also can be held against the incision by the practitioner or patient.

    b. Instruct the patient to breathe two or three times in through the nose and out through the mouth.

    c. Instruct the patient to take in as deep a breath as possible and to perform a normal cough.

    d. If the patient cannot cough normally because of pain, a serial or huff cough can be performed.

Teach the following cough techniques to the patient with obstructive airways disease:

    a. Avoid an ineffective, shallow, hacking cough.

    b. Position the patient in a sitting position, bent slightly forward, with feet on the floor or supported. The patient who must lie in bed can be positioned on the preferred side with the legs flexed at the knees and hips.

    c. Instruct the patient to perform a midinspiratory cough:

       1. Breathe two or three times in through the nose and out through the mouth.

       2. Breathe in to a comfortable volume larger than the tidal volume (V_T) but not as deeply as possible.

       3. Briefly hold the breath.

       4. Cough hard or perform a serial cough at relatively low flows. This should help to raise secretions without causing airway collapse.

       5. Squeezing the knees and thighs together at the instant of coughing helps to increase the airflow and volume.

Coaching is important because patients in pain or suffering from chronic lung disease tend to be uncooperative and will not try hard. Give positive reinforcement when the patient does well. Correct any problems the patient is having with following the instructions. Demonstrations are often useful so that the patient can copy a good example.

MODULE B
Incentive spirometry

1. Teach the patient the proper techniques for incentive spirometry and evaluate the patient's ability to perform it (WRE code: IIID1a) [Difficulty: Ap]

Incentive spirometry (IS) is a technique whereby a patient is encouraged to breathe deeply by seeing his or her inhaled volume on the spirometry device. The patient receives positive feedback by seeing that the volume gradually increases as his or her condition improves. IS is indicated in any patient in whom atelectasis has developed or is likely to develop and can perform the procedure. Examples of conditions in which atelectasis is likely to be seen include postoperative thoracic or upper abdominal surgery cases, the aged, the obese, and patients with airway obstruction, inadequate sigh, and cardiopulmonary disease.

> **Exam Hint**
>
> **R**emember that incentive spirometry is the preferred treatment choice for atelectasis in patients who can perform it properly.

Because the goal of IS is to prevent or treat atelectasis, the patient should inhale a near-normal inspiratory capacity (IC). The patient can benefit more by holding the IC for several seconds, which is referred to as sustained maximal inspiration (SMI). Before the operation, the cooperative surgical patient should have the IC measured at the bedside or calculated from a pulmonary function test in which vital capacity (VC) is measured (review Chapter 4 for IC information). The IC is measured again postoperatively.

Before starting the instruction, make sure that the patient is alert and cooperative enough to follow instructions. The patient's respiratory rate should be less than 25 breaths/min to perform the procedure properly. Use the following steps in teaching IS:

a. Have the patient sit in semi-Fowler's position, on the edge of the bed, or up in a chair.

b. Set an initial goal of twice the patient's V_T.

c. Tell the patient the purpose of the treatment and how to perform it properly.

d. Simulate the procedure for the patient.

e. Put the unit within easy reach and keep it upright.

f. Have the patient exhale normally (to functional residual capacity), seal the lips around the mouthpiece, and inspire maximally through the unit. The patient must inspire in a slow, controlled effort.

g. Have the patient hold the IC for *at least* 3 sec before exhaling (the SMI) but no longer than 15 sec.

h. Proceed to increase the patient's goal as tolerated and indicated earlier.

i. The patient should perform the deep breath at least 10 times per hour while awake. A rest period with normal breathing should take place between each large breath.

Monitor your patient's progress in the following ways:

a. If the patient cannot meet the initial goal, reconsider whether this is the best form of treatment. Intermittent positive-pressure breathing (IPPB) might be a better choice to provide a deep breath.

b. Stop the treatment temporarily if the patient has signs of hyperventilation, such as dizziness or tingling of the fingertips. A few minutes of normal breathing should result in a normal feeling again. Have the patient take longer rest periods between maximal breaths.

c. Stop the treatment if the patient complains of acute chest pain. It is possible to cause pulmonary barotrauma by breathing in as deeply as possible. Evaluate the patient's pulmonary condition, and call the physician if indicated.

2. Modify the incentive spirometry device to increase or decrease the patient's incentive spirometry goal (WRE code: IIIF2) [Difficulty: An]

See Table 7-1 for IS guidelines. The following guidelines are also suggested:

TABLE 7-1 Guidelines for the Use of Incentive Spirometry

Postoperative Bedside Spirometry	Treatment Modality
IC > 80% of the preoperative value	No treatment needed unless radiographic or clinical evidence of atelectasis exists
IC at least 33% of the preoperative value or FVC of at least 10 mL/kg	IS is indicated
IC < 33% of the preoperative value or FVC < 10 mL/kg	IPPB is indicated

FVC, Forced vital capacity; IC, inspiratory capacity; IPPB, intermittent positive-pressure breathing; IS, incentive spirometry.

a. Set the initial IC goal at twice the V_T.

b. Increase the goal in 200-mL increments as the patient tolerates.

c. Set a final IC goal of greater than 12 mL/kg of ideal body weight, or set a forced vital capacity (FVC) goal of greater than 15 mL/kg of ideal body weight.

d. A normal person should have an IC of about 75% of his or her FVC. For example, a predicted FVC of 5.166 L was calculated for a male patient in Chapter 4. His predicted IC would be calculated as 5.166 L × 0.75 = 3.875 L. However, because of natural variations in persons, he might inhale only 80% of this (3.1 L) and still be considered within normal limits. Use this as a guideline for anticipating a patient's maximal IC, and do not expect your patient to inhale a greater IC than is physically possible.

Consider increasing the IS goal if the patient is easily able to reach the set goal, or if the patient's breath sounds are diminished in the bases. Consider decreasing the IS goal if the patient cannot reach the set goal because it is too large, the patient is frustrated and discouraged at his or her inability to reach the set goal, or excessive surgical site pain prevents the patient from reaching the set goal.

MODULE C
Incentive spirometry equipment

1. Get the necessary equipment for the procedure (WRE code: IIA12) [Difficulty: Ap]

2. Put the equipment together, make sure that it works properly, and identify and fix any problems with it (WRE code: IIA12) [Difficulty: Ap]

Two basic types of IS equipment exist: flow-displacement and volume-displacement units.

a. Flow displacement

Flow-displacement units work by having the patient breathe in a flow great enough to raise one or more

Fig. 7-2 Triflo II incentive deep-breathing exerciser. *(From Eubanks DH, Bone RC: Comprehensive respiratory care, ed 2, St Louis, 1990, Mosby.)*

Fig. 7-3 Volume incentive breathing exerciser. *(From Eubanks DH, Bone RC: Comprehensive respiratory care, ed 2, St Louis, 1990, Mosby.)*

plastic balls in calibrated cylinders (Fig. 7-2). The patient is encouraged to try to keep the ball (or balls) suspended by breathing in more deeply. Encourage the patient to breathe in *slowly* to suspend the balls for as long as possible. Have the patient watch as the balls are held up by the inspired breath to provide positive reinforcement for doing a good job. The patient is not helped by breathing in a fast, short breath and having the balls pop up and down. Volume is calculated by multiplying the flow per second needed to suspend the balls by the number of seconds that the balls are suspended. For example,

$$600 \text{ cc/sec} \times 2 \text{ sec} = 1200 \text{ cc IC}$$

Assembly is performed by attaching the flow tube to the unit and the mouthpiece to the flow tube.

b. Volume displacement

Volume-displacement units work by having the patient breathe in a preset volume goal from the reservoir bellows (Fig. 7-3). Many of these units have a whistle built into them to warn if the breath is too fast. Patients who cannot generate enough inspiratory flow to use a flow-displacement unit should use a volume-displacement unit instead.

Some units also have a small built-in leak so that the patient must continue inspiring to keep the bellows suspended. Have the patient watch as the bellows is suspended to provide positive reinforcement for doing a good job. Volume is marked on the bellows container. If the unit has a built-in leak, multiply the volume inspired by the time the bellows is suspended. For example,

$$800 \text{ mL} \times 3 \text{ sec} = 2400 \text{ mL IC}$$

Assembly is performed by attaching the flow tube to the unit and the mouthpiece to the flow tube.

3. Troubleshoot any problems with the equipment (WRE code: IIA12) [Difficulty: Ap]

In either type of incentive spirometer, an obstruction to the flow tube or mouthpiece or a built-in leak in the calibrated cylinders stops airflow. With a flow-displacement unit, no balls will rise despite the patient's inspiratory effort. With a volume-displacement unit, the bellows will not rise despite the patient's inspiratory effort. Clearing the obstruction or sealing the leak allows either unit to work properly.

MODULE D
Respiratory care plan

1. Analyze the available information to determine the patient's pathophysiologic state (CSE code: IIIH1)

2. Determine the appropriateness of the prescribed therapy and goals for the identified pathophysiologic state (CSE code: IIIH3)

    a. Review the interdisciplinary patient and family plan (WRE code: IIIH1b) [Difficulty: An]

IS is the easiest and least expensive way to treat atelectasis if the patient can properly perform the procedure. See Table 7-1 for guidelines on the indications for IS or IPPB.

    b. Review the planned therapy to establish the therapeutic plan (WRE code: IIIH1a) [Difficulty: An]

c. Recommend changes in the therapeutic plan if supportive data exist (WRE code: IIIH2) [Difficulty: An]

The following should be considered in evaluating the patient's response:

1. The opening of atelectatic areas would be signaled by the return of normal rather than diminished or absent breath sounds.
2. Acute chest pain could be the result of a pneumothorax from barotrauma. A chest radiograph film would be needed to confirm or deny the presence of a pneumothorax. Stop the treatment if a pneumothorax is suspected.
3. Be prepared to measure V_T, VC, and IC to determine the patient's goals and evaluate his or her progress.
4. The patient may have an increase in sputum production if the deep-breathing exercises and IS open up atelectatic areas. The patient may have a more productive cough because of a greater VC.

d. Stop the treatment if the patient has an adverse reaction to it (CSE code: IIIF1)

Be prepared to stop the current treatment if the patient is having an adverse reaction to it. Usually incentive spirometry is a safe procedure. However, some patients will hyperventilate during it and feel dizzy or lightheaded. If this should happen, the patient should be told to stop the treatment for a few minutes. The dizziness should go away, and the patient should be able to resume the IS procedure. Direct the patient to continue to inhale deeply but at a slower rate.

e. Discontinue the patient's incentive spirometry treatment based on the patient's response (WRE code: IIIG1e) [Difficulty: An]

A treatment can be discontinued for three reasons: first, a serious adverse reaction or complication to the treatment. For example, stop the treatment if the patient complains of chest pain. It may be the result of a pneumothorax. Inform the physician if clinical evidence of this is noted. The treatment also may be discontinued if the patient repeatedly hyperventilates during the IS procedure. Other reasons to terminate the treatment include inadequate pain control, exacerbation of bronchospasm, hypoxemia from the removal of the patient's oxygen mask, and fatigue. If these problems are corrected, it may be possible to begin the IS treatment again.

Second, the treatment is no longer effective. If the patient cannot perform a proper IS treatment, another way to treat the atelectasis should be found. This could include IPPB. See Chapter 14 for the discussion.

Third, the patient has recovered and no longer needs the treatment. As the postsurgical patient recovers, can walk about, and can perform proper coughing and deep-breathing exercises, any atelectasis will be corrected. In many cases, IS can be stopped within a week after surgery.

3. Respiratory care protocols

a. Develop the outcomes of the hyperinflation therapy protocol (WRE code: IIIH4b) [Difficulty: An]

b. Apply the hyperinflation therapy protocol (WRE code: IIIH6) [Difficulty: Ap, An]

c. Explain planned therapy and goals to the patient in understandable (nonmedical) terms to achieve the best results from the treatment (WRE code: IIIA6) [Difficulty: An]

d. Monitor the outcome of the hyperinflation therapy protocol (WRE code: IIIH5) [Difficulty: An]

e. Communicate the outcomes of therapy and change the treatment based on the protocol (WRE code: IIIA5) [Difficulty: An]

Review Table 7-1 for guidelines on the use of incentive spirometry. These and the previous discussion on adjusting the IS goal can be used to develop and implement a protocol and to evaluate its outcomes. It may be possible to use a simpler patient care plan such as cough and deep-breathing exercises with ambulation, or it may be necessary to switch to IPPB.

> **Exam Hint**
>
> Understand the indications for IS compared with those for IPPB. Be prepared to recommend a change in the IS volume or to change from IS to IPPB.

4. Record and evaluate the patient's response to the treatment(s) or procedure(s), including the following:

a. Record and interpret the following: heart rate and rhythm, respiratory rate, blood pressure, body temperature, and pain level (WRE code: IIIA1b, IIIA1c) [Difficulty: An]

b. Record and interpret the patient's breath sounds (WRE code: IIIA1a) [Difficulty: An]

If IS is effective, the patient's breath sounds should improve. Areas of atelectasis, with diminished breath sounds, should now be heard as normal.

c. Record and interpret the type of cough the patient has and the nature of the sputum (WRE code: IIIA1a) [Difficulty: An]

If IS is effective, the patient should be able to take in a deeper breath. This should result in a more effective cough and the ability to cough out secretions. Always note the nature of the patient's secretions.

d. Recheck any math work and make note of incorrect data (WRE code: IIIA2) [Difficulty: An]

Errors made in charting must be corrected by drawing a single mark through the error and writing in the correct information. Some prefer that the error be further clarified by writing in "error" next to it and adding initials. *Never* erase or use any covering material over an error.

5. Communicate information relevant to coordinating patient care and discharge planning (e.g., scheduling, avoiding conflicts, and sequencing of therapies) (WRE code: IIIA3) [Difficulty: An]

Common scheduling problems include eating times and when the patient must go to another department, such as radiology or physical therapy.

BIBLIOGRAPHY

American Association for Respiratory Care: Clinical practice guideline: incentive spirometry, *Respir Care* 36(12):1402, 1991.

Cairo JM: Lung expansion devices. In Cairo JM, Pilbeam SP, editors: *Mosby's respiratory care equipment,* ed 2, St. Louis, 2004, Mosby.

Douce FH: Incentive spirometry and other aids to lung inflation. In Barnes TA, editor: *Core textbook of respiratory care practice,* ed 2, St Louis, 1994, Mosby.

Eubanks DH, Bone RC: *Comprehensive respiratory care, a learning system,* ed 2, St Louis, 1990, Mosby.

Fink JB: Volume expansion therapy. In Burton GG, Hodgkin JE, Ward JJ, editors: *Respiratory care: a guide to clinical practice,* Philadelphia, 1997, Lippincott-Raven.

Fink JB: Bronchial hygiene and lung expansion. In Fink JB, Hunt GE, editors: *Clinical practice in respiratory care,* Philadelphia, 1999, Lippincott Williams & Wilkins.

Fink JB, Hess DR: Secretion clearance techniques. In Hess DR, MacIntyre NR, Mishoe SC: *Respiratory care principles and practice,* Philadelphia, 2002, WB Saunders.

Johnson NT, Pierson DJ: The spectrum of pulmonary atelectasis: pathophysiology, diagnosis, and therapy, *Respir Care* 31:1107, 1986.

Mang H, Obermayer A: Imposed work of breathing during sustained maximal inspiration: comparison of six incentive spirometers, *Respir Care* 34:1122, 1989.

Scuderi J, Olsen GN: Respiratory therapy in the management of postoperative complications, *Respir Care* 34:281, 1989.

Shapiro BA, Kacmarek RM, Cane RD, et al: *Clinical application of respiratory care,* ed 4, St Louis, 1991, Mosby.

Rutkowski JA: Hyperinflation therapy. In Wyka KA, Mathews PJ, Clark WF, editors: *Foundations of respiratory care,* Albany, NY, 2002, Delmar.

Wilkins RL: Lung expansion therapy. In Wilkins RL, Stoller JK, Scanlan CL, editors: *Egan's fundamentals of respiratory care,* ed 8, St Louis, 2003, Mosby.

Wojciechowski WV: Incentive spirometers, secretion evacuation devices, and inspiratory muscle training devices. In Barnes TA, editor: *Core textbook of respiratory care practice,* ed 2, St Louis, 1994, Mosby.

SELF-STUDY QUESTIONS

1. A previously healthy 27-year-old woman had an emergency appendectomy 2 days ago. After a few minutes of incentive spirometry, she complains of tingling in her fingers and feeling dizzy. What should the respiratory therapist do?
   A. Stop the treatment and chart the patient's complaint.
   B. Have her inhale at a slower rate.
   C. Reduce her IS volume goal.
   D. Have her inhale a deeper volume.

2. A patient with advanced COPD is anxious and feeling short of breath after returning from a medical procedure. What should the respiratory therapist tell the patient to do?
   A. Turn up the oxygen flow rate to his nasal cannula.
   B. Inhale through his PFLEX inspiratory muscle trainer.
   C. Use pursed-lip breathing.
   D. Exhale through his flutter valve unit.

3. You are the respiratory therapist assigned to teach a postoperative abdominal surgery patient about incentive spirometry. How would you explain the purpose of the treatment?
   A. It will prevent bilateral basilar microatelectasis.
   B. It will help the surgical wound heal faster.
   C. It will treat pneumonia.
   D. It will keep areas of the lungs from collapsing.

4. A 40-year-old cooperative female patient had her gallbladder removed 2 days ago. She is now slightly feverish, and her chest radiograph shows signs of atelectasis in the right lower lobe. What should be the first treatment procedure to treat the problem?
   A. Incentive spirometry
   B. Positive expiratory pressure (PEP) therapy
   C. Nasotracheal suctioning
   D. Intermittent positive-pressure breathing (IPPB) therapy

5. A patient is recovering from a neuromuscular disease, and the physician wishes to speed the process of strengthening his inspiratory muscles. What technique should the respiratory therapist recommend?
   A. PFLEX inspiratory muscle trainer
   B. Maximal inspiratory pressure (MIP)
   C. Maximal expiratory pressure (MEP)
   D. Trendelenburg positioning.

6. As the lead respiratory therapist, you are in charge of developing an incentive spirometry protocol for an obese postoperative open-heart surgery patient with bilateral atelectasis. All of the following could be outcome measures EXCEPT:
   A. Normal lung fields on chest radiograph
   B. Increased arterial oxygen level
   C. Increased cardiac output
   D. Improved breath sounds

7. A 150-pound (70-kg) patient with a recent stroke has complications of atelectasis and bronchitis. His inspiratory capacity is measured at 40% of his predicted value. What therapy would be most appropriate initially?
   A. Incentive spirometry with sustained maximal inspiration
   B. Intermittent positive-pressure breathing (IPPB) therapy

C. Positive expiratory pressure therapy
D. Postural drainage with percussion and vibration

8. Your patient is using a flow-displacement–type of incentive spirometer at a rate of 20 times per minute. She is able to suspend the ball marker for 1 second at her targeted inspiratory capacity. How could the treatment be improved upon?
   A. Increase her target volume by 500 mL.
   B. Have her breathe at a slower rate and hold the volume longer.
   C. Have her exhale more rapidly.
   D. Lower her target volume by 100 mL and increase her respiratory rate to 25 times per minute.

9. You are called to evaluate a patient who has been using a volume-displacement–type incentive spirometer for 2 days since her cholecystectomy procedure. She has been following a patient-directed protocol and is easily able to inspire the 1.5-L goal set on the unit. What would you recommend?
   A. Increase her goal to 3 L.
   B. Switch her to a flow-displacement–type unit with a 1.5-L goal.
   C. Increase her volume goal to 2 L.
   D. Stop the protocol, and begin IPPB treatments.

ANSWER KEY

1. **B.** Rationale: The patient's symptoms indicate that she is hyperventilating. Having her inhale at a slower rate will cause her to retain more carbon dioxide while still taking in the desired deep breath. It is not necessary, at this time, to stop the treatment. However, it may be necessary if the hyperventilation symptoms return while she is breathing more slowly. Reducing her IS volume goal will not expand her lungs as deeply. The patient is more likely to hyperventilate if she breathes in a deeper volume at the original rate.

2. **C.** Rationale: Pursed-lip breathing should help the patient regain control over his breathing and be able to calm down. The patient should not be encouraged or allowed to change his own oxygen flow. This is potentially dangerous. The PFLEX unit is only indicated to help strengthen inspiratory muscles. It will not help to reduce dyspnea. The variable backpressure created by blowing through the flutter valve unit will only help to mobilize secretions. It will not help to reduce dyspnea.

3. **D.** Rationale: It is best to use common language when describing the basic purpose of a treatment. The phrase *bilateral basilar microatelectasis* is too technical for the average patient to understand. Limit technical discussions to other health care professionals. No evidence exists that incentive spirometry will make a

surgical wound heal faster. The topic of pneumonia should not be brought up at this time because the patient does not have it yet, and there is no need to cause concern about a potential problem at this time in the teaching process.

4. **A.** Rationale: Incentive spirometry is the simplest and least expensive way to correct a limited case of atelectasis. PEP therapy is indicated when a patient has difficulty mobilizing secretions. Nasotracheal suctioning is limited to unconscious, uncooperative patients who cannot cough out their secretions. IPPB would be needed only if the patient could not adequately perform incentive spirometry. It is not needed yet.

5. **A.** Rationale: The PFLEX unit (and other similar units by other manufacturers) is specifically designed to help strengthen the inspiratory muscles. Maximal inspiratory pressure (MIP) and maximal expiratory pressure (MEP) are bedside spirometry tests to identify a patient's respiratory accessory muscle strength at that time. Neither is intended to exercise the patient's muscles to increase their strength over time. Trendelenburg positioning is used in some surgical procedures and in some postural-drainage positions. Although the patient may have to work harder to breathe with his or her head down, this position is not used to increase respiratory muscle strength.

6. **C.** Rationale: No evidence suggests that IS will increase cardiac output. Outcome measures indicating that IS is improving lung function include normal lung fields on chest radiograph, increased arterial oxygen level, and improved breath sounds. All would indicate the opening of atelectatic alveoli.
7. **A.** Rationale: According to Table 7-1, IS is indicated in this patient at this time. In addition, a sustained maximal inspiration effort should be helpful. IPPB should be tried only if IS is found not to be effective. No evidence suggests that either positive expiratory pressure therapy or postural drainage with percussion and vibration is needed at this time to help in mobilizing secretions.
8. **B.** Rationale: By inhaling at a slower rate, she should be able to hold the inspiratory capacity longer. If her inspiratory-capacity target is appropriate, she will not be able to inhale an additional 500 mL. No advantage exists in having her exhale faster. No therapeutic reason suggests lowering her target volume by 100 mL and increasing her respiratory rate to 25 times per minute. IS is most effective at treating atelectasis when the inspiratory capacity is inhaled slowly and sustained for several seconds.
9. **C.** Rationale: It is best to increase her goal by 500 mL because she can easily reach her current volume goal. Doubling her volume goal is too large a step. It is best to increase volume goals gradually, as the patient improves, so that progress can be seen. No benefit is gained by switching to a flow-displacement device with the same volume goal. The patient seems to be doing well with the self-directed protocol, so no reason exists to change to IPPB at this time.

8 Humidity and Aerosol Therapy

Note 1: The National Board for Respiratory Care (NBRC) has released the *RRT Examination Matrix* (covering the testable items on the Written Registry Exam) and the *CSE Examination Matrix* (covering the testable items on the Clinical Simulation Exam). Turn to the appendices at the back of this book for both publications in their original format. This book is intended to cover all of the testable items in these two publications. This chapter (and all others) uses the abbreviation "WRE" for the coded items testable on the Written Registry Exam and Clinical Simulation Exam. The listed difficulty (R, Recall; Ap, Application; An, Analysis) relates to the question difficulty on the Written Registry Exam. The abbreviation "CSE" is used for the coded items testable on *only* the Clinical Simulation Exam. Because no question difficulty level is given for this exam, be prepared for anything.

Note 2: A review of the most recent Written Registry Examinations has shown an average of two questions (2% of the exam) that cover humidity and aerosol therapy. The Clinical Simulation Exam is comprehensive and may include everything that should be known or performed by an advanced level respiratory therapist.

MODULE A
Humidity and aerosol generators and administrative devices

1. Humidity delivered through small bore tubing
   a. Bubble-type humidifiers
      1. Get the necessary equipment for the procedure (WRE code: IIA3) [Difficulty: An]

The bubble-type humidifiers are used on patients with a normal upper airway who need some supplemental humidity because of the dryness of medical oxygen. These devices are not usually heated and deliver gas cooled to less than room temperature. They provide around 40% relative humidity (RH) at the delivered gas temperature. The rest of the humidity has to be made up by the patient (Figs. 8-1 and 8-2). It is possible to add a wrap-around type of heater if it is clinically indicated to raise the temperature of the delivered gas and reduce the patient's humidity deficit.

Three different types of these humidifiers are designed to add some humidity to dry oxygen delivered through small-bore tubing: tradition bubble humidifiers, jet humidifiers, and underwater jet humidifiers.

Bubble humidifiers. Bubble humidifiers use a perforated capillary tube or porous diffusion head to break the oxygen into small bubbles (see Fig. 8-2). This allows more surface area contact of the oxygen with the water and increases the RH by evaporation. It is important to keep the water level in the reservoir within the manufacturers' specifications and, if possible, as full as possible. The lower the water level, the lower the RH, because there is less time for evaporation. The faster the oxygen flow, the lower the RH.

Jet humidifiers. Jet humidifiers create an aerosol that is baffled out of the delivered gas flow. The RH is increased by evaporation of some of the aerosol droplets. These units deliver a higher RH than do the bubble humidifiers. They have the additional advantage of delivering the same RH at higher flow levels and as the water level drops.

Underwater jet humidifiers. Underwater jet humidifiers create water vapor and an aerosol. The aerosol is not baffled out as it is in the jet humidifiers. Because of this, these units deliver the highest RH. They can deliver the same humidity level at high gas flows and as the water level drops. The aerosol particles can carry pathogens, so stricter infection-control standards must be met to protect the patient. The water and humidifier must be changed at least every 24 hours. If the patient needs the highest possible delivered RH, a jet humidifier or underwater jet humidifier is a better choice than a bubble type.

      2. Put the equipment together and make sure that it works properly (WRE code: IIA3) [Difficulty: An]
      3. Troubleshoot any problems with the equipment (WRE code: IIA3) [Difficulty: An]

Many of the simple bubble humidifiers come prepackaged with sterile water. They can be used for many short-term patients (e.g., those in the recovery room) or for a single long-term patient. When the water runs low, they are

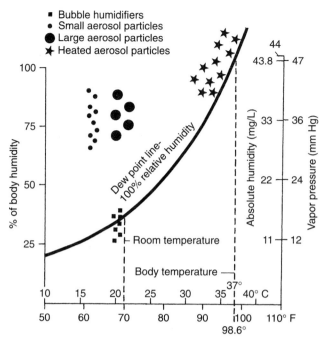

- ■ Bubble humidifiers
- • Small aerosol particles
- ● Large aerosol particles
- ★ Heated aerosol particles

Fig. 8-1 Comparison of humidity content by bubble-type humidifiers and various nebulizers.

discarded. The bubble and other types of humidifiers consist of a reservoir jar for the water and a Diameter Index Safety System (DISS) oxygen-connector lid that screws on. Turn on the flowmeter, and make sure that oxygen flows through the delivery tube and bubbles into the water. Failure to bubble usually indicates that the lid and jar are not screwed together tightly or the delivery tube is plugged. If the tube cannot be cleared, it must be replaced.

Most of the newer bubble-type units have a pop-off type of high-pressure relief valve that is released if the pressure builds up to either 40 mm Hg or 2 psi. Pinch closed the small-bore tubing to build up pressure and test the pop-off valve. Feel for the gas to escape from the valve. Many units whistle to signal a gas leak. Do not use a unit whose pop-off valve does not open under pressure.

b. Nasal cannula

Current guidelines state that humidity does not need to be added to these devices if the flow is 4 L/min or less. However, some patients complain of nasal dryness and discomfort if the cannula's oxygen is not humidified. The physician and practitioner may believe that the patient's discomfort warrants the addition of a bubble-type humidifier. There is agreement that humidity should be added to flows of greater than 4 L/min. See Fig. 8-3 for a humidified nasal cannula setup.

c. Oxygen masks

It is not believed to be necessary to add humidity to any oxygen mask that has an oxygen flow of 4 L/min or less. Humidity should be added to any mask that has more than 4 L/min of oxygen added. This includes simple oxygen masks at higher flows, higher oxygen percentage air entrainment masks, partial rebreathing masks, and non-rebreathing masks.

2. Humidity delivered through large bore tubing

Most of these patients have had their upper airway bypassed by an endotracheal or tracheostomy tube. Because of this, they cannot humidify inspired gas in the

Fig. 8-2 Oxygen leaving outlet of the bubble-type humidifier is cooler than room temperature because of evaporation. Some warming toward room temperature occurs as the oxygen travels through the tubing to the patient. *(From Scanlan CL: Humidity and aerosol therapy. In Scanlan CL, Spearman CB, Stoller JK, editors: Egan's fundamentals of respiratory care, ed 5, St Louis, 1990, Mosby.)*

Fig. 8-3 Adult wearing a nasal cannula delivering oxygen humidified by a bubble-type humidifier. *(From Guidelines for disinfection of home equipment,* Respir Care *33:801–808, 1988.)*

normal manner. In some other cases, humidity is added because the patient is receiving dry medical oxygen. Therefore it is recommended that a heated humidifier be used with these patients. It should be set to deliver gas between 31°C and 35°C to the patient and should be able to provide 80% to 100% RH in this temperature range.

All of the following humidity and aerosol-generating devices deliver the conditioned gas to the patient through large-bore (22-mm inner diameter [ID]) tubing.

a. Large volume humidifiers: cascade, wick, and passover-type

1. Get the necessary equipment for the procedure (WRE code: IIA3) [Difficulty: An]

All of these humidifiers have an adjustable heater so that the water in the reservoir is at or greater than body temperature. This enables them to provide up to 100% of the patient's body humidity. It is necessary with all of these units to measure the temperature of the inspired gas near the patient. The gas temperature is usually kept the same as the patient's or a few degrees cooler (Fig. 8 4).

The Bennett Cascade is the most well known, but now obsolete, example of these types of humidifiers (Fig. 8-5). The Cascade-type humidifier is most commonly used with a mechanical ventilator but can be used with other types of systems for delivering humidity with or without oxygen. Its basic principle of operation is an efficient bubble-type humidifier. The inspiratory gas must flow through the water for evaporation to occur. A variety of similar devices are now on the market.

The wick-type heated humidifier uses a wick, often made of sponge or paper, to soak up water for evaporation. The water, wick, or both are heated so that 100% RH can be delivered. These units also are used with mechanical ventilators or other systems, including air entrainment devices. This is because they have very little resistance to the gas flowing through them as evaporation occurs.

Fig. 8-4 Gases leaving outlet of heated humidifier are hot and saturated with water vapor. As cooling occurs in tubing, vapor condenses and absolute humidity (AH) decreases while relative humidity (RH) remains 100% (saturated). Note that almost half of the original vapor is "lost" to condensate in this example. *(From Fink JB, Scanlan CL: Humidity and bland aerosol therapy. In Scanlan CL, Wilkins RL, Stoller JK, editors:* Egan's fundamentals of respiratory care, *ed 7, St Louis, 1999, Mosby.)*

Fig. 8-5 Cascade-type humidifier. *(From Scanlan CL: Humidity and aerosol therapy. In Scanlan CL, Spearman CB, Stoller JK, editors: Egan's fundamentals of respiratory care, ed 5, St Louis, 1990, Mosby.)*

Passover-type humidifiers simply have the patient's gas passing over the surface of a reservoir of hot water. They are sometimes called "hot pots." By themselves, these units are probably the least effective at humidifying gas. When they are used on ventilators, other features such as copper mesh in a heated inspiratory tube are used to increase the surface area for evaporation.

2. Put the equipment together and make sure it works properly (WRE code: IIA3) [Difficulty: An]

3. Troubleshoot any problems with the equipment (WRE code: IIA3) [Difficulty: An]

It is important that the humidifiers be properly assembled. This is especially important when they are used to humidify a mechanical ventilator. Any loose connections will result in an air leak and loss of tidal volume. Make sure that the water level is properly maintained.

As the heated gas passes through the large-bore tubing, some cooling occurs. This results in condensation that must be drained out. Placing a water trap in the lowest point of the tubing drains the water and helps keep the tubing clear. Remember to continue to look periodically for water puffing or sloshing back and forth in the tubing. Make sure that any condensate is drained out of the tubing and thrown away. Do not drain the condensate back into the water reservoir. This is because any microorganisms in the tubing or condensate could reproduce in the reservoir.

b. Heat-moisture exchanger
1. Get the necessary equipment for the procedure (WRE code: IIA3) [Difficulty: An]

A heat-moisture exchanger (HME) contains a highly absorbent material that is warmed and moistened when a patient's exhaled breath passes through it. The patient's next inspiration is warmed and humidified by the HME. In effect, the patient is rebreathing his or her own exhaled water vapor. These units are not as efficient as the previously described humidifiers and are not able to provide 100% of the body humidity to a patient.

Many brands of HME exist, but only two main types. The first type is designed to be added to the outer part of a tracheostomy tube. It has a 15-mm ID opening to attach to the tube; the other end of the HME is open to room air. They are small and convenient to use for many patients with a permanent tracheostomy and increase a patient's mobility. The second type is used with patients who require mechanical ventilation. The patient end of the HME has a 15-mm ID to attach to the endotracheal or tracheostomy tube. The other end of the HME has an opening to attach to the ventilator circuit. See Chapter 15 for more detail.

2. Put the equipment together and make sure it works properly (WRE code: IIA3) [Difficulty: An]
3. Troubleshoot any problems with the equipment (WRE code: IIA3) [Difficulty: An]

HMEs typically come preassembled by the manufacturer. The 15-mm ID opening must be placed over the patient's endotracheal or tracheostomy tube. Secretions coughed into the HME present a significant problem because they can obstruct the flow of gas. This makes it difficult or impossible for the patient to breathe. The HME must be removed and discarded if it becomes obstructed. Replace it with a new one. Ideally, an HME should not be used with a patient known to cough out large amounts of secretions.

3. Nebulizers and related delivery systems
a. Ultrasonic nebulizers
1. Get the necessary equipment for the procedure (WRE code: IIA3) [Difficulty: An]

Ultrasonic units are often chosen for delivering bland solutions to the lower airways because of the small particle size and the high output. Ultrasonic nebulizers work by converting electrical energy into very high frequency sound energy that creates aerosol particles. The frequency is vital because it results in a stable aerosol with a mean particle size of about 3 mm in diameter. This is an ideal size to penetrate deeply into the lungs to the smallest airways. The only control on these units is for amplitude (power) to control the aerosol output. The range is usually up to 3 to 6 mL/min, depending on the model. This output is greater than most pneumatic nebulizers can produce. The aerosol can be carried to the patient by a built-in fan or by an outside oxygen source (Fig. 8-6). The patient's humidity deficit is minimized by the warm aerosol that is created.

The ultrasonic nebulizer should not be chosen for upper airway aerosol deposition or for administering pharmacologically active medications such as bronchodilators, mucolytics, and antibiotics. These medications may not nebulize at the same rate as the saline diluent, which creates the risk of delivering a very concentrated dose at the end of the treatment. Some of the medications also may be mechanically broken down by the high-frequency vibration and made useless.

2. Put the equipment together and make sure that it works properly (WRE code: IIA3) [Difficulty: An]
3. Troubleshoot any problems with the equipment (WRE code: IIA3) [Difficulty: An]

Always follow the manufacturer's instructions when setting up the system. Fig. 8-6 shows the common features, and Table 8-1 describes how to troubleshoot many common problems. Many of the clinical difficulties have to do with keeping the proper fluid levels in the couplant chamber and the solution cup. If the sterile water in the couplant chamber is too low, the vibration cannot reach the solution cup, and no aerosol will be produced. If the saline level in the solution cup is either too low or too high, the vibrational energy will not focus properly on the surface of the saline solution, and no aerosol will be

Fig. 8-6 Functional diagram of the ultrasonic nebulizer. *A,* Electric current generator. *B,* Cable. *C,* Piezoelectric crystal. *D,* Couplant chamber. *E,* Solution cup. *F,* Carrier gas inlet. *G,* Aerosol outlet. *(From Barnes TA, editor: Core textbook of respiratory care practice, ed 2, St Louis, 1994, Mosby.)*

TABLE 8-1 Ultrasonic Nebulizer Troubleshooting		
Symptom	**Possible Problem**	**Suggested Check**
Unit installed and connected as specified, but pilot light does not turn on when switch is turned to the "on" position	Electrical outlet defective Circuit breaker tripped Fuse blown	Check outlet with lamp or other appliance Reset the circuit breaker, or change fuse on the power switch; if the circuit breaker continues to trip or the fuse blows again, service is needed
Unit installed and connected as specified; power pilot light turns on, normal ultrasonic activity visible in nebulizer chamber, but no aerosol output occurs	Nebulizer chamber contaminated	Wash nebulizer chamber; decontaminate
Unit installed and connected as specified; power pilot light turns on, but little ultrasonic activity is visible in the nebulizer chamber, and aerosol output is low (even when on the no. 10 power setting)	Couplant water excessively aerated Nebulizer module and couplant water too cold Diaphragm distorted, permitting air bubbles to interfere with proper transmission of vibrational energy into the nebulizer chamber	Wait for deaeration Use warmer couplant water Check to see that diaphragm is properly shaped and installed; be sure the concave (recessed) side faces the interior of the chamber Clean couplant compartment and replace couplant water
Same as symptom described above but at a lower power setting	Power setting too low to start and establish nebulization	Turn output control knob to maximum power setting, then reduce to desired setting
Unit installed and connected as specified, and power pilot light turns on; "Add couplant" light is on, and no ultrasonic activity is visible in the nebulizer chamber	Insufficient couplant water	Add water to the couplant compartment
Unit installed and connected as specified, and power pilot light turns on; "Add couplant" light is off, but no ultrasonic activity is visible in the nebulizer chamber	Power supply overheated and its thermostatic control opened	The cooling air has been restricted, or cooling fins need cleaning; the switch will reset when the equipment returns to room temperature
Liquid reservoir filled and properly connected to nebulizer chamber, but chamber does not fill (for continuous-feed system only)	Foreign material or air bubbles in feed tubes Liquid level control in nebulizer chamber plugged with foreign material Air leaks at tube connection or reservoir cap	Flush the system Clean or flush the system Tighten all connections by pushing tubes into fittings

From Op't Holt T: Aerosol generators and humidifiers. In Barnes TA, editor: *Respiratory care practice*, St Louis, 1988, Mosby.

produced. Water should not be allowed to condense out and fill any low points in the large-bore tubing. If this were to occur, the ultrasonic particles would liquefy as the carrier gas is forced to pass through the condensate. The exiting gas would be humidified through evaporation but carry no aerosol particles. If the carrier gas is oxygen that is blended with air through an air-entrainment system, any backpressure might result in an increase in the oxygen percentage and a decrease in the total flow. Remember to always measure the oxygen percentage near the patient.

b. Large volume, pneumatic nebulizers
1. Get the necessary equipment for the procedure (WRE code: IIA3) [Difficulty: An]

Large volume, pneumatically powered nebulizers all share the common feature of having a liquid reservoir of at least

250 mL. Commonly, they also entrain room air to increase the total gas flow. They share these common features

 a. All are powered by air or oxygen delivered through a flowmeter. As the gas flow decreases, the aerosol output decreases.

 b. All make use of Bernoulli's principle with a jet that is used to entrain liquid, room air, or both into the main gas flow.

 c. All have a capillary tube that allows the liquid to flow *up* to the jet for nebulization. (Remember that with the bubble-type humidifiers, the oxygen flows *down* the capillary tube.)

 d. All have a baffle against which the aerosol is sprayed to create a more uniform particle size.

Many, but not all, of the pneumatic nebulizers allow for a changeable inspired oxygen percentage. Provided that the jet is powered by oxygen, the air entrainment ports can be opened up more to increase air entrainment (reducing the inspired oxygen percentage), or closed down to decrease air entrainment (increasing the inspired oxygen percentage). The oxygen percentage usually can be varied from 35% to 100%. Remember always to analyze the inspired oxygen percentage near the patient, because water in the aerosol tubing and backpressure decrease the entrained air and increase the oxygen percentage.

2. Put the equipment together, and make sure that it works properly (WRE code: IIAe) [Difficulty: An]
3. Troubleshoot any problems with the equipment (WRE code: IIA3) [Difficulty: An]

Most pneumatic nebulizers look similar to the bubble-type humidifiers. The key components include a large reservoir jar and a top with a DISS oxygen connector and capillary tube to the jet. These units allow for variable oxygen percentages. Keep the capillary tube and jet clear of debris, or the aerosol output will decrease. Keep the air entrainment ports open so that proper gas mixing occurs and the desired oxygen percentage is provided (Fig. 8-7). Heating of the water or aerosol or both is accomplished in one of the following ways:

 a. A heated metal rod is immersed into the reservoir water through a port in the top of the nebulizer. A dial is used to control the temperature of the rod. The water temperature varies depending on how deep it is, so as the water level drops, the remaining water becomes hotter. It is very important to measure the gas temperature near the patient and keep the water level stable to prevent burning the airway. The heated rod presents a risk of burns to a practitioner who accidentally touches it while it is still hot. It must be disinfected between patients and changed as often as the nebulizer is.

 b. Two other systems are variations on the previously mentioned idea of directly heating the water in the reservoir jar. The first heats the water as it passes through the capillary tube. All have the advantage of a short warm-up time when compared with all of the other systems. Some units have an external temperature probe to place in the aerosol tubing. It acts as a servocontroller of the heating unit for better temperature regulation. Some types directly heat only a small amount of the reservoir water just before it is aerosolized.

 c. A flexible heater is wrapped around the outside of the reservoir. A dial is used to control the temperature of the heater. The water temperature increases as the water level drops. Monitor the gas temperature near the patient for safety purposes.

 d. A clip-on heating base plate can be added to special reservoir jars with a metal plate. These are preferable

Fig. 8-7 Large volume air entrainment nebulizer. *(From Shapiro BA, Kacmarek RM, Cane RD, et al, editors: Clinical application of respiratory care, ed 4, St Louis, 1991, Mosby.)*

to the previously mentioned types because they ensure a constant temperature to the aerosol as the water level drops.

Heating the water or aerosol reduces the patient's humidity deficit and is usually done if the secretions are thick. See Fig. 8-1 for the location of the aerosol particles and their relation to the dew point and the patient's body humidity.

4. Aerosol delivery systems

Large bore tubing (also known as *aerosol tubing* or *corrugated tubing*) is needed to connect the aerosol generator with the patient. This tubing is 22 mm in inner diameter (ID).

a. Aerosol masks

The aerosol mask looks similar to the simple oxygen mask except that it has larger side ports for exhalation and has a 22-mm outer diameter (OD) adapter for the large-bore tubing to attach to (Fig. 8-8). This is often considered a low-flow oxygen mask because the ports are open to room air. Because of this, it is difficult to ensure that the patient receives the oxygen percentage that has been set. If the flow is high enough that aerosol mist can be seen flowing out of the side ports during an inspiration, little room air is being inspired. It is best to analyze the oxygen percentage inside the mask to be sure. Any of the previously mentioned humidity or aerosol devices can be used and powered by compressed air or oxygen.

b. Face tents, tracheostomy masks/collars, and Brigg's adapter/T-piece

Face tents, tracheostomy masks and collars, and Brigg's adapter (T-piece) are discussed in Chapter 6. Any of the

Fig. 8-8 Adult wearing an aerosol mask receiving supplemental oxygen and aerosol from a heated large volume nebulizer. *(From Guidelines for disinfection of home equipment,* Respir Care *33:801-808, 1988.)*

previously mentioned humidity or aerosol devices can be used with them and powered by compressed air or oxygen.

5. Medication-delivery systems
a. Small volume, pneumatic nebulizers
1. Get the necessary equipment for the procedure (WRE code: IIA4) [Difficulty: An]

A small volume nebulizer (SVN) is designed to hold a relatively small volume of fluid (typically 3 to 5 mL) and to nebulize liquid medications such as bronchodilators, mucolytics, or antibiotics for inhalation. Either compressed air or oxygen can be used to generate the aerosol. These units operate under the same physical principles as the large volume nebulizers described earlier.

Two different types of SVNs exist: mainstream and sidestream. *Mainstream nebulizers* are designed so that the main flow of gas to the patient flows through the aerosol as it is produced. A second high-pressure gas flow is used to power the jet to create the aerosol (Fig. 8-9). *Sidestream nebulizers* are designed so that the aerosol is produced out of the main flow of gas and added to it by the jet's gas flow (Fig. 8-10). Many manufacturers produce disposable medication SVN nebulizers for intermittent positive-pressure breathing (IPPB) circuits or handheld circuits. Most of these are the sidestream type. Select the nebulizer that produces a particle size that matches the therapeutic target.

See Fig. 8-11 for a typical handheld nebulizer circuit. The nebulizer can be powered by either air or oxygen.

Exam Hint

Typically, an exam question covers troubleshooting problems with aerosol delivery equipment. Examples include but are not limited to (1) incorrect water level in an ultrasonic so that no aerosol is produced; (2) plugged capillary line in a jet nebulizer so that no aerosol is produced; (3) missing baffle in a jet nebulizer so that no aerosol is produced; and (4) water in the large-bore tubing preventing aerosol from traveling through it. It is important to remember that with an oxygen-powered jet nebulizer system, the inspired oxygen percentage increases if condensate water fills the low point of the aerosol tubing. This is because the backpressure on the jet and air entrainment ports prevents room air from being drawn in (see Fig. 8-8).

Fig. 8-9 Mainstream-type small volume nebulizer for medications. *(From Shapiro BA, Kacmarek RM, Cane RD, et al, editors:* Clinical application of respiratory care, *ed 4, St Louis, 1991, Mosby.)*

Fig. 8-10 Sidestream-type small volume nebulizer for medications. *(From Shapiro BA, Kacmarek RM, Cane RD, et al, editors:* Clinical application of respiratory care, *ed 4, St Louis, 1991, Mosby.)*

Fig. 8-11 Handheld small volume nebulizer for medications with added components. *(Adapted from Guidelines for disinfection of home equipment,* Respir Care *33:801–808, 1988.)*

Typically, flows of 4 to 6 L/min are used to nebulize 3 to 5 mL of medication in about 10 minutes. The nebulizer finger control allows the patient to power the nebulizer by covering the open hole in the "T." Uncovering the hole permits the gas to exit, and the medication is not nebulized and wasted. The reservoir tube serves to hold oxygen and medication for the next inspiration.

Practitioners face two possible risks when using SVNs. First, any aerosolized medications that escape into the room air may be inhaled. It is possible that the practitioner, or anyone else who happens to be near, may have an allergic or other adverse reaction. Second, nebulized secretions from the patient's airway and lungs may be inhaled. This may place the practitioner or others at risk of acquiring a pulmonary infection from the patient. Although it is unlikely that many actual problems like this occur, it is a possibility. If either of these situations is a concern, a small volume nebulizer with one-way valves and a downstream particle filter should be used. This filter acts as a scavenging system and traps any exhaled aerosol droplets (Fig. 8-12). A filtered SVN is recommended for use when nebulizing pentamidine isethionate (NebuPent). A filtered SVN can be used for any other antibiotic or medication that should not contaminate the room air.

Fig. 8-12 Diagram of the Respirgard II small volume nebulizer system showing one-way valves and expiratory filter to scavenge exhaust aerosol. *(From Rau JL Jr: Respiratory care pharmacology, ed 5, St Louis, 1998, Mosby.)*

2. Put the equipment together and make sure that it works properly (WRE code: IIA4) [Difficulty: An]

3. Troubleshoot any problems with the equipment (WRE code: IIA4) [Difficulty: An]

Most small volume nebulizers consist of a medication reservoir and a top piece that contains a capillary tube and baffle. The top piece screws onto the reservoir and holds a mouthpiece and aerosol reservoir tube. Small-bore oxygen tubing connects the SVN to the flowmeter. If any small volume nebulizer fails to generate an aerosol, make sure that the pieces are properly assembled and the capillary tube is not plugged with debris. Sometimes the capillary tube can be cleared by running it under water or pushing a needle through the channel. Make sure that the liquid in the reservoir is at the proper depth (typically 3 to 5 mL). Do not use a nebulizer that does not generate an aerosol.

b. Metered dose inhalers

1. Get the necessary equipment for the procedure (WRE code: IIA19) [Difficulty: Ap]

2. Put the equipment together, and make sure that it works properly (WRE code: IIA19) [Difficulty: An]

3. Troubleshoot any problems with the equipment (WRE code: IIA19) [Difficulty: An]

Metered dose inhalers (MDIs) are designed to dispense a premeasured amount of medication into the airway. Each activation increases the amount of medication taken by the patient. The available medications include adrenergic and anticholinergic bronchodilators, corticosteroid drugs, and an antibiotic (see Chapter 9 for details on the medications). All MDIs operate in the same way. They have several milliliters of medication and either a compressed chlorofluorocarbon (CFC) gas or hydrofluoroalkane (HFA) gas contained inside of a metal container with a built-in jet nozzle. Because of environmental concerns, the CFC gas units will be replaced by the HFA gas units by the end of 2008.

The metering chamber is filled with medicine by tipping it over and back upright. A plastic actuator opens the jet when pressed into the container (Fig. 8-13). The patient can inhale the medication through the built-in mouthpiece. Adapters allow the medication to be sprayed into a mechanical ventilator circuit or through a bronchoscopy adapter to an endotracheal tube. A specific amount of medication is nebulized with each actuation of the device.

Make sure when assembling the MDI that the medication canister nozzle fits into the jet of the actuator. Patients should be instructed to use warm, soapy water daily to wash out the actuator and keep open the jet channel.

c. Spacer and holding chamber for a metered dose inhaler

1. Get the necessary equipment for the procedure (WRE code: IIA19) [Difficulty: An]

2. Put the equipment together and make sure that it works properly (WRE code: IIA19) [Difficulty: An]

Fig. 8-13 The effect of a spacer on aerosol particle size and velocity from a metered-dose inhaler. *(From Rau JL Jr: Respiratory care pharmacology, ed 5, St Louis, 1998, Mosby.)*

3. Troubleshoot any problems with the equipment (WRE code: IIA19) [Difficulty: An]

It has been shown that the addition to some sort of spacer or holding chamber between the actuator and the patient's mouth increases the amount of inhaled medication. These devices slow the aerosol so that less impact occurs on the back of the throat. This should result in fewer systemic side effects, such as the risk of oral thrush (*Candidiasis* fungal infection) with an MDI-powered corticosteroid. The patient with poor hand and breathing coordination wastes less medication.

A spacer is a simple open extension tube between the actuator and the patient. Its main advantage over inhaling directly from the MDI mouthpiece is that the aerosol plume expands and slows so that more medication is inhaled (see Fig. 8-13). The patient should be told not to exhale through the spacer because any remaining medication will be blown out and wasted. Some spacers are designed for use with a ventilator circuit when an MDI-based medication is to be given. A holding chamber holds the medication, as a spacer, but also has valves. These valves prevent the medicine from being exhaled and allow the patient to inhale several times to get more medication. This is especially helpful for children or small adults with small tidal volumes. Some of the holding chambers have a built-in whistle that sounds if the patient is inhaling too quickly (Fig. 8-14). Several types of spacers or holding chambers exist. Some spacers are designed to fit with only one actuator, whereas others adapt to fit to any actuator. A face mask comes attached to some holding chambers so that pediatric patients or uncooperative adults can be given the medication.

Patients must be instructed to wash out the spacer or holding chamber on a daily basis. Warm, soapy water and a thorough rinsing are usually adequate for home use. However, a disinfecting liquid such as Cidex is preferable if the patient can afford it. Acetic acid (white vinegar) also may be used to save money.

d. Dry powder inhalers
1. **Get the necessary equipment for the procedure (WRE code: IIA20) [Difficulty: Ap]**
2. **Put the equipment together and make sure that it works properly (WRE code: IIA20) [Difficulty: An]**
3. **Troubleshoot any problems with the equipment (WRE code: IIA20) [Difficulty: An]**

Dry powder inhalers (DPIs) dispense a dry medicinal powder into the patient's airways and lungs when inhaled. A growing number of respiratory medications are now available in the DPI form. Currently medications in the following categories are available in a DPI: adrenergic bronchodilators, anticholinergic bronchodilators, and corticosteroids. See Chapter 9 for more information on the specific medications. The drug manufacturer sells both the medication and the dispenser to the patient. The three representative DPI types discussed here describe the different ways that the medications may be dispensed.

The Rotahaler (Fig. 8-15, *A*) is designed to break in half a single gelatin capsule containing a powdered form of albuterol or beclomethasone. Care must be taken with the Rotahaler to hold it horizontally after the capsule has been broken, or the medication will spill out. A fast inhalation with a breath hold is recommended to deliver the medication to the airways.

The Spinhaler (Fig. 8-15, *B*) is used to pierce a single gelatin capsule holding cromolyn sodium and dispense it into the patient's airway. As the patient inhales rapidly (a flow rate of at least 40 to 60 L/min is needed on any DPI), the plastic rotor blades spray the powder into the inhaled stream of air. The patient should inhale as deeply as possible and hold the breath for maximum deposition in the small airways. Care must be taken to hold the unit upright when the capsule is pierced and the powder is inhaled, or it will spill. Cromolyn sodium is used to prevent the onset of an asthma attack and is useless after an attack has begun.

Multidose dispensers contain many doses of a medication within a drug reservoir (Fig. 8-15, *C*) or on a blister pack. A single dose is then loaded into the dispenser by the patient. A fast inhalation with breath hold is needed. These dispensers are more convenient to use than the single-dose units discussed previously. The following are currently available: Turbuhaler (terbutaline sulfate or budesonide), Rotadisk (albuterol or salmeterol), and Diskus (salmeterol). Some practice is needed in using the Spinhaler and Rotahaler units. The two main pieces must be unscrewed so that the capsule can be placed in the holding chamber. With the Spinhaler, the plastic slide must be moved up and down once to pierce the capsule. With the Rotahaler, the mouthpiece is twisted around to break open the capsule. The medication is then forcefully inhaled. Unscrew both units to remove the empty capsule.

Fig. 8-14 Five types of MDI reservoirs (holding chambers). **A,** Aerochamber (Monaghan Medical Corp); **B,** MediSpacer (Allegiance Healthcare, Inc); **C,** Aerosol Cloud Enhacer, ACE (DHD, Inc); **D,** InspirEase (Schering, Inc); **E,** OptiHaler (Healthscan, Inc). *(From Rau JL Jr: Respiratory care pharmacology, ed 5, St Louis, 1998, Mosby.)*

Fig. 8-15 Three types of dry powder inhaler. The Rotahaler **(A)** and Spinhaler **(B)** must have an individual medication capsule loaded for each inhalation. The Turbuhaler **(C)** has a drug reservoir that holds many doses of medication. *(From Rau JL Jr: Respiratory care pharmacology, ed 5, St Louis, 1998, Mosby.)*

6. Aerosol (mist) tents

a. Get the necessary equipment for the procedure (WRE code: IIA11) [Difficulty: Ap]

The aerosol or mist tents are essentially like the oxygen tents discussed in Chapter 6. The main difference is that no supplemental oxygen is used because the patient does not need it. The top of the canopy can now be left open for better flow-through ventilation. Aerosol tents are sometimes used to treat an active infant with an upper respiratory tract problem such as laryngotracheobronchitis (LTB or pediatric croup). The tent is used because a small, active child will not keep an aerosol mask in place. A tent is not indicated for an older child or adult who will keep an aerosol mask in place that will easily provide the needed aerosol to the patient.

b. Put the equipment together and make sure that it works properly (WRE code: IIA11) [Difficulty: Ap]

c. Troubleshoot any problems with the equipment (WRE code: IIA11) [Difficulty: Ap]

At least 10 L/min of compressed air should still be run through the nebulizer to make sure that no carbon dioxide buildup occurs. The nebulizer or ultrasonic system should be cared for as described earlier to ensure that enough aerosol is formed to treat the condition.

If the child has LTB, a cool aerosol is clinically preferred because it reduces airway edema. Never use so much aerosol that the child cannot be seen inside the tent. Be wary of fluid overloading the young patient who is in the tent for a prolonged period.

MODULE C

Modify the patient's breathing pattern so that a medication is properly deposited (WRE code: IIIFA3) [Difficulty: An]

1. Upper airway deposition

Particles 10 μm or larger are more likely to impact on the upper airway (oropharynx, larynx, trachea, and mainstem bronchi) when the patient is coached to
   a. Inhale at a normal or faster speed. The flow should be greater than 30 L/min.
   b. Inhale a normal tidal volume.
   c. Breathe in a normal pattern.

2. Lower airway and alveolar deposition

Particles 2 to 5 μm are more likely to deposit on the smaller airways (respiratory bronchioles) and in the alveoli when the patient is coached to
   a. Inhale at a slow speed. The flow should be less than 30 L/min.
   b. Inhale an inspiratory capacity.
   c. Hold the full breath in for 10 seconds if possible before exhaling.

Obviously, all patients will not be able to perform these techniques perfectly, but to the extent that they can, the medication will be deposited where it is needed, and the treatment will be more effective.

Exam Hint

One question has regularly dealt with recognizing that a patient is hyperventilating during a nebulizer treatment. Signs of hyperventilation include dizziness, lightheadedness, and tingling fingers. The patient should be told to breathe slower and less deeply.

MODULE D

Respiratory care plan

1. Analyze available information to determine the patient's pathophysiologic state (CSE code: IIIH1)

If a patient has retained secretions, humidity or aerosol therapy is indicated. Review Chapter 1 and this chapter for information on assessing breath sounds, etc., to determine whether the patient has a secretion-management problem.

2. Determine the appropriateness of the prescribed therapy and goals for the identified pathophysiologic state (CSE code: IIIH3)

Know the indications, advantages, and disadvantages of the types of humidity and aerosol therapy devices described in this chapter. Be prepared to make a recommendation to change humidity or aerosol therapy equipment.

3. Administer aerosol therapy (WRE code: IIIC3) [Difficulty: An]

The patient with a secretion problem should be helped by the addition of a bland aerosol or mucolytic medication and is better able to clear them out effectively. This should result in the patient feeling better, as well as having improved vital signs, oxygenation, breath sounds, and spirometry values. The use of a bland aerosol therapy can cause bronchospasm in some asthmatic patients. Patients with viscous, thick, dry secretions can have their airways occluded if aerosol therapy causes the secretions to take in water and swell. The patient must be able to cough out the thinned secretions, or suctioning equipment must be available to remove them.

In general, a cool humidity or aerosol system is used with patients with the following conditions:
   1. Pediatric croup
   2. Upper airway irritation such as after extubation or a bronchoscopy procedure

In general, a body temperature humidity or aerosol system is used with patients with the following conditions:
   1. Bypassed upper airway (endotracheal or tracheostomy tube)

2. Thick (viscous) secretions
3. Hypothermia
4. Neonate to maintain a neutral thermal environment

Neonates are sensitive to overhydration. Long-term aerosol therapy for them should be avoided or minimized. Adult patients with heart failure or pulmonary edema also should not be given long-term aerosol therapy. Instead, a Cascade-type humidifier can be used.

The adult patient who has thick secretions may be aided by long-term aerosol therapy of a dense mist at body temperature. The secretions are often liquefied and made easier to cough or suction out. An ultrasonic nebulizer is often used for this purpose. The child with croup is usually given a dense mist of a cool, bland aerosol in a mist tent. This therapy is usually needed for only a few days. Be wary of fluid overload if the mist is needed for a longer period.

a. Stop the treatment or procedure if the patient has an adverse reaction to it (CSE code: IIIF1)

In some asthmatic patients, bronchospasm may develop in reaction to aerosol therapy. Be prepared to stop the aerosol therapy if this should happen. The patient may need to be given an inhaled bronchodilator medication before aerosol therapy can be continued.

b. Discontinue treatment based on the patient's response (WRE code: IIIG1e) [Difficulty: An]

Be prepared to discontinue aerosol therapy if the patient has a persistent bronchospasm reaction to the treatment despite being given an inhaled bronchodilator medication. Also be prepared to stop aerosol therapy if the patient has an increase in secretions and cannot cough them out. The therapist may need to perform endotracheal suctioning to remove the secretions.

> **Exam Hint**
>
> **P**ast exams have had a question that deals with stopping aerosol therapy when a patient demonstrates reactive bronchospasm by the development of wheezing.

4. Record and evaluate the patient's response to the treatment(s) or procedure(s), including the following:
a. Record and interpret the patient's breath sounds (WRE code: IIIA1a) [Difficulty: An]

Interpretation of breath sounds is discussed in Chapter 1. It should be expected that bland aerosol administration will result in the patient's secretions becoming thinner (less viscous), so that they can be coughed or suctioned out more easily. However, some patients with a history of

asthma may react to inhaled saline solutions by developing bronchospasm.

b. Record and interpret the type of cough the patient has and the nature of the sputum (WRE code: IIIA1a) [Difficulty: An]

Find out from the patient approximately how much sputum is produced in a day. Also find out whether certain times of the day are more productive or less productive. Try to relate this to breathing treatments, medications, activities, meals, and allergies.

It is important to monitor the patient's sputum quantity and consistency to know whether the humidity or aerosol therapy is effective. Again, try to relate this to breathing treatments, medications, activities, meals, and allergies. It may be necessary to suggest a change in bland aerosol therapy administration based on the patient's condition. For example, change from normal saline to hypertonic saline for a sputum induction. See Chapter 9 for information on the saline solutions used as mucolytics.

> **Exam Hint**
>
> **B**e prepared to change the type of humidity- and aerosol delivery system, from among those discussed in this chapter based, on the patient's condition. Review the indications, contraindications, uses, and limitations of the various systems.

BIBLIOGRAPHY

Adams DA: Humidity and aerosol therapy. In Wyka KA, Mathews PJ, Clark WF, editors: *Foundations of respiratory care,* Albany, NY, 2002, Delmar.

American Association for Respiratory Care: Aerosol consensus statement, *Respir Care* 36:916, 1991.

American Association for Respiratory Care: Clinical practice guideline: selection of aerosol delivery device, *Respir Care* 37:891, 1992.

American Association for Respiratory Care: Clinical practice guideline: selection of aerosol delivery device for neonatal and pediatric patients, *Respir Care* 40:1325, 1995.

American Association for Respiratory Care: Clinical practice guideline: bland aerosol administration, *Respir Care* 38:1196, 1993.

American Association for Respiratory Care: Clinical practice guideline: bland aerosol administration–2003 revision & update, *Respir Care* 48:529, 2003.

American Association for Respiratory Care: Clinical practice guideline: delivery of aerosols to the upper airway, *Respir Care* 39(8):803, 1994.

Barnes TA, editor: *Core textbook of respiratory care practice,* ed 2, St Louis, 1994, Mosby.

Branson RD, Hess DR, Chatburn RL, editors: *Respiratory care equipment,* ed 2, Philadelphia, 1999, Lippincott Williams & Wilkins.

Fink JB: Humidity. In Fink JB, Hunt GE, editors: *Clinical practice in respiratory care,* Philadelphia, 1999, Lippincott-Raven.

Fink JB, Dhand R: Aerosol drug therapy. In Fink JB, Hunt GE, editors: *Clinical practice in respiratory care,* Philadelphia, 1999, Lippincott-Raven.

Fink JB, Hess DR: Humidity and aerosol therapy. In Hess DR, MacIntyre NR, Mishoe SC, et al, editors: *Respiratory care principles and practices,* Philadelphia, 2002, WB Saunders.

Fink JB, Scanlan CL: Aerosol drug therapy. In Scanlan CL, Wilkins RL, Stoller JK, editors: *Egan's fundamentals of respiratory care,* ed 7, St Louis, 1999, Mosby.

Fink JB: Humidity and bland aerosol therapy. In Wilkins RL, Stoller JK, Scanlan CL, editors: *Egan's fundamentals of respiratory care,* ed 8, St Louis, 2003, Mosby.

Hess D: The delivery of aerosolized bronchodilator to mechanically ventilated intubated adult patients, *Respir Care* 35:399, 1990.

Hess D: Aerosol therapy. In Dantzker DR, MacIntyre NR, Bakow ED, editors: *Comprehensive respiratory care,* Philadelphia, 1995, WB Saunders.

Rau JL Jr: *Respiratory care pharmacology,* ed 5, St Louis, 1998, Mosby.

Shapiro BA, Kacmarek RM, Cane RD, et al, editors: *Clinical application of respiratory care,* ed 4, St Louis, 1991, Mosby.

Ward JJ, Hess D, Helmholz HF Jr: Humidity and aerosol therapy. In Burton GC, Hodgkin JE, Ward JJ, editors: *Respiratory care: a guide to clinical practice,* ed 4, Philadelphia, 1997, Lippincott-Raven.

Whitaker K: *Comprehensive perinatal and pediatric respiratory care,* ed 2, Albany, NY, 1997, Delmar.

White GC: *Equipment theory for respiratory care,* ed 3, Albany, NY, 1999, Delmar.

Wissing DR: Humidity and aerosol therapy. In Cairo JM, Pilbeam SP, editors: *Mosby's respiratory care equipment,* ed 7, St. Louis, 2004, Mosby.

SELF-STUDY QUESTIONS

1. Ten minutes into a handheld nebulizer treatment to deliver albuterol (Proventil), the patient complains of dizziness and tingling fingers. What should be done?
   A. Advise the patient to breathe in the same pattern.
   B. Change the medication.
   C. Tell the patient to breathe more slowly.
   D. Advise the patient to breathe deeper and faster.

2. An adult patient is receiving 40% oxygen by way of a heated large volume nebulizer to a face mask. While making equipment rounds, the therapist notices that puffs of aerosol are coming into the patient's face mask. What could be causing this?
   A. Water has collected in the aerosol tubing.
   B. The nebulizer should have water added to it.
   C. The nebulizer has too much water in its reservoir.
   D. The puffs of aerosol are caused by the patient's breathing pattern.

3. The physician wants more aerosol inside the mist tent of a 3-year-old child. What would be the best way to do this?
   A. Cut a hole in the top of the tent.
   B. Close the hole on the top of the tent.
   C. Lower the temperature on the refrigeration unit.
   D. Increase the gas flow to the nebulizer.

4. An entry level respiratory therapist calls you when he has analyzed 40% oxygen for an infant inside an oxygen tent. This is despite his attempt to get the ordered 50% oxygen by setting the nebulizer's entrainment port at 60% and the oxygen blender to the nebulizer at 50%. What would you recommend?
   A. Increase the flow by 5 L/min.
   B. Set the blender to 100%.

   C. Check the accuracy of the oxygen analyzer.
   D. Set the entrainment port on the nebulizer to 100%.

5. A humidity or aerosol system delivering body temperature gas is used in all the following situations *except*:
   A. Patient with a tracheostomy
   B. Twenty-month-old infant with laryngotracheobronchitis
   C. Chronic obstructive pulmonary disease patient with thick secretions
   D. Newborn receiving oxygen inside an oxygen hood

6. A T-piece is being used to deliver 40% oxygen and heated aerosol to the tracheostomy tube of an adult patient. While checking the patient's pulse oximeter reading, you notice that it is only 88%, and with each inspiration the aerosol cannot be seen coming from the end of the T-piece. What action would you recommend?
   I. Increase the oxygen flow to the nebulizer.
   II. Increase the delivered oxygen to 45%.
   III. Increase the temperature to the heated aerosol system.
   IV. Add 100 mL of aerosol tubing to the open end of the T-piece.
   V. Change the patient to a tracheostomy mask.
   A. I and II
   B. I and IV
   C. III and IV
   D. II and V

7. When doing patient rounds, you notice that very little aerosol is going to a new patient's tracheostomy mask. Which of the following could be the problem?

I. The water level is above the refill line on the nebulizer's reservoir jar.

II. The nebulizer is not tightly screwed into the DISS connector on the flowmeter.

III. The nebulizer jet is obstructed.

IV. The water level is below the refill line on the nebulizer's reservoir jar.

V. The capillary tube is obstructed.
A. II, III, IV, and V
B. I and II
C. III and IV
D. III and V

ANSWER KEY

1. **C.** Rationale: The patient's signs and symptoms indicate hyperventilation. The easiest way to correct this situation is to have the patient breathe more slowly (and/or less deeply). If the patient continues to breathe in the same pattern, the hyperventilation will continue. Although albuterol may cause tachycardia, it is unlikely to cause dizziness and tingling fingers in the patient. If the patient is advised to breathe deeper and faster, the hyperventilation will get worse.

2. **A.** Rationale: Condensation forms when a heated aerosol cools as it goes through aerosol tubing. This condensed water will accumulate at the low point in the tubing. The force of gas coming through the tubing makes the water flow back and forth. This results in the puffs of aerosol seen coming from the patient's aerosol mask. Neither the water level in the nebulizer reservoir nor the patient's breathing pattern will cause puffs of aerosol.

3. **D.** Rationale: Increasing the gas flow on the nebulizer will increase the total amount of water that is nebulized and delivered to the mist tent. Mist tents are supposed to have a hole at the top of the tent canopy to allow the excess gas and aerosol to exit. Only oxygen tents, not mist tents, have the hole closed on the top of the tent canopy. This is to ensure that the oxygen tent has the highest possible oxygen percentage. Remember, a mist tent does not deliver supplemental oxygen. Lowering the temperature on the refrigeration unit will further cool the infant but will not affect the amount of aerosol delivered into the mist tent.

4. **D.** Rationale: It is necessary to set the entrainment ports on the nebulizer to 100% source gas (50% blended oxygen) to prevent room air from being entrained. This way only 50% oxygen will power the nebulizer and be delivered into the oxygen tent. Increasing the flow to the nebulizer by 5 L/min will increase the flow through the nebulizer to increase aerosol production but will not change the oxygen percentage. Setting the blender to 100% oxygen will not close the air-entrainment ports on the nebulizer. Therefore 60% oxygen will be delivered into the tent, not the ordered 50%. No indication is found that the oxygen analyzer is inaccurate. The problem is an incorrect equipment setup.

5. **B.** Rationale: An infant with laryngotracheobronchitis (LTB or croup) is usually best managed with a *cool*, bland aerosol. This helps to reduce the swelling in the large airways. Body temperature aerosol is delivered to a patient with a tracheostomy, thick (viscous) secretions, or a newborn in an oxygen hood to minimize the patient's humidity deficit.

6. **B.** Rationale: Increasing the oxygen flow to the nebulizer will better match the patient's inspired tidal volume. Adding 100 mL of aerosol tubing to the open end of the T-piece will act as a reservoir to help to make sure that the patient inhales only 40% oxygen from the nebulizer. Enough flow and reservoir tubing should be used to make sure that aerosol can be seen exiting the end of the reservoir tubing during inspiration. This ensures that only humidified 40% oxygen is inhaled. No order is needed to increase the delivered oxygen to 45% if these items are done. The patient's pulse oximeter reading is 88% because room air is being inhaled to dilute the set 40% oxygen. Increasing the temperature to the heated aerosol system will not affect the inspired oxygen percentage. No need is seen to change the patient to a tracheostomy mask. It will not ensure that the patient gets 40% oxygen because it is an open system, and the patient can inhale room air.

7. **A.** Rationale: Any of the following will result in less or no aerosol being delivered: (1) If the nebulizer is not tightly screwed into the DISS connector on the flowmeter, the gas will leak and not go through the nebulizer. (2) If the nebulizer jet is obstructed, no aerosol will be created. (3) If the water level is *below* the refill line on the nebulizer's reservoir jar, no water will be drawn up the capillary tube to the jet and baffle; therefore no aerosol will be created. (4) If the capillary tube is obstructed, the water in the reservoir jar will not be drawn up to the jet and baffle. However, if the water level is *above* the refill line on the nebulizer's reservoir jar water, water will be drawn up the capillary tube to the jet and baffle. Aerosol will be generated if everything else is functioning normally.

9 Pharmacology

Note 1: The National Board for Respiratory Care (NBRC) has released the *RRT Examination Matrix* (covering the testable items on the Written Registry Exam) and the *CSE Examination Matrix* (covering the testable items on the Clinical Simulation Exam). Turn to the appendices at the back of this book for both publications in their original formats. This book is intended to cover all of the testable items in these two publications. This chapter (and all others) uses the abbreviation "WRE" for the coded items testable on the Written Registry Exam *and* Clinical Simulation Exam. The listed difficulty (R, Recall; Ap, Application; An, Analysis) relates to the question difficulty on the Written Registry Exam. The abbreviation "CSE" is used for the coded items testable on *only* the Clinical Simulation Exam. Because no question difficulty level is given for this exam, be prepared for anything.

Note 2: A review of the most recent Written Registry Examinations has shown an average of six questions (6% of the exam) that cover pharmacology. The Clinical Simulation Exam is comprehensive and may include everything that should be known or performed by an advanced level respiratory therapist.

MODULE A
Recommend or administer medications

1. Bronchodilators

The bronchodilators are medications designed to relax the bronchial smooth muscles so that the airways dilate, airway resistance is reduced, and breathing is easier. The first two classes of medications in this group are widely given by respiratory therapists.

a. Inhaled adrenergic (sympathomimetic) agents
1. Recommend their use (WRE code: IIIG4a) [Difficulty: An]
2. Administer the prescribed medication (WRE code: IIIC3, IIID4a) [Difficulty: An]

This group of medications is often called *catecholamines, sympathomimetic amines, sympathomimetic bronchodilators,* or *β (beta)-adrenergic bronchodilators.* They have the effect of stimulating the body's sympathetic nerves, which results in bronchodilation and other effects. Patients with asthma are most effectively treated with drugs from this group.

A brief review of the autonomic nervous system helps in understanding how these medications (and the following group of medications) work and some side effects that may occur. The autonomic nervous system is not under voluntary control. It is an automatic system designed to regulate metabolism and the vital signs. This system is made up of two branches: the sympathetic nervous system and the parasympathetic nervous system. The lungs, heart, and most other organs are innervated by both branches. The blood vessels in the mucous membranes are innervated only by the sympathetic branch. The parasympathetic nervous system is usually dominant and keeps the body functioning normally. The sympathetic nervous system is an "emergency" system that is dominant during great stress (sometimes called the "fight or flight" system). Adrenaline (or epinephrine) is released by the adrenal glands in these emergencies. Adrenaline causes a number of effects, including one that many respiratory patients need: bronchodilation. The sympathetic nervous system has the following three types of receptors that are located in different organs and are affected by adrenaline and related medications:

a. α_1-Receptors are located in the blood vessels of the mucous membranes (other tissues are not included in this discussion). Vasoconstriction results when α_1-receptors are stimulated.
b. β_1-Receptors are located in the heart. Tachycardia, increased stroke volume, and possibly arrhythmias result when β_1-receptors are stimulated.
c. β_2-Receptors are located in the airways. Bronchodilation results when β_2-receptors are stimulated.

Aerosolized sympathomimetic bronchodilators are usually recommended under one of the three following situations:

Acute bronchospasm with severe shortness of breath. This patient needs rapid relief. Recommend a fast-acting medication such as albuterol. The current asthma-management guidelines list albuterol and similar medications as "rescue" agents. When the patient is recovered, a medication listed as a "controller" agent should be prescribed. Table 9-1 lists the peak onset times and duration for the

TABLE 9-1 Inhaled Adrenergic Bronchodilator Agents Currently Available in the United States

Drug	Brand Name	Receptor Preference	Adult Dosage	Time Course (Onset, Peak, Duration)
Albuterol	Proventil, Proventil HFA, Ventolin	β_2	SVN: 0.5% solution, 0.5 ml (2.5 mg) tid, qid MDI: 90 μg/puff, 2 puffs tid, qid DPI: 200 μg capsule, 1 capsule q4-6h Tab: 2 mg, 4 mg tid, qid Syrup: 2 mg/5 mL, 1-2 tsp tid, qid	*Onset:* 15 min *Peak:* 30-60 min *Duration:* 5-8 hr
Bitolterol	Tornalate	β_2	SVN: 0.2% solution, 1.25 mL (2.5 mg) bid-qid MDI: 370 μg/puff, 2 puffs q8h	*Onset:* 3-4 min *Peak:* 30-60 min *Duration:* 5-8 hr
Epinephrine	Adrenalin Cl	α, β	SVN: 1% solution (1:100), 0.25-0.5 mL (2.5-5.0 mg) qid MDI: 0.2 mg/puff, puffs as ordered or needed	*Onset:* 3-5 min *Peak:* 5-20 min *Duration:* 1-3 hr
Formoterol	Foradil	β_2	DPI: 12 μg/inhalation bid	*Onset:* 15 min *Peak:* 30-60 min *Duration:* 12 hr
Isoetharine	Isoetharine HCl	β_2	SVN: 1% solution, 0.25-0.5 mL (2.5-5.0 mg) qid	*Onset:* 1-6 min *Peak:* 15-60 min *Duration:* 1-3 hr
Isoproterenol	Isuprel, Isuprel Mistometer	β	SVN: 0.5% solution (1:200), 0.25-0.5 mL (1.25-2.5 mg) qid MDI: 103 μg/puff, 2 puffs qid	*Onset:* 2-5 min *Peak:* 5-30 min *Duration:* 0.5-2 hr
Levalbuterol	Xopenex Xopenex HFA	β_2	SVN: 0.31 mg/3 mL tid; 0.63 mg/3 mL tid; or 1.25 mg/3 mL tid MDI: 45 μg/puff, 2 puffs q4-6h, ≥ 4 yrs old	*Onset:* 15 min *Peak:* 30-60 min *Duration:* 5-8 hr
Metaproterenol	Alupent	β_2	SVN: 5% solution, 0.3 mL (15 mg) tid, qid MDI: 650 μg/puff, 2-3 puffs tid, qid Tab: 10 or 20 mg, 20 mg tid, qid Syrup: 10 mg/5 mL, 2 tsp tid, qid	*Onset:* 1-5 min *Peak:* 60 min *Duration:* 2-6 hr
Pirbuterol	Maxair	β_2	MDI: 200 μg/puff, 2 puffs q4-6h	*Onset:* 5 min *Peak:* 30 min *Duration:* 5 hr
Racemic epinephrine	MicroNefrin, AsthmaNefrin	α, β	SVN: 2.25% solution, 0.25-0.5 mL (5.63-11.25 mg) qid	*Onset:* 3-5 min *Peak:* 5-20 min *Duration:* 0.5-2 hr
Salmeterol	Serevent	β_2	MDI: 25 μg/puff, 2 puffs bid DPI: 50 μg/blister bid	*Onset:* 20 min *Peak:* 3-5 hr *Duration:* 12 hr
Terbutaline	Brethaire	β_2	MDI: 200 μg/puff, 2 puffs q4-6h Tab: 2.5 or 5 mg, 5 mg q6h Inj: 1 mg/mL, 0.25 mg SC	*Onset:* 5-30 min *Peak:* 30-60 min *Duration:* 3-6 hr

DPI, Dry powder inhaler; MDI, metered dose inhaler; SVN, small volume nebulizer.
Modified from Rau JL Jr: *Respiratory care pharmacology,* ed 6, St Louis, 2002, Mosby.

various medications. Avoid drugs with unnecessary α_1 and β_1 effects or long onset and peak times.

Chronic but stable bronchospasm with moderate shortness of breath. These patients need a dependable medication of longer duration such as salmeterol or formoterol. They are considered to be controller agents with a long onset time and a duration of up to 12 hours. It is very important

that the patient also have a prescription for a fast-acting drug in case of sudden bronchospasm. Several newer medications also come in both oral and aerosol preparations. The oral forms are especially helpful when taken in the evening to help the patient get a good night's sleep. Table 9-1 lists information on the administration method, strength, and dosages.

Laryngeal edema or bleeding from a bronchoscopy biopsy site. The laryngeal edema problem requires the administration of a medication that reduces the swelling of the mucous membrane of the larynx and epiglottis. If bleeding results from a biopsy during a bronchoscopy, the cut blood vessels must be made to constrict and to form clots. In both cases, racemic epinephrine (MicroNefrin, AsthmaNefrin) is the medication of choice because it stimulates α_1 receptors. This results in vasoconstriction of the mucosal and deeper blood vessels. Therefore the laryngeal edema swelling is reduced, and biopsy bleeding stops.

Most of the medications listed in this section are chemically derived from adrenaline. They are somewhat different in their structures so that the desired effects and side (unwanted) effects vary. Box 9-1 lists the side effects of the sympathomimetic bronchodilators. Clinically, the most dangerous of these side effects are palpitations, tachycardia, and hypertension.

Exam Hint

Recommend a fast-onset medication (albuterol, Proventil, Ventolin; levalbuterol, Xopenex) to treat a patient with acute bronchospasm. Recommend a long-duration medication (salmeterol, Serevent or formoterol, Foradil) to treat a patient with chronic bronchospasm. Recommend a vasoconstricting medication (racemic epinephrine, MicroNefrin, AsthmaNefrin) to treat airway edema or bleeding.

Exam Hint

The NBRC rarely asks questions with specific drug doses. However, the following drug doses should be known. The standard adult dose of albuterol (Proventil) for a small volume nebulizer (SVN) is 0.5 mL (2.5 mg), three or four times a day. The standard adult dose of levalbuterol (Xopenex) for an SVN is 1.25 mg, three times a day.

---

b. Inhaled anticholinergic (parasympatholytic) agents
1. Recommend their use (WRE code: IIIG4a) [Difficulty: An]
2. Administer the prescribed medication (WRE code: IIID4a) [Difficulty: An]

This group of medications works to promote bronchodilation by suppressing the action of the parasympathetic nervous system. This results in the sympathetic nervous system dominating and causing bronchial smooth

---

BOX 9-1 Clinically Observed Side Effects of Sympathomimetic Aerosolized Bronchodilators from the Most Commonly Seen to the Least Commonly Seen

Tremor: gentle, uncontrollable, involuntary muscle shaking
Palpitations and tachycardia: irregular heartbeats and fast heart rate
Headache
Increased blood pressure: possibly from both the α-1 effect on blood vessels and tachycardia
Nervousness and irritability
Dizziness
Nausea
Decreased Pao_2 level from a worsening of the ventilation/perfusion ratio

Pao_2, Partial pressure of O_2 in arterial blood.

---

muscle relaxation. The parasympatholytic (anticholinergic) group has been found to be more effective in helping patients with chronic obstructive pulmonary disease (COPD) (e.g., emphysema, chronic bronchitis) than in helping patients with asthma. However, it is often best to treat COPD and asthma patients with medications from both the sympathomimetic and parasympatholytic groups. Combivent and DuoNeb combine a sympathomimetic and a parasympatholytic medication. The newest drug in this group, tiotropium bromide (Spiriva), provides the patient with 24 hours of medication effect. See Table 9-2 for information on the parasympatholytic medications.

c. Recommend a theophylline agent (WRE code: IIIG4a) [Difficulty: An]

The family of drugs called xanthines includes theophylline and caffeine. They have been used in a variety of situations. A theophylline agent (Aminophylline, Elixophyllin, Theo-Dur, etc.) is sometimes used to aid the breathing of a status asthmaticus patient or a patient with moderate to severe COPD. Current guidelines indicate that theophylline agents should be given to these patients only if optimal doses of inhaled bronchodilators and corticosteroid drugs have not been able to manage the patient's problem. Then intravenous theophylline ethylenediamine (Aminophylline) can be given. However, it should be used with caution. It is very difficult to regulate the proper serum level, and serious side effects have been seen with it.

Caffeine citrate (Cafcit) has been approved for oral or intravenous administration to a neonate with apnea of prematurity. It has been shown to stimulate the breathing of these neonates.

TABLE 9-2	Inhaled Anticholinergic Bronchodilator Agents			
Drug	Brand Name	Adult Dosage		Time Course (Onset, Peak, Duration)
Ipratropium bromide	Atrovent	MDI: 18 µg/puff, 2 puffs qid SVN: 0.02% solution (0.2 mg/mL), 500 µg tid, qid Nasal spray: 0.03%, 0.06%; 2 sprays per nostril 2 to 4 times daily (dosage varies)		*Onset*: 15 min *Peak*: 1–2 hr *Duration*: 4–6 hr
Ipratropium bromide and albuterol	Combivent	MDI: ipratropium 18 µg/puff and albuterol 90 µg/puff, 2 puffs qid		*Onset*: 15 min *Peak*: 1–2 hr *Duration*: 4–6 hr
	DuoNeb	SVN: ipratropium 0.5 mg and albuterol 3.0 mg (equal to 2.5 mg albuterol base)		
Tiotropium bromide	Spiriva	DPI: 18 µg/inhalation, 1 inhalation daily		*Onset*: 30 min *Peak*: 3 hr *Duration*: 24 hr

DPI, Dry powder inhaler; MDI, metered dose inhaler; SVN, small volume nebulizer.
A holding chamber is recommended with MDI administration to prevent accidental eye exposure.
Modified from Rau JL Jr: *Respiratory care pharmacology*, ed 6, St Louis, 2002, Mosby.

2. Antiinflammatory agents

a. Recommend use of nonsteroidal antiinflammatory drugs (WRE code: IIIG4b) [Difficulty: An]

Nonsteroidal antiinflammatory drugs (NSAIDs) include several different types of over-the-counter medications. None is as powerful an antiinflammatory as the corticosteroid drugs. Note the other clinical uses of acetylsalicylic acid and ibuprofen.

1. Acetylsalicylic acid (Bayer aspirin, etc.): antiinflammatory, mild analgesia, antipyretic, blocks platelet formation
2. Ibuprofen (Advil, Motrin): antiinflammatory, mild analgesia, antipyretic
3. Antihistamine (Claritin): antiinflammatory

b. Inhaled corticosteroids

1. **Recommend use of corticosteroids (WRE code: IIIG4b) [Difficulty: An]**
2. **Administer the prescribed medication (WRE code: IIIC3, IIID4a) [Difficulty: An]**

Corticosteroids affect the respiratory system in two ways: they potentiate the effects of the sympathomimetic agents, and they stop the inflammatory response seen in the airways of asthmatic patients after exposure to an allergen. This prevents mucosal edema from developing. The patient with chronic airflow obstruction, such as asthma or asthmatic bronchitis, should be given inhaled corticosteroids. When they are used as directed, little systemic (bodily) absorption occurs. Table 9-3 shows specific strength and dosage information for the inhaled corticosteroids. The patient who is using any of these medications must gargle and rinse out his or her mouth after each use. If not, the patient runs the risk of developing a fungal infection of the mouth and throat.

The patient who is diagnosed with status asthmaticus should have systemic corticosteroids promptly given by the intravenous (IV) route. Examples of commonly used systemic corticosteroids include methylprednisolone (Medrol and Solu-Medrol), prednisone (Deltasone), prednisolone (Meticortelone and Delta-Cortef), cortisone (Cortone), and hydrocortisone (Cortef and Solu-Cortef). These drugs can be lifesavers if used properly. However, prolonged use of large oral or IV doses can lead to serious systemic complications such as immunosuppression and adrenal gland insufficiency. If a patient has been taking systemic corticosteroids for an extended time, he or she should be gradually weaned from them after an inhaled corticosteroid has been started. It is dangerous to suddenly stop an oral or intravenous corticosteroid that has been used for a prolonged time.

3. Nonsteroidal antiasthma agents

a. Recommend the use of cromolyn sodium (WRE code: IIIG4b) [Difficulty: An]

Cromolyn sodium (Intal) is indicated to prevent an asthma attack. It does this by coating the mast cells found in the airways so that they do not rupture. Without cromolyn sodium, the mast cells of asthmatic patients would rupture when they are exposed to immunoglobin E (IgE) from their allergen(s). This mast cell rupture would result in the spilling of leukotriene agents, histamine, and other chemical mediators that cause the bronchospasm, airway edema, and increased airway secretions of an asthma attack. When cromolyn

TABLE 9-3	Corticosteroids Available by Aerosol for Oral Inhalation*	
Drug	**Brand Name**	**Formulation and Dosage**
Beclomethasone dipropionate	Beclovent, Vanceril	MDI:42 µg/puff Adults: 2 puffs tid or qid Children: 1–2 puffs tid or qid
	Vanceril 84µg Double Strength	MDI: 84 µg/puff Adults and children ≥ 6 yr: 2 inhalations bid
Beclomethasone dipropionate HFA	QVAR	MDI: 40µg/puff and 80µg/puff Adults ≥ 12 yr: 40 to 80 µg twice daily,† or 40 to 160 µg twice daily‡
Budesonide	Pulmicort Turbuhaler	DPI: 200 µg/actuation Adults: 200–400 µg bid,† 200–400 µg bid,‡ 400–800 µg bid¶ Children ≥ 6 yr: 200 µg bid
	Pulmicort Respules	SVN: 0.25 mg/2 mL, 0.5 mg/2 mL Children 1 to 8 yr: 0.5 mg total dose given once daily, or twice daily in divided doses†,‡; 1 mg given as 0.5 mg bid or once daily¶
Flunisolide	AeroBid, AeroBid-M	MDI: 250 µg/puff Adults: 2 puffs bid Children: 2 puffs bid
Fluticasone propionate	Flovent	MDI: 44 µg/puff, 110 µg/puff, 220 µg/puff Adults ≥ 12 yr: 88 µg bid,† 88–220 µg bid,‡ or 880 µg bid¶
	Flovent Rotadisk	DPI: 50 µg, 100 µg, 250 µg Adults: 100 µg bid,† 100–250 µg bid,‡ 1000 µg bid¶ Children 4–11 yr; 50 µg twice daily
Fluticasone propionate/ salmeterol	Advair Diskus	DPI: 100 µg fluticasone/50 µg salmeterol, 250 µg fluticasone/50 µg salmeterol, or 500 µg fluticasone/ 50 µg salmeterol Adults and children ≥ 12 yr: 100 µg fluticasone/50 µg salmeterol, 1 inhalation twice daily, about 12 hours apart (starting dose if not currently on inhaled corticosteroids) Maximum recommended dose is 500 µg fluticasone/50 µg salmeterol twice daily
Mometasone furoate	Asmanex	DPI: 220 µg mg‡ actuation Adults and children ≥ 12 yr: 1–2 inhalations/day
Triamcinolone acetonide	Azmacort	MDI: 100 µg/puff Adults: 2 puffs tid or qid Children: 1–2 puffs tid or qid

*Individual agents are discussed subsequently in a separate section. Detailed information on each agent should be obtained from manufacturer's drug insert.
†Recommended starting dose if on bronchodilators alone.
‡Recommended starting dose if on inhaled corticosteroids previously.
¶Recommended starting dose if on oral corticosteroids previously.
Modified from Rau JL Jr: *Respiratory care pharmacology,* ed 6, St Louis, 2002, Mosby.

sodium, or nedrocromil sodium, is inhaled at least a week before exposure to the allergen, the asthmatic reaction is prevented or reduced. Cromolyn was first made available through a dry powder inhaler and is now available by metered dose inhaler or SVN. Nedrocromol sodium (Tilade) is similar to cromolyn in its use and effects. It is available in a metered dose inhaler. See Table 9-4 for detailed information on both medications.

It is very important to understand that both drugs are taken for prophylactic purposes to prevent an asthma attack. They are contraindicated during an asthma attack. A patient experiencing acute bronchospasm should be treated with a fast sympathomimetic bronchodilator, as previously discussed.

b. Recommend the use of leukotriene modifiers (WRE code: IIIG4b [Difficulty: An]

Leukotrienes are chemicals found in mast cells that are released during an asthma attack. These released leukotriene chemicals stimulate bronchospasm, airway edema, and increased airway secretions. The leukotriene-modifier medications work to reduce the number of leukotriene chemicals that are released or block the effect of leukotrienes on the airways. By doing this, the patient's asthma symptoms are reduced or eliminated. See Table 9-4 for detailed information on all four medications in this group.

As with cromolyn sodium, it is very important to understand that all of these drugs are taken for prophylactic

TABLE 9-4 Nonsteroidal Antiasthma Medications, with Brand and Generic Names, Formulations, and Usual Recommended Dosages*

Drug	Brand Name	Formulation and Dosage
CROMOLYN-LIKE (MAST CELL STABILIZERS)		
Cromolyn sodium†	Intal	MDI: 800 µg/actuation
		Adults and children ≥ 5 yr: 2 inhalations 4 times daily
		SVN: 20 mg/amp or 20 mg/vial
		Adults and children ≥ 2 yr: 20 mg inhaled 4 times daily
	Nasalcrom	Spray: 40 mg/mL (4%)
		Adults and children ≥ 6 yr: 1 spray each nostril, 3-6 times daily every 4-6 hr
Nedocromil sodium	Tilade	MDI: 1.75 mg/actuation
		Adults and children ≥ 12 yr: 2 inhalations 4 times daily
ANTI-LEUKOTRIENES		
Montelukast	Singulair	Tablets: 10 mg, 4 mg, and 5 mg cherry-flavored chewable
		Adults and children ≥ 15 yr: one 10 mg tab each evening
		Children 6-14 yr: one 5 mg chewable tablet each evening
		Children 2-5 years: one 4 mg chewable tablet each evening
Omalizumab	Xolair	Adults and children ≥ 12 years: subcutaneous injection every 4 weeks at 150 to 300 mg per dose; or subcutaneous injection every 2 weeks at 225, 300, or 375 mg per dose. Doses of more than 150 mg should be divided among more than one injection site.
Zafirlukast	Accolate	Tablets: 20 mg
		Adults and children ≥ 12 yr: 20 mg (1 tab) twice daily, without food
Zileuton	Zyflo	Tablets: 600 mg
		Adults and children ≥ 12 yr: one 600 mg tablet 4 times a day

*Detailed prescribing information should be obtained from the manufacturer's package insert.
†Note: Cromolyn sodium is also available in an oral concentrate giving 100 mg in 5 mL (Gastrocrom), for treatment of systemic mastocytosis, and as an ophthalmic 4% solution (Opticrom, 40 mg/mL) for treatment of vernal keratoconjunctivitis.
Modified from Rau JL Jr: *Respiratory care pharmacology*, ed 6, St Louis, 2002, Mosby.

purposes to prevent an asthma attack. They are contraindicated *during* an asthma attack. A patient experiencing acute bronchospasm should be treated with a fast sympathomimetic bronchodilator, as previously discussed.

4. Mucolytics or proteolytic agents

a. Recommend the use of mucolytics or proteolytic agents (WRE code: IIIG4c) [Difficulty: An]

b. Administer the prescribed medication (WRE code: IIIC3, IIID4a) [Difficulty: An]

Acetylcysteine (Mucomyst) is a mucolytic drug that has been widely used with patients who have thick (viscous) mucus or mucus plugs. Its bad odor (rotten eggs) may lead to nausea and vomiting in some patients. Of greater concern is the stimulation of bronchospasm in some asthmatic patients. Therefore it is often wise either to pretreat the patient with an aerosolized sympathomimetic bronchodilator or to mix one with the acetylcysteine before it is nebulized for the patient. Any fast onset bronchodilator can be used in the usual dose. Mucomyst is usually administered with a handheld nebulizer or with

intermittent positive-pressure breathing (IPPB). Most adult patients are given 3 to 5 mL of the 20% solution or 6 to 10 mL of the 10% solution. The 20% solution is often diluted with an equal volume of normal saline solution. Direct instillation of 1 to 2 mL of the drug into the trachea also helps to liquefy secretions. The manufacturer recommends that all medication in a vial be used within 96 hours or discarded. It should be stored in the refrigerator. A slightly purple color is commonly seen after the vial has been opened, but it can still be used safely.

Dornase alfa (Pulmozyme; The NBRC refers to this drug as recombinant human deoxyribonuclease [RhDNAse].) is a proteolytic drug that has been approved for use in the treatment of patients with cystic fibrosis. It works by breaking up strands of DNA found in the secretions of these patients with a pulmonary infection. Usually a single daily dose of 2.5 mL of solution (containing 2.5 mg of dornase alfa) is inhaled by SVN. Store the drug in a refrigerator, and protect it from strong light. It has no serious side effects. See Table 9-5 for detailed information on Mucomyst, Pulmozyme, and the saline solutions (discussed subsequently).

TABLE 9-5 Mucoactive Agents Available for Aerosol Administration

Drug	Brand Name	Adult Dosage	Use
Acetylcysteine 10%	Mucomyst	SVN: 3–5 mL	Bronchitis; efficacy not proven
Acetylcysteine 20%	Mucosil-10		
Aqueous aerosols: water,	N/A	SVN: 3–5 mL	
saline (0.45%, 0.9%,		SVN: 3–5 mL, as ordered	Sputum induction, secretion
5%–10%)		USN: 3–5 mL, as ordered	mobilization
Dornase alfa	Pulmozyme	SVN: 2.5 mg/ampule one ampule daily*	Cystic fibrosis
Mucosil-20	Mucomyst		

*Use recommended nebulizer system (see package insert).
N/A, Not applicable; SVN, small volume nebulizer; USN, ultrasonic nebulizer.
From Rau JL Jr: *Respiratory care pharmacology,* ed 6, St Louis, 2002, Mosby.

5. Saline solutions
a. Recommend the use of saline solutions (WRE code: IIIG4c) [Difficulty: An]
b. Administer the prescribed medication (WRE code: IIIC3) [Difficulty: An]

The various saline solutions (and sterile water) are known collectively as "bland" aerosols, because they have no direct pharmacologic effect on the lungs and airways. When they are inhaled as aerosols, however, a vagal nerve mediated reflex causes the bronchial/sub-mucosal glands to release more watery secretions. Therefore a saline aerosol is commonly used to help liquefy secretions and induce a patient to cough out sputum. See Table 9-5 and Box 9-2 for information on the various saline solutions.

6. Recommend the use of diuretic agents (WRE code: IIIG4f) [Difficulty: An]

Diuretics are most commonly indicated in patients with edema or hypertension. Edema is usually a result of heart failure or fluid overload. Examples of diuretics used to treat these problems follow:

a. Furosemide (Lasix)
b. Ethacrynic acid (Edecrin)
c. Chlorothiazide (Diuril)

These are some of the most powerful diuretics in use. They produce a rapid increase in urine output. They basically prevent the kidneys from retaining sodium so that water is excreted. A side effect of their use is a loss of potassium through the kidneys.

Another category of diuretic is used in patients who have an increased intracranial pressure (ICP). The increased ICP is usually due to cerebral edema from a head injury. Examples of medications used to treat an increased ICP include the following:

a. Mannitol (Osmitrol)
b. Sterile urea (Ureaphil, Urevert)

These medications have a large molecular weight and, through osmosis, "pull" fluid from the brain into the bloodstream. Therefore they are sometimes called *osmotic*

diuretics. The medication, after crossing into the kidney, prevents the reabsorption of water and increases urine output.

> **Exam Hint**
>
> A diuretic drug such as furosemide (Lasix) tends to cause the loss of potassium through the kidneys. Know to check the serum potassium level. Remember that the normal potassium level is 3.5 to 5.5 mEq/L. If the patient has the signs of dangerous hypokalemia (see Chapter 1), know to recommend that replacement potassium be given.

7. Recommend the use of sedative agents (WRE code: IIIG4d) [Difficulty: An]

Sedatives are medications that affect the brain to induce calming in a patient who can be either simply anxious or very agitated and uncooperative. A patient would be given a sedative in the following situations: (1) when he or she is struggling against a necessary intubation or the mechanical ventilator, thus worsening his or her condition; (2) when he or she is displaying self-destructive behavior because of a drug reaction; and (3) before a medical procedure, for so-called conscious sedation. The effects on the patient are dose related. Low to moderate doses calm the patient, and higher doses induce sleep. Three different groupings of these types of medications exist. The most widely used are the benzodiazepines, because they have fewer side effects, fewer drug interactions, and are less likely to cause addiction than are the barbiturate drugs. The benzodiazepine agents can be pharmacologically reversed. The barbiturates are widely used during general anesthesia to induce sleep rapidly. Commonly used examples of the sedative agents include the following:

a. Benzodiazepine minor tranquilizers: midazolam (Versed), diazepam (Valium), chlordiazepoxide (Librium), alprazolam (Xanax), triazolam (Halcion), flurazepam (Dalmane)

BOX 9-2   Saline Solutions Used as Mucolytics

NORMAL SALINE SOLUTION, 0.9% SALINE
Direct instillation into the airway:
   Infants may be given about 1 mL several times before suctioning.
   Adults may be given about 3-5 mL several times daily before suctioning.
Aerosol: most medication nebulizers hold 3-5 mL that is nebulized several times daily.
Miscellaneous:
   Usually is well tolerated because it is isotonic to the body.
   Particle size is fairly stable as nebulized.

HYPOTONIC SALINE SOLUTION, 0.45% SALINE
Direct instillation into the airway: same as with normal saline solution.
Aerosol: same as with normal saline solution; many practitioners use this concentration in ultrasonic nebulizers.
Miscellaneous: particles tend to shrink because of evaporation, which results in smaller particles than nebulized that are closer to
   isotonic; impaction is more likely in the smaller airways.

HYPERTONIC SALINE SOLUTION, 1.8%-20% SALINE
Aerosol: some practitioners use a large-reservoir nebulizer with a heater to generate the aerosol.
   Hypertonic saline solution is most commonly used to induce a cough and sputum sample for cytology (lung cancer) or fungal or
   mycobacteria (tuberculosis) culture; it should not be used for a general bacteria culture because the high salt concentration
   inhibits the growth of most bacteria.
Miscellaneous:
   Particles tend to enlarge because of the absorption of water vapor, which results in larger particles than nebulized that are closer
   to isotonic; impaction is more likely in the upper airway.
   This concentration is the most likely to cause bronchospasm in asthma patients because it is the furthest from isotonic and,
   therefore, the most irritating.

---

   b. Nonbarbiturate sedative-hypnotics: ethchlorvynol (Placidyl), meprobamate (Miltown), glutethimide (Doriden), chloral hydrate (Noctec)
   c. Barbiturate sedative-hypnotics: pentobarbital sodium (Nembutal), secobarbital sodium (Seconal), phenobarbital (Luminol), thiopental sodium (Pentothal)

The benzodiazepine antagonist drug flumazenil (Romazicon) is indicated in the reversal of benzodiazepine agents such as Valium and Librium. Unconscious patients usually awaken quickly once the proper dose of flumazenil is given. Watch the patient for signs of seizure activity related to the rapid reversal of the benzodiazepine medication. The patient should be observed for 2 hours in case resedation occurs. If so, flumazenil can be given again.

8. Recommend the use of analgesic agents (WRE code: IIIG4e) [Difficulty: R, Ap, An]

Analgesics are medications that control or block pain after an injury or a surgical procedure. Morphine or similar narcotic-type analgesic drugs are indicated to control moderate to severe pain. Morphine also is indicated to treat the pain of a myocardial infarction and to produce vasodilation in the patient with pulmonary edema. Additionally, pain-relieving agents, when given in large enough doses, will sedate or induce sleep. The patient who is both in pain and agitated may be treated with a combination of an analgesic and a sedative (e.g., moderate doses of morphine and diazepam). The two drugs potentiate each other. The physician may instead decide to give the patient a larger dose of morphine rather than both drug types. Examples of commonly used analgesics include the following:
   a. Morphine sulfate (Duramorph) injection; Oramorph SR, tablets
   b. Codeine phosphate (methylmorphine)
   c. Hydromorphone (Dilaudid)
   d. Meperidine (Demerol)
   e. Propoxyphene (Darvon)

Patients receiving sedatives or analgesics or both must be closely monitored. Each can cause respiratory center depression if given in great enough doses. The patient may hypoventilate and even experience apnea and death. Narcotic analgesic agents (e.g., morphine) and some other analgesic medications can become habit forming or addictive if used for a prolonged period.

The narcotic antagonist drug naloxone (Narcan) counteracts the effects of narcotic agents, such as morphine, heroin, and codeine. Narcan does *not* reverse benzodiazepine or barbiturate drugs. Remember that the patient who was given an accidental overdose of morphine to control pain will feel pain again when Narcan is given.

9. Recommend the use of neuromuscular blocking agents (WRE code: IIIG1b) [Difficulty: An]

Neuromuscular blocking agents are used to cause a pharmacologic paralysis. These medications block nerve transmission from reaching skeletal (voluntary) muscles, and complete paralysis follows. They are most commonly used as part of balanced anesthesia before major thoracic or abdominal surgery. These drugs also are used in the intensive care unit to stop a patient from fighting against an intubation or to prevent the patient from struggling against the mechanical ventilator. All are given intravenously and act rapidly. Obviously, in all these cases, the patient stops breathing and must receive mechanical ventilation. Examples of the commonly used neuromuscular blocking agents include the following:

a. Depolarizing blocker: succinylcholine chloride (Anectine, Quelicin)
b. Nondepolarizing blockers: pancuronium bromide (Pavulon; preferred), vecuronium bromide (Norcuron), gallamine triethiodide (Flaxedil), atracurium besylate (Tracrium)

The nondepolarizing blockers (e.g., Pavulon) are preferred for their longer duration of action. Although all these agents induce complete paralysis of all voluntary muscles, they have little or no effect on the involuntary muscles or autonomic nervous system. Some patients may have a minor, passing change in heart rate and blood pressure. Remember that they are able to hear, able to feel pain, and are completely awake and alert to their surroundings. Care must be taken to sedate the patient for anxiety and give analgesics for pain. Talk to the patient normally, and move the patient periodically to prevent pressure sores.

The nondepolarizing neuromuscular blocking agents can be reversed so that the patient can breathe and move again. These intravenous medications include neostigmine bromide (Prostigmin; preferred) and edrophonium (Tensilon). It should be noted that these reversing agents cause an outpouring of oral and bronchial secretions. Atropine is given to prevent this. The reversing agents have no effect on the depolarizing neuromuscular blocker succinylcholine chloride. Patients given this drug usually regain movement within 15 minutes after the medication is stopped.

10. Recommend the use of surfactant agents (WRE code: IIIG4g) [Difficulty: R, Ap, An]

Surfactant has been approved for the prevention or treatment of infant respiratory distress syndrome (RDS) in premature neonates. These neonates have immature lungs that lack natural surfactant. As a result, atelectasis develops. These four surfactant agents have been approved for instillation into the airways to treat this problem and are widely used:

a. Colfosceril palmitate, cetyl alcohol, and tyloxapol (Exosurf)
b. Beractant (Survanta)
c. Poractant alfa (Curosurf)
d. Calfactant (Infasurf)

Dosages for all of the medications are based on the infant's weight. Be prepared to make rapid changes in the neonate's mechanical ventilator settings as the lungs rapidly become more compliant.

MODULE B
Drug dosage calculations (math review)

$$\frac{1 \text{ mL active ingredient}}{100 \text{ mL total solution}} =$$

$$\frac{\text{unknown active ingredient or } x}{0.5 \text{ mL solution}} \text{ (cross multiply)}$$

100 x = 0.5 mL (Divide both sides of the equation by 100.)

x = 0.005 mL = 0.005 g = 5 mg of active ingredient

2. How much active ingredient would be in 0.25 mL of Alupent? (Alupent is 5.0% active ingredient.)

A 5% drug concentration means that there are 5 parts of active ingredient in 100 parts of the solution, or 5 mL or 5 g of active ingredient in 100 mL or 100 g of the solution. This can be set up in the following proportion:

$$\frac{5 \text{ mL active ingredient}}{100 \text{ mL total solution}} =$$

$$\frac{\text{unknown active ingredient or } x}{0.25 \text{ mL solution}} \text{ (cross multiply)}$$

100 x = 1.25 mL (Divide both sides of the equation by 100.)

x = 0.0125 mL = 0.0125 g = 12.5 mg of active ingredient

Thus the *amount of active ingredient* can be calculated if the drug concentration is given in either a fractional or percentage form.

The next two examples deal with calculating the *volume of medication solution* needed to deliver a desired amount of active ingredient. With these types, it is necessary to convert to consistent units, usually converting grams to milligrams.

3. How much 0.5% Proventil would be needed to give a patient 2.5 mg of active ingredient by SVN?

A 0.5% (1:200) drug concentration means that there is 1 part of active ingredient in 200 parts of the solution, or 1 mL or 1 g of active ingredient in 200 mL or 200 g of the solution. This converts to 1000 mg/200 mL. Set up the following proportion:

$$\frac{1000 \text{ mg active ingredient}}{200 \text{ mL total solution}}$$

$$= \frac{2.5 \text{ mg (cross multiply)}}{x \text{ mL solution}}$$

1000 x = 500 mL (Divide both sides of the equation by 1000.)

x = 0.5 mL of Proventil should be given.

4. How much 4% Xylocaine would be needed to give a patient 100 mg of active ingredient by handheld nebulizer before a bronchoscopy?

A 4% drug concentration means that 4 parts of active ingredient are in 100 parts of the solution, or 4 mL or 4 g of active ingredient in 100 mL or 100 g of the solution. This converts to 4000 mg/100 mL. Set up the following proportion:

$$\frac{4000 \text{ mg active ingredient}}{100 \text{ mL total solution}}$$

$$= \frac{100 \text{ mg (cross multiply)}}{x \text{ mL solution}}$$

4000 x = 10,000 mL (Divide both sides of the equation by 4000.)

x = 2.5 mL of Xylocaine should be given.

Thus the *volume of medication solution* needed to deliver a given amount of active ingredient can be calculated if the drug concentration is given in either a fractional or percentage form.

MODULE C
Respiratory care plan

1. **Analyze the available information to determine the patient's pathophysiologic state (CSE code: IIIH1)**

The respiratory therapist should be able to determine whether the patient is having cardiopulmonary problems. Review, if needed, information presented in Chapters 1, 3, 4, and 5 that deals with bedside assessment, blood gases, pulmonary function tests, and advanced cardiopulmonary monitoring.

2. **Determine the appropriateness of the prescribed therapy and goals for the identified pathophysiologic state (CSE code: IIIH3)**
   a. **Review the interdisciplinary patient and family care plan (WRE code: IIIH1b) [Difficulty: An]**
   b. **Review the planned therapy to establish the therapeutic plan (WRE code: IIIH1a) [Difficulty: An]**

If the patient has a pulmonary infection, the correct antimicrobial drug should be used to treat the problem. See Table 9-6 for the common respiratory pathogens and Table 9-7 for the commonly used microbial agents.

Past examinations have expected the respiratory therapist to make the following recommendations:
1. Penicillin (Penicillin G, Ampicillin, etc.) to treat gram-positive bacteria
2. Gentamicin (Garamycin) to treat gram-negative bacteria
3. Aerosolized Tobramycin (TOBI) to treat *Pseudomonas* pneumonia in children with cystic fibrosis

TABLE 9-6	Common Respiratory Pathogens in Approximate Order of Frequency		
	GRAM POSITIVE	**GRAM NEGATIVE**	**CELL WALL DEFICIENT**
			Mycoplasma
Bacteria:	Streptococcus pneumoniae	Hemophilus influenzae	**ACID-FAST**
	Staphylococcus aureus*	Klebsiella pneumoniae	Mycobacterium tuberculosis*
	Streptococcus faecalis (enterococcus)	Pseudomonas aeruginosa*	
		Serratia species*	
Viruses:	Rhinovirus	Varicella virus*	
	Adenovirus	Herpes simplex virus*	
	Respiratory syncytival virus	Cytomegalovirus*	
Fungi:	Candida albicans*	Histoplasma capsulatum (Ohio Valley)	
	Aspergillus species*	Coccidioides immitis (Southwest U.S.)	
	Pneumocystis carinii		
Protozoa:	Toxoplasma gondii*		
	Cryptosporidium*		

*Seen most frequently in debilitated or immunosuppressed hosts.

4. Aerosolized pentamidine isethionate (NebuPent) for prophylactic treatment of *Penumocystis carinii*
5. Aerosolized ribavirin (Virazole) to treat *respiratory syncytial virus* (RSV) in young children
6. Isoniazid (INH) to treat *Mycobacterium tuberculosis* (TB)

c. Recommend changes in the therapeutic plan if supportive data exist (WRE code: IIIH2) [Difficulty: An]

This chapter discusses medications that can be used to help treat many commonly seen cardiopulmonary conditions. When these medications are used properly on the appropriate patient problem, there is a good chance of recovery. The patient's vital signs and other clinical indicators will improve. The patient will report feeling better.

However, if the patient's signs and symptoms do not indicate improvement, be prepared to recommend a change in the medication. This may be a dose change or switching to another medication. Stop any medication to which the patient is having an allergic reaction. Tell the patient's physician about the problem, and ask for further orders.

d. Conduct disease management education programs (WRE code: IIIH7) [Difficulty: Ap, An]

The most recent Written Registry Exams have had questions that relate to the management and education of the patient with asthma. It also is recommended that the management and education of a patient with COPD be studied. The bibliography includes information on standard references on these two subjects.

e. Stop the treatment or procedure if the patient has an adverse reaction to it (CSE code: IIIF1)

As mentioned earlier, Box 9-1 lists the side effects most often seen with adrenergic (sympathomimetic) bronchodilators. The most serious problem is tachycardia. In some cases, patients may have cardiac arrhythmias. A common clinical guideline calls for the treatment to be stopped if the patient's heart rate increases by more than 20% during the treatment. The patient should be monitored to confirm that the heart rate slows. Chart the information, and notify the nurse.

> **Exam Hint**
>
> Expect to see a question in which the decision has to be made to stop the bronchodilator treatment because the patient's heart rate increases by more than 20% from the baseline.

f. Discontinue treatment based on the patient's response (WRE code: IIIG1e) [Difficulty: An]

The physician discontinues treatment for one of two reasons. First, the patient has recovered and no longer needs a medication. Some asthma patients may fully recover and not need any medications. However, it is more common to find the right medications to control the condition so that the patient does not need to use rescue medications. Patients with emphysema or chronic bronchitis (COPD) or both are likely to always need medications.

TABLE 9-7	Classification of Antibiotic Agents Commonly Used Against Pulmonary Infections		
Class or Group	**Agents**	**Spectrum**	**Major Toxicity**
Aminoglycosides	Streptomycin	Primarily tuberculostatic	Vestibular, renal
	Tobramycin, TOBI	*Pseudomonas aeruginosa* lung infection in cystic fibrosis patients	Auditory, renal
	gentamicin, Garamycin	Gram-negative rods, including *Pseudomonas* and *Proteus*	Vestibular, renal
Antifungal agents	ketoconazole, Nizoral	Major agent for systemic fungal disease	Gastrointestinal upset
	Amphotericin B	Major agent for systemic fungal disease	Renal, gastrointestinal
Antituberculosis agents	isonicotinic acid hydrazide (INH), Isoniazid	Used for both prophylaxis and treatment	Hepatic
	Ethambutol, Rifampin	Used for tuberculostatic therapy	Retinal (maculapathy), hepatic
Antiviral agents	AZT, Retrovir	Stops reproduction in retroviruses; used against HIV	Anemia
	ribavirin, Virazole	Same spectrum, used against respiratory syncytial virus; experimental against HIV	
Cephalosporine	Cephalothin, Keflin	Like penicillin, with antistaphylococcal effects	Renal (usually not severe)
Chloramphenicol	Chloromycetin	Broad spectrum; used for *Haemophilus* if it is Ampicillin-resistant or if patient is allergic	Bone marrow
Macrolide	erythromycin, Erythrocin	Like penicillin (used in penicillin allergy); drug of choice for *Mycoplasma*	Gastrointestinal
Penicillin	Penicillin G	Gram-positive organisms; *Staphylococcus aureus* often resistant	Allergy
Semisynthetic penicillins	Ampicillin, Omnipen	Gram-positive organisms, Gram negative *Haemophilus influenzae*; variable against gram-negative rods	Diarrhea and rash, especially with viral disease (mononucleosis)
	Oxacillin, Prostaphlin	Like penicillin, with antistaphylococcal effects	Allergy
	Carbenicillin, Geopen	Like penicillin, with antipseudomonas effects	Sodium overload-congestive failure
Sulfonamides	pentamidine isethionate, NebuPent, Pentam 300	Prophylaxis against *Pneumocystis carinii*	Impaired renal and liver function
	trimethaprim and sulfamethoxazole, Bactrim	Used against *Pneumocystis carinii*	Impaired renal and liver function
Tetracyclines	tetracycline, Achromycin	Broad spectrum; useful against *Haemophilus* and *Mycoplasma* infections	Fungal overgrowth in bowel or vagina; hepatic with large IV doses

Second, the patient has a serious adverse reaction to the medication. As discussed earlier, Table 9-1 lists the adverse reactions to the adrenergic (sympathomimetic) bronchodilators. Repeated episodes of tachycardia or cardiac arrhythmias or both could lead to the physician discontinuing their use.

3. Make a recommendation to change the dosage or concentration of an aerosolized medication (WRE code: IIIG2b) [Difficulty: An]

a. Bronchodilators

Make a recommendation to increase the amount of medication if the patient's bronchospasm is not reversed and no adverse side effects are present. Make a recommendation to decrease the amount of medication if the patient is having serious side effects such as tachycardia or palpitations. The current guidelines on the pharmacologic management of asthma list the medications that should be used, depending on how the patient's asthmatic condition is categorized. All asthmatic patients should have an inhaled, short-acting, rapid-onset β-adrenergic bronchodilator. The medications albuterol (Proventil, Ventolin) and levalbuterol (Xopenex) are widely used for quick relief. For persistent asthma, several additional medications are taken for long-term control. These include an inhaled corticosteroid (beclomethasone, triamcinolone), an inhaled long-acting β-adrenergic bronchodilator (salmeterol), and a preventive agent (cromolyn sodium or zafirlukast). Patients with the most severe persistent asthma also require a corticosteroid medication by syrup or pill and sustained-release theophylline. It is recommended that the National Institutes of Health guidelines, as listed in the bibliography, be reviewed for complete information.

b. Mucomyst or saline solutions

Make a recommendation to increase the amount of medication if the patient's secretions are still too thick to cough out or suction and if no adverse side effects to the medication exist. Make a recommendation to decrease the amount of medication if the patient's secretions are watery enough for expectoration or suctioning or if side effects to the drug (e.g., bronchospasm) exist.

4. Change the dilution of a medication used in aerosol therapy (WRE code: IIIFc3) [Difficulty: An]

The various saline solutions and sterile water are known collectively as *bland* aerosols, because they have no direct pharmacologic effect on the lungs and airways. They are used to increase the volume of liquid in an SVN after the medication has been added. Most of these nebulizers work most efficiently when they hold about 3 to 5 mL of liquid. Usually a normal saline solution (0.9% sodium chloride) is added.

Adding little or no saline to the medication results in the patient inhaling a very concentrated solution or the nebulizer not functioning properly. The nebulizer will aerosolize the medication within a few minutes, and the patient should quickly feel the beneficial effects of the treatment. However, depending on the nature of the medication, the patient might find it to be quite irritating to the airway. Coughing or bronchospasm could result. Side effects (e.g., tachycardia) should be watched for with sympathomimetic agents, because the medication enters the bloodstream so quickly.

If more saline is added, the solution will be less concentrated. The nebulizer will take longer to aerosolize the medication because of the added volume, and relief of symptoms will take longer. However, it will be less likely to irritate the airway. Side effects with sympathomimetic agents could be less severe, because the drug is given over a longer period. However, remember that increasing the amount of saline makes no difference on the total amount of medication in the nebulizer for the patient. Tachycardia or other side effects may still be seen if the total amount of medication is given.

Saline-only aerosol treatments, as for induced sputum, are more effective at higher concentrations of saline. See Box 9-2 for complete information on the saline solutions.

5. Respiratory care protocols
a. Develop the outcomes of respiratory care protocols (WRE code: IIIH4b) [Difficulty: An]
b. Apply respiratory care protocols to patient care situations (WRE code: IIIH6) [Difficulty: Ap]

Respiratory therapists should be familiar with two widely used respiratory disease and medication protocols.

Patients with asthma should be managed as described in National Asthma Education and Prevention Program, Expert Panel Report II: *Guidelines for the diagnosis and management of asthma*. Patients with emphysema and chronic bronchitis should be managed as described in "Global Initiative for Chronic Obstructive Lung Disease (GOLD), Workshop Report: Global strategy for the diagnosis, management, and prevention of COPD." The bibliography lists the complete information on these two documents. They are too long to list here.

The guidelines for asthma and COPD rank both conditions in four categories by the severity of the illness, and medications are given based on the severity ranking.

c. Explain planned therapy and goals to the patient in understandable (nonmedical) terms to achieve the best results from the treatment or procedure (WRE code: IIIA6) [Difficulty: An]
d. Monitor the outcomes of respiratory care protocols (WRE code: IIIH5) [Difficulty: An]

Both guidelines list key things to monitor for patient success. Goals of therapy for the *asthma patient* include
1. Minimal or no chronic symptoms day or night
2. Minimal or no episodes
3. No limitations on activities; no school or work missed
4. Peak expiratory flow greater than 80% of personal best
5. Minimal use of inhaled short-acting β_2 agonist medication (fewer than one per day)
6. No or minimal adverse effects from medications

Goals of therapy for the *COPD patient* include
1. Prevent disease progression
2. Relieve symptoms (dyspnea, cough, fatigue)
3. Improve exercise tolerance
4. Improve health status
5. Prevent and treat complications
6. Prevent and treat exacerbations
7. Reduce mortality

e. Communicate the outcomes of therapy, and change the therapy based on the protocol (WRE code: IIIA5) [Difficulty: An]

Inform the patient's nurse or physician and the supervising therapist if any serious question or problem occurs with the patient. Routine communication should occur as needed between these people and any other caregiver.

6. Record and evaluate the patient's response to the treatment(s) or procedure(s), including the following

a. Record and interpret the following: heart rate and rhythm, respiratory rate, blood pressure, body temperature, and pain level (WRE code: IIIA1b, IIIA1c) [Difficulty: An]

With many treatment protocols, the practitioner must count the patient's heart rate before, at least one time during, and after an aerosolized bronchodilator is given because of the risk of tachycardia. It is generally acceptable to count for 30 seconds and multiply by 2 to get a 1-minute count. Record the various heart rates and determine the heart rhythm as the pulse is measured. A stethoscope can be used to determine an abnormality. Treatment is usually stopped if the patient's pulse increases by more than 20% from the initial level.

b. Record and interpret the patient's breath sounds (WRE code: IIIA1a) [Difficulty: An]

Listen for a reduction in wheezing after the administration of an aerosolized bronchodilator as proof of an effectively reduced bronchospasm. If the patient were given an aerosolized bronchodilator for bronchospasm, the patient's spirometry results would be expected to move toward more normal values as the bronchospasm is reduced. The two most important bedside spirometry values to monitor are the peak flow and forced expiratory volume in 1 second. A 15% to 20% improvement in either one or both after the inhalation of an aerosolized bronchodilator indicates that the medication works, and the patient has reversible bronchospasm. A patient with stable asthma may be given a drug such as cromolyn sodium (Intal) or nedocromil sodium (Tilade) by inhalation to prevent a future asthma attack. Remember that these drugs are not to be used during an asthma attack.

c. Record and interpret the type of cough the patient has and the nature of the sputum (WRE code: IIIA1a) [Difficulty: An]

Listen for a reduction in airway secretions after a productive cough. The mucolytics should be helpful in making the secretions less thick.

d. Recheck any math work and make note of incorrect data (WRE code: IIIA2) [Difficulty: An]

Errors made in charting must be corrected by drawing a single mark through the error and writing in the correct information. Some prefer that the error be further clarified by writing in "error" next to it and adding initials. *Never* erase or use any covering material over an error.

BIBLIOGRAPHY

Au JP, Ziment I: Drug therapy and dosage adjustment in asthma, *Respir Care* 31:415, 1986.

Bills GW, Soderberg RC: *Principles of pharmacology for respiratory care*, ed 2, Albany, NY, 1998, Delmar.

Carter C, Solberg C: Respiratory pharmacology. In Hess DR, MacIntyre NR, Mishoe SC, et al, editors: *Respiratory care: principles and practices*, Philadelphia, 2002, WB Saunders.

Colbert BJ, Mason BJ: *Cardiopulmonary drug guide*, Upper Saddle River, NJ, 2003, Prentice Hall.

Colbert BJ, Mason BJ: *Integrated cardiopulmonary pharmacology*, Upper Saddle River, NJ, 2002, Prentice Hall.

Cottrell GP, Surkin HB: *Pharmacology for respiratory care practitioners*, Philadelphia, 1995, FA Davis.

Global Initiative for Chronic Obstructive Lung Disease (GOLD): *Workshop report: global strategy for the diagnosis, management, and prevention of COPD*, Bethesda, MD, 2000, National Heart, Lung, and Blood Institute and the World Health Organization.

Hill F: *Delmar's respiratory care drug reference*. Albany, NY, 1999, Delmar.

Howder CL: *Cardiopulmonary pharmacology: a handbook for respiratory practitioners and other allied health personnel*, ed 2, Baltimore, 1996, Williams & Wilkins.

Levine SR, McLaughlin AJ: *Pharmacology in respiratory care*, New York, 2001, McGraw-Hill.

Malmeister M: Pharmacology associated with respiratory care. In Fink JB, Hunt GE, editors: *Clinical practice in respiratory care,* Philadelphia, 1999, Lippincott-Raven.

McLaughlin AJ, Levine SR: *Respiratory care drug reference,* Gaithersburg, Md, 1997, Aspen.

National Asthma Education and Prevention Program, Expert Panel Report II: *Guidelines for the diagnosis and management of asthma,* Bethesda, Md, 1997, National Institutes of Health.

National Institutes of Health: *Practical guide for the diagnosis and management of asthma,* Pub. No. 97-4053, Bethesda, Md, 1997, NIH.

Physicians' desk reference, ed 57, Montvale, NJ, 2003, Thomson PDR.

Rau JL: *Respiratory care pharmacology,* ed 6, St Louis, 2002, Mosby.

Rau JL: Airway pharmacology. In Wilkins RL, Stoller JK, Scanlan CL, editors: *Egan's fundamentals of respiratory care,* ed 8, St Louis, 2003, Mosby.

Tashkin DP: Dosing strategies for bronchodilator aerosol delivery, *Respir Care* 36:977, 1991.

Witek TJ, Schachter EN: *Pharmacology and therapeutics in respiratory care,* Philadelphia, 1994, WB Saunders.

Ziment I: Drugs used in respiratory care. In Burton GG, Hodgkin JE, Ward JJ, editors: *Respiratory care: a guide to clinical practice,* ed 4, Philadelphia, 1997, Lippincott-Raven.

SELF-STUDY QUESTIONS

1. You are called to help assess a premature neonate. The patient is having difficulty breathing, and respiratory distress syndrome is suspected. You would recommend all of the following *except:*
   A. Flumazenil (Romazicon)
   B. Beractant (Survanta)
   C. Calfactant (Infasurf)
   D. Proactant alpha (Curosurf)

2. A 2-month-old infant has periods of apnea that result in bradycardia and cyanosis. What medication should be recommended to treat the apnea periods?
   A. Lidocaine (Xylocaine)
   B. Neostigmine (Prostigmin)
   C. Theophylline (Aminophylline)
   D. Isoetharine (Bronkosol)

3. An anxious 10-year-old asthma patient is being given a breathing treatment with levalbuterol (Xopenex). His initial heart rate of 110 breaths/minute has now increased to 120 breaths/minute. What do you recommend be done?
   A. Continue the treatment.
   B. Stop the treatment.
   C. Change to albuterol and continue the treatment.
   D. Cut the medication dose in half and continue.

4. A mechanically ventilated patient who has been paralyzed with a neuromuscular blocking agent should be given a sedative agent for what reason?
   A. To sustain the paralysis
   B. To control pain
   C. To keep the patient synchronized with the ventilator
   D. To relieve the patient's anxiety

5. A patient had a bronchoscopy procedure and biopsy taken of a suspected lung tumor. After the biopsy, uncontrolled bleeding occurs. What would you recommend to control the bleeding?
   A. Instill epinephrine through the bronchoscopy at the site of the bleeding.
   B. Administer heparin by intravenous line.

   C. Nebulize albuterol (Proventil) by small volume nebulizer.
   D. Administer lidocaine (Xylocaine) by intravenous line.

6. Your 48-year-old patient has large amounts of thick secretions related to chronic bronchitis from smoking. No sign of infection is present. What should be administered to help manage the secretion problem?
   A. Salmeterol (Serevent)
   B. Dornase alfa (Pulmozyme)
   C. Normal (0.9%) saline
   D. Acetylcysteine (Mucomyst)

7. A home care patient with asthma has finished her standard dose of albuterol (Ventolin). After waiting 15 minutes, she performs a peak flow measurement, which shows 65% of her personal best. What should be recommended to the physician?
   A. Decrease the dose of albuterol.
   B. Add an intravenous corticosteroid to the patient's medications.
   C. Maintain the present therapy.
   D. Increase the dose of albuterol.

8. A 14-year-old patient with cystic fibrosis and a pulmonary infection has many thick secretions. What should be recommended to help manage the secretion problem?
   I. Nebulize acetylcysteine (Mucomyst)
   II. Intravenous fluticasone (Flovent)
   III. Nebulize dornase alfa (Pulmozyme)
   IV. Intravenous flumazenil (Romazicon)
      A. I and III
      B. I and II
      C. III and IV
      D. I, III, and IV

9. An adult patient is panicking and fighting against the mechanical ventilator. All of the following may be used to control the patient on the ventilator *except:*
   A. Flumazenil (Romazicon)
   B. Pancuronium bromide (Pavulon)

C. Succinylcholine (Anectine)

D. Morphine sulfate (Duramorph)

10. A patient is in shock from an allergic reaction to a bee sting. In addition, she has inspiratory stridor from laryngeal edema. What is the best medication to use to help raise her blood pressure and help her breathing?

A. Intravenous epinephrine (Adrenaline)

B. Oral ibuprofen (Advil)

C. Nebulized racemic epinephrine (MicroNefrin)

D. Intravenous naloxone (Narcan)

11. A 12-year-old patient with cystic fibrosis has been admitted with a pulmonary infection. She is being treated with a systemic antibiotic and inhaled mucolytic and bronchodilator medications. She has complained of muscle soreness from coughing and has a fever of 101°F. What additional medication should she be given?

A. Acetylsalicylic acid (aspirin)

B. Meperidine (Demerol)

C. Ibuprofen (Advil, Motrin)

D. Midazolam (Versed)

ANSWER KEY

1. **A.** Rationale: Flumazenil (Romazicon) is used to reverse the effects of the benzodiazepine-type sedative agents (Valium, Versed). There is no indication that the patient had been given a sedative. The other three drugs (Survanta, Infasurf, Curosurf) are used in surfactant replacement therapy in neonates with respiratory distress syndrome.

2. **C.** Rationale: Theophylline (Aminophylline) is known to be a respiratory-center stimulant in infants and will stimulate breathing. This should help to prevent the apnea spells. Xylocaine is a local anesthetic agent. It is used to numb an injury or to stop cardiac arrhythmias, such as premature ventricular contractions (PVCs). Prostigmin is used to reverse the paralyzing effects of the nondepolarizing neuromuscular blocking agents like Pavulon. Bronkosol is a fast acting sympathomimetic bronchodilator. It does not simulate breathing.

3. **A.** Rationale: The patient's treatment can be continued because his heart rate has not increased by at least 20% from the baseline. The therapist cannot change a medication or decrease a medication amount without the physician's approval.

4. **D.** Rationale: A sedative agent will have a calming effect on a patient anxious about being unable to move or communicate while paralyzed on the ventilator. A sedative will not control pain or sustain a pharmacologic paralysis. Although a high enough dose of a sedative will put a patient to sleep and therefore prevent "fighting" the ventilator, that is not its primary purpose. In addition, if the patient is pharmacologically paralyzed, no need exists for any other medication to control the patient's breathing efforts.

5. **A.** Rationale: Epinephrine has vasoconstricting properties (as well as properties causing bronchodilation and tachycardia) and should help to stop bleeding at the biopsy site. Intravenous heparin is contraindicated because it increases clotting time and will likely increase the bleeding. Albuterol (Proventil) is a very effective bronchodilator but has no effect on peripheral blood vessels. Lidocaine (Xylocaine) is used to stop cardiac arrhythmias but has no effect on peripheral blood vessels.

6. **D.** Rationale: Acetylcysteine (Mucomyst) is very effective at decreasing the viscosity (thickness) of mucoid secretions. Dornase alfa (Pulmozyme) is not indicated in this patient because purulent (infected) secretions with DNA strands are not present. Normal (0.9%) saline has been shown to be helpful in decreasing the thickness of pulmonary secretions. However, it is not as effective as acetylcysteine (Mucomyst).

7. **D.** Rationale: Increasing the dose of albuterol should improve the patient's bronchodilation and result in an improved peak flow. Because the patient's peak flow is only 65% of personal best, the albuterol dose should not be maintained or decreased. Adding an intravenous corticosteroid to the patient's medications would require the home care patient to travel to the physician's office for injections. This is not a practical solution. In addition, no clear indication exists that intravenous corticosteroids are needed at this time.

8. **A.** Rationale: Nebulize acetylcysteine (Mucomyst) and dornase alfa (Pulmozyme) to decrease the viscosity (thickness) of mucoid and purulent secretions. Fluticasone (Flovent) is an inhaled corticosteroid; it has no effect on secretions. Flumazenil (Romazicon) is used to reverse the effects of the benzodiazepine-type sedative drugs like Valium or Versed. It has no effect on pulmonary secretions.

9. **A.** Rationale: Flumazenil (Romazicon) is used to reverse the effects of benzodiazepine-type sedative agents (Versed, Valium). Rather than calming a patient, flumazenil is used to reverse the effects of oversedation. Pancuronium bromide (Pavulon) and succinylcholine (Anectine) are medications used to paralyze a patient. This will certainly result in the patient's breathing being controlled by the ventilator. Morphine sulfate (Duramorph) is given to control pain and will have a secondary benefit of sedating the patient if enough is given.

10. **A.** Rationale: Adrenaline will cause vasoconstriction of the systemic blood vessels to raise the blood pressure

and of the laryngeal blood vessels to open the larynx. In addition, it is a bronchodilator. Advil has some anti-inflammatory properties but will not have any effect on the patient's low blood pressure. Nebulized racemic epinephrine (MicroNefrin) is useful with upper airway edema but will not have enough systemic effect to raise the blood pressure significantly. Narcan is a reversing agent for the narcotic-type analgesics.

11. **C.** Rationale: Advil or Motrin will relief her minor muscle pain and reduce her fever. Aspirin will do the same thing. However, it also will affect her clotting time. It is not recommended in children because of the risk of Reye syndrome as a complication of its use. Demerol is a more powerful pain-relieving drug than is needed in this case. It will not have any effect on the patient's fever. No indication exists to give the sedative Versed to the patient. It will have no effect on her pain or fever.

10 Bronchopulmonary Hygiene Therapy

Note 1: The National Board for Respiratory Care (NBRC) has released the *RRT Examination Matrix* (covering the testable items on the Written Registry Exam) and the *CSE Examination Matrix* (covering the testable items on the Clinical Simulation Exam). Turn to the appendices at the back of this book for both publications in their original format. This book is intended to cover all of the testable items in these two publications. This chapter (and all others) uses the abbreviation "WRE" for the coded items testable on the Written Registry Exam *and* Clinical Simulation Exam. The listed difficulty (R, Recall; Ap, Application; An, Analysis) relates to the question difficulty on the Written Registry Exam. The abbreviation "CSE" is used for the coded items testable on *only* the Clinical Simulation Exam. Because no question difficulty level is given for this exam, be prepared for anything.

Note 2: A review of the most recent Written Registry Examinations has shown an average of three questions (3% of the exam) that cover bronchopulmonary hygiene issues. The Clinical Simulation Exam is comprehensive and may include everything that should be known or performed by an advanced level respiratory therapist.

MODULE A
Postural drainage therapy

Postural drainage therapy (PDT) also is known as chest physiotherapy, chest physical therapy, bronchopulmonary drainage, postural drainage and percussion, and percussion and vibration.

1. Recommend starting bronchopulmonary hygiene procedures (WRE code: IIIG1a) [Difficulty: An]

2. Instruct and encourage bronchopulmonary hygiene techniques (WRE code: IIIC4) [Difficulty: An]

The directed cough is one of the simplest, yet most important bronchopulmonary hygiene procedures to teach a patient with retained secretions. Ideally, the surgical patient is taught proper coughing techniques before surgery. If not, it is necessary to teach them postoperatively:

  a. Minimize traction or tension on the incision, to decrease the pain, by placing either your hands or the patient's hands on both sides of the incision. A pillow also can be held against the incision by the practitioner or patient.

  b. Instruct the patient to breathe 2 or 3 times in through the nose and out through the mouth.

  c. Instruct the patient to take in as deep a breath as possible and to perform a normal cough.

  d. If the patient cannot cough normally because of pain, a serial or huff cough can be performed.

Teach the patient with chronic obstructive pulmonary disease the following cough techniques:

  a. Avoid an ineffective, shallow, hacking cough.

  b. Position the patient in a sitting position, bent slightly forward, with feet on the floor or supported. The patient who must lie in bed can be positioned on the preferred side with the legs flexed at the knees and hips.

  c. Instruct the patient to perform a midinspiratory cough.
    1. Breathe two or three times in through the nose and out through the mouth.
    2. Breathe in to a comfortable volume larger than the tidal volume but not as deeply as possible.
    3. Briefly hold the breath.
    4. Cough hard or perform a serial cough at relatively low flows. This should help to raise secretions without causing airway collapse.
    5. Squeezing the knees and thighs together at the instant of coughing helps to increase the airflow and volume.

Coaching is important because patients in pain or suffering from chronic lung disease tend to be uncooperative and do not try hard. Give positive reinforcement when the patient does well. Correct any problems the patient is having following the instructions. Demonstrations are often useful so that the patient can copy a good example.

If the patient cannot cough effectively, other secretion clearance procedures will be needed. PDT and other procedures follow. The American Association for Respiratory Care (AARC) clinical practice guideline on PDT was used to help develop the following information. See Box 10-1 for indications for turning, postural drainage, and percussion and vibration. Contraindications are listed in Box 10-2, and recommended actions for problems are listed in Box 10-3. Beyond the patient assessment issues listed in

227

BOX 10-1 Indications for Turning, Postural Drainage, and Percussion and Vibration

TURNING

- Patient is unable to change his or her body position (e.g., the patient has a cerebral injury or neuromuscular disease, is being mechanically ventilated, or has been medicated to cause sedation or paralysis)
- Atelectasis or the potential for its development
- Hypoxemia associated with a particular position; if one-sided lung disease is present, the patient is typically turned so that the affected lung is superior
- Patient with an artificial airway

POSTURAL DRAINAGE

- Mobilize retained secretions so that they can be coughed or suctioned out; patient has difficulty coughing out secretions but produces more than 25–30 mL/day; evidence or indications that a patient with an artificial airway has retained secretions
- Atelectasis that is known or is believed to be caused by mucus plugging
- Patient diagnosed with cystic fibrosis, bronchiectasis, or cavitating lung disease
- Foreign body in an airway
- Removal of aspirated foreign body or stomach contents

PERCUSSION AND VIBRATION

- Patient receiving postural drainage who has a large volume of thick sputum; this suggests that external manipulation of the thorax would assist gravity in its movement toward a more central airway

---

Based on information found in American Association for Respiratory Care: Clinical practice guidelines: postural drainage therapy, *Respir Care* 36:1418, 1991.

Box 10-4, the following should be evaluated to determine whether PDT is needed:

a. PDT is not indicated if an optimally hydrated patient is coughing out less than 25 mL/day with the procedure.

b. A dehydrated patient should have apparently ineffective PDT continued for at least 24 hours after the patient is rehydrated. The combination of rehydration and PDT may help to mobilize previously thick secretions.

c. PDT is not indicated in a patient producing more than 30 mL of secretions daily (if the PDT treatments do not increase the sputum production) because the patient is already able to cough out the sputum effectively.

3. Perform postural drainage (WRE code: IIIC1a) [Difficulty: An]

Turning involves rotating the patient's body in the longitudinal (head-to-toe) axis to promote unilateral or bilateral lung expansion. Patients can be turned from the back to one side, side to side, or one side to back to other side, depending on their need. The bed may be moved to any head-up or head-down position, as the patient needs and tolerates. Patients should be turned every 1 to 2 hours as tolerated. The patient can turn himself or herself, be turned by a caregiver, or be placed in a bed that is motorized and programmed to change positions in a set pattern.

Postural drainage (bronchopulmonary drainage) is performed to clear secretions or prevent the accumulation of secretions. The patient is positioned so that the bronchus of a particular segment is as vertical as possible. Gravity pulls the secretions toward a major bronchus or the trachea; the secretions are then either coughed or suctioned out. The anatomy of the pulmonary lobes with their segments and respective bronchi should be reviewed (Fig. 10-1).

Note that each segment and its bronchus adjoin the right or left mainstem bronchus at a particular angle. This critical angle determines the positioning that must be used to drain the various segments. Obviously, putting the patient in the wrong position does nothing to drain the desired segment. Auscultation, palpation, and percussion of the chest should lead the practitioner to know where the secretions are located.

Individual segments should be drained when the physician's order specifies them or when the practitioner determines that secretions are present. Individual segments are generally drained for 3 to 15 minutes. Drainage may be provided for a longer period in special situations. Postural drainage and the external manipulation of the patient's thorax (percussion and vibration) can be very strenuous or contraindicated in some patients. Watch for hypoxemia or an increase in dyspnea. If the patient normally has supplemental O_2, it should be kept on while in the drainage positions. Some patients need supplemental O_2 only when in certain positions, and it must be made available to them.

Coughing should be encouraged after each segment is drained. The patient should not cough in a head-down position, however, because of the risk of increased intracranial pressure. Have the patient sit up to cough vigorously.

1. Pulmonary drainage positions
Lower lobes

a. Posterior basal segment (Fig. 10-2)
   1. The patient lies face down on the bed. A pillow is placed beneath the hips.
   2. The foot of the bed is elevated 18 inches or 30 degrees.
   3. If ordered, perform percussion or vibration over the lower ribs near the spine on either or both sides, depending on whether one or both segments are to be drained. Note the shaded areas in Fig. 10-2.

BOX 10-2 Contraindications for Turning/Postural Drainage and Percussion and Vibration

TURNING/POSTURAL DRAINAGE*
ALL POSITIONS ARE CONTRAINDICATED FOR
PATIENTS WITH THE FOLLOWING:
1. Unstabilized head or neck injury, or both (absolute)
2. Active hemorrhage and hemodynamic instability (absolute)
3. ICP greater than 20 mm Hg
4. Recent spinal surgery, such as a laminectomy, or acute spinal injury
5. Active hemoptysis
6. Empyema
7. Bronchopleural fistula
8. Pulmonary edema as a result of congestive heart failure
9. Large pleural effusions
10. Advanced age, anxiety, or confusion and intolerance of position changes
11. Fractured rib(s) with or without flail chest
12. Healing tissue or surgical wound

TRENDELENBURG POSITION IS CONTRAINDICATED
IN PATIENTS WITH THE FOLLOWING:
1. ICP greater than 20 mm Hg
2. Sensitivity to increased ICP (e.g., neurosurgery, cerebral aneurysms, eye surgery)
3. Uncontrolled hypertension
4. Distended abdomen
5. Esophageal surgery
6. Recent gross hemoptysis (especially if associated with lung cancer that was recently treated surgically or by radiation therapy)
7. Uncontrolled airway if at risk for aspiration (recent meal or tube feeding); many authors consider < 1 hr after eating as a contraindication

REVERSE TRENDELENBURG POSITION IS
CONTRAINDICATED IN PATIENTS WHO ARE:
1. Hypotensive
2. Receiving a vasoactive medication

PERCUSSION AND VIBRATION
1. All of the previously listed contraindications
2. Subcutaneous emphysema (several authors list an untreated pneumothorax as an absolute contraindication)
3. Spinal anesthesia or recent epidural spinal infusion for pain control
4. Recent thoracic skin grafts or skin flaps
5. Thoracic burns, open wounds, or skin infections
6. Recently placed transvenous or subcutaneous pacemaker (especially true if a mechanical percussor/vibrator is to be used)
7. Suspicion of pulmonary tuberculosis
8. Lung contusion
9. Bronchospasm
10. Osteomyelitis of the ribs
11. Osteoporosis
12. Clotting disorder (coagulopathy)
13. Complaints of chest wall pain

IN ADDITION, A NUMBER OF AUTHORS HAVE
LISTED THE FOLLOWING AS CONTRAINDICATIONS
TO PERCUSSION AND VIBRATION:
1. Not over bare skin
2. Not over buttons, zippers, folded clothes, or seams of clothing
3. Not over female breast tissue
4. Not over the spine, sternum, or kidneys
5. Not over an area with a known lung tumor

*These are relative contraindications except those marked as absolute.
ICP, Intracranial pressure.
Based on information found in American Association for Respiratory Care: Clinical practice guidelines: postural drainage therapy, *Respir Care* 36:1418, 1991.

---

b. Lateral basal segment (Fig. 10-3)
  1. The patient is shown in a position to drain the right lateral basal segment. The left lateral basal segment would be drained by placing the patient the same way on the opposite side.
  2. The patient lies one-fourth turn up from the face-down position. A pillow may be placed in front of the patient for support or between the knees for comfort.
  3. The foot of the bed is elevated 18 inches or 30 degrees.
  4. If ordered, percussion or vibration would be performed over the posterolateral areas of the lower ribs. See the shaded areas in Fig. 10-3.
c. Anterior basal segment (Fig. 10-4)
  1. The patient is shown in a position to drain the left anterior basal segment. (Note: This combined segment is the anatomic equivalent of the medial basal segment and anterior basal segment of the right lung.) The right anterior basal and medial basal segments would be drained by placing the patient the same way on the opposite side.
  2. The patient lies straight up on his or her side. Pillows may be used in front or behind the patient (or both) for positioning or between the knees for comfort.
  3. The foot of the bed is elevated 18 inches or 30 degrees.
  4. If ordered, percussion or vibration would be performed over the lower ribs below the axilla. See the shaded areas in Fig. 10-4.
d. Superior segment (Fig. 10-5)
  1. The patient lies face down on the bed. A pillow is placed beneath the hips.

BOX 10-3 Hazards/Complications, with Recommended Actions, and Limitations of Postural Drainage and Percussion and Vibration

HAZARDS/COMPLICATIONS

- *Hypoxemia.* The patient known to be hypoxic or prone to hypoxemia during the procedure should be given a higher inspired O_2 percentage. Give 100% O_2 to any patient who becomes hypoxic during the procedure. Stop the treatment, return the patient to the original resting position, make sure ventilation is adequate, and consult with the physician before continuing.
- *Increased intracranial pressure or acute hypotension during the procedure.* If either of these happens, stop the treatment, return the patient to the original resting position, and consult with the physician before continuing.
- *Pulmonary hemorrhage.* If this happens, stop the treatment, return the patient to the original resting position, and call the physician immediately. Give the patient supplemental O_2 and keep an open airway until the physician responds.
- *Pain or injury to the patient's muscles, ribs, or spine.* Stop the therapy that seems to be causing the problem. Carefully move the patient to a more comfortable position, and call the physician before continuing.
- *Vomiting and aspiration.* Stop the treatment, apply suction as needed to clear the airway, give supplemental O_2, maintain a patent airway, return the patient to the original resting position, and call the physician immediately.
- *Bronchospasm.* If this happens, stop the treatment, return the patient to the original resting position, and give or increase the supplemental O_2 while calling the physician. Give the patient any aerosolized bronchodilators that the physician orders.
- *Arrhythmias.* If this happens, stop the treatment, return the patient to the original resting position, and give or increase supplemental O_2 while calling the physician.

LIMITATIONS

- Be careful to give postural drainage therapy only to those patients who would benefit from it. Do not rely on past experiences with other patients when you judge current situations.
- Patients with ineffective coughs may be unable to clear their airways as well as desired.
- Critically ill patients are difficult to position optimally.

Based on information found in American Association for Respiratory Care: Clinical practice guidelines: postural drainage therapy, *Respir Care* 36:1418, 1991.

---

2. The bed is flat.
3. If ordered, percussion or vibration would be performed over the middle of the back below the scapula on either or both sides of the spine, depending on whether one or both segments are to be drained. See the shaded areas in Fig. 10-5.

BOX 10-4 Assessment of the Patient's Needs for Postural Drainage Therapy (PDT)*

- Excessive production of sputum
- Ineffectiveness of cough
- Patient history of PDT that was helpful in treating past problem (e.g., bronchiectasis, cystic fibrosis, lung abscess)
- Abnormal breath sounds (e.g., decreased breath sounds, crackles, or rhonchi, suggesting airway secretions)
- Change in the patient's vital signs
- Abnormal chest radiograph finding consistent with infiltrates, atelectasis, or mucus plugging

---

*These problems should be assessed *together* to evaluate the patient's need for PDT. Not all patients experience all of these problems. The seriousness of these problems should be assessed by the clinician in determining which patients will benefit from PDT.

Based on information found in American Association for Respiratory Care: Clinical practice guidelines: postural drainage therapy, *Respir Care* 36:1418, 1991.

Right middle lobe and left lingula
a. Right lateral and medial segments (Fig. 10-6)
   1. The same position is used to drain both segments.
   2. The patient lies one-fourth turn up from the back-down position. A pillow may be placed in back of the patient for support or between the flexed knees for comfort.
   3. The foot of the bed is elevated 14 inches or 15 degrees.
   4. If ordered, percussion or vibration would be performed below the right nipple area in a male patient. See the shaded area in Fig. 10-6. Percussion and vibration may not be possible on a female patient.
b. Left superior and inferior lingula segments (Fig. 10-7)
   1. The same position is used to drain both segments.
   2. The patient lies one-fourth turn up from the back-down position. A pillow may be placed in back of the patient for support or between the flexed knees for comfort.
   3. The foot of the bed is elevated 14 inches or 15 degrees.
   4. If ordered, percussion or vibration would be performed below the left nipple area in a male patient. See the shaded area in Fig. 10-7. Percussion and vibration may not be possible on a female patient.

Upper lobes
a. Posterior segment (Fig. 10-8)
   1. The patient leans forward 30 degrees. This can be over the back of a chair (as shown in Fig. 10-8) or in bed. A pillow can be used to lean against or support the chest.

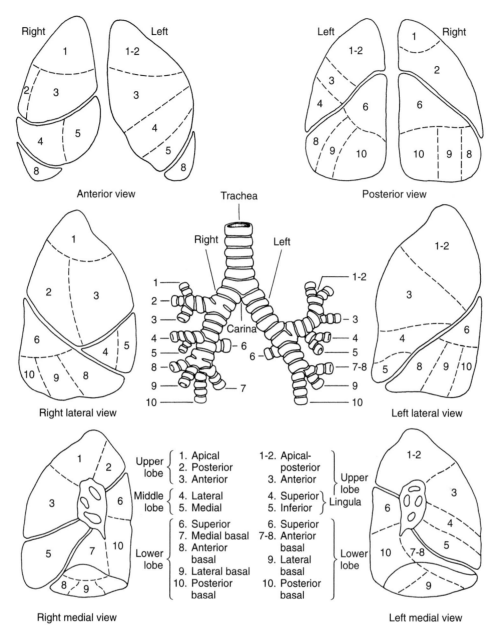

Right   Left

Anterior view

Trachea

Left   Right

Posterior view

Right   Left

Right lateral view

Carina

Left lateral view

Right medial view

Upper lobe { 1. Apical 2. Posterior 3. Anterior

Middle lobe { 4. Lateral 5. Medial

Lower lobe { 6. Superior 7. Medial basal 8. Anterior basal 9. Lateral basal 10. Posterior basal

1-2. Apical-posterior 3. Anterior } Upper lobe

4. Superior 5. Inferior } Lingula

6. Superior 7-8. Anterior basal 9. Lateral basal 10. Posterior basal } Lower lobe

Left medial view

Fig. 10-1 Names and locations of the lung segments and their respective bronchi. *(From Shibel EM, Moser KM, editors:* Respiratory emergencies, *St Louis, 1977, Mosby.)*

2. If ordered, percussion or vibration would be performed over the upper portion of the back on either or both sides of the spine, depending on whether one or both segments are being drained. See the shaded areas in Fig. 10-8.
b. Apical segment (Fig. 10-9)
   1. The patient leans backward 30 degrees. This can be done in bed (as shown in Fig. 10-9) or in a chair. A pillow can be leaned against to support the lower portion of the back.

2. If ordered, percussion or vibration would be performed between the clavicle and the top of the scapula on either or both sides, depending on whether one or both segments are being drained. See the shaded areas in Fig. 10-9.
c. Anterior segment (Fig. 10-10)
   1. The patient lies supine in bed with a pillow placed under the knees. This enables the abdominal muscles to relax so that the patient can breathe more easily.

Fig. 10-2 Drainage position for the posterior basal segments of both lower lobes. *(From Eubanks DH, Bone RC: Comprehensive respiratory care, ed 2, St Louis, 1990, Mosby.)*

Fig. 10-4 Drainage position for the anterior basal segment of the left lower lobe. The same segment in the right lung would be drained by positioning the patient similarly on the left side. *(From Eubanks DH, Bone RC: Comprehensive respiratory care, ed 2, St Louis, 1990, Mosby.)*

2. If ordered, percussion or vibration would be performed between the clavicle and the nipple of a male patient on either or both sides, depending on whether one or both segments are being drained. See the shaded areas in Fig. 10-10. Percussion and vibration may not be possible on a female patient.

Some authors may list slightly different positions or several additional positions. The most commonly accepted postural drainage positions have been presented. The postural drainage positions in the infant are basically the same as in the adult. Positioning can be accomplished more easily by using pillows. Fig. 10-11 shows the various segmental drainage positions.

> ### Exam Hint
>
> **T**he examination usually contains at least one question that deals with knowing the correct position to drain a particular lobe. The lower lobes are usually tested. The question may give information on an opaque area seen on the chest radiograph. The therapist is expected to know what segment or lobe needs to be drained. Review Fig. 1-8 for a drawing showing areas of consolidation.

Fig. 10-3 Drainage position for the lateral basal segment of the right lower lobe. The same segment in the left lung would be drained by positioning the patient similarly on the right side. *(From Eubanks DH, Bone RC: Comprehensive respiratory care, ed 2, St Louis, 1990, Mosby.)*

Fig. 10-5 Drainage position for the superior segments of both lower lobes. *(From Eubanks DH, Bone RC: Comprehensive respiratory care, ed 2, St Louis, 1990, Mosby.)*

Fig. 10-6 Drainage position for the lateral and medial segments of the right middle lobe. *(From Eubanks DH, Bone RC: Comprehensive respiratory care, ed 2, St Louis, 1990, Mosby.)*

4. Perform percussion (WRE code: IIIC1a) [Difficulty: An]

Percussion (also known as *clapping, cupping,* and *tapotement*) is the act of rhythmically striking the patient's chest with cupped hands over an area with secretions. The secretions are vibrated to flow more quickly down the vertical bronchus. Percussion will not work to move secretions if the patient is not in the proper postural drainage position. It is performed throughout the breathing cycle and can be done with one or both hands. A properly cupped hand traps air against the chest and

causes a popping sound. The wrists, elbows, and shoulders should be kept as loose as possible to enable the practitioner to keep the proper loose waving motion of the hand and minimize fatigue (Fig. 10-12). Percussion should not be painful to the patient. As an added precaution, most authors recommend that the chest be covered lightly with the patient's gown or towel. Percussion should not be done over buttons or zippers or female breast tissue.

Percussion is recommended for 5 minutes or longer in each position. Some patients, however, may not tolerate this length of treatment; 1 minute seems to be the shortest time for some therapeutic benefit. No agreement exists on the ideal rate of percussion. The practitioner must vary the rate, depending on how the patient feels and what seems to produce the best clearance of secretions.

Infants can be percussed by putting the index, middle, and ring fingers together into a kind of three-sided tent. This enables the practitioner to percuss a small area of the chest wall. Mechanical percussors/vibrators and other devices may be used to supplement manual percussion and are discussed later in this chapter.

Fig. 10-8 Drainage position for the posterior segments of both upper lobes. *(From Eubanks DH, Bone RC:* Comprehensive respiratory care, *ed 2, St Louis, 1990, Mosby.)*

Fig. 10-7 Drainage position for the superior and inferior segments of the lingula. *(From Eubanks DH, Bone RC: Comprehensive respiratory care, ed 2, St Louis, 1990, Mosby.)*

Fig. 10-9 Drainage position for the apical segments of both upper lobes. *(From Eubanks DH, Bone RC: Comprehensive respiratory care, ed 2, St Louis, 1990, Mosby.)*

5. Perform vibration (WRE code: IIIC1a) [Difficulty: R, Ap]

Vibration is the gentle, rapid shaking of the chest wall directly over the lung segment that is being drained. It may be performed alone or with percussion. The practitioner places his or her hands side by side if the chest area is large enough or one on the other for a smaller chest area. The elbows are locked with the arms straight (Fig. 10-13). The patient's chest is gently but effectively shaken during exhalation. The patient should exhale at least the complete tidal volume (V_T) as the chest wall is vibrated. Blowing out the expiratory reserve volume should help to clear out more secretions. A vibration rate of 200 per minute (about three per second) has been recommended as ideal to help move secretions. The literature differs as to how the patient should exhale during the procedure. Both breathing out slowly through pursed lips and breathing out forcefully through an open mouth have been recommended. A pursed-lip exhalation pattern seems reasonable if the patient has a problem with bronchospasm and air trapping. A patient without this problem should exhale forcefully because this helps to clear more secretions. Vibration should be performed for several expiratory efforts or until it is no longer effective in helping to mobilize secretions.

6. Modify the postural drainage therapy (WRE code: IIIF6) [Difficulty: An]
a. Change the length of treatment time

Lung segments should generally be drained for 3 to 15 minutes. If the patient is tolerating the position, and secretions are still being cleared, the position can be held longer. Stop the treatment if the patient is showing any signs of intolerance.

The total time of the procedure is recommended to be no longer than 30 to 40 minutes because the patient may become exhausted by the various position changes. If so, the practitioner must select the worst segments to be drained first. Several drainage sessions may be needed to get to all of the involved segments.

b. Change the treatment techniques used

Be prepared to modify the postural drainage, percussion, and vibration procedures, depending on how the patient tolerates them. For example:

1. Some patients cannot tolerate certain positions, especially head down, because of pain, shortness of breath (SOB), hypoxemia, or elevated blood pressure.
2. Percussion rate, pressure, and hand position may need to be modified, depending on the patient's tolerance, chest size, and secretion clearance.

Fig. 10-10 Drainage position for the anterior segments of both upper lobes. *(From Eubanks DH, Bone RC: Comprehensive respiratory care, ed 2, St Louis, 1990, Mosby.)*

Fig. 10-11 Drainage positions in infants. **A,** Apical segment of upper lobes. **B,** Posterior segments of upper lobes. **C,** Anterior segments of upper lobes. **D–F,** Superior segments of lower lobes. **G** and **H,** Anterior basal segments of both lower lobes (*H* on right and left sides). **I,** Segments of the right middle lobe and lingula (shown). **J,** Posterior basal segments of the lower lobes. *(From Crane LD: Physical therapy for the neonate with respiratory disease. In Irwin S, Tecklin JS, editors:* Cardiopulmonary physical therapy, *ed 3, St Louis, 1995, Mosby.)*

3. It may not be possible to percuss or vibrate female patients in the right middle lobe and left lingular positions because of breast tissue.
4. Hypoxemia should be prevented with supplemental O_2 in those patients who need it. Pulse oximetry could be performed before and during the procedure to monitor the patient's O_2 saturation.
5. Cardiac patients should have their heart rate, heart rhythm, and blood pressure monitored.

Check the heart rate before the procedure and with each position change.
6. Postoperative or trauma patients may not tolerate certain positions or percussion or vibration because of pain.
7. Patients with copious secretions that cannot be coughed out (e.g., those who are not alert or have a tracheostomy) should not be put in a compromising situation. Suctioning equipment must be available.

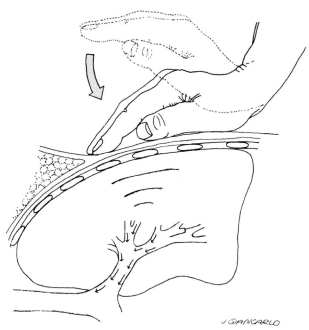

Fig. 10-12 Movement of the cupped hand at the wrist during chest percussion. *(From Shapiro BA, Kacmarek RM, Cane RD, et al: Clinical application of respiratory care, ed 4, St Louis, 1991, Mosby.)*

8. Very obese patients may not tolerate any head-down positions because of increased SOB.

c. Organize the sequence of drainage positions and treatment techniques

Differences of opinion exist as to the sequence in which the segments should be drained. Some authors state that an apices-to-bases approach is better, whereas others state that a bases-to-apices pattern is preferred. It makes sense to take an apices-to-bases approach for a first

Fig. 10-13 Vibration of the chest during postural drainage therapy. *(From Eubanks DH, Bone RC: Comprehensive respiratory care, ed 2, St Louis, 1990, Mosby.)*

treatment when all lobes are to be drained. This pattern gives the patient time to get used to the whole procedure. It also may be safer because the practitioner can evaluate the patient through a sequence of positions that progresses from the least to the most stressful.

If the patient can tolerate all positions without any difficulties, and the lower lobes are the worst in terms of secretions, drain the lower lobes first. If time permits, work up through the middle lobe and lingula to the upper lobes.

d. Change the postural drainage therapy position based on the patient's response

During the treatment, the patient's secretions may be found to be more effectively drained if he or she is repositioned from what would seem to be the ideal angle. The patient's airway anatomy may be different from what is expected. Patients with chronic lung disease, such as cystic fibrosis or bronchiectasis, often know what positions and angles are best for draining their lungs. Follow their advice if it produces good results.

Some patients cannot tolerate being properly placed because their underlying lung or heart disease is aggravated by the unnatural body position. This is most commonly seen in the head-down positions to drain the lower lobes. Watch for signs of hypoxemia and SOB. The patient may have to be put in a better-tolerated but less-desirable position. As long as some downward angle to the bronchus exists, mucus will drain. Each patient must be evaluated on an individual basis.

7. Stop the treatment if the patient has an adverse reaction to it (CSE code: IIIF1)

Be prepared to stop the treatment if the patient has an adverse reaction. Often this results when a patient is placed into a head-down position. Review Box 10-3 for hazards and complications of postural drainage, percussion, and vibration.

Exam Hint

Be prepared to stop the treatment if the patient becomes short of breath, becomes hypoxic, develops a headache or dizziness, or needs to cough.

---

8. Postural drainage therapy equipment: percussors and vibrators

a. Get the necessary equipment for the procedure (WRE code: IIA13) [Difficulty: Ap]

The terms *percussor* and *vibrator* are sometimes used interchangeably. Several manufacturers produce either electrically or pneumatically powered percussors/vibrators. Some

Fig. 10-14 An electrically powered mechanical percussor/vibrator. *(From Eubanks DH, Bone RC: Comprehensive respiratory care, ed 2, St Louis, 1990, Mosby.)*

Fig. 10-15 Right-angle adapter for Vibramatic chest percussor. The percussion adapter must be tightly screwed into the ring adapter, and the various patient applicators must be tightly screwed into the percussion adapter. *(Courtesy of General Physiotherapy, Inc., St Louis, Mo.)*

are large enough to be wheeled into the patient's room (Fig. 10-14). Obviously, electrically powered units need a standard electrical outlet for power, and the pneumatically powered units must be plugged into a 50-psi O_2 or air source.

Battery-powered pediatric units must be smaller to focus accurately on the much smaller target area of the infant's chest. Some practitioners find that an electric toothbrush with padded bristles works very well. Manual percussion of infants can be aided by using soft rubber palm cups that come in several pediatric sizes.

b. Put the equipment together and make sure that it works properly (WRE code: IIA13) [Difficulty: Ap]

Because various devices are powered by wall electrical output, 50-psi source gas, or batteries, check the power source if the device fails to work. Some units have different patient applicators and connectors. These must be fastened properly so that the vibrating action does not cause them to loosen or fall off. For example, the Vibramatic has several patient applicators that must be screwed into the percussion adapter, which is then screwed into the ring adapter (Fig. 10-15).

Some electrically powered units use a rubber belt and different sized wheels to change gears and produce several vibration rates. Others electrically vary the motor speed to change the vibration rate. Some pneumatically driven units can have their percussion force and rate varied.

c. Troubleshoot any problems with the equipment (WRE code: IIA13) [Difficulty: Ap]

Pneumatically powered units would suddenly fail if the high-pressure hose to the wall gas outlet or the O_2 tank were to become disconnected. Electrically powered units would fail if the electrical cord were unplugged or the batteries were depleted.

MODULE B
Positive expiratory pressure therapy

1. Positive expiratory pressure therapy equipment
a. Get the necessary equipment for the procedure (CSE code: IIA16)

Currently, several positive expiratory pressure (PEP) systems are available for selection, based on the patient's needs. Fig. 10-16 shows a unit that provides only expiratory pressure.

Fig. 10-16 Drawing of the DHD TheraPEP device. *1,* Patient mouthpiece. *2,* Hose to connect the mouthpiece to the pressure generator. *3,* One-way inlet valve for inspiration. *4,* Pressure generator the patient exhales through to create positive expiratory pressure. *(From Myslinski MJ, Scanlan CL: Bronchial hygiene therapy. In Wilkins RL, Stoller JK, Scanlan CL, editors: Egan's fundamentals of respiratory care, ed 8, St Louis, 2003, Mosby.)*

Fig. 10-17 shows a unit that can use either a mouthpiece or face mask for delivering expiratory pressure. In addition, this unit can have a small volume nebulizer (SVN) added to it for medication delivery during the PEP treatment. The PEP mask should be transparent, flexible, and fit the patient's facial contours so that no air will leak out as the pressure is increased. The following equipment is needed for PEP therapy, as shown in Fig. 10-17.

a. Appropriate size PEP mask or mouthpiece and nose clips, or universal airway (elbow) adapter for attachment to an endotracheal or tracheostomy tube

b. Expiratory resistor

c. Pressure manometer calibrated in centimeters of water

d. Small-bore oxygen tubing to connect the expiratory resistor to the pressure manometer

e. Basin and tissues to collect and dispose of sputum

f. Gloves, mask, goggles, and gown for the practitioner

The following *additional* equipment is needed to deliver an aerosolized medication, as shown in Fig. 10-17:

a. SVN

b. T-piece and female adapter to connect the nebulizer to the expiratory resistor

c. Large bore aerosol tubing to act as medication reservoir

b. Put the equipment together and make sure that it works properly (CSE code: IIA16)

As shown in Figs. 10-16 and 10-17, the component pieces must be properly put together. Make sure that all connections are airtight. If a leak is present, the desired PEP goal will not be reached or maintained. In addition, if an air leak is present, it may be felt or a high-pitched sound may be heard. If a nebulizer is added for aerosolizing medications, ensure that it works properly. Connect the SVN into the system as shown. Add the medication, and run a flow of oxygen or air at 4 to 6 L/min through the nebulizer (as is customary).

c. Alter the positive expiratory pressure therapy equipment (WRE code: IIIC4) [Difficulty: An]

Be prepared to adjust the expiratory resistance to meet the clinical goal of PEP therapy. The Resistex unit has four fixed-orifice settings to choose from. The orifice diameters are 4 mm, 3.5 mm, 3 mm, and 2.5 mm interior diameter.

Fig. 10-17 Positive expiratory pressure (PEP) mask components. The basic PEP assembly necessitates a transparent mask or mouthpiece, expiratory resistor (this shows the Resistex), and pressure manometer with connecting oxygen tubing. If a nebulized medication is added, the following also are needed: small volume nebulizer with T-piece, oxygen tubing to flowmeter, and large bore tubing for an aerosol reservoir. *(From Malmeister MJ, Fink JB, Hoffman GL, et al: Positive-expiratory-pressure mask therapy: theoretical and practical considerations and a review of the literature,* Respir Care 36[11]:1218, 1991.)

The PEP mask made by Astra Meditec uses a series of different sized pediatric endotracheal tube adapters. They are fitted into an adapter through which the patient exhales. With either unit, the patient should be started out with the largest opening to breathe out through. The TheraPEP device allows the expiratory pressure to be adjusted as well.

d. Troubleshoot any problems with the equipment (CSE code: IIA16)

Any leaks in the system will prevent the PEP goal from being reached. Tighten any loose connections. If the one-way valves in the Resistex unit are put together backward, the patient will inspire against a resistance instead of exhaling against it. Observe the one-way valves in use, and ask the patient if he or she finds it easy to inhale but more difficult to exhale. Move the valves to their proper positions if incorrectly placed. If no mist is seen coming from the nebulizer, check the capillary tube or baffle for an obstruction; clear it by running tap water or a sterile needle through it. See Chapter 8, if necessary, for more information on fixing problems with SVNs.

2. Alter the treatment duration and positive expiratory pressure therapy techniques as needed (WRE code: IIIF6) [Difficulty: An]

PEP therapy involves having a spontaneously breathing patient exhale against a fixed-orifice resistor to create expiratory pressures between 10 and 20 cm H_2O. This therapy also is called *PEP mask therapy* because many pediatric patients use a face mask to deliver the pressure to the airways. Box 10-5 lists indications for PEP therapy. In patients with air trapping because of small-airways disease, PEP therapy acts like pursed-lips breathing to keep the small airways from collapsing. This allows the trapped alveolar gas to be more completely exhaled. Patients with atelectasis or at risk for developing atelectasis respond well to PEP therapy. PEP seems to push air through the Kohn pores of open alveoli into adjacent areas of atelectasis to force the alveoli open. The other indications are discussed later.

Box 10-6 lists relative contraindications to PEP therapy. No absolute contraindications exist. Box 10-7 lists hazards or complications of PEP therapy. These should be weighed against the benefits to the patient when making the recommendation to start PEP therapy. Other considerations include the patient's history of pulmonary disease and the response to postural drainage therapy, ineffective cough to clear retained secretions, and breath sounds and chest radiograph findings of secretions.

PEP therapy has proven effective in helping patients with chronic, copious amounts of secretions, primarily children aged 4 years or older with cystic fibrosis. It also helps patients with chronic bronchitis, bronchiectasis, or bronchiolitis obliterans. Clinical evidence indicates that the PEP dilates the small airways so that air is able to get past obstructing secretions. This fills the alveoli and, on expiration, tends to force the secretions into the larger airways for coughing or suctioning out. See Fig. 10-16 for an example of a PEP therapy system.

PEP therapy also seems to increase the effectiveness of inhaled aerosolized bronchodilators. As shown in Fig. 10-17, the component pieces must be gathered and

---

BOX 10-6 Relative Contraindications to Positive Expiratory Pressure Therapy

- Untreated pneumothorax
- Intracranial pressure > 20 mm Hg
- Active hemoptysis
- Recent trauma or surgery to the skull, face, mouth, or esophagus
- Patient with asthma attack or acute worsening of chronic obstructive pulmonary disease who cannot tolerate increased work of breathing
- Acute sinusitis or epistaxis
- Tympanic membrane rupture or other known or suspected middle ear pathology
- Nausea

BOX 10-5 Indications for Positive Expiratory Pressure Therapy

- To reduce air trapping in patients with emphysema, bronchitis, and asthma
- To prevent or reverse atelectasis
- To help mobilize retained secretions in patients older than 4 years who have cystic fibrosis, chronic bronchitis, bronchiectasis, or bronchiolitis obliterans
- To maximize the delivery of aerosolized medications, such as bronchodilators, to patients receiving bronchial hygiene therapy

---

BOX 10-7 Hazards or Complications of Positive Expiratory Pressure Therapy

- Pulmonary barotrauma
- Increased intracranial pressure
- Myocardial ischemia or decreased venous return to the heart
- Increased work of breathing
- Air swallowing that can lead to vomiting
- Discomfort from mask or skin breakdown from mask pressure
- Claustrophobia

properly put together. Make sure that all connections are airtight. If a leak is present, the desired PEP goal will not be reached or maintained. In addition, an air leak may be felt or a high-pitched sound may be heard. The SVN must be tested to ensure that it works properly. Connect the SVN into the system, as shown in Fig. 10-17. Add the medication and run a flow of O_2 or air at 4 to 6 L/min through the nebulizer (as is customary). The slowed exhalation during PEP breathing should promote better deposition of medication into the small airways.

The patient must be old enough to understand instructions and be able to perform the procedure. Box 10-8 lists the steps in performing a proper PEP therapy treatment. Be prepared to adjust the expiratory resistance to meet the clinical goal of PEP therapy. Initially the pressure or resistance to exhalation should be kept low. As the training continues, the resistance or pressure the patient breathes against can be increased. The goal is to maintain a PEP of 10 to 20 cm H_2O with an inspiratory/expiratory (I:E) ratio of about 1:3. If the pressure is too high or the expiratory time too long, the patient will likely become fatigued. If the orifice is too large, the pressure will not be high enough to be of any benefit. The patient will probably become tired if the total treatment time lasts longer than 20 minutes.

3. Coordinate the sequence of therapies to modify bronchial hygiene (WRE code: IIIF6) [Difficulty: An]

Coordinate PEP therapy with effective "huff" cough techniques, PDT, or aerosolized medication delivery. As listed in Box 10-8, PEP breaths should be alternated with huff coughs to clear secretions. Huff coughs are not full, deep coughs; rather, they are performed as follows:

a. Have the patient inhale a slow, deep breath but not to total lung capacity (TLC).

b. Hold the breath in for 1 to 3 seconds.

c. Perform several quick, forced exhalations with an open epiglottis.

d. Small children may be taught to say "huff" with each quick exhalation. It also may help to have the young patient perform a "chicken breath" by flapping his or her arms against the sides of the chest during the exhalation.

PDT may be used before or after PEP therapy, or it may be alternated with PEP therapy, to help in the removal of secretions. Likewise, aerosolized medications may be inhaled before or simultaneously with PEP therapy. Bronchodilators and mucolytic agents should be very helpful with PEP therapy to mobilize secretions. Evaluate sputum for quantity, color, odor, and thickness.

4. Stop the treatment if the patient has an adverse reaction to it (CSE code: IIIF1)

During the treatment, ask the patient if he or she feels dyspnea, pain, or chest discomfort. Also monitor the

---

BOX 10-8 Steps in Performing Positive Expiratory Pressure (PEP) Therapy

1. Put the equipment together as shown in Figs. 10-16 and 10-17.
2. Have the conscious patient sit up straight, rest elbows on a table, and hold the PEP mask comfortably but tightly over the nose and mouth. The patient may use a mouthpiece and nose clips if preferred.
3. The patient should inhale a deeper-than-normal breath, but not to total lung capacity, by using the diaphragm. The unconscious patient will inhale only a tidal volume breath.
4. The conscious patient should exhale to functional residual capacity fast enough to generate 10–20 cm H_2O in the manometer. Have the patient look at the pressure manometer to judge how fast to exhale. The unconscious patient will exhale passively but will still benefit from the increased baseline pressure.
5. The patient should have an expiratory time that is about three times longer than the inspiratory time (an inspiratory/expiratory ratio of 1:2 to 1:4 is acceptable). The clinician can accomplish this by changing the expiratory resistor and/or having the patient change the force of exhalation.
6. Between 10 and 20 proper PEP breaths should be performed.
7. The patient should now perform two or three "huff"-type coughing efforts to raise secretions.
8. Repeat steps 2 to 7 between four and eight times (for ~ 10–20 min) for a full PEP treatment.

Patients in the intensive care unit can perform PEP therapy as often as every hour or as rarely as every 6 hr. They should be reevaluated for treatment effectiveness every 24 hr. Patients in the acute care or home care setting can perform PEP therapy between two and four times each day. The acute care patient should be reevaluated every 72 hr; the home care patient can be evaluated at longer intervals or when a change in pulmonary status occurs.

patient's breath sounds, blood pressure, heart rate, and breathing pattern and rate. Monitor oxygenation by pulse oximetry, mental clarity, and skin color. Be prepared to stop the treatment if necessary. Review the contraindications listed in Box 10-6 and hazards listed in Box 10-7.

MODULE C
High frequency airway oscillation

1. Flutter valve and Acapella unit
a. Get the necessary equipment for the procedure (CSE code: IIA17)

The Flutter valve (Fig. 10-18) is a pipe-shaped device with a steel ball nesting loosely inside the bowl. The Flutter valve has been used with cystic fibrosis patients to help them loosen their secretions. It is believed that the high-frequency oscillations of backpressure on the airway caused by the fluttering steel ball help to dislodge thick (viscous) secretions. The more recent Acapella device uses an adjustable counterweighted lever and magnet to produce variable frequency and amplitude of the expiratory pressure. It has the same clinical indications as the Flutter valve.

b. Put the equipment together and make sure it works properly (CSE code: IIA17)

The Flutter valve comes preassembled by the manufacturer. A perforated cap should be over the bowl to keep the ball from falling while letting exhaled air escape. The Acapella has an adjustable knob at the opposite end of the unit from the patient's mouthpiece. As the knob is rotated, a magnet is moved closer to or farther from a counterweighted lever. Rotate the knob, as needed, to set the patients expiratory frequency and amplitude pressure.

Fig. 10-18 A, Patient correctly holding the Flutter valve for an exhalation. **B,** Cross-section drawing of the Flutter valve showing how the steel ball is lifted by the patient's exhaled tidal volume. When the ball drops back down, the backpressure is transmitted to the airways. *(From Fink JB, Hess DR: Secretion clearance techniques. In Hess DR, MacIntyre NR, Mishoe SC, et al, editors:* Respiratory care principals and practice, *Philadelphia, 2002, WB Saunders.)*

c. Troubleshoot any problems with the equipment (CSE code: IIB2l)

The patient must keep the Flutter valve in the proper position with the perforated cap in the upright position. This keeps the patient's exhaled air blowing through the device to push up the steel ball. If a patient should cough secretions into the unit, it will become clogged. Air will not flow through it. Try clearing the obstruction from the mouthpiece with a cotton swab or by running warm water through the unit. If necessary, the cap can be unscrewed and ball removed to remove secretions. Be sure to put them back together properly.

With the Acapella, if the adjustable knob cannot move or the frequency and amplitude pressure cannot be adjusted, the unit may be obstructed or defective. If a secretion obstruction cannot be removed, the unit must be replaced.

2. Alter the treatment duration and technique for the vibratory positive expiratory pressure (Flutter valve) devices (WRE code: IIIF6) [Difficulty: An]

The Flutter valve has been used with cystic fibrosis patients to help them loosen their secretions. The high-frequency oscillations of backpressure on the airway caused by the fluttering steel ball are believed to help dislodge viscous secretions. The Flutter valve is a pipe-shaped device with a steel ball nesting loosely inside the bowl. A perforated cap over the bowl keeps the ball from falling out but allows exhaled air to escape. Make sure that the components are properly assembled, as shown in Fig. 10-18. If the ball does not move loosely, it may be stuck by secretions. In this case, unscrew the cap, take out the ball, and clean out the secretions. Once reassembled, the ball should move loosely within the bowl.

Because of its simplicity, both small children and adults can be instructed in its use. The patient is taught to take a deeper-than-usual breath, hold the flutter valve with the cap up, and blow out through the mouthpiece. The exhaled breath pushes the ball up in the bowl, air briefly escapes, and the ball falls back down again. When the ball falls back, more pressure is exerted against the patient's airway. The airway pressure generated during the exhalation varies from 10 to 25 cm H_2O, depending on how fast the patient blows out. The rate at which the ball flutters up and down is about 15 Hz (hertz or cycles/sec) and varies with the angle of the bowl.

3. Coordinate the sequence of therapies to modify bronchial hygiene (WRE code: IIIF6) [Difficulty: An]

If inhaled bronchodilator or mucolytic medications are ordered for the patient, they should be taken before the Flutter valve treatment. Typically the patient repeats the

Flutter valve maneuver for 10 to 20 breaths. The patient should then perform two or three huff-type coughs. The cycle of Flutter valve exhalations and huff coughs is repeated four to eight times. Total treatment time should not be longer than 20 minutes.

4. Stop the treatment if the patient has an adverse reaction to it (CSE code: IIIF1)

It is unlikely that a patient will have an adverse reaction from using the Flutter valve. However, it is possible that some patients will not like the feeling of increased pressure in the lungs. In this case, it may be better to stop the treatment and switch to another method of secretion management.

Exam Hint

Expect to see at least one question about PEP therapy. Be prepared to recommend it in a patient with a secretion problem. PEP therapy may have to be modified to maximize secretion mobilization, or PEP therapy may be added to another treatment such as incentive spirometry, an SVN for medications, or high frequency chest wall oscillation to help the patient mobilize and clear secretions.

---

5. High frequency chest wall oscillation equipment
a. Get the necessary equipment for the procedure (WRE code: IIA14) [Difficulty: R, Ap]

High-frequency chest wall oscillation (HFCWO) is indicated to help mobilize and clear secretions. This equipment may be used in patients who do not tolerate other secretion mobilization procedures. For example, a cystic fibrosis patient may have an adverse effect when put into head-down positions for postural drainage therapy. Currently, two HFCWO devices are available. The Vest (Fig. 10-19) consists of a nonstretchable inflatable vest that covers the entire torso, an electrically powered pumping and control system, and two connecting hoses. The controls allow an adjustable air pulse rate of 5 Hz (Hertz; cycles/second) that produces a vest pressure of 25 mm Hg and 25 Hz, which produces a vest pressure of 40 mm Hg.

The Hayek Oscillator (Fig. 10-20) consists of a flexible chest cuirass, an electrically powered pumping and control panel, and a connecting hose. This machine can deliver both positive and negative pressure to the patient's chest throughout the breathing cycle. Added negative pressure around the patient's chest will increase inspiration. Added positive pressure around the patient's chest will increase expiration. The therapist can adjust an oscillation rate of 8 to 999 oscillations/min, with an I:E ratio of 6:1 to 1:6, and inspiratory and expiratory pressures of up to +70 cm water.

Fig. 10-19 The Vest high-frequency chest wall oscillation device with its pumping and control unit, air hoses, inflatable vest, and foot control. *(Courtesy Hill-Rom Services, Inc.)*

With either unit, it is believed that the pressure on the outside of the chest is transmitted internally to increase expiratory airflow and push secretions from small to larger airways. HFCWO has been found to help cystic fibrosis patients mobilize retained secretions.

b. Put the equipment together and make sure that it works properly (WRE code: IIA14) [Difficulty: R, Ap]
c. Troubleshoot any problems with the equipment (WRE code: IIA14) [Difficulty: R, Ap]

Follow the manufacturer's guidelines to assemble the components, as shown in Figs. 10-19 and 10-20. The patient should be instructed to sit up during the treatment, put on the inflatable vest or cuirass, and connect the air hose(s) between the vest/cuirass and the pumping unit. A general recommendation is to have the patient set whatever oscillation rate results in the greatest production of secretions. Common sense indicates that it is appropriate to start at the lowest rate and pressure and progress to a faster rate and higher pressure as the patient tolerates. Treatments typically last 30 minutes and can be repeated up to six times per day. This procedure cannot be used in a patient with a chest wall injury such as broken ribs.

One problem area could relate to the vest/cuirass not fitting properly. If the vest/cuirass is too large, air will leak, and the desired pressures will not be reached. Adjust the unit for a tighter fit, or place pads between the patient and the vest/cuirass to seal the leak. Too tight a vest/cuirass could rub on the skin and be uncomfortable. Loosen the vest/cuirass or add more padding over the skin. If the hose(s) come loose from the vest/cuirass or the

Cuirass
Cuirass short tubes
Pressure sensor tubing
Keyboard/control unit
Power unit
Cuirass Y-connector
Wide bore tube

Fig. 10-20 Drawing of the Hayek Oscillator with its pumping and control unit, air hose, and patient cuirass. *(From McIntyre NR, Mishoe SC: Respiratory care: principles and practice, St Louis, 2002, WB Saunders. Modified from materials courtesy of Breasy Medical Equipment, Stanford, Conn.)*

pumping unit, the air will leak out, and no pressure will be generated. Reattach the hose(s).

MODULE D
Respiratory care plan

1. Analyze the available information to determine the patient's pathophysiologic state (CSE code: IIIH1)

The patient's breath sounds should be auscultated before the treatment begins to determine which segments are normal or have secretions. Auscultate each segment after the treatment and after the patient has coughed. Listen for air moving into formerly silent areas or areas that are cleared of secretions.

Make a recommendation for a chest radiograph examination to find specific areas for PDT. A white shadow on a chest radiograph film over what should be normal lung may indicate areas of atelectasis or infiltrates that can be targeted for treatment. Chest radiograph examinations should be repeated to look for an improvement in the lungs. The resolution may be slow or dramatic, depending

on the original problem and how it responds to the various treatments used on it.

2. Record and interpret the type of cough the patient has and the nature of the sputum (WRE code: IIIA1a) [Difficulty: An]

All of the procedures discussed in this chapter are done to improve the patient's cough and increase sputum production. If they are ineffective, another procedure must be tried.

3. Record and interpret the patient's breath sounds (WRE code: IIIA1a) [Difficulty: An]

The patient's breath sounds should improve if retained secretions are coughed out.

4. Determine the appropriateness of the prescribed therapy and goals for the identified pathophysiologic state (CSE code: IIIH3)
  a. Review the interdisciplinary patient and family care plan (WRE code: IIIH1b) [Difficulty: An]
  b. Review the planned therapy to establish the therapeutic plan (WRE code: IIIH1a) [Difficulty: An]
  c. Recommend changes in the therapeutic plan if supportive data exist (WRE code: IIIH2) [Difficulty: An]

The AARC clinical practice guideline recommends that the following be evaluated to determine whether PDT is needed:
  1. PDT is usually not indicated if an optimally hydrated patient is coughing out less than 25 mL/day with the procedure.
  2. A dehydrated patient should have apparently ineffective PDT continued for at least 24 hours after the patient is rehydrated. The combination of rehydration and PDT may help to mobilize previously thick secretions.
  3. PDT is not indicated in a patient producing more than 30 mL of secretions per day if the treatments do not increase the sputum production. The patient is already able to cough out the sputum effectively.

For any of the previously discussed procedures, be prepared to measure the patient's blood pressure, heart rate, and respiratory rate before, during, and after a change in therapy. Minor changes (less than 20%) can be expected. The patient's oxygenation should improve as secretions and mucus plugs are removed and atelectatic areas open. The patient's breath sounds should be auscultated before and after any treatment procedure. Listen for air moving into formerly silent areas and for secretions being cleared.

Ask the patient how he or she feels before, during, and after the treatment. PDT should not be performed for at least 1 hour after a patient has eaten to minimize the chances of nausea from the head-down positions.

PEP therapy has been indicated in patients who have retained secretions that are difficult to cough out. Increase or decrease the PEP level to help the patient without causing fatigue or complications. If PEP therapy does not increase the amount of sputum produced per day in a patient who already produces more than 30 mL, PEP may not be needed. It does not make sense to continue an ineffective treatment.

d. Conduct patient education and disease management programs (WRE code: IIIH7) [Difficulty: An]

The previously discussed procedures are used primarily with cystic fibrosis or chronic bronchitis patients. All have been shown to help in the mobilization of secretions. However, each patient may find that one procedure works better than another. Be prepared to make recommendations to change the type of procedure and the way each procedure is conducted. In addition, other respiratory care procedures (e.g., O_2 therapy) and inhaled bronchodilators and mucolytic medications may have to be modified as the patient's condition warrants.

5. Discontinue treatment based on the patient's response (WRE code: IIIG1e) [Difficulty: An]

Review the previous discussion for indications that the patient has recovered and no longer needs bronchopulmonary hygiene procedures. For example, the secretions have decreased or can be easily coughed out by the patient, or both. Review Boxes 10-2 and 10-3 for contraindications and hazards/complications of postural drainage and percussion and vibration. Review Boxes 10-6 and 10-7 for contraindications and hazards/complications of PEP therapy.

BIBLIOGRAPHY

American Association for Respiratory Care: Clinical practice guideline: directed cough, *Respir Care* 38(5):495, 1993.

American Association for Respiratory Care: Clinical practice guideline: postural drainage therapy, *Respir Care* 36:1418, 1991.

American Association for Respiratory Care: Clinical practice guideline: use of positive airway pressure adjuncts to bronchial hygiene therapy, *Respir Care* 38(5):516, 1993.

Branson RD, Hess DR, Chatburn RL: *Respiratory care equipment,* ed 2, Philadelphia, 1999, Lippincott Williams & Wilkins.

Cairo JM: Lung expansion devices. In Cairo JM, Pilbeam SP, editors: *Mosby's respiratory care equipment,* ed 7, St Louis, 2004, Mosby.

Campbell TC, Ferguson N, McKinlay RGC: The use of a simple self-administered method of positive expiratory pressure (PEP) in chest physiotherapy after abdominal surgery, *Physiotherapy* 72(10):498, 1986.

Eid N, Buchheit J, Neuling M, et al: Chest physiotherapy in review, *Respir Care* 36(4):270, 1991.

Eubanks DH, Bone RC: *Comprehensive respiratory care,* ed 2, St Louis, 1990, Mosby.

Fink JB: Bronchial hygiene therapy and lung expansion. In Fink JB, Hunt GE, editors: *Clinical practice in respiratory care,* Philadelphia, 1999, Lippincott-Raven.

Fink JB: Volume expansion therapy. In Burton GC, Hodgkin JE, Ward JJ, editors: *Respiratory care: a guide to clinical practice,* ed 4, Philadelphia, 1997, Lippincott-Raven.

Fink JB, Hess DR: Secretion clearance techniques. In Hess DR, MacIntyre NR, Mishoe SC, et al, editors: *Respiratory care principals and practice,* Philadelphia, 2002, WB Saunders.

Frownfelter DL: Chest physical therapy and airway care. In Barnes TA, editor: *Core textbook of respiratory care practice,* ed 2, St Louis, 1994, Mosby.

Hess DR, Branson RD: Chest physiotherapy, incentive spirometry, intermittent positive-pressure breathing, secretion clearance, and inspiratory muscle training. In Branson RD, Hess DR, Chatburn RL, editors: *Respiratory care equipment,* ed 2, Philadelphia, 1999, Lippincott Williams & Wilkins.

Hill KV: Bronchial hygiene therapy. In Aloan CA, Hill TV, editors: *Respiratory care of the newborn and child,* ed 2, Philadelphia, 1997, Lippincott-Raven.

Hoffman GL, Cohen NH: Positive expiratory pressure therapy, *NBRC Horizons* 19(2):1, 1993.

Johnson NT, Pierson DJ: The spectrum of pulmonary atelectasis: pathophysiology, diagnosis, and therapy, *Respir Care* 31(11):1107, 1986.

Kacmarek RM, Dimas S, Mack CW: *The essentials of respiratory care,* ed 4, St Louis, 2005, Mosby.

Malmeister MJ, Fink JB, Hoffman GL: Positive-expiratory-pressure mask therapy: theoretical and practical considerations and a review of the literature, *Respir Care* 36(11):1218, 1991.

Myslinski MJ, Scanlan CL: Bronchial hygiene therapy. In Wilkins RL, Stoller JK, Scanlan CL, editors: *Egan's fundamentals of respiratory care,* ed 8, St Louis, 2003, Mosby.

Oberwaldner PT, Evans JC, Zach MS: Forced expirations against a variable resistance: a new chest physiotherapy method in cystic fibrosis, *Pediatr Pulmonol* 2(6):358, 1986.

Rutkowski JA: Pulmonary hygiene and chest physical therapy. In Wyka KA, Mathews PJ, Clark WF, editors: *Foundations of respiratory care,* Albany, NY, 2002, Delmar.

Scott AA, Koff PB: Airway care and chest physiotherapy. In Koff PB, Eitzman D, Neu J, editors: *Neonatal and pediatric respiratory care,* ed 2, St Louis, 1993, Mosby.

Shapiro BA, Kacmarek RM, Cane RD, et al, editors: *Clinical application of respiratory care,* ed 4, St Louis, 1991, Mosby.

Sobush DC, Hilling L, Southorn PA: Bronchial hygiene therapy. In Burton GC, Hodgkin JE, Ward JJ, editors: *Respiratory care: a guide to clinical practice,* ed 4, Philadelphia, 1997, Lippincott-Raven.

White GC: *Equipment theory for respiratory care,* ed 3, Albany, NY, 1999, Delmar.

Wojciechowski WV: Incentive spirometers, secretion evacuation devices, and inspiratory muscle training devices. In Barnes TA, editor: *Core textbook of respiratory care practice,* ed 2, St Louis, 1994, Mosby.

SELF-STUDY QUESTIONS

1. A patient who is being instructed in positive expiratory pressure (PEP) therapy complains that it is taking too long to breathe out. What would you do?
   A. Tell the patient to blow out harder.
   B. Change the expiratory resistance to a larger diameter orifice.
   C. Change the expiratory resistance to a smaller diameter orifice.
   D. Increase the flow of oxygen to the system.

2. Your patient is 40 years old and had upper abdominal surgery 2 days ago. He is showing signs of atelectasis and retained secretions. Your instructions for a directed cough would include all of the following *except*:
   A. Take in as deep a breath as possible.
   B. Support the incision.
   C. Perform a serial cough at low air flows.
   D. Inhale and exhale several times before coughing.

3. A 56-year-old patient has been in the Trendelenburg position for 10 minutes receiving percussion and vibration. Tachycardia and dyspnea develop. Which of the following should the respiratory therapist do?
   A. Continue for 5 minutes with gentle percussion.
   B. Turn the patient to the other side.
   C. Give the patient oxygen.
   D. Have the patient sit up.

4. A 12-year-old patient with cystic fibrosis has had PEP therapy started at 5 cm water. After a few minutes of use, the patient fails to cough productively. What should be done now?
   A. Increase the PEP level to 10 cm water.
   B. Increase the PEP level to 15 cm water.
   C. Change to incentive spirometry.
   D. Discontinue the treatment.

5. After several days of receiving postural drainage and percussion therapy to all lobes in the left lung, the patient's chest radiograph shows improvement except for the left lower lobe. What position should he now be placed in for postural drainage?
   A. Right side down with the head of the bed down 30 degrees
   B. Right side down with the bed flat
   C. Left side down with the head of the bed down 30 degrees
   D. Flat on his back with the bed flat and a pillow beneath the knees

6. A physician has ordered PEP therapy with albuterol. All of the following are needed to start the treatment *except*:
   A. Variable orifice resistor
   B. Pressure manometer

   C. Bedside spirometer
   D. Nebulizer with reservoir

7. The patient benefits from using the Flutter valve by which of the following?
   I. Increased transpleural pressure
   II. Airway vibrations
   III. Increased intrapleural pressure
   IV. Rapid variation in airway pressure
   A. I and II
   B. II and III
   C. III and IV
   D. II and IV

8. A 48-year-old woman has had her gallbladder removed. What is most effective in preventing postoperative atelectasis?
   A. Blow bottles
   B. PEP therapy
   C. Mechanical chest percussor
   D. Inspiratory muscle training

9. A patient is being started on high-frequency chest wall oscillation (HFCWO) to help mobilize secretions. Which of the following instructions should the patient be given for the initial treatment?
   I. Lie on the side with the most secretions.
   II. Sit up straight.
   III. Set the controls at a low rate and pressure.
   IV. Set the controls at a high rate and pressure.
   V. Set the unit for maximum nebulization during inspiration.
   A. II and III
   B. I and III
   C. II, IV, and V
   D. I, III, and V

10. A 70-year-old patient who had a stroke has aspirated and now has a fever and pulmonary secretions. The respiratory therapist notices on the anteroposterior (AP) and right lateral chest radiographs that the posterior basal area of the right lung is opaque. What postural drainage position should be used with this patient?
    A. On the right side, head down 30 degrees, one-fourth turn up from face-down
    B. On the left side, head down 30 degrees, one-fourth turn up from face-down
    C. Head down 15 degrees, pillow behind the right side to turn one-fourth turn up from flat
    D. Head down 15 degrees, pillow behind the left side to turn one-fourth turn up from flat

11. A patient is using the Flutter valve and coughs productively. Later, the patient tries to use the device but finds that no air will go through it. What should be done?
    A. Have the patient breathe in harder.
    B. Check for an obstruction.

C. Remove the steel ball to reduce the backpressure.

D. Have the patient blow out harder.

12. A mechanical percussor is ordered to assist with secretion clearance in a patient receiving PDT. The patient is positioned to drain the posterior basal segments of both lower lobes. The percussor is activated and applied to the patient's lower back. After a minute, the patient complains of skin discomfort. What should the respiratory therapist do?

A. Have the patient sit up.

B. Apply oxygen and check the pulse-oximeter value.

C. Increase the speed on the percussor.

D. Change to another type of pad on the percussor.

13. A 10-year-old patient with cystic fibrosis has large amounts of secretions. He cannot tolerate PDT because of nausea when he is tipped down. He is receiving aerosolized bronchodilator and mucolytic medications. To improve his condition, the respiratory therapist could recommend all of the following *except*:

A. PEP therapy

B. Flutter valve or Acapella unit

C. High-frequency chest wall oscillation

D. Continuous positive airway pressure (CPAP) at 10 cm water

ANSWER KEY

1. **B.** Rationale: By changing the expiratory resistance to a larger diameter orifice, the patient will be able to exhale more quickly. See Fig. 10-1. Telling the patient to blow out harder will increase the pressure within the system. This could increase the patient's discomfort. Changing the expiratory resistance to a smaller diameter orifice will further increase the expiratory time, not decrease it. Although a PEP system can have oxygen added to it to power the nebulizer, no mention of one is made in the question. In addition, the use of supplemental oxygen to a nebulizer does not have any effect on the expiratory time of the patient.

2. **C.** Rationale: Initially the patient should be taught to cough out as hard as possible. If that is not possible because of pain, a serial cough with low flows can be tried. The patient should be given a pain medication so that a strong cough can be tolerated. It is important that the patient inhale deeply to have an effective cough. Pain will be lessened if the incision is supported with the patient's hands or a pillow. Inhaling and exhaling several times before coughing helps the patient to build up to a large breath and prepare for the coughing effort.

3. **D.** Rationale: The patient should sit up because tachycardia and dyspnea are definite indications of intolerance of the head-down position. It could be dangerous for the patient to continue in the head-down position for even 5 more minutes. The treatment should be stopped, and the patient should sit up rather than being turned to the other side. Give the patient supplemental oxygen only if needed after having the patient sit up and finding that he or she is hypoxic.

4. **A.** Rationale: It is reasonable to increase the PEP level from 5 to 10 cm water. Have the patient try this moderately increased pressure for several minutes, and evaluate the effectiveness of the patient's cough effort. The PEP level should not be increased to 15 cm water unless 10 cm water has been shown to be ineffective.

Incentive spirometry is indicated for atelectasis or the prevention of atelectasis. It is not indicated for secretion clearance, as is PEP therapy. It is too early in the treatment to determine that PEP therapy should be discontinued.

5. **A.** Rationale: To drain the left lower lobe, the patient must be placed with the right side down on the bed and the head of the bed down 30 degrees. The other positions will not properly drain the left lower lobe. Review the postural drainage positions if needed.

6. **C.** Rationale: A bedside spirometer is not needed because the patient's exhaled volume does not need to be measured. In addition, a spirometer cannot be connected to the unit for volume measurement. All of the other listed items are needed. The variable orifice resistor is needed to set the level of expiratory resistance. A pressure manometer is needed to determine that the expiratory pressure is kept in the 10- to 20-cm water range. A small volume nebulizer with reservoir is needed to deliver the albuterol.

7. **D.** Rationale: The Flutter valve is designed to cause rapid airway vibrations. These vibrations result in a rapid variation in airway pressure. This results in the airways rapidly dilating and then contracting to their resting diameter. These changes seem to loosen secretions so that they can be coughed out more easily by the patient. Neither increased transpleural pressure nor increased intrapleural pressure have any effect on the mobilization of secretions.

8. **B.** Rationale: PEP therapy will increase end expiratory lung pressure. This should increase alveolar volume and prevent the development of atelectasis. Blow bottles are no longer in use because they have been shown not to be effective in the management of atelectasis. A mechanical chest percussor can be used with PDT to help mobilize secretions. However, it does not have any benefit in preventing atelectasis. Inspiratory muscle

training is beneficial in patients with chronic obstructive lung disease because they are usually deconditioned. This should be part of a general conditioning program. However, inspiratory muscle training has no direct effect on atelectasis and should not be confused with use of an incentive spirometer.

9. **A.** Rationale: The patient must sit up straight because the vest is ridged. To work best, it should have even contact with the patient's entire chest wall. This would not happen if the patient were lying on a side. It is best to have the patient start at the lowest rate and pressure to gain confidence in the unit and not risk injury. The HFCWO unit does not have a nebulizer.

10. **B.** Rationale: The position described would be used to drain secretions from the patient's lateral basal segment of the right lower lobe. See Fig. 1-8 for the area of consolidation and Fig. 10-3 for the postural drainage position.

11. **B.** Rationale: It is likely that the patient coughed secretions into the unit. Check for an obstruction. If one is present, it must be cleaned out. A cotton swab or warm running water should clear out any secretions. The Flutter valve is designed to be blown out through, not breathed in through. It is not an incentive spirometer device. Removing the steel ball from the device will prevent it from working as intended. If the patient blows out hard, the obstruction may be blown deeper into the unit.

12. **D.** Rationale: Try another type of pad on the percussor to determine whether it is more comfortable for the patient. A flat one is probably best for the lower back. The patient is not having a reaction to the head-down position and does not need to sit up. No indication exists that the patient is hypoxic. Increasing the speed on the percussor is likely to increase the skin irritation.

13. **D.** Rationale: CPAP is indicated to increase a patient's functional residual capacity to improve oxygenation. It has no effect on secretions. PEP therapy, the Flutter valve, Acapella unit, and HFCWO have all been shown to be effective at mobilizing secretions.

11 Cardiac Monitoring and Cardiopulmonary Resuscitation

Note 1: The National Board for Respiratory Care (NBRC) has released the *RRT Examination Matrix* (covering the testable items on the Written Registry Exam) and the *CSE Examination Matrix* (covering the testable items on the Clinical Simulation Exam). Turn to the appendices at the back of this book for both publications in their original format. This book is intended to cover all of the testable items in these two publications. This chapter (and all others) uses the abbreviation "WRE" for the coded items testable on the Written Registry Exam *and* Clinical Simulation Exam. The listed difficulty (R, Recall; Ap, Application; An, Analysis) relates to the question difficulty on the Written Registry Exam. The abbreviation "CSE" is used for the coded items testable on *only* the Clinical Simulation Exam. Because no question difficulty level is given for this examination, be prepared for anything.

Note 2: A review of the most recent Written Registry Examinations has shown an average of five questions (5% of the examination) that cover cardiac monitoring and cardiopulmonary resuscitation (CPR) issues. The Clinical Simulation Exam is comprehensive and may include everything that should be known or performed by an advanced level respiratory therapist.

MODULE A
Cardiac monitoring

1. **Cardiac electrodes**
   a. **Get the necessary equipment for the procedure (WRE code: IIA16) [Difficulty: Ap]**
   b. **Put the equipment together and make sure that it works properly (WRE code: IIA16) [Difficulty: Ap]**
   c. **Troubleshoot any problems with the equipment (WRE code: IIA16) [Difficulty: Ap]**

NOTE: The NBRC does not specifically list cardiac electrodes on it content outlines. However, recent Written Registry Exams have had questions about troubleshooting problems with electrodes when performing an electrocardiogram (ECG).

Cardiac electrodes, or leads, pick up the electrical signal from a heart contraction and conduct it to the electrocardiogram machine. Several different types of leads are distinguished by their placement on the patient and how long they are used.

The first type of lead is used for a period of hours or days for basic rhythm monitoring or Holter monitoring. They are usually called *chest leads* (or *chest electrodes*) and consist of four parts: (1) a conducting wire coated with an electrically neutral plastic, (2) an adapter at one end of the wire that plugs into the electrocardiograph machine, (3) a different adapter at the opposite end of the wire that attaches to a patient electrode, and (4) the patient electrode (Fig. 11-1). Conducting jelly is added to the surface of the electrode to reduce the skin's resistance to the heart's electrical signal. An adhesive ring holds the electrode tightly to the skin. The conducting wire snaps or clips onto the back of the electrode. Typically, three of these chest leads are used for rhythm monitoring. Holter monitoring involves using chest leads and long-term precordial leads.

The second type of cardiac electrode is often used for only a few minutes during a diagnostic ECG. They come in two sets of electrodes for different placements. Limb leads come as a group of four with one for each limb (Fig. 11-2). Precordial leads came in a group of six and are placed on the chest in the positions shown in Fig. 11-3. Long-term precordial leads must be used for a Holter monitor. A conducting and adhesive jelly is used to reduce the skin's resistance and to hold the lead in place. The limb leads are longer, and they may need to be held in place by a rubber strap. With all types of cardiac leads, bad skin contact, dried conducting jelly, or a disconnected wire results in a distorted or absent electrical signal.

2. **Electrocardiograph**
   a. **Get the necessary equipment for the procedure (WRE code: IIA16) [Difficulty: Ap]**
   b. **Put the equipment together and make sure that it works properly (WRE code: IIA16) [Difficulty: Ap]**

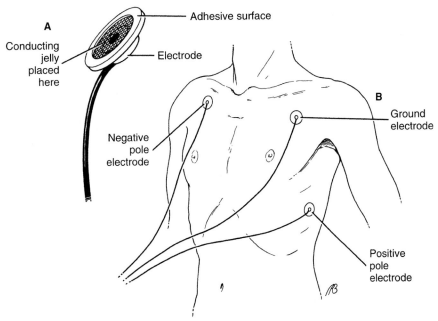

Fig. 11-1 A, Close-up of the features of a prepackaged monitoring electrode or lead. **B,** Standard electrode placements for lead II monitoring. This results in the traditional-looking electrocardiogram waveform with upright P, QRS, and T waves. (Note: The electrodes are often labeled as right arm [RA] instead of negative pole, left arm [LA] instead of ground electrode, and left leg [LL] instead of positive electrode.) *(From Eubanks DH, Bone RC: Comprehensive respiratory care, ed 2, St Louis, 1990, Mosby.)*

c. Fix any problems with the equipment (WRE code: IIA16) [Difficulty: Ap]

Twelve-lead electrocardiogram test for diagnostic purposes. A 12-lead ECG test requires a machine capable of receiving electrical input from the four limb leads and six precordial leads (see Figs. 11-2 and 11-3). The operator can manually select the combinations needed to get the 12 different combinations for a 12-lead ECG tracing, or they can be done automatically. The various ECG combinations are printed out on ECG paper. Modern units also store the patient's information on a self-contained computer.

Fig. 11-2 Limb electrodes or leads properly placed on all four of the patient's limbs. Make sure that the right leg lead is placed on the right leg, the right arm lead is placed on the right arm, and so forth. The electrode cables are then plugged into the electrocardiograph machine to record the ECG tracings. *(From Eubanks DH, Bone RC: Comprehensive respiratory care, ed 2, St Louis, 1990, Mosby.)*

Cable line

Fig. 11-3 Proper placement of the six precordial leads. (See Table 10-1 for a description of the locations.) *(From Eubanks DH, Bone RC: Comprehensive respiratory care, ed 2, St Louis, 1990, Mosby.)*

Basic bedside rhythm monitoring. A bedside rhythm monitoring unit usually receives input from only three or four chest leads. That collective signal is sent to an oscilloscope (video display terminal) for a real-time display of the patient's rhythm. These ECG machines have several additional features. They continuously display the patient's heart rate. High and low heart rate alarm settings can be set. If the high or low setting is reached, an audible and visual alarm is triggered. The patient's heart rhythm can be recorded on ECG paper manually by pushing a record button or automatically when an alarm setting is reached. These units are often seen mounted at the patient's bedside in the intensive care unit.

Cardiopulmonary resuscitation cart. Cardiopulmonary resuscitation (CPR) "crash" carts have electrocardiographs and oscilloscopes mounted on them. These are connected to the defibrillator. This allows synchronous defibrillation (cardioversion). Crash carts have other features that are similar to those seen on bedside rhythm monitoring units. Portable versions of these units are used when the patient must be transported. They operate by battery power when unplugged from the wall electrical outlet.

Holter monitoring. Holter monitoring involves recording a patient's complete ECG for 1 to 3 days through the use of a portable, battery-powered monitor. In addition, the patient keeps a diary of any episodes of chest pain, dyspnea, and so forth. The whole system includes the recording device, magnetic tape to record the patient's ECG, a set of chest leads (and precordial leads if needed), a carrying bag for the recording device, and a patient activity diary (Fig. 11-4).

Successful ECG monitoring requires that the right electrodes be chosen, put together properly, attached to the patient as indicated, and connected to the correct ECG machine. Any errors will result in an electrical signal that is distorted or absent. Recheck all patient electrodes and wire connections if a problem is seen.

3. Begin electrocardiogram monitoring (WRE code: IB7a) [Difficulty: Ap]

Holter monitoring is done to evaluate noncritical patients with a suspected cardiac problem. Because the patient will be mobile for at least 1 day, the limb leads are placed on the upper and lower chest area. Precordial leads are placed normally. The patient wears a tight-fitting undershirt or netlike dressing to keep the leads in place. The patient cannot bathe while the leads are on.

Emergency ECG monitoring is done on any patient with a serious cardiopulmonary problem. If a possibility exists that the patient will experience serious changes in heart rate or rhythm, he or she should be continuously monitored. In this case, use bedside rhythm monitoring. This unit should have an oscilloscope for viewing the rhythm and additional features for counting the heart rate, setting high and low heart rate alarms, and recording the rhythm on standard ECG paper for a permanent record.

The most common chest electrode pattern used for rhythm monitoring is called *lead II*. The three chest electrodes are placed as shown in Fig. 11-1, *B*. The negative (right arm, RA) electrode is on the right upper chest. The positive (left leg, LL) electrode is placed on the left lateral chest. The ground (left arm, LA) electrode is placed on the left upper chest. With this electrode configuration, known as the Einthoven triangle, the heart's electrical signal is followed as it flows from the right atrium to the left ventricle. This results in the so-called normal ECG tracing with upright P, R, and T waves, as shown in Figs. 11-5 and 11-6. Table 11-1 shows the sequential electrical events of the normal cardiac rhythm that correspond with those in Fig. 11-5.

Fig. 11-4 Holter monitoring system for ambulatory electrocardiography. *(From Pagana K, Pagana TJ: Mosby's manual of diagnostic and laboratory tests, St Louis, 1998, Mosby.)*

Fig. 11-5 Sequence of electrical events of the cardiac cycle during normal sinus rhythm. (See Table 10-2 for the description of each event.) *(From Phillips RE, Feeney MK: The cardiac rhythms: a systematic approach to interpretation, ed 3, Philadelphia, 1990, WB Saunders.)*

TABLE 11-1	Electrophysiologic Events Represented by the Electrocardiogram
Sequential Electrical Events of the Cardiac Cycle	**Electrocardiographic Representation**
1. Impulse from the sinus node	Not visible
2. Depolarization of the atria	P wave
3. Depolarization of the atrio-ventricular node	Isoelectric
4. Repolarization of the atria	Usually obscured by the QRS complex
5. Depolarization of the ventricles	QRS complex
a. Intraventricular septum	a. Initial portion
b. Right and left ventricles	b. Central and terminal portions
6. Quiescent state of the ventricles immediately after depolarization	ST segment: isoelectric
7. Repolarization of the ventricles	T wave
8. Afterpotentials following repolarization of the ventricles	U wave

From Phillips RE, Feeney MK: *The cardiac rhythms: a systematic approach to interpretation,* ed 3, Philadelphia, 1990, WB Saunders.

4. Perform an electrocardiogram (WRE code: IB7a) [Difficulty: Ap]

A diagnostic 12-lead ECG is indicated if the patient is suspected of having cardiac problems. Symptoms such as syncope, angina pectoris, sudden crushing chest pain, shortness of breath, or unstable heart rate and blood pressure point to a heart problem. Growing evidence indicates that men and women have different signs and symptoms during an acute myocardial infarction (AMI or MI). Men tend to have crushing central chest pain that may radiate

down the left arm or the left side of the neck, diaphoresis, cold extremities, shortness of breath, and a feeling of impending doom. Women tend to experience pain in the lower back and the abdominal area. A diagnostic ECG is indicated to document the nature of the cardiac problem or rule out the heart as a source of the symptoms.

The 12-lead ECG test involves the use of an electrocardiograph machine with heat-sensitive ECG recording paper, four limb leads, and six precordial leads (see Figs. 11-2 and 11-3). Table 11-2 describes the locations of the precordial leads and the positive and negative electrode combinations that are used to record the heart's electrical signal through the 12 different leads. Each lead individually records the heart's electrical activity, but does so from a different position in relation to the heart. These 12 leads give the physician a three-dimensional impression of how the cardiac conduction system and the myocardium are functioning. Abnormal functioning can be diagnosed. Review the normal anatomy and physiology of the heart and its conduction system if necessary.

Clinical experience is important in performing a diagnostic ECG. Improper placement of the precordial or limb leads can easily result in a misleading ECG tracing and a misdiagnosis. For example, reversing the arm leads causes the QRS to be reversed in lead I. Technical errors in grounding the patient and not keeping the patient still during the ECG also result in useless tracings because of electrical interference and an unstable baseline.

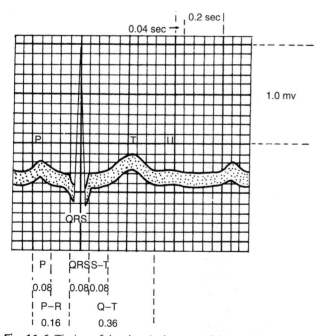

Fig. 11-6 Timing of the electrical events of the cardiac cycle during normal sinus rhythm. *(From Spearman CB, Sheldon RL, Egan DF: Egan's fundamentals of respiratory therapy, ed 4, St Louis, 1982, Mosby.)*

TABLE 11-2 Standard Electrocardiogram Leads					
	Leads	**Positive Electrode**			**Negative Electrode**
Bipolar	1. I	Left arm		and	Right arm
	2. II	Left leg		and	Right arm
	3. III	Left leg		and	Left arm
Unipolar	4. aV_R	Right arm			
	5. aV_L	Left arm			Central terminal*
	6. aV_F	Left leg			
Precordial	7. V_1	Right of sternum in 4th intercostal space (4th ICS)			
	8. V_2	Left of sternum in 4th ICS			
	9. V_3	Midway between V_2 and V_4			Central terminal*
	10. V_4	Midclavicular line in 5th ICS			
	11. V_5	Midway between V_4 and V_6			
	12. V_6	Lateral chest in 5th ICS			

*The *central terminal* is a combination of electrode potentials, producing a summation effect. This serves as the single negative or *indifferent* electrode. The specific combination of electrodes for each lead is automatically determined in the lead selector switch.

aV, augmented voltage; ICS, intercostal space.

From Phillips RE, Feeney MK: *The cardiac rhythms: a systematic approach to interpretation*, ed 3, Philadelphia, 1990, WB Saunders.

Exam Hint

Usually one or two questions require the respiratory therapist to recognize possible signs of a myocardial infarction and recommend either ECG monitoring or the performance of a diagnostic 12-lead ECG.

MODULE B
Cardiopulmonary resuscitation equipment

1. Manual resuscitator (bag valve)

a. Get the necessary equipment for the procedure (WRE code: IIA5) [Difficulty: An]

The first consideration when deciding which manual resuscitator to select is the size of the patient. Although the volume of the reservoir bag and the tidal volume expelled from it vary among the types of bags, three basic sizes are available. An infant or newborn unit typically has a reservoir bag volume of about 250 mL. A pediatric unit usually has a reservoir bag volume of about 250 to 500 mL, and an adult unit typically has a reservoir bag volume of 1500 to 2000 mL. In addition to all of these reusable units, a number of disposable units are thrown away after one patient use. They also come in comparable infant, pediatric, and adult reservoir bag volumes.

Any unit should deliver 100% oxygen at the flow rate of 15 L/min. An oxygen reservoir system must be added to the basic unit to achieve these oxygen percentages. The valve to the patient must be clearable within 20 seconds if it becomes fouled by vomitus, sputum, or blood.

Neonatal and pediatric units must have a pressure release (pop-off) valve that opens at 40 cm H_2O pressure. The pressure may be adjustable. If an adult unit has a pressure release valve, it must have an override system that is easy to operate.

b. Put the equipment together and make sure that it works properly (WRE code: IIA5) [Difficulty: An]

Fig. 11-7 shows line drawings of a complete set of Laerdal infant, pediatric, and adult manual resuscitators. The following steps should be taken when the function of a manual resuscitator is evaluated:

1. Squeeze and release the bag to see if the nonrebreathing valve and air/oxygen reservoir intake valve open and close properly.
2. Feel the air leave the outlet port of the nonrebreathing valve when the bag is squeezed.
3. Occlude the outlet port, and squeeze the bag. No gas should leak out. If present, the pop-off valve should open at the correct pressure.
4. The face mask should fit onto the 22-mm outer diameter (OD) fitting and have its cushion properly inflated. The mask is selected based on the size of the patient's face. As can be seen in Fig. 11-7, the masks come in pediatric, infant, and adult sizes.

c. Troubleshoot any problems with the equipment (WRE code: IIA5) [Difficulty: An]

Check for a reversed or improperly seated one-way valve if the gas does not enter or exit the unit as it should. In clinical use, mucus, vomitus, and blood can foul the

Fig. 11-7 A, Adult Laerdal resuscitator. **B,** Pediatric Laerdal resuscitator. **C,** Infant Laerdal resuscitator. These features are found on all modern units: *A,* self-filling reservoir bag; *B,* elation valve that does not jam at an oxygen flow of 15 L/min or in subfreezing temperatures (it must be clearable of debris within 20 seconds); *C,* intake valve for adding draw room air or supplemental oxygen into the reservoir bag; *D,* transparent mask that easily conforms to the patient's face; *E,* pressure relief (pop-off) valve that is set to open at 40 cm water; *F,* standard 15-mm inner diameter/22-mm outer diameter connector for the endotracheal tube or face mask; *G,* oxygen enrichment/reservoir system. In addition, some units have an adjustable positive end-expiratory pressure valve (not shown) attached to the elation valve. *(From Eubanks DH, Bone RC: Comprehensive respiratory care, ed 2, St Louis, 1990, Mosby.)*

nonrebreathing valve system and must be cleared within 20 seconds. Do this by disconnecting the unit from the patient, aiming the adapter into a neutral area, and squeezing the bag to blow out the obstruction. Replace a unit that cannot be promptly cleared.

2. Mouth-to-valve mask resuscitator
a. Get the necessary equipment for the procedure (WRE code: IIA5) [Difficulty: An]

The following are important considerations when selecting the best device for the victim:

1. The mask must fit the victim's face so that no air leak is present. Infant, child, and adult sizes should be available.
2. The mouthpiece should be designed so that it fits only one way into the mask. Some units include a short length of aerosol tubing between the mouthpiece and mask for greater flexibility.
3. The one-way (nonrebreathing) valve should be designed to ensure that all of the rescuer's breath is

directed into the victim, and the victim's exhaled breath is vented to room air rather than back at the rescuer. Some units include a bacteria filter in the one-way valve between the rescuer and victim.

4. It should be possible to add supplemental oxygen through a T-piece or nipple on the mask. This is important for hospital or ambulance use. If a T-piece is added, it must be designed to easily fit between the mouthpiece and face mask. An oxygen administration nipple should have a cap over it when not in use to prevent any leakage of the delivered breath.

b. Put the equipment together and make sure that it works properly (WRE code: IIA5) [Difficulty: An]

Mouth-to-valve resuscitators are relatively simple devices. Most have only two or three pieces: a face mask, a mouthpiece with a one-way valve, and possibly an oxygen T-piece (Fig. 11-8). The "male" and "female" connections are designed to fit together in only one way. When they are

Fig. 11-8 Proper positioning to use a mouth-to-valve mask resuscitator. The top rescuer has added supplemental oxygen to the device. The bottom rescuer is ventilating without the use of added oxygen. *(Courtesy Laerdal Medical Corporation, Wappingers Falls, NY.)*

properly assembled, no air leaks should occur when the breath is delivered to the victim.

c. Troubleshoot any problems with the equipment (WRE code: IIA5) [Difficulty: An]

If the breath cannot be delivered, check the one-way valve to make sure that it has not been put together backward. Reverse it, if necessary, and ventilate the victim's airway. Keep the oxygen nipple on the mask or T-piece capped off if it is not being used. Air will leak out during the delivered breath if the cap is left off the nipple.

Exam Hint

Usually an exam question deals with a malfunctioning manual resuscitator or mouth-to-valve resuscitator. Often the question involves identifying that the patient's chest does not rise despite the ventilating device being used to deliver a breath. Fixing the problem can involve clearing an obstruction or properly assembling a one-way valve. If the unit cannot be quickly repaired, it should be replaced. A gas-powered pneumatic (demand valve) resuscitator should not be used.

MODULE C

Perform cardiopulmonary resuscitation and related functions

1. Basic cardiac life support (WRE code: III I1a) [Difficulty: An]

The key steps of basic cardiac life support (BCLS) include the following:

a. Establish that the patient is unresponsive and needs cardiopulmonary resuscitation

Observing a patient who *appears* to be dead does not prove that the patient needs CPR. Clinical death must be proved before CPR is begun. Adults should be tapped or gently shaken while you shout, "Are you okay?" Infants should have the bottom of their feet gently slapped while you shout, "Wake up!" The rescuer also can clap his or her hands together loudly to wake a sleeping infant. CPR should never be started on a person who does not need it.

b. Call out for help

Call out for help if the victim does not respond to any attempts at arousal. The second rescuer should be told to call in the cardiac arrest team. Many hospitals have a cardiac arrest button in each patient's room. If this is the case, the first rescuer can push the button while calling out for help. Dial 911 if the victim is found at home.

c. Open the airway

The head-tilt/chin-lift maneuver is the procedure of choice for opening the airways of all victims except those with a known or suspected cervical (neck) spine injury. The victim is gently positioned on his or her back. In an adult, the head is firmly pushed back with one hand, and the jaw is pulled upward with the fingers of the other hand (Fig. 11-9). In an infant, it is not necessary to tilt the head back beyond a neutral position. Children may need to have the head pushed back slightly beyond neutral.

Fig. 11-9 Opening the adult's airway. *Top,* Airway obstruction produced by the tongue and epiglottis. *Bottom,* Relief by head-tilt/chin-lift method. *(From Standards and guidelines for cardiopulmonary resuscitation [CPR] and emergency cardiac care [ECC], JAMA 268:2186, 1992.)* Copyright © 1992, American Medical Association. All rights reserved.

Fig. 11-10 Opening the adult's airway by the jaw-thrust method. *(From Watson MA: Cardiopulmonary resuscitation. In Barnes TA, editor: Respiratory care practice, St Louis, 1988, Mosby.)*

The jaw-thrust maneuver is the procedure of choice for opening the airway of all victims with a known or suspected cervical spine injury. The rescuer's elbows are rested on the ground, and the hands are placed on either side of the victim's jaw. Lifting of the jaw usually opens the airway and eliminates the need to tilt the head back. See Fig. 11-10 for the adult maneuver.

Any obstruction that can be seen in the mouth or throat should be removed. The cross-finger technique can be used to open the mouth wide enough so that a finger or suction device can be inserted to remove a blockage (Fig. 11-11). An oral airway should be used only in an unconscious patient to keep the tongue from falling back and blocking the airway.

d. Determine that the patient is not breathing

The rescuer places his or her face close to the victim's face to *look* for rising and falling of the chest, *listen* for victim's

Fig. 11-11 The cross-finger method of opening the victim's mouth to look for an obstruction. *(From Watson MA: Cardiopulmonary resuscitation. In Barnes TA, editor: Respiratory care practice, St Louis, 1988, Mosby.)*

Fig. 11-12 Determining breathlessness by looking, listening, and feeling. *(From Standards and guidelines for cardiopulmonary resuscitation [CPR] and emergency cardiac care [ECC], JAMA 268:2187, 1992.)* Copyright © 1992, American Medical Association. All rights reserved.

movement, and *feel* any air movement from the victim's breathing (Fig. 11-12). The entire procedure should not take longer than 10 seconds.

e. Ventilate the patient
1. Mouth-to-mouth breathing

The first rescuer should begin mouth-to-mouth breathing as soon as possible if no spontaneous breathing by the victim occurs once the airway is opened. No matter the age of the victim, an effective seal must be present between the rescuer and the victim. The adult victim's nose must be pinched closed; often the infant's nose can be blocked by the cheek of the rescuer. The mouth of the rescuer can cover both the nose and mouth of an infant. Alternative methods of ventilation include mouth-to-nose and mouth-to-stoma (Fig. 11-13).

In an adult, two breaths large enough to raise the victim's chest should be given. An adequate volume of 500 to 600 mL may be given. Blow into the victim's mouth for more than 1 second. This is to ensure a large enough volume without having to use much pressure. Keeping the ventilating pressure as low as possible minimizes the risk of forcing air into the stomach. Ensure that the victim exhales completely by watching the chest fall and feeling the air escape against your cheek. Rescue breathing should be performed at a rate of 10 to 12 times per minute (every 4 to 5 seconds) if the victim has a pulse but is apneic.

In a child, two breaths large enough to raise the victim's chest should be given. A child obviously needs less volume than an adult. All of the same considerations apply as in the adult. Rescue breathing should be performed at a rate of 20 per minute (every 3 seconds) in an infant and a child. A newly born infant should be ventilated at a rate of 40 to 60 per minute.

If the victim's airway cannot be ventilated, reposition the head and attempt to ventilate again. Failure to ventilate a second time means that the victim has an obstructed airway. The following steps should be taken:

Unconscious adult obstructed airway maneuvers.
a. Position: Place the victim on his or her back.
b. Heimlich maneuver: Perform the Heimlich maneuver (also known as abdominal thrusts) several times, if needed, by kneeling astride the victim, placing the heel of one hand midline on the abdomen slightly above the navel, but well below the xiphoid process. The other hand is placed on top, and both are quickly thrust upward toward the chest (Fig. 11-14). The markedly obese or obviously pregnant victim can have chest thrusts performed on them. The rescuer's hands should be placed on the lower half of the sternum as with cardiac compressions. Several compressions should be performed slowly but similarly to a cardiac compression.
c. Finger sweep: Attempt to clear out any foreign body with a finger sweep. First, grasp the victim's tongue and jaw between your thumb and fingers, and lift the jaw open. Next, insert the index finger of the other hand along the inside of the victim's cheek and down the back of the throat so as to hook and remove food, gum, dentures, and so on.

Fig. 11-13 Adult mouth-to-mouth, mouth-to-nose, and mouth-to-stoma ventilation. *(From Standards and guidelines for cardiopulmonary resuscitation [CPR] and emergency cardiac care [ECC], JAMA 268:2188, 1992.)*

Fig. 11-14 Administering the Heimlich maneuver to an unconscious adult victim of an airway obstruction. *(From Standards and guidelines for cardiopulmonary resuscitation [CPR] and emergency cardiac care [ECC], JAMA 268:2193, 1992.)*

Unconscious child (1 year old and older) obstructed airway maneuvers.

a. Position: Same as the adult position previously described.

b. Heimlich maneuver: Same as the adult maneuver but with up to five thrusts performed if needed. Chest thrusts are not used.

c. Finger sweep: Same as the adult, except that the index finger is inserted only when a foreign body has been seen. Blindly inserting the index finger may push a foreign body farther down the throat.

Unconscious infant obstructed airway maneuver.

a. Position: The infant is straddled over the rescuer's forearm. The infant's jaw and head are held by the rescuer's hand. The infant's head should be lower than the body. Five firm back blows are delivered between the shoulder blades with the heel of the rescuer's other hand (Fig. 11-15).

b. Heimlich maneuver: The infant is sandwiched by the rescuer's other arm, and the head and body are supported and turned to a supine position. The head should remain lower than the body. Five chest thrusts are performed in the same location and manner as cardiac compressions but at a slower rate. Steps a and b can be done by placing the infant on the rescuer's lap.

c. Finger sweep: Same as finger sweep in the unconscious child, mentioned previously.

2. Manual resuscitator (bag valve)

A manual resuscitator should be used during hospital-based CPR as soon as one is available. The resuscitation mask must be held to the victim's face so that no air leak occurs during the forced inspiration (Fig. 11-16). An assistant can hold the mask tightly to the face so that the rescuer who is pumping the resuscitation bag can use both hands. This has been shown to produce a larger tidal volume. If the victim's airway contains an endotracheal tube or tracheostomy tube, the valve adapter fits directly over the tube adapter. Rescue breathing continues with the previously mentioned considerations for volume and rate. After an adult victim has had an endotracheal tube placed, the tidal volume goal is 500 to 600 mL over a 1-second period to produce a visible chest rise.

3. Mouth-to-valve mask ventilation

A mouth-to-valve mask device (or *pocket mask*) combines a resuscitation mask with a one-way valve mouthpiece. It is used to ventilate an apneic patient rather than perform mouth-to-mouth breathing. Concerns about protecting the rescuer from patient infections such as acquired immunodeficiency syndrome (AIDS) and hepatitis have led to their widespread acceptance. As shown in Fig. 11-8, the patient's neck is hyperextended, the mask is applied over the mouth and nose to get an airtight seal, and the

Fig. 11-15 Administering **(A)** back blows and **(B)** chest thrusts to an infant victim of an obstructed airway. *(From Standards and guidelines for cardiopulmonary resuscitation [CPR] and emergency cardiac care [ECC], JAMA 268:2258, 1992.)* Copyright © 1992, American Medical Association. All rights reserved.

rescuer breathes into the mouthpiece. It is best if the rescuer is positioned at the victim's head so that the chest can be seen to rise with each delivered breath. The one-way valve is designed so that the victim's exhaled gas is vented out to the room air. Some units have a nipple adapter so that supplemental oxygen can be added to the delivered breath. Simply attach oxygen tubing between the nipple and oxygen flowmeter, and turn the flowmeter on to the manufacturer's recommended flow. When this type of device is used with an adult victim, the tidal volume goal is 500 to 600 mL over a 1-second period to produce a

Fig. 11-16 Ventilation of an adult with a manual resuscitation bag and mask. *(From Eubanks DH, Bone RC: Comprehensive respiratory care, ed 2, St Louis, 1990, Mosby.)*

visible chest rise. These devices should be replaced by a manual resuscitator as soon as possible.

f. Add supplemental oxygen (WRE code: IIIF2a) [Difficulty: An]

The victim should be given 100% oxygen as soon as possible. There is no contraindication for giving pure oxygen during a resuscitation effort. This can be done easily if a manual resuscitator is used to ventilate the victim. All modern units are capable of giving 100% oxygen if the oxygen flow is high enough and a reservoir is added.

g. Determine pulselessness

The carotid pulse is felt for in all victims except children younger than 1 year. The carotid pulse is found by gently feeling with two or three fingers in the groove between the larynx and the sternocleidomastoid muscle on either side of the neck (Fig. 11-17). Check for 5 to 10 seconds to be sure that the victim is pulseless and not just bradycardic. In addition, check for other signs of circulation such as spontaneous breathing, coughing, and movement. An infant younger than 1 year should have the pulse felt in the brachial artery; the carotid artery is difficult to find in such young children because they have short, chubby necks.

The femoral pulse can be felt for as an alternative site in victims in the hospital who are wearing few clothes. Once the CPR team has arrived and two-person CPR is instituted, the femoral pulse may be most accessible for monitoring the pulse and the effectiveness of the chest compressions.

h. Perform external chest compressions

The absence of a palpable pulse confirms a cardiac arrest. Blood must be pumped by external chest compressions

Fig. 11-17 Determining pulselessness by checking the carotid pulse of an adult. *(From Standards and guidelines for cardiopulmonary resuscitation [CPR] and emergency cardiac care [ECC], JAMA 268:2189, 1992.)*

of the heart. The victim must be supine on a hard surface. A CPR backboard is placed behind a victim who is in bed.

In adults and large children or those older than 8 years, the heel of the rescuer's hand is placed over the lower half of the sternum. This is found by placing the middle finger of one hand in the notch where the ribs meet the sternum, placing the index finger next to it, and placing the other hand next to the finger. The first hand is placed over it, the elbows are locked, and the shoulders are directly over the hands. This creates the most efficient pumping action (Fig. 11-18). The rescuer pivots from the hips, with half of the time spent pumping down and half of the time releasing pressure. The hands should always touch the victim's chest. The sternum must be compressed 4 to 5 cm (1.5 to 2.0 inches) in an adult at a rate of 100 compressions per minute for an actual rate of more than 80 per minute.

In a child 8 years old or younger, hand position is found as in the adult. The child's sternum must be compressed with *one* hand to a depth of 2.5 to 4 cm (1 to 1.5 inches). Half of the time should be spent on compression,

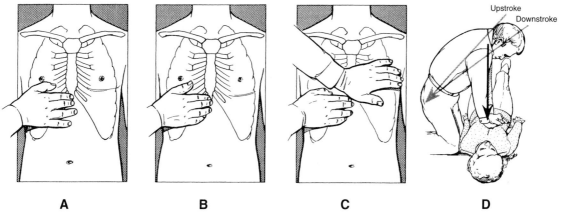

Fig. 11-18 Cardiac compression of an adult. **A,** Locate tip of xiphoid process. **B,** Place two fingertips at xiphoid process. **C,** Place palm of other hand on sternum next to fingers. **D,** Arm and body positions for cardiac compression. *(From Barnes TA, editor:* Respiratory care practice, *St Louis, 1988, Mosby.)*

Fig. 11-19 The preferred way to provide chest compressions on a newly born neonate is called two thumbs–encircling hands. This method is best when one rescuer can provide chest compressions and another can ventilate the patient. **A,** Side-by-side thumb placement for most newborns. **B,** Overlapping thumbs for very small newborns. *(From Aloan CA, Hill TV, editors:* Respiratory care of the newborn and child, *ed 2, Philadelphia, 1997, Lippincott-Raven.)*

and half on relaxation. The rate should be 100 compressions per minute for a rate of more than 80 per minute between ventilations.

In newly born infants and older infants, the preferred methods of chest compressions is called the two thumbs–encircling hands technique (Fig. 11-19). This method works best when a second rescuer can ventilate the infant. It also is acceptable to compress with two or three fingers placed over the middle of the sternum one finger's width below an imaginary line drawn between the nipples (Fig. 11-20). This method is easier when one rescuer must provide ventilations and compressions. In either case, the child's sternum must be compressed to a depth of 1.3 to 2.5 cm (0.5 to 1 in.). Half the time should be spent on compression, and half the time on relaxation. A newly born infant should have a rate of at least 120 compressions per minute to achieve an actual rate of 90 per minute.

The steps for one- and two-person CPR follow.

1. Adult one-rescuer CPR

a. Assess the victim's need for CPR.
b. Call out for help.

c. Open the airway.
d. Assess the victim's lack of breathing.
e. Give two rescue breaths.
f. Assess the victim's lack of a pulse.
g. Perform 30 chest compressions at a rate of 100 compressions per minute.
h. Reopen the airway, and give two breaths of more than 1 second duration to produce visible chest rise.
i. Repeat this cycle (30:2 ratio) a total of 5 times.
j. Check the victim's carotid pulse for less than 10 seconds. If it has not returned, give two breaths, and continue with compressions.
k. If the pulse has returned, check on the return of breathing. If it has not returned, give 12 breaths per minute.
l. If CPR is continued, check for the return of a heartbeat and breathing after five cycles.

2. Adult hospital based two-rescuer CPR

a. Perform steps a to f, as previously described, for adult one-rescuer CPR.

Fig. 11-20 Locating the proper finger position for chest compressions on an infant. *(From Standards and guidelines for cardiopulmonary resuscitation [CPR] and emergency cardiac care [ECC], JAMA 268: 2256, 1992.)* Copyright © 1992, American Medical Association. All rights reserved.

b. After the victim has had an endotracheal tube inserted, the compression/ventilation ratio changes. The compressing rescuer delivers continuous chest compressions at a rate of 100 per minute without pausing for ventilation.

c. The second rescuer gives 8 to 10 breaths per minute (about every 6 seconds). A manual resuscitator with 100% oxygen is used to ventilate the victim.

d. Provide breathing, circulation, or both, as needed. If CPR is continued, check for the return of a heartbeat and breathing every few minutes.

e. Switch positions whenever one rescuer becomes tired. Make the switch at the end of a cycle, check the victim for a return of pulse or breathing, and continue as needed.

3. Infant and child hospital based one- and two-rescuer CPR

a. Perform steps a to l, as described for adult one-rescuer CPR.

b. After the victim has had an endotracheal tube inserted, the compression/ventilation ratio changes. The compressing rescuer delivers continuous chest compressions at a rate of 100 per minute without pausing for ventilation.

c. The second rescuer gives 8 to 10 breaths per minute (about every 6 seconds). A manual resuscitator with 100% oxygen is used to ventilate the victim.

d. Provide breathing and circulation or both as needed. If CPR is continued, check for the return of a heartbeat and breathing every few minutes.

e. Switch positions whenever one rescuer becomes tired. Make the switch at the end of a cycle, check the victim for a return of pulse or breathing, and continue as needed.

4. Neonatal one and two-rescuer CPR

a. Perform steps a to d as described for adult one-rescuer CPR.

b. If the patient is apneic or if breathing is inadequate, provide ventilation at a rate of 40 to 60 per minute. In the hospital setting, provide bag-mask ventilation with 100% oxygen.

c. Check the pulse.

d. Begin chest compressions if the heart rate is less than 60 beats per minute despite assisted ventilation with supplemental oxygen for 30 seconds.

e. The ratio of chest compressions to ventilations is 3:1. These are delivered at a rate of 90 compressions per minute and 30 breaths per minute.

f. Assess the patient's heart rate, respirations, and color about every 30 seconds.

g. Continue CPR efforts until the spontaneous heart rate is at least 60 beats per minute.

h. Continue assisted ventilation with oxygen at a rate of 40 to 60 per minute, if needed.

Exam Hint

Past exam questions have focused on basic cardiac life support procedures. However, occasional advanced CPR questions have been included. Discussion of key advanced CPR procedures is included here and in other areas of this text.

---

2. Advanced cardiac life support (WRE code: III I1b) [Difficulty: An]

It is beyond the scope of this text to present advanced cardiac life support (ACLS) in detail. The following items relate to procedures that are important in the care of adult, pediatric, and neonatal patients needing advanced resuscitation.

a. Interpret the results of the electrocardiogram

Before discussing ECG interpretation, it is important to understand how ECG paper is designed so that the heart's electrical signal traced on it can be understood. This special paper is heat sensitive and, after exiting the ECG machine, shows a black line from the heated stylus. Fig. 11-21 shows the grid markings on the paper and how to interpret the ECG tracing for voltage and time. Each large square box is 5 mm in height and represents 0.5 millivolts (mV) of the heart's electrical force. The large square box is divided into five smaller boxes that are 1 mm in height and represent 0.1 mV. Timing of the ECG tracing is determined by the speed with which the paper passes under the heated stylus. Normally, this is 25 mm/sec. At this speed, each

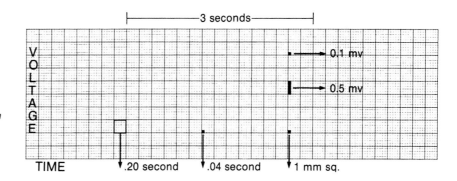

Fig. 11-21 ECG paper with added details on how to interpret time and voltage. *(From Patel JM, McGowan SG, Moody LA: Arrhythmias: detection, treatment, and cardiac drugs, Philadelphia, 1989, WB Saunders.)*

large square box is .20 seconds, and each of the five small boxes is 0.04 seconds; 300 large boxes compose 1 minute's time (0.20 seconds × 300 = 60 seconds).

The following 10 features should be examined in every ECG:

1. Heart rate
2. Rhythm
3. P wave
4. PR interval
5. QRS interval
6. QRS complex
7. ST segment
8. T wave
9. QT interval
10. U wave

The systematic evaluation of these factors usually results in a clear understanding of the patient's cardiac function. All of these factors are discussed and illustrated in this chapter.

The *heart rate* can be most accurately found by counting it for 1 minute; however, this time-consuming method is not always practical. An approximate heart rate can be quickly found. First, find a heartbeat tracing in which the R wave is on a heavy vertical line. Then count the number of large boxes between this first R wave and the next R wave (see Fig. 11-22 for an example). Approximate heart rates can be estimated as follows:

Two large boxes = 150 beats/min (300 divided by 2)
Three large boxes = 100 beats/min (300 divided by 3)
Four large boxes = 75 beats/min (300 divided by 4)
Five large boxes = 60 beats/min (300 divided by 5)
Six large boxes = 50 beats/min (300 divided by 6)

Obviously, the normal cardiac rhythm must be understood to distinguish it from the abnormal rhythms. The normal adult's cardiac rhythm is usually called *normal sinus rhythm* (NSR) and has these characteristics:

a. Heart rate between 60 and 100 beats/min while at rest
b. Rhythm that varies by no more than ±10% between QRS complexes
c. P wave before every QRS complex and upright in lead II
d. A QRS complex follows every P wave
e. Proper timing of the components of the ECG rhythm

Fig. 11-6 shows the normal timing of the components of the ECG tracing.

1. Abnormal cardiac rhythms

The following list of abnormal cardiac rhythms (usually called arrhythmias or dysrhythmias) includes many of those that are commonly encountered in clinical practice. It is beyond the scope of this text to discuss all possible arrhythmias. Instead, those that are either frequently seen or dangerous are described. Each of the following cardiac irregularities is (a) defined, (b) exemplified, (c) described, (d) discussed in terms of its clinical significance, and (e) accompanied by a treatment (if any) description.

a. Arrhythmias with a sinoatrial node origin

The following three arrhythmias all originate from the sinoatrial (SA) node. The electrical signal follows the

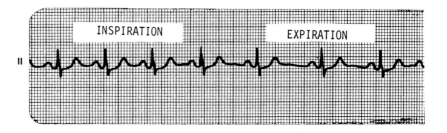

Fig. 11-22 Sinus arrhythmia showing slightly increased heart rate during inspiration and slightly decreased heart rate during exhalation. *(From Goldberger AL: Clinical electrocardiography: a simplified approach, ed 6, St Louis, 1999, Mosby.)*

normal pathway and results in contraction of both atria and ventricles, as expected. They are distinguished from NSR by the differences in rate and regularity of the impulses.

Sinus arrhythmia. This arrhythmia is characterized by normal complexes, but is a heart rate that varies with the respiratory cycle (see Fig. 11-22 for an example). Notice how the QRS complexes are closer together on inspiration than on expiration. This is because the increased venous return to the heart during inspiration causes the heart to fill more quickly, so that the pulse rate quickens. The opposite rhythm effect is sometimes seen with a patient on a mechanical ventilator. No cardiac treatment is needed. The mechanically ventilated patient should have every attempt made to lower the intrathoracic pressure.

Sinus tachycardia. Sinus tachycardia in the adult is defined as a heart rate of more than 100 beats/min while at rest. All complexes are normal, and the rate is seldom more than 140 (see Fig. 11-23 for an example). Causes include caffeine, anxiety, fever, pain, or hypotension. Correction of the problem results in the heart rate decreasing to the normal range. Cardiac drugs are not needed.

Sinus bradycardia. Sinus bradycardia is defined as a heart rate of less than 60 beats/min while at rest (Fig. 11-24). All complexes remain normal. This is commonly seen in well-trained athletes during rest and in patients receiving digitalis or morphine. Cardiac drugs are not needed.

If sinus bradycardia is associated with a myocardial infarct, it may result in fainting or congestive heart failure (pulmonary edema). The patient must be treated not only for the heart attack but also to increase the heart rate. Atropine with or without isoproterenol (Isuprel) is commonly used to speed the heart rate. A pacemaker is needed if the patient does not respond to medications and continues to have symptoms.

b. Arrhythmias with an abnormal atrial origin

The following three arrhythmias originate in either one or both atria from a source other than the SA node. The electrical signal travels through the atria, which results in their contraction. It then moves on to the atrioventricular (AV) node and the ventricles, which contract normally. All of these arrhythmias result in faster than normal atrial contraction and often in a faster than normal ventricular contraction.

Paroxysmal atrial tachycardia. Paroxysmal atrial tachycardia (PAT) (also known as paroxysmal supraventricular tachycardia [PSVT]) is a series of three or more premature atrial contractions. It is characterized by a heart rate between 140 and 250 beats/min with an average rate of 180. The ECG tracing will show a normal QRS complex after each P wave (Fig. 11-25). Notice the abnormal origin of the P wave seen during the PAT episode. The recommended term for any abnormal origin to a heartbeat is *focus*. The term *foci* refers to more than one abnormal site to a heartbeat.

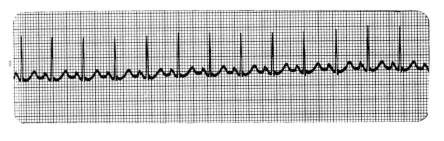

Fig. 11-23 Sinus tachycardia. *(From Goldberger AL: Clinical electrocardiography: a simplified approach, ed 6, St Louis, 1999, Mosby.)*

Fig. 11-24 Sinus bradycardia. *(From Goldberger AL: Clinical electrocardiography: a simplified approach, ed 6, St Louis, 1999, Mosby.)*

Fig. 11-25 A short run of paroxysmal trial tachycardia (PAT). Although a short run is probably not dangerous, a long run should be treated. *(From Wilkins RL, Krider SJ, Sheldon RL: Clinical assessment in respiratory care, ed 4. St Louis, 2000, Mosby.)*

ATRIAL FLUTTER

A

B

Fig. 11-26 Two examples of atrial flutter. **A**, Note the variable appearance of the flutter waves in different leads. This example shows a 2:1 ratio between atrial contractions and ventricular contractions. **B**, This shows how the ventricular rate is decreased after carotid sinus pressure is applied. The "F" letterings show flutter waves from a single focus. The "R" letterings mark R waves when the electrical signal traveled through the atrioventricular node to stimulate the ventricles. *(From Goldberger AL: Clinical electrocardiography: a simplified approach, ed 6, St Louis, 1999, Mosby.)*

Patients with long runs of PAT usually complain of a sudden onset of pounding or fluttering in the chest. This is often associated with breathlessness, weakness, and angina pectoris in patients with coronary artery disease. Because of these problems, long runs of PAT must be treated. Treatment usually progresses in the following sequence: (1) give a sedative, (2) stimulate the vagus nerve by rubbing the carotid sinus (Fig. 11-26), (3) give propranolol (Inderal) or a similar medication, and (4) perform synchronized cardioversion. (This last procedure is described in Chapter 18.) Obviously, if the patient responds to one treatment method, no need exists to go on to the next.

Atrial flutter. Atrial flutter is characterized by a single, fast, abnormal atrial focus that fires at a rate of about 250 to 350 beats/min. This rate is so fast that the AV node does not pass all of them along to the ventricles. On an ECG, a ratio between the fast flutter waves and the QRS complex is seen. Usually this ratio is 2:1, but it may be 3:1, 4:1, or more. (See Fig. 11-26 for several example ECG tracings of atrial flutter.) As with PAT, the fast ventricular rate found in atrial flutter is not well tolerated. An attempt must be made to suppress the abnormally fast atrial focus. Carotid sinus pressure, digoxin (Lanoxin), and synchronized cardioversion are the preferred treatments to slow the heart rate.

Atrial fibrillation. This condition is identified by the variably shaped fibrillation waves and the irregular spacings between the QRS complexes. Each focus is seen on the ECG as a separately shaped wave. As with atrial flutter, the AV node does not pass the electrical current from each fibrillation wave through to the ventricles. However, with atrial fibrillation, the ratio is not set, and variable spacing is seen between the QRS complexes and an inconsistent rate (Fig. 11-27). Patients with atrial fibrillation do

Fig. 11-27 Atrial fibrillation. Note the variable shapes to the fibrillation waves, indicating their different origins. Also note how the distances between the R waves change considerably. This depends on when an electrical signal from the atria passes through the atrioventricular node to the ventricles. *(From Wilkins RL, Krider SJ, Sheldon RL: Clinical assessment in respiratory care, ed 4, St Louis, 2000, Mosby.)*

A

B

Fig. 11-28 First degree atrioventricular block results in a PR interval that is longer than the normal interval of five small blocks or .20 seconds. ECG strip **A** shows a PR interval of 0.30 seconds. ECG strip **B** shows a PR interval of 0.24 seconds. *(From Conover MB: Understanding electrocardiography, arrhythmias, and the 12-lead ECG, ed 4, St Louis, 1984, Mosby.)*

not completely empty their atria. Often this results in the formation of blood clots that become pulmonary or cerebral emboli. Digitalis and synchronized cardioversion usually are effective treatments. Heparin or coumadin may be added to prolong the blood-clotting time.

c. Arrhythmias with an atrioventricular node origin

Both of the following arrhythmias originate in an AV node. The patient may or may not have a normal SA node, atria, and ventricles.

Atrioventricular block. AV block is most commonly caused by digitalis toxicity, arteriosclerosis, or myocardial infarction. The latter two may result in scarring,

inflammation, or edema. These causes slow or prevent the transmission of the electrical signal from the SA node through the AV node and to the ventricles. *First-degree* AV block is seen with an increased PR interval of at least 0.20 seconds. Each P wave is followed by a normal QRS complex (Fig. 11-28). It does not require any treatment. *Second-degree* AV block results in some P waves being blocked out completely with no ventricular response. This more serious condition comes in two different variations. Wenckebach (also known as Mobitz type I) is characterized by a progressively longer PR interval until a P wave is not conducted through at all. Then the cycle starts over again and continues to repeat itself. (See Fig. 11-29 for examples.) Medications such as

WENCKEBACH (MOBITZ TYPE I) SECOND-DEGREE AV BLOCK

WENCKEBACH (MOBITZ TYPE I) SECOND-DEGREE AV BLOCK

Fig. 11-29 Two examples of Wenckebach (Mobitz type I) second-degree atrioventricular block. Note how the PR interval progressively lengthens with each beat until one P wave is not conducted through at all. The cycle then repeats itself. *(From Goldberger AL: Clinical electrocardiography: a simplified approach, ed 6, St Louis, 1999, Mosby.)*

Fig. 11-30 Mobitz type II second-degree heart block. Note how some P waves are conducted through the atrioventricular node with a resulting QRS complex, and other P waves are not conducted. *(From Aehlert B:* ECGs made easy, *St Louis, 1995, Mosby.)*

atropine or isoproterenol may be used to increase the heart rate. Mobitz type II is seen on the ECG as a rhythm in which the PR interval is normal for those that result in a QRS complex, but some P waves are completely blocked (Fig. 11-30). The ratio between those P waves that conduct and those that are blocked off may be 2:1, 3:1, or 4:1. Mobitz type II is a sign of severe conduction-system disease. The usual treatment is to place a cardiac pacemaker into the patient. *Third-degree* AV block also is known as complete heart block (Fig. 11-31). No P waves are conducted through to the ventricles. The ventricles beat about 40 times per minute based on the intrinsic rate of the bundle of His and Purkinje fibers. Obviously, a heartbeat this slow is not normal or healthy. Patients have no stamina and frequently faint. A cardiac pacemaker must be placed into these patients.

Junctional premature beats. A junctional premature beat is also known as a premature AV nodal contraction (PNC), nodal beat, or junctional beat (Fig. 11-32). This arrhythmia involves the AV node sending out a premature electrical signal and becoming the primary pacemaker instead of the SA node. The ventricles contract normally with the expected QRS complex.

d. Arrhythmias with a ventricular origin Myocardial infarction

A myocardial infarction (MI) or acute myocardial infarction (AMI), commonly known as a heart attack, is an occlusion of a coronary artery that results in the death of some segment of the heart muscle. Often the patient with partial or complete coronary artery occlusion has symptoms of shortness of breath, central chest pain, pain that radiates down the left arm or up the left side of the neck,

THIRD-DEGREE (COMPLETE) AV BLOCK

THIRD-DEGREE (COMPLETE) AV BLOCK

Fig. 11-31 Two examples of third-degree (complete) heart block. Both show P waves that have no relation with the QRS complexes. The top example has QRS complexes of the normal width, indicating that the atrioventricular (AV) junction is acting as the pacemaker. The bottom example has QRS complexes that are wider than normal because the ventricles are being paced from below the AV junction. Instead, an idioventricular pacemaker is determining the patient's heart rate. *(From Goldberger AL:* Clinical electrocardiography: a simplified approach, *ed 6, St Louis, 1999, Mosby.)*

Fig. 11-32 Two electrocardiogram tracings of junctional premature beats. They are from the same patient but from different leads. *Arrows,* Retrograde P waves of opposite polarity from normal. *(From Goldberger AL, Goldberger E: Clinical electrocardiography, St Louis, 1981, Mosby.)*

or a feeling of stomach upset. If an ECG is performed, it may show ST-segment depression as a sign of myocardial hypoxia (Fig. 11-33). If the patient is properly treated, an MI may be prevented by opening the blocked artery.

Often, however, the patient comes to the hospital too late, and an MI with heart damage is present. If the damaged area is large enough, the heart fails to pump adequately, and the patient dies. A smaller infarct weakens the heart. In addition, the damaged or dying tissue acts as an abnormal focus for the arrhythmias discussed next. The series of ECG changes that occurs during the acute stage of an MI and as the heart heals are shown in Fig. 11-34 and are listed here:

1. The initial ECG may be normal. This happens about 15% of the time. The patient should be admitted for observation and cardiac enzyme studies if symptoms are present.
2. The first sign of an MI is an elevated ST segment. This occurs within a few hours of the injury.
3. Next the T wave inverts. This happens within hours to days of the infarct.

4. The ST segment returns to the normal baseline position within days to weeks.
5. After a period of weeks to months, the T wave becomes upright again. A lasting ECG change is an enlarged Q wave as shown.

Premature ventricular contraction. A premature ventricular contraction (PVC) is an abnormal, fast contraction of the ventricles that originates from a focus below the AV node (Fig. 11-35). This is usually a sign of a diseased or hypoxic ventricle. Pathologic causes include arteriosclerotic heart disease or MI. An example of an isolated PVC is shown in Fig. 11-36 and has these traits:

1. It is premature and happens before the normal heartbeat.
2. No P wave is present.
3. The QRS complex is bizarre looking and more than 0.12 seconds wide.
4. The T wave is inverted.
5. Usually, a fully compensatory pause occurs before the next normal heartbeat.

Fig. 11-33 An electrocardiogram tracing showing ST segment depression. This is usually caused by myocardial hypoxia and can lead to a myocardial infarction if not promptly treated. *(From Wilkins RL, Krider SJ, Sheldon RL: Clinical assessment in respiratory care, ed 4, St Louis, 2000, Mosby.)*

Fig. 11-34 The sequence of electrocardiogram rhythms commonly seen after a myocardial infarction. See the text for a description of each step in the sequence.

R₁-R₂
520 msec   R₃-R₄
1040 msec

Fig. 11-36 Premature ventricular contractions (PVCs) cause a fully compensatory pause. Note that the interval between the two sinus beats that surround the PVC (R₃ and R₄ in this case) is exactly two times the normal interval between the sinus beats R₁ and R₂. Notice that the P waves come on time, except that the third P wave is interrupted by the PVC and therefore does not conduct normally through the atrioventricular junction. The next (fourth) P wave also comes on time. The fact that the sinus node continues to pace despite the PVC results in the fully compensatory pause. *(From Goldberger AL: Clinical electrocardiography: a simplified approach, ed 6, St Louis, 1999, Mosby.)*

Fig. 11-35 Premature ventricular contraction (PVC; *arrows*) is detected when an impulse is propagated from a ventricular focus before the next normal beat is due. The QRS complex is commonly widened and not preceded by a P wave. A longer than usual (compensatory) pause follows. Retrograde activation of the atria may occur after a premature contraction, or the normal sinus P waves may continue. The sinus P waves after the PVC are blocked by conduction-system refractoriness. *(From Stein E: Clinical electrocardiography: a self-study course, Philadelphia, 1987, Lea & Febiger.)*

A single PVC is not dangerous unless it originates during the T wave, when the heart is especially vulnerable to electrical stimulation. Then it can cause ventricular fibrillation. Patients with PVCs should be watched more closely and probably treated when their PVCs are seen more frequently than 1 in 10 beats, seen in groups of two or three, or seen in multiple configurations. For example, two different-looking PVCs mean that two different ventricular foci are firing prematurely (Fig. 11-37). Bigeminy occurs when every second beat is a PVC; trigeminy is when every third beat is a PVC. Dangerous PVCs must be rapidly treated. Lidocaine (Xylocaine) is given intra-

venously if the heart rate is more than 60 beats/min. If that does not work, procainamide hydrochloride (Pronestyl) is added.

Ventricular tachycardia. Ventricular tachycardia (VT or V tach) is a serious consequence of untreated premature ventricular contractions (Fig. 11-38). VT is defined as a series of three or more consecutive PVCs. Runs of VT may be fairly short or prolonged. The rate counted during VT is between 110 and 250 beats/min. Cardiac output decreases dramatically during this arrhythmia. If the patient has a stable blood pressure, VT is treated with lidocaine as an antiarrhythmic. Synchronized cardioversion is needed if the lidocaine is ineffective. If the VT is sustained and the patient is unresponsive, pulseless, hypotensive, or in pulmonary

Fig. 11-37 An electrocardiogram tracing showing multifocal premature ventricular contractions (PVCs). Counting from the left, after the normal beat, note that the next beat and sixth beat are PVCs. Because they look different, they do not originate at the same abnormal focus. Therefore the patient has multifocal PVCs. This dangerous situation should be quickly corrected. *(From Wilkins RL, Krider SJ, Sheldon RL: Clinical assessment in respiratory care, ed 4, St Louis, 2000, Mosby.)*

Fig. 11-38 Electrocardiogram tracing showing normal sinus rhythm that suddenly converts to ventricular tachycardia. This can happen if a premature ventricular contraction occurs early in the heart's repolarization process and is called the R-on-T phenomenon. If ventricular tachycardia is not treated promptly, it will deteriorate into ventricular flutter or ventricular fibrillation. *(From Wilkins RL, Krider SJ, Sheldon RL: Clinical assessment in respiratory care, ed 4, St Louis, 2000, Mosby.)*

Fig. 11-39 Example of an electrocardiogram showing ventricular flutter. If this arrhythmia is not treated promptly, it will deteriorate into ventricular fibrillation. *(From Kacmarek RM, Mack CW, Dimas S: The essentials of respiratory care, ed 3, St Louis, 1990, Mosby.)*

edema, unsynchronous cardioversion is necessary. If left untreated, VT usually progresses to either ventricular flutter (Fig. 11-39) or ventricular fibrillation (discussed next). Ventricular flutter looks similar on the ECG to VT except that the rate is usually faster, and the rhythm less regular. Its treatment is the same as that for VT and, if left untreated, will progress to ventricular fibrillation. Both of these arrhythmias originate from a single fast ventricular focus, as shown in Fig. 11-35.

Ventricular fibrillation. Ventricular fibrillation (VF or V fib) is caused when multiple, fast ventricular foci are firing (see Fig. 11-40 for the electrical pathways). When several ventricular foci are firing in an uncoordinated manner, the rhythm is chaotic and without any pattern. Virtually no cardiac output occurs. The patient is pulseless and without any blood pressure. This is a true medical emergency. If it is not treated immediately, brain death will occur within minutes. CPR must be started to provide oxygen to the brain. The treatment of choice for VF is defibrillation as quickly as possible. No attempt is made to synchronize the electrical shock. Fig. 11-41 shows the usual position of the defibrillator paddles. It is hoped that with prompt CPR efforts and electrical defibrillation, the patient's heartbeat will return to normal sinus rhythm (see Fig. 11-5).

Ventricular asystole. Ventricular asystole (or asystole) occurs when no cardiac electrical signal and no myocardial activity are present. The ECG tracing shows a flat line, indicating the absence of cardiac electrical activity. The presence of this arrhythmia is ominous. When seen after a full attempt at CPR, it indicates a nonfunctioning

heart. The patient will almost assuredly die. Some physicians may elect to defibrillate the patient in asystole in an attempt to generate some sort of rhythm. Because of the dire consequences of ventricular asystole,

Fig. 11-40 Multiple disorganized contractions of the ventricles characterize ventricular fibrillation and represent cardiac arrest. It may be of sudden onset or may follow premature ventricular contractions, ventricular tachycardia, or ventricular flutter. *(From Stein E: Clinical electrocardiography: a self-study course, Philadelphia, 1987, Lea & Febiger.)*

Fig. 11-41 Schematic drawing of automated external defibrillator and its attachment to the patient. *(Modified from Cummins RO: Advanced cardiac life support, American Heart Association, 1994, Dallas, Tex.)*

it is wise to double-check all the equipment. This includes the ECG leads or defibrillator paddles being used to check the rhythm, all electrical connections, and the functioning of the ECG monitor to be sure that no technical error can be found.

> **Exam Hint**
>
> A CPR related question may include an ECG tracing. Usually it is of ventricular tachycardia or ventricular fibrillation. The question usually includes the patient being pulseless or without a blood pressure. The therapist must realize that the situation is life threatening and requires CPR or defibrillation as necessary.

b. Make a recommendation for an arterial blood gas measurement (WRE code: IC3) [Difficulty: An]

Blood for arterial blood gas (ABG) determination is usually drawn in any hospital-based CPR effort. It should not be done at the expense of time that should be spent starting effective ventilations and chest compressions or defibrillating the heart. The blood gas values give important information on the patient's oxygenation and whether the patient is acidotic. Changes in the ventilation efforts and medications such as bicarbonate are based on information from the ABGs.

The femoral site is usually the best to draw from in a CPR situation because it is the largest artery and the easiest to hit. It is far enough from the chest that blood can be

drawn without interfering in the chest compression efforts.

c. Interpret the results of arterial blood gas analysis (WRE code: IB8e) [Difficulty: An]

The full discussion of ABG interpretation is presented in Chapter 3. During a CPR attempt, the key things to look for are the patient's Pao_2 and $Paco_2$, because they relate to the adequacy of ventilations and chest compressions. If the patient has an acidotic pH and a normal or low $Paco_2$, the patient has an uncorrected metabolic acidosis. Intravenous (IV) sodium bicarbonate is indicated.

d. Endotracheal intubation

Oral endotracheal intubation is usually performed during a CPR attempt. See Chapter 12 for a complete discussion of endotracheal tubes, intubation equipment, and the process of performing intubation.

e. Make the recommendation to defibrillate the patient

Defibrillation sends a specific amount of direct electrical current (DC) through the patient's chest wall and heart. Its purpose is to stimulate the entire cardiac muscle and electrical system so that the source of an abnormal signal will be suppressed. The SA node usually then takes over as the normal pacemaker. Chapter 18 includes a table listing the stepped progression of power used in defibrillation.

Synchronized defibrillation (cardioversion) (see Chapter 18) should be performed under the following circumstances: atrial flutter, PAT, atrial fibrillation, and ventricular tachycardia unless the patient is pulseless, unresponsive, hypotensive, or in pulmonary edema.

Unsynchronized defibrillation should be performed under the following circumstances: ventricular fibrillation or ventricular tachycardia when the patient is pulseless, unresponsive, hypotensive; or in pulmonary edema. Some physicians also may administer a cardiac shock to a patient in ventricular asystole.

> **Exam Hint**
>
> Usually one question requires the therapist to identify the indications for defibrillation and recommend the procedure.

f. Recommend medications during an emergency

Cardiotonic (positive inotropic) drugs. Positive inotropic agents are used to increase the contractility of the heart muscle. Two classes of drugs do this, and both are used in patients who have a weak or damaged myocardium. They increase the patient's myocardial contractility. This results in increased cardiac output, increased blood pressure, and increased urine output. The best-known, older group consists of cardiac glycosides and is commonly referred to as "digitalis." The cardiac glycosides increase the level of intramuscular sodium and calcium to increase the contraction of the heart muscle. Of these, Lanoxin (digoxin) is the preferred medication for a patient with congestive heart failure.

The newer group includes synthetic catecholamine agents. The catecholamine agents are similar to adrenaline and stimulate β receptors in the heart. Dobutamine hydrochloride (Dobutrex) is used as a short-term agent in adult patients who have organic heart disease or who have had heart surgery. Its use results in an increase in contraction with only a minor increase in heart rate. Epinephrine (Adrenaline) is used during a cardiac arrest to increase heart rate and contractility.

Antiarrhythmic drugs. Bradycardia is defined as a heart rate of less than 60 beats/min in an adult at rest. If the patient has symptoms such as light-headedness or low blood pressure, the heart rate should be increased. Common medications that increase the heart rate include atropine (atropine sulfate), isoproterenol (Isuprel), and epinephrine (Adrenaline chloride).

Tachycardia (a resting adult heart rate of greater than 100 beats/min) and abnormal, fast heartbeats originating from the atria or ventricles are potentially very dangerous. Fast tachycardia and dangerous arrhythmias must be controlled with medications that slow the heart's conduction system or suppress the generation of abnormal electrical signals. Common medications that do this include propranolol (Inderal), lidocaine (Xylocaine), and procainamide (Pronestyl).

Vasoconstricting drugs. Vasoconstrictors are medications that cause the peripheral blood vessels to constrict so that blood flow is reduced through them. Many medications do this by stimulating the alpha-1 (α_1 receptors on the vessels. They are chiefly used in a hypotensive patient. Hypotension is usually defined as a systemic blood pressure of less than 80 mm Hg in an adult and less than 70 mm Hg in a child. A pressure of less than this does not adequately perfuse the kidneys. Urine output decreases dramatically or stops altogether. Cerebral blood flow also is greatly reduced. When hypotension is caused by vasodilation, as in allergic anaphylaxis or sepsis, it usually has to be treated by inducing vasoconstriction. Hypotension from heart failure or an MI often also must be treated with a vasoconstrictor. Common examples of medications that cause vasoconstriction to increase blood pressure include dopamine hydrochloride (Intropin) and norepinephrine (Levophed, Levarterenol).

The effects of dopamine are dose related. At relatively low doses, an increase in renal blood flow is noted, and urine output increases, with no change in blood pressure. At medium doses, an increase in myocardial contractility and a progressive peripheral vasoconstriction is found. These effects increase the blood pressure without decreasing renal blood flow. At high doses, the total systemic vascular resistance further increases. However, renal blood flow and urine output both decrease. Current practice indicates that dopamine works best in patients with moderate hypotension. A patient who does not respond to dopamine probably needs norepinephrine (Levophed or Levarterenol) to increase the blood pressure. Any time a hypotensive patient is given a vasoconstricting agent, the blood pressure, peripheral blood flow, and urine output must be watched closely. The prognosis is grim for patients who do not respond to these medications or for attempts to correct the underlying condition.

Vasodilating drugs. Hypertension in the adult is defined as a blood pressure of greater than 140 to 150/90 mm Hg. The higher the blood pressure, the greater the strain on the heart. It also increases the risk of vessel rupture and stroke.

A wide variety of medications in a number of drug categories are used to reduce blood pressure. They range from diuretics to reduce blood volume, to calcium and sympathomimetic blockers that reduce heart rate and vasodilate, to angiotensin-converting enzyme (ACE) inhibitors. Medications in these categories are used to treat moderate, chronic hypertension.

The patient in a hypertensive crisis (blood pressure greater than 200/120 mm Hg) must be treated quickly and effectively. The following medications are commonly given by the IV route to control severe hypertension:

a. Nitroprusside (Nipride)
b. Diazoxide (Hyperstat)
c. Trimethaphan (Arfonad)

Nitroprusside also is given to reduce the afterload in a patient with left ventricular failure after an MI. Any patient who is receiving a powerful vasodilator must have frequent blood pressure monitoring.

Bicarbonate (sodium bicarbonate). According to the most recent guidelines, bicarbonate (sodium bicarbonate) should be used, if at all, only after all other CPR procedures have been instituted. Bicarbonate may then be used if a diagnosis has been made and the patient has a preexisting metabolic acidosis, hyperkalemia, or tricyclic or phenobarbital overdose. Bicarbonate also may be beneficial if the patient has been in prolonged arrest or if CPR has been performed for an extended time.

When used, bicarbonate should be given initially at a dose of 1 mEq/kg; a half dose is then given every 10 minutes. If available from ABG results, use the calculated base deficit or bicarbonate concentration as a guideline for giving more bicarbonate. Do not completely correct the base deficit to avoid accidentally making the patient alkalotic.

g. Recommend the instillation of medications through the endotracheal tube during an emergency situation

Cardiac medications may be instilled down the endotracheal tube when a resuscitation attempt is under way and the patient does not have a functional central or peripheral IV line. The following medications may be instilled into all patients: lidocaine, epinephrine, and atropine. Adults should be given a dose 2 to 2.5 times the normal IV amount. The medication should be diluted by adding 10 mL of normal saline or distilled water. Pediatric patients may be given a dose that is up to 0.1 mg/kg. It should be diluted with 1 to 2 mL of normal or half-normal saline.

h. Instill the ordered medication down the endotracheal tube

The following steps for instillation are recommended:
1. Disconnect the manual resuscitator from the endotracheal tube and stop the chest compressions.
2. Pass a suction catheter or feeding tube past the distal tip of the endotracheal tube.
3. Quickly inject the drug solution down the catheter.
4. Withdraw the suction catheter.
5. Reconnect the manual resuscitator to the endotracheal tube and give the patient several deep breaths. This helps to force the medication down to the alveolar level or causes aerosolization so that faster absorption occurs.
6. Resume chest compressions and ventilation.

> **Exam Hint**
>
> **E**pinephrine (Adrenaline) is the first-line drug used in a CPR attempt because it increases the heart's rate and contraction and causes vasoconstriction.

i. Observe the size of the patient's pupils and their reaction to light

Normally the pupils react to a light being shined into them by constricting. The pupils dilate within 30 to 40 seconds after cardiac arrest and do not constrict normally when the brain is hypoxic. If CPR is being done properly to deliver oxygen to the brain, the pupils should constrict normally. Fixed (nonreactive) and dilated pupils are an ominous sign. Even if the heart can be restarted, the brain has probably had irreversible damage.

In several conditions, the pupils do not react as expected. The pupils remain constricted if the victim has received morphine sulfate or other opiates. The pupils are dilated if the victim has received atropine, quinidine, or epinephrine. Hypothermia also causes the pupils to dilate.

j. Recommend capnography or exhaled carbon dioxide measurement to evaluate the adequacy of resuscitation

The general discussion of capnography was presented in Chapter 5 and exhaled carbon dioxide monitors in Chapter 12. Either can be used to help confirm that the endotracheal tube is properly located in the trachea. It also is helpful if the patient is being transported or the endotracheal tube is being repositioned. The presence of exhaled carbon dioxide confirms that the tube is properly positioned in the trachea. In addition, clinical evidence suggests that monitoring the exhaled carbon dioxide level during a CPR attempt is helpful in evaluating the patient's response. In general, if chest compressions and assisted ventilation are effective, carbon dioxide is removed from the tissues and circulated to the lungs for exhalation. If the CPR efforts are ineffective, little exhaled carbon dioxide is measured.

> **Exam Hint**
>
> **T**he Written Registry Exam usually has one ACLS level question. Review the advanced CPR procedures such as life-threatening arrhythmia recognition, intubation, and defibrillation.

3. Pediatric advanced life support (WRE code: III I1c) [Difficulty: An]

The general steps and procedures related to pediatric advanced life support (PALS) are covered in this chapter and Chapter 12.

4. Neonatal resuscitation program (WRE code: III I1d) [Difficulty: An]

A neonatal resuscitation program (NRP) provides training in resuscitating a newborn at birth in the delivery room. In addition to the basic and advanced CPR steps discussed in this chapter and Chapter 12, the person trained in NRP is prepared to perform the following:
a. Dry the newborn and keep it warm.
b. Suction the airway to remove amniotic fluid and meconium.
c. Evaluate the newborn to determine the need for 100% oxygen, bag-mask ventilation, intubation, and chest compressions.

It is beyond the scope of this text to cover all aspects of ACLS, PALS, and NRP training. The bibliography lists helpful sources of information.

Exam Hint

Usually one question relates to PALS or NRP. Recognize that if a newborn has a low Apgar score, is apneic, has bradycardia, or has hypotension, action must be taken. A child who is apneic, has bradycardia, or has hypotension also must be treated quickly. Past questions have required the therapist to begin bag-mask ventilation with oxygen.

MODULE D
Respiratory care plan

1. Analyze available information to determine the patient's pathophysiologic state (CSE code: IIIH1)

It is critically important that the respiratory therapist be able to recognize the need to start CPR procedures. Discussion in this chapter should be helpful in preparing for this possibility.

2. Determine the appropriateness of the prescribed therapy and goals for the identified pathophysiologic state (CSE code: IIIH3)

BCLS, ACLS, PALS, and NRP are all CPR-related protocols. CPR should be started, adjusted, and terminated based on these protocols and the patient's recovery.

a. Stop the treatment or procedure if the patient has an adverse reaction to it. (CSE code: IIIF1)

The practitioner should make a recommendation to the physician to stop a procedure being performed as an adjunct to CPR if the patient is having an adverse reaction to it. For example, bag and mask ventilation may force air into the stomach; recommend intubation. Always notify the physician of any change in the patient's condition or if a complication to any CPR-related procedure is seen.

b. Discontinue treatment based on the patient's response (WRE code: IIIG1e) [Difficulty: An]

The physician will make the decision to stop futile CPR activities that are taking place in the hospital.

BIBLIOGRAPHY

Abedin Z, Conner RP: *12-Lead ECG interpretation: the self-assessment approach,* Philadelphia, 1989, WB Saunders.

Aloan CA, Hill TV, editors: *Respiratory care of the newborn and child,* ed 2, Philadelphia, 1997, Lippincott-Raven.

American Association for Respiratory Care: Clinical practice guideline: resuscitation and defibrillation in the health care setting: 2004 revision and update, *Respir Care* 49(9):1085, 2004.

American Association for Respiratory Care: Clinical practice guideline: resuscitation in acute care hospitals, *Respir Care* 38(11):1179, 1993.

American Association for Respiratory Care: Clinical practice guideline: defibrillation during resuscitation, *Respir Care* 40(7):744, 1995.

American Association for Respiratory Care: Clinical practice guideline: management of airway emergencies, *Respir Care* 40(7):749, 1995.

American Heart Association: *ACLS provider manual,* Dallas, Tex, 2001, American Heart Association.

American Heart Association: *PALS provider manual,* Dallas, Tex, 2002, American Heart Association.

Barnes TA, editor: *Core textbook of respiratory care practice,* ed 2, St Louis, 1994, Mosby.

Barnes TA, Boudin KM: Cardiopulmonary resuscitation. In Burton GG, Hodgkin JE, Ward JJ, editors: *Respiratory care: a guide to clinical practice,* ed 4, Philadelphia, 1997, Lippincott-Raven.

Barnes TA, Hess DR: Cardiopulmonary resuscitation. In Hess DR, MacIntyre NR, Mishoe SC, editors: *Respiratory care principles and practice,* Philadelphia, 2002, WB Saunders.

Barnhart SL, Czervinske MP: *Perinatal and pediatric respiratory care,* Philadelphia, 1995, WB Saunders.

Branson RD, Hess DR, Chatburn RL, editors: *Respiratory care equipment,* ed 2, Philadelphia, 1999, Lippincott Williams & Wilkins.

Burton GC, Hodgkin JE, Ward JJ, editors: *Respiratory care: a guide to clinical practice,* ed 4, Philadelphia, 1997, Lippincott-Raven.

Butler HH: How to read an ECG, *RN* 36(1):35, 1973.

Butler HH: How to read an ECG, *RN* 36(2):49, 1973.

Butler HH: How to read an ECG, *RN* 36(3):50, 1973.

Cairo JM, Pilbeam SP: *Mosby's respiratory care equipment,* ed 6, St Louis, 1999, Mosby.

Davis D: *Differential diagnosis of arrhythmias,* Philadelphia, 1991, WB Saunders.

Durbin CG: Airway management. In Cairo JM, Pilbeam SP, editors: *Mosby's respiratory care equipment,* ed 7, St. Louis, 2004, Mosby.

Eubanks DH, Bone RC: *Comprehensive respiratory care,* ed 2, St Louis, 1990, Mosby.

Fink JB, Hunt GE, editors: *Clinical practice in respiratory care,* Philadelphia, 1999, Lippincott-Raven.

Fluck RR: Emergency medicine. In Wyka KA, Mathews PJ, Clark WF, editors: *Foundations of respiratory care,* Albany, NY, 2002, Delmar.

Goldberger AL, Goldberger E: *Clinical electrocardiography,* St Louis, 1981, Mosby.

Harwood R: *Exam review and study guide for perinatal/pediatric respiratory care,* Philadelphia, 1999, FA Davis.

Hess D, Goff G, Johnson K: The effect of hand size, resuscitator brand, and use of two hands on volumes delivered during adult bag-valve ventilation, *Respir Care* 34:805, 1989.

Kacmarek RM, Mack CW, Dimas S: *The essentials of respiratory care,* ed 3, St Louis, 1990, Mosby.

Madama VC: Safe mouth-to-mouth resuscitation requires adjunct equipment, caution, *Occup Health Saf* 60(1):56, 1991.

Marriott HJL: *Practical electrocardiography,* ed 7, Baltimore, 1983, Williams & Wilkins.

Marshak AB: Emergency life support. In Wilkins RL, Stoller JK, Scanlan CL, editors: *Egan's fundamentals of respiratory therapy,* ed 8, St Louis, 2003, Mosby.

Pagana K, Pagana TJ: *Mosby's manual of diagnostic and laboratory tests,* St Louis, 1998, Mosby.

Part 4: Adult basic life support. *Circulation* 112:IV18–IV34, 2004.

Part 11: Pediatric basic life support. *Circulation* 112:IV156–IV166, 2005.

Part 13: Neonatal resuscitation guidelines. *Circulation* 112:IV188–IV195, 2005.

Patel JM, McGowan SG, Moody LA: *Arrhythmias: detection, treatment, and cardiac drugs,* Philadelphia, 1989, WB Saunders.

Phillips RE, Feeney MK: *The cardiac rhythms: a systematic approach to interpretation,* ed 3, Philadelphia, 1990, WB Saunders.

Shapiro BA, Kacmarek RM, Cane RD, et al, editors: *Clinical application of respiratory care,* ed 4, St Louis, 1991, Mosby.

Stein E: *Clinical electrocardiography: a self-study course,* Philadelphia, 1987, Lea & Febiger.

Sweetwood HM: *Clinical electrocardiography for nurses,* Rockville, Md, 1983, Aspen Systems.

Whitaker K: *Comprehensive perinatal and pediatric respiratory care,* ed 2, Albany, NY, 1997, Delmar.

White GC: *Equipment theory for respiratory care,* ed 3, Albany, NY, 1999, Delmar.

SELF-STUDY QUESTIONS

1. A normal sinus rhythm can be identified by:
   I. A resting rate of 60 to 100 beats/min in an adult
   II. A P wave before every QRS complex
   III. A regular rhythm
   IV. A QRS complex after every P wave
   V. An upright T wave in lead II
   A. II and IV
   B. II, III, and IV
   C. I, II, III, and V
   D. I, II, III, IV, and V

2. Your ventilator-dependent patient is set up for routine ECG monitoring. Because of refractory hypoxemia, the physician orders 10 cm water of positive end-expiratory pressure (PEEP). Shortly after the PEEP therapy is added, you notice that sinus arrhythmia has developed. Which of the following is the best course of action to follow?
   A. Recommend the administration of atropine.
   B. Recommend synchronized cardioversion.
   C. Recommend decreasing the PEEP from 10 to 5 cm water.
   D. Make a record of the rhythm and inform the nurse and physician of your observation.

3. Electrocardiogram monitoring is important with an intensive care unit in all of the following situations *except:*
   A. If it is used to evaluate peripheral perfusion.
   B. The patient has an electrolyte disturbance.
   C. The patient has a history of arrhythmias.
   D. The patient is being given a rapid infusion of potassium.

4. After an exercise routine, a 59-year-old man experiences sudden chest pain with shortness of breath. ECG monitoring in the Emergency Department reveals the following rhythm strip. What should the respiratory therapist recommend?
   I. Synchronized cardioversion
   II. 12-lead ECG
   III. Defibrillation
   IV. Administer oxygen
   V. Angioplasty
   A. I and V
   B. II and IV
   C. II, III, and IV
   D. I, II, IV, and V

(Wilkins RL, Krider SJ, Sheldon RL: Clinical assessment in respiratory care, *ed 4, St Louis, 2000, Mosby.)*

5. A mouth-to-valve resuscitation device is being used on an apneic patient. The respiratory therapist delivers a breath, but the patient's chest does not rise. What should be done next?
   A. Begin chest compressions.
   B. Request a lateral neck radiograph.
   C. Check the valve for proper position.
   D. Perform abdominal thrusts.

6. Which of the following medications can be administered down the endotracheal tube during a CPR attempt?
   I. Epinephrine
   II. Potassium chloride
   III. Atropine
   IV. Lidocaine
      A. I
      B. II and III
      C. I and IV
      D. I, III, and IV

7. Two respiratory therapists respond to a cardiopulmonary-arrest call and begin CPR procedures on an adult patient. On looking at the ECG monitor, the following rhythm strip is seen.

(*Goldberger AL, Goldberger E:* Clinical electrocardiography, *ed 4, St Louis, Mosby.*)

What should be recommended in this situation?
   A. Defibrillate the patient.
   B. Increase the oxygen flow to the manual resuscitation bag and mask.
   C. Change ventilation and chest compression duties.
   D. Intubate the patient.

8. CPR steps have been under way for 15 minutes when an arterial blood gas sample is drawn and sent off for analysis. The following results are obtained with 100% oxygen being used to ventilate the patient:
   pH, 6.97
   $PaCO_2$, 30 torr
   PaO_2, 210 torr
   HCO_3^-, 8 mEq/L
   What should the therapist recommend at this time?
   A. Decrease the oxygen percentage.
   B. Decrease the respiratory rate.
   C. Administer intravenous sodium bicarbonate.
   D. Add mechanical dead space to the manual resuscitator.

9. During a CPR attempt on a 50-year-old patient, the respiratory therapist successfully intubates the patient and begins ventilating with a manual resuscitator. The physician is unable to start an IV line. How should the CPR drugs be given?
   A. Intraosseous injection
   B. Endotracheal instillation
   C. Intracardiac injection
   D. Nasal spray

10. A 59-year-old patient is brought to the hospital with a complaint of sudden, severe substernal chest pain and dyspnea. What initial thing should the respiratory therapist recommend?
    A. Begin ECG monitoring.
    B. Draw an ABG sample.
    C. Get a chest radiograph.
    D. Get a capnometer value.

11. Defibrillation should be done immediately in which of the following patient situations?
    A. Second degree heart block
    B. Atrial flutter
    C. Pulseless ventricular tachycardia
    D. Sinus tachycardia

12. You are the respiratory therapist attending the delivery of a preterm neonate. His vital signs are:
    Respiratory rate, 12 per minute
    Heart rate, 70 beats/min
    In addition, he has peripheral cyanosis and is responding minimally to stimulation. What should be done?
    A. Direct supplemental oxygen to his face.
    B. Begin chest compressions.
    C. Begin manual ventilation with 100% oxygen.
    D. Continue to stimulate the newborn to breathe more deeply.

ANSWER KEY

1. **D.** Rationale: All of the listed options are found in the normal sinus rhythm. See the text for the discussion, Fig. 11-5 for a tracing, and Table 11-1 for a review if necessary.

2. **D.** Rationale: Sinus arrhythmia is shown in Fig. 10-8. Review the associated discussion if needed. In a patient receiving mechanical ventilation and PEEP, it is possible to put too much pressure on the heart, which reduces venous return. If the returning blood volume is decreased, the cardiac output also will decrease. The patient should be monitored and key people informed. It is too early to decide whether the PEEP level is too high and should be reduced. The physician should be consulted before making any change. Atropine will increase the patient's heart rate and is not indicated in this situation. No indication suggests that the patient has an arrhythmia that requires synchronized cardioversion.

3. **A.** Rationale: ECG monitoring will not provide any useful information about peripheral perfusion. The patient could have a normal heart rhythm and have altered perfusion. Electrolyte disturbances, especially the potassium (K^+) level, can alter the heart's electrical conduction system. It is wise to monitor a patient with a known history of arrhythmias in case they return. Fast or excessive infusion of potassium can lead to serious arrhythmias that justify ECG monitoring.

4. **B.** Rationale: The rhythm strip shows two identical premature ventricular contractions (PVCs). This, combined with the patient's history of sudden chest pain and shortness of breath, suggests a heart problem. A 12-lead ECG is indicted for the physician to be able to determine the patient's cardiac condition. Oxygen is indicated for the shortness of breath. In addition, the oxygen will help the heart if it is hypoxic. The patient's condition is not life threatening, and no need is seen for either synchronized cardioversion or defibrillation. A cardiac catheterization procedure is needed to identify any coronary artery blockages before angioplasty is indicated.

5. **C.** Rationale: It is easy and quick to check the valve for proper position. Fix the valve if necessary, and attempt to ventilate the patient again. Because the patient's pulse has not yet been checked, no indication is seen that chest compressions are needed. Getting a lateral neck radiograph will greatly delay (probably fatally) ventilating the patient. There is not yet an indication that the patient needs abdominal thrusts to clear an airway obstruction. If the patient cannot be ventilated by the fixed mouth-to-valve resuscitation device, check for an obvious obstruction in the mouth or throat. Reposition the

head, and attempt to ventilate again. If the patient still cannot be ventilated, then perform abdominal thrusts.

6. **D.** Rationale: Current ACLS guidelines state that atropine, epinephrine (both for bradycardia), and lidocaine (to suppress ventricular arrhythmias) can be given via the endotracheal tube during a CPR attempt if the patient does not have a functioning IV line. Potassium chloride can be given only intravenously.

7. **A.** Rationale: The rhythm strip shows ventricular fibrillation. The best way to treat this dangerous arrhythmia is to defibrillate the patient immediately. All of the other listed options are reasonable in a CPR attempt when appropriate. However, they are all secondary to treating the patient's ventricular fibrillation.

8. **C.** Rationale: Interpretation of the patient's ABG results shows hyperventilation with a metabolic acidosis. Intravenous sodium bicarbonate should be given to correct the patient's acidosis. It is appropriate to keep the patient's PaO_2 at 210 torr during the CPR attempt to try to oxygenate the brain. Decreasing the respiratory rate or adding mechanical dead space to the manual resuscitator will result in the patient's carbon dioxide increase and a further reduction of the pH.

9. **B.** Rationale: Current ACLS guidelines state that atropine, epinephrine, and lidocaine can be given via the endotracheal tube during a CPR attempt if the patient does not have a functioning IV line. Intraosseous (within the bone) injection of CPR drugs is approved for neonatal resuscitation attempts. Intracardiac injection of CPR drugs is no longer performed. Currently CPR drugs are not given by nasal spray.

10. **A.** Rationale: The patient's symptoms indicate a cardiac problem. It is wise to begin ECG monitoring quickly in case the patient has an arrhythmia. An ABG sample can be drawn after ECG monitoring is started. A chest radiograph also can be done after ECG monitoring is started. A capnometer value to check the patient's exhaled carbon dioxide value is not indicated at this time.

11. **C.** Rationale: Pulseless ventricular tachycardia is a life-threatening arrhythmia (see Fig. 11-38). If the rate is so fast that a pulse cannot be felt, the cardiac output and blood pressure will be very low. The patient must be defibrillated as soon as possible to restore normal sinus rhythm. Second degree heart block is treated with drugs or a pacemaker to speed the heart rate. Atrial flutter and sinus tachycardia are fast, but not life-threatening arrhythmias that are first treated with medications to slow the heart rate.

12. **C.** Rationale: The newborn's vital signs and other clinical findings point to the need for manual ventilation with oxygen. Although directing oxygen to the neonate's face will be helpful, it does not go far enough to ensure adequate ventilation. It is too early to begin chest compressions. They will not be needed if the supplemental ventilation and oxygen cause the heart rate to increase. The neonate is in significant trouble, and additional stimulation will not be enough to improve its breathing.

12 Airway Management

Note 1: The National Board for Respiratory Care (NBRC) has released the *RRT Examination Matrix* (covering the testable items on the Written Registry Exam) and the *CSE Examination Matrix* (covering the testable items on the Clinical Simulation Exam). Turn to the appendices at the back of this book for both publications in their original formats. This book is intended to cover all of the testable items in these two publications. This chapter (and all others) uses the abbreviation "WRE" for the coded items testable on the Written Registry Exam *and* Clinical Simulation Exam. The listed difficulty (R, Recall; Ap, Application; An, Analysis) relates to the question difficulty on the Written Registry Exam. The abbreviation "CSE" is used for the coded items testable on *only* the Clinical Simulation Exam. Because no question difficulty level is given for this exam, be prepared for anything.

Note 2: A review of the most recent Written Registry Examinations has shown an average of six questions (6% of the exam) that cover airway management issues. The Clinical Simulation Exam is comprehensive and may include everything that should be known or performed by an advanced level respiratory therapist.

MODULE A

Care for artificial airways and equipment to maintain a patent airway

1. Recommend the insertion of an artificial airway or a change of the type of artificial airway (WRE code: IIIG1c) [Difficulty: An]

An artificial airway is indicated in any patient who cannot protect his or her airway. The patient could be at risk of obstructing the upper airway by the tongue falling back, have facial trauma or surgery, be at risk of vomiting and aspirating, or need mechanical ventilation for assisted breathing. A number of possible airways are available; select the best one based on the patient's needs.

An oropharyngeal airway is used in an unconscious patient at risk of obstructing the airway with his or her tongue or of having seizure activity. It prevents the tongue from being bitten during a seizure. It should not be used in a conscious patient because it may cause gagging. (See the additional discussion and illustrations in the chapter.)

A nasopharyngeal airway is used to keep the tongue from blocking the airway when an oropharyngeal airway cannot be used. This would include conscious patients or patients with oral trauma or surgery. It also is used as a guide to pass a catheter for tracheal suctioning. (See the additional discussion and illustrations in the chapter.)

An endotracheal tube is indicated when a patent airway is required for endotracheal suctioning or mechanical ventilation. Aspiration also is prevented when the cuff is inflated. An oral endotracheal tube is indicated in most emergency situations because it is faster and easier than placing a nasal endotracheal tube. A nasal endotracheal tube is indicated when the patient has oral trauma or when a cervical spine injury prevents the neck from being hyperextended for placing the oral tube. (See the additional discussion and illustrations in the chapter.)

A tracheostomy tube is indicated for long-term airway management or when facial trauma or surgery prevents the use of an oral or nasal endotracheal tube. This tube also provides a patent airway for suctioning and mechanical ventilation and prevents aspiration. In addition, it is more comfortable than an endotracheal tube and allows the patient to eat and drink. The so-called "talking" tracheostomy tubes permit the patient to vocalize with the aid of an additional source of air flow through the vocal cords. (See the additional discussion and illustrations in the chapter.)

A laryngeal mask airway (LMA) is used by an anesthesiologist to provide a way to ventilate an anesthetized patient without placing an endotracheal tube (Fig. 12-1). The LMA comes in six sizes for insertion into patients ranging in weight from a small child to an adult. The distal end has a cuff that surrounds and seals the larynx when it is inflated. The proximal end of the attached tube has a standard adapter for ventilation with a manual resuscitator or an anesthesia machine. The LMA does not absolutely protect against aspiration, and tidal volume gas can leak if mechanical ventilation pressures greater than 20 cm water are needed.

Fig. 12-1 Laryngeal mask airway. It features an inflatable mask that creates a seal around the patient's larynx. The proximal end of the tube can be connected to a resuscitation bag, anesthesia machine, or mechanical ventilator. *(From Laryngeal Mask Company Limited, Seychelles.)*

Exam Hint

Know the uses, advantages, and disadvantages of the various airway devices. Be prepared to make a recommendation for which to use or when to change to a different airway device, as necessary.

---

2. Properly position the patient to maintain a patent airway and minimize hypoxemia (WRE code: IIID5) [Difficulty: Ap]

Positioning of the head to open the airway is discussed in Chapter 11. In brief, use the head-tilt/chin-lift maneuver to hyperextend the neck of an adult, and slightly extend the neck of a child to open the airway. You can place a small pad behind the neck and head to put the patient in the "sniff" position. Always keep the head in line with the body. If the patient has a known or suspected cervical spine injury, the neck cannot be hyperextended. Instead, open the airway with the jaw-thrust maneuver. Keep the head in line with the body.

The patient may be supine during the airway opening procedures just mentioned. Frequently, however, the patient is positioned with the head and body elevated. An unconscious patient is less likely to vomit and aspirate in either the Fowler or semi-Fowler position. The combination of either of these body positions and the head and neck hyperextended into the sniff position will probably keep the airway open, minimize the risk of aspiration of vomitus, and minimize the patient's work of breathing (WOB). This should help to minimize hypoxemia.

3. Humidify an artificial airway (WRE code: IIIB3b) [Difficulty: An]

Patients with an endotracheal or tracheostomy tube in place should ideally be provided 100% relative humidity at body temperature. If not, secretions in the airway may dry and result in mucus plugs. Patients with an oropharyngeal or nasopharyngeal airway also may be given supplemental humidity by a simple aerosol mask to help prevent drying of secretions. See Chapter 8 for a complete discussion of humidity and aerosol therapy and administrative devices. It may be necessary to change from a heat-moisture exchanger to a cascade-type humidifier if the patient has thick secretions that are difficult to remove by coughing or suctioning.

4. Oropharyngeal airways
a. Get the necessary equipment (WRE code: IIA7a) [Difficulty: Ap]

The oropharyngeal airway (or bite block) is made of plastic that is hard enough to withstand any patient's biting force. This airway is indicated in two situations. First, it is used in an unconscious, supine patient who is experiencing upper airway obstruction because the tongue is falling back and blocking the oropharynx. Second, the oropharyngeal airway is used in a patient who is unconscious and biting down hard when having a seizure. This can cause injury to the patient or pinch off an oral endotracheal tube if one is present.

A properly sized and placed oropharyngeal airway lifts the tongue forward from the posterior portion of the oropharynx to keep a patent airway and make suctioning oral secretions easier. An oropharyngeal airway is poorly tolerated in a conscious patient and can cause gagging and even vomiting. Oropharyngeal airways come in a variety of sizes from infant to adult. The proper size is found by holding the airway against the patient's face with the flange against the lips. The end of the airway should reach the angle of the jaw (Fig. 12-2). Too large an airway can block the oropharynx by extending past the tongue. Too small an airway can push the tongue back into the oropharynx rather than pulling the tongue forward as it should. Fig. 12-3 shows a properly placed and sized oropharyngeal airway.

A number of manufacturers make oropharyngeal airways, which fall into two basic types: hollow center and I-beam (Fig. 12-4).

Fig. 12-2 Procedure for measuring the proper size of the oropharyngeal airway. *(From Eubanks DH, Bone RC: Comprehensive respiratory care, ed 2, St Louis, 1990, Mosby.)*

Fig. 12-3 Cross section through the head showing the proper position of an oropharyngeal airway. *(From Eubanks DH, Bone RC: Comprehensive respiratory care, ed 2, St Louis, 1990, Mosby.)*

1. Hollow center

Hollow center types have an oval or rectangular shape in cross section and are hollow in the center. A suction catheter can be easily placed through the hollow center so that the back of the throat can be cleared of secretions. Some types have an outer tube that can be attached by a practitioner to provide a mouthpiece for rescue breathing. If rescue breathing must be performed, it is probably more effective to ventilate with a mask and manual resuscitator when one becomes available.

2. I-beam

I-beam types are shaped like an I-beam in cross section. A suction catheter can easily be guided along the groove on either side of the I-beam to the back of the throat so that secretions can be cleared out.

Fig. 12-4 Close-ups of hollow and I-beam types of oropharyngeal airways.

b. Put the equipment together and make sure that it works properly (WRE code: IIA7a) [Difficulty: Ap]

Most oropharyngeal airways are single units with nothing to assemble. Some hollow center types have an attachable outer part. The outer part is snapped onto the oropharyngeal airway when the practitioner must perform rescue breathing. It has a wide flange so that the lips can be covered and sealed to prevent a leak.

c. Troubleshoot any problems with the equipment (WRE code: IIA7a) [Difficulty: Ap]

Make sure that the channel in the hollow center types is patent. If a unit is plugged by secretions, blood, or a foreign substance, the patient cannot breathe through the opening and a suction catheter cannot be passed through. Remove an airway that the patient cannot breathe through.

d. Insert the correct oropharyngeal airway (WRE code: IIIB1) [Difficulty: An]

Two widely used methods exist to insert an oropharyngeal airway.

1. First method
   a. Open the patient's mouth with the cross-finger technique. Insert the airway backward into the patient's mouth until it reaches the palate. Some authors recommend inserting it past the uvula.
   b. Twist the airway 180 degrees, and insert it the rest of the way until the tongue is supported by the curved body.
   c. The flange should rest at the lips (Fig. 12-5).

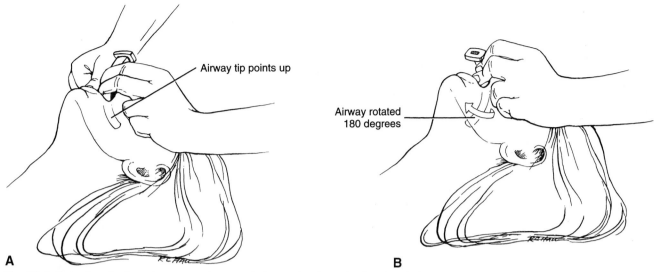

Fig. 12-5 Procedure for inserting an oropharyngeal airway. **A,** Airway is placed with the tip pointing toward the palate. **B,** Airway is rotated 180 degrees to support the tongue. (*From Eubanks DH, Bone RC:* Comprehensive respiratory care, *ed 2, St Louis, 1990, Mosby.*)

2. Second method
   a. Open the patient's mouth with the cross-finger technique. Insert the airway into the mouth with the curved body rotated toward a cheek.
   b. Twist the airway 90 degrees, and insert it the rest of the way so that the tongue is supported by the curved body.
   c. The flange should rest at the lips.

5. Nasopharyngeal airways

a. Get the necessary equipment (WRE code: IIA7a) [Difficulty: Ap]

Nasopharyngeal airways (also known as nasal airways, nasal trumpets, or nasal stents) are made of a relatively soft and pliable plastic or rubber. This decreases the chances of damaging the delicate mucous membranes of the nasal turbinate opening it passes through and the nasopharynx. A nasopharyngeal airway is often used in a supine patient to ensure a patent airway by pushing the tongue forward off of the posterior portion of the oropharynx. The nasopharyngeal airway is probably not as effective in keeping the tongue forward as is the oropharyngeal airway. However, it is better tolerated in a semiconscious or alert patient.

It is also commonly used to provide a secure channel through which to pass a suction catheter or bronchoscope. The nasopharyngeal airway protects the patient's mucous membranes from the trauma of repeatedly passed catheters. Another use is in a patient with trauma to the jaw or in a patient with seizures with a tightly closed jaw. In these cases, an oropharyngeal airway cannot be used. The nasopharyngeal airway can be passed into the patient's oropharynx to push the tongue forward and maintain an airway.

Several manufacturers make the two basic types of nasopharyngeal airways, the *blunt tip* and the *beveled tip*. The beveled-tip types come with right-sided and left-sided cut bevels. If possible, get the airway with the bevel cut that opens toward the patient's oropharynx (toward the nasal septum). For example, if the airway is going to be inserted into the left naris, the bevel should be cut on the right side of the tube so that it is open to the patient's oropharynx. If you were inserting the tube into the right nostril, you would want the bevel cut on the left side of the tube.

See Fig. 12-6 for a close-up of a nasopharyngeal airway. All nasopharyngeal airways have a flange that fits up close to the patient's nostril. This prevents the entire tube from being pushed into the patient. All nasopharyngeal airways have a cannula with a channel for breathing or passing a suction catheter through. Nasopharyngeal airways come in a variety of sizes for adults. They can be properly sized by measuring from the tip of the nose to the tragus of the ear and adding 2 to 3 cm (Fig. 12-7).

b. Put the equipment together and make sure that it works properly (WRE code: IIA7a) [Difficulty: Ap]

All nasopharyngeal airways are made up of a single piece with nothing to assemble.

c. Troubleshoot any problems with the equipment (WRE code: IIA7a) [Difficulty: Ap]

Make sure that the tube is not plugged by dried secretions, blood, or a foreign body. If it is plugged, the patient cannot breathe through it, and a suction catheter cannot be passed through it. Remove a plugged nasopharyngeal airway.

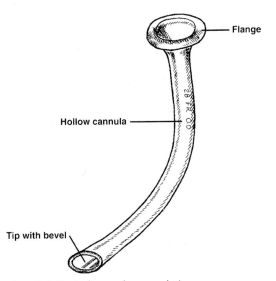

Fig. 12-6 Typical nasopharyngeal airway.

Fig. 12-7 Procedure for measuring the proper size of the nasopharyngeal airway. *(From Eubanks DH, Bone RC: Comprehensive respiratory care, ed 2, St Louis, 1990, Mosby.)*

d. Insert the correct nasopharyngeal airway (WRE code: IIIB1) [Difficulty: An]

The following steps are used for nasopharyngeal airway insertion:

1. Select the most patent nostril. Check the patient's chart for a history of a broken nose, deviated septum, or current head cold. Interview the conscious patient to see whether one nostril is more open than the other. Place your finger in front of the patient's nostrils to feel which one has greater airflow. Avoid forcing the airway into a nostril and nasal passage that may be damaged by the procedure.
2. Lubricate the proper size airway with a sterile, water-soluble lubricant such as K-Y jelly. Place the lubricant on a sterile, 4 × 4-in gauze pad, and then smear it over the length of the airway.
3. Tell the patient what you are going to do.
4. Gently place the airway into the nostril. It should be directed straight back parallel to the hard palate.

Stop if you feel any resistance. Try a different angle if resistance is felt. Do not force the airway. Try the other nostril if necessary.

5. Check the placement by looking into the patient's mouth with a flashlight and tongue depressor. A properly placed nasopharyngeal airway can be seen in the oropharynx and extends behind the tongue (Figs. 12-8 and 12-9).
6. Secure the airway by sticking a safety pin through the flange and taping the pin to the bridge of the

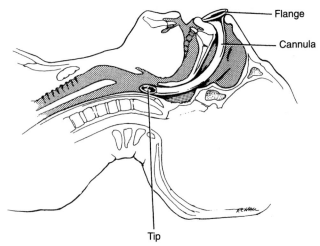

Fig. 12-8 Proper position of the nasopharyngeal airway behind the tongue can be determined by looking into the mouth. The tube is secured by placing a safety pin through the flange and taping it to the cheek.

Fig. 12-9 Cross section of head showing the proper position of the nasopharyngeal airway. *(From Ellis PD, Billings DM: Cardiopulmonary resuscitation: procedures for basic and advanced life support, St Louis, 1980, Mosby.)*

patient's nose or cheek (see Fig. 12-8). This helps prevent the airway from being accidentally pulled out or pushed in.

7. Rotate the airway to the other nostril, if possible, on a regular basis. This helps prevent ulceration of the mucous membrane. Some authors recommend rotation at least every 48 hours, whereas others recommend rotation at much shorter time intervals.

6. Standard and fenestrated tracheostomy tubes

a. Get the necessary equipment (WRE code: IIA7c) [Difficulty: An]

The tracheostomy tube offers the same uses as the endotracheal tube, such as maintaining a secure airway, providing a direct suctioning route to the lungs, preventing aspiration, and assuring a safe route to provide mechanical ventilation. In addition, it is placed in the patient who has an upper airway obstruction or facial trauma that makes intubation impossible. A tracheostomy tube is often placed in a patient who requires long-term mechanical ventilation or who needs a permanent artificial airway. In the long term, a tracheostomy is said to be more comfortable than an endotracheal tube, even though it requires a surgical procedure. An additional advantage of a tracheostomy tube over an endotracheal tube is that it allows the patient to eat and drink.

These tubes come in a variety of sizes for patients of all ages from neonate to adult. See Table 12-1 for tracheostomy tube sizes based on patient age. Most modern tracheostomy tubes are constructed of a hard polyvinyl chloride plastic and have a high-volume, low-pressure cuff. Some specialty tubes are made of silver, rubber, or latex. The older, silver tubes have a cuff that may be removed. Specific information on three types of tubes is given in the following text.

b. Put the equipment together and make sure that it works properly (WRE code: IIA7c) [Difficulty: An]

The following are commonly seen examples of tracheostomy tube styles:

1. Standard tracheostomy tube

The majority of patients have a standard tube placed after the tracheostomy procedure. Refer to Fig. 12-10 for these features of a typical tracheostomy tube:

a. The cannula is the airway through which the patient breathes. The proximal end is outside of the patient's stoma and attached to an adjustable flange. The angle of the flange can be adjusted so that the distal end of the cannula fits properly into the patient's trachea. Soft, cloth tracheostomy tie strings are tied to the ends of the flange. The loose ends are tied behind the patient's neck to hold the

TABLE 12-1 Endotracheal and Tracheostomy Tube Sizes Based on Patient Age*			
Age	ID (mm)	Approximate OD (mm)	Fr size (OD)
NEWBORN			
<1000 g	2.5	4.0	12
1000–2000 g	3.0	5.0	14
2000–3000 g	3.5	5.5	16–18
3000 g to 6 mo old	3.5–4.0		
PEDIATRIC			
18 mo	4.0	6.0	18
3 yr	4.5	6.5	20
5 yr	5.0	7.0	22
6 yr	5.5	8.0	24
8 yr	6.0	9.0	26
ADULT			
16 yr	7.0	10.0	30
Normal sized woman	7.5–8.0	11.0	32–34
Normal sized man	8.0–8.5	12.0	34–36
Large adult	9.0–10.0	13.0–14.0	38–42

*Two notes: First, it is important always to use the largest tube that can be placed into the patient without causing any harm during the intubation. This is because the larger the ID of the tube, the less airway resistance it causes. Be prepared to insert a tube that is one size larger or smaller than anticipated based on individual variances. Second, the mathematical relation between the OD in millimeters and Fr size can be easily calculated. The Fr size is determined by multiplying the OD in millimeters by 3. The OD in millimeters is found by dividing the Fr size by 3.
ID, Inner diameter; OD, outer diameter; Fr, French.

tube in place. The distal end of the cannula has a small area where radiopaque material is imbedded. As with an endotracheal tube, this allows the end of the cannula to be seen on a chest radiograph. The cuff is a high residual volume, low-pressure type. Air is put into and taken out of the cuff by an inflation tube with a pilot balloon and one-way valve.

b. The obturator is slid into the outer cannula opening before it is inserted into the patient's stoma. The obturator has a rounded end that protrudes from the end of the cannula. This prevents any tissue trauma during the insertion. The obturator is removed as soon as the cannula is in place.

c. An inner cannula is slid into the outer cannula opening and locked into place with a clockwise twist. This completes the airway. The proximal end has a standard 15-mm outer diameter (OD) adapter

Tracheostomy tie strings

Flange

Outer cannula

15-mm adapter

Cuff

Inflation tube

Hollow inner cannula

Pilot balloon

Obturator

One-way valve   Rounded tip

Fig. 12-10 Typical tracheostomy tube with its component parts and features.

so that all respiratory care equipment fits onto it. The distal end is flush with the end of the outer cannula. Some practitioners believe that the inner cannula should be periodically removed and cleaned so that secretions do not build up. Other practitioners believe that this is unnecessary if the airway is properly humidified and suctioning is performed as needed.

2. Fenestrated tracheostomy tube

A fenestrated tube is often placed in a patient who can breathe spontaneously and who is being considered for a complete removal of the tracheostomy tube. If the patient does well with this tube, it can probably be removed safely.

If the patient has difficulty, the plug can be removed, the inner cannula can be replaced, and the patient's airway can be suctioned or mechanically ventilated.

Refer to Fig. 12-11 when reviewing these features of the fenestrated tracheostomy tube:

a. The outer cannula has an opening called the fenestration (Dutch for window). The rest of the cannula, cuff, inflation tube, and flange are the same as already discussed.

b. The inner cannula functions as discussed earlier. When it is in place, the tube functions as the standard model does.

c. The outer cannula plug is used to prevent the patient from breathing through the proximal end of the tube. The plug does not cover the fenestration; therefore the patient is able to breathe through the upper airway. The patient can now talk and cough out any secretions.

> ### Exam Hint
>
> A standard tracheostomy tube should be replaced with a fenestrated tube when a patient is improving and can breathe spontaneously (off of the ventilator) for an extended period. Remove the inner cannula so that the patient can breathe through the upper airway. Replace the inner cannula when mechanical ventilation is resumed.

c. Troubleshoot any problems with the equipment (WRE code: IIA24) [Difficulty: An]

Most tubes have cuffs that must be inflated before insertion into the patient to make sure that the cuff is sealed and the one-way valve does not leak. Do not use a tube with a leaking cuff or leaking one-way valve. Make sure that the obturator, inner cannula, and plug all fit properly into the outer cannula. They all should easily snap into place and be easily removable. Check this before inserting the tube into the patient.

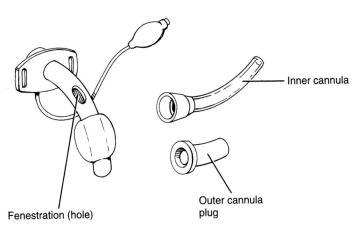

Inner cannula

Fenestration (hole)

Outer cannula plug

Fig. 12-11 Fenestrated tracheostomy tube with its component parts and features. *(From Eubanks DH, Bone RC: Comprehensive respiratory care, ed 2, St Louis, 1990, Mosby.)*

7. Speaking tubes and valves

a. Use speaking tubes and valves (WRE code: IIA23) [Difficulty: R, Ap, An]

Speaking tracheostomy tubes and valves are indicated in a patient who cannot or should not be inhaling through the nose or mouth but can exhale through the natural upper airway. Commonly, these are patients with a neuromuscular disease. Their condition causes them to have a small tidal volume, which results in a large percentage of dead space ventilation. Placing a tracheostomy tube into these patients improves their dead space to tidal volume ratio (review the discussion in Chapter 5, if necessary) and improves their blood gas values. Most commonly, a speaking tracheostomy tube is indicated in a patient who requires support on a mechanical ventilator but is conscious and wishes to speak.

b. Get the necessary equipment (WRE code: IIA23) [Difficulty: R, Ap, An]

Table 12-1 has the standard sizes of tracheostomy tubes. Speaking tracheostomy tubes come only in adult sizes. See Fig. 12-12 for the features of the speaking tracheostomy tube. The cannula is the standard type except that an additional tube has been added to carry a compressed gas through a hole in the back of the cannula. This gas flows up through the vocal cords and allows the patient to speak. The voice is not as strong as normal but should be understandable. Improved communication ability is a great help to the patient's psychological well-being. The patient can still be mechanically ventilated and suctioned and can eat and drink as usual.

c. Put the equipment together and make sure that it works properly (WRE code: IIA23) [Difficulty: R, Ap, An]

A Y-connector is added to the compressed gas tube. Usually about 4 to 6 L/min of compressed air or oxygen is

Fig. 12-12 Pitt tracheostomy tube permits the patient to speak. Note its special feature that directs outside gas flow past the vocal cords. *(From Simmons KF: Airway care. In Scanlan CL, Spearman CB, Sheldon RL, editors:* Egan's fundamentals of respiratory care, *ed 5, St Louis, 1990, Mosby.)*

set by a flowmeter to run to the Y. Closing off the other opening in the Y with a finger diverts the gas into the patient's larynx for speaking. A little experimentation with flows helps the patient find the flow that works best for speaking.

d. Troubleshoot any problems with the equipment (WRE code: IIA24) [Difficulty: An]

See the earlier discussion on care of the standard or fenestrated tracheostomy tubes. The same problems can occur with the speaking tubes.

8. Tracheostomy buttons
a. Get the necessary equipment (WRE code: IIA7c) [Difficulty: An]

A tracheostomy button is a hard plastic tube that is placed into the patient's stoma to keep it open after the tracheostomy tube has been removed. The patient is able to eat, talk, and cough normally. Yet in case the patient has difficulty or needs a breathing treatment, the airway can be reestablished quickly. In general, the patient sizes for tracheostomy buttons match the sizes for tracheostomy tubes listed in Table 12-1. Kistner and Passey-Muir are common types of tracheostomy buttons.

b. Put the equipment together and make sure that it works properly (WRE code: IIA7a) [Difficulty: An]

Refer to Fig. 12-13 when reviewing these features of the tracheostomy button:

1. The hollow outer cannula has a slightly flared proximal end. This keeps the button from slipping entirely into the patient. The distal end is flanged and split into several flexible "grippers."
2. A closure plug fits into the outer cannula and snaps into the flexible grippers on the end of the outer cannula. This seals the button so that the patient breathes through the upper airway.
3. A hollow inner cannula can be inserted into the outer cannula instead of the plug. This inner cannula has a standard 15-mm OD so that a T-piece/Briggs adapter or other respiratory care equipment can be attached if needed. The patient also can be suctioned.
4. Spacers of various widths are used to make sure that the inner cannula is placed at the right depth. The end of the tube should enter the trachea but not obstruct it. See the airway picture in Fig. 12-13 for the proper position.

As discussed in the previous section, special tracheostomy buttons are used with patients who are not to inspire through their upper airway but may breathe out through it. In patients with a very small tidal volume, breathing in through one of these valves reduces the

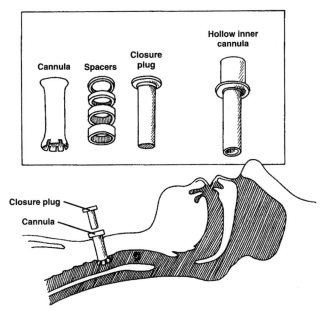

Fig. 12-13 Typical tracheostomy button properly positioned in patient. Insert shows its component parts.

patient's upper airway anatomic dead space. Because expiration is through the upper airway, the patient can speak normally. Refer to Fig. 12-14 when reviewing these features of the Kistner tracheostomy tube:

1. The hollow plastic cannula keeps the stoma open. The distal end is flanged so that it is not likely to be pulled out of the trachea accidentally.
2. The proximal end of the cannula is capped with a one-way valve. The valve allows the patient to breathe in room air or an oxygen- and aerosol-enriched gas source. Expiration is through the upper airway. The patient can talk, eat, and cough normally.

c. Troubleshoot any problems with the equipment (WRE code: IIA7c) [Difficulty: An]

Make sure that all component pieces of these tracheostomy buttons fit together properly and can be easily disconnected if necessary. The cannula must be kept clear of any secretions, blood, or foreign debris. A suction catheter should be passable through the hollow opening in the cannula. If the button is obstructed and the patient is having trouble breathing through the upper airway, the button should be removed and replaced with another button or a tracheostomy tube.

9. Intubation equipment: laryngoscope and blades
a. Get the necessary equipment (WRE code: IIA7d) [Difficulty: An]

The laryngoscope is made up of two basic parts: a handle and a blade. The most commonly seen handle is made of

Fig. 12-14 Kistner tracheotomy button. *(From Eubanks DH, Bone RC:* Comprehensive respiratory care, *ed 2, St Louis, 1990, Mosby.)*

stainless steel; some newer units are made of plastic. The handle contains two C-cell batteries to power the light source in the blade. They all have a common base with a hooking bar so that the blades can be attached (Figs. 12-15 and 12-16).

Blades come in a variety of sizes from pediatric to adult. They all have a common hook so that they can be snapped and locked in place on the handle. The stainless steel handles use stainless steel blades. The newer plastic handles use plastic blades. The two different sets of handles and blades are not interchangeable. The blades come in two different shapes. The Miller blades are straight, and MacIntosh blades are curved (see Fig. 12-15). The intubating person may specify a particular style of blade as well as blade size.

b. Put the equipment together and make sure that it works properly (WRE code: IIA7d) [Difficulty: An]

See Fig. 12-16 for the steps in fastening the blade to the handle:

1. Hold the handle in the left hand and the blade in the right hand.
2. Place the hook on the blade over the hooking bar on the base of the handle.
3. Pull the blade down so that it snaps into place on the handle. The handle and blade should fit together at a 90 degree angle.
4. Make sure that the light bulb in the stainless steel blade is tight.

c. Troubleshoot any problems with the equipment (WRE code: IIA7d) [Difficulty: An]

The light source shines when the handle and blade are properly connected because an electrical circuit has been

Fig. 12-15 Laryngoscope handle with a MacIntosh (curved) blade attached. A Miller (straight) blade is shown for comparison. Note component parts and features.

Fig. 12-16 Motions to attach a laryngoscope to a handle.

completed. Failure of the light source to shine may result from any of the following problems:

1. The handle and blade are not properly connected and snapped into place. Disconnect them by performing the opposite motions and reconnect them properly.
2. Stainless steel and plastic components are cross-connected. Stainless steel handles go only with stainless steel blades, and plastic handles go only with plastic blades.
3. The batteries are low, as shown by the bulb failing to glow or glowing with a yellow instead of a white light. Unscrew the cap from the handle. Replace the old batteries with two new C-cell batteries. When reassembled, the bulb should glow with a white light.
4. The batteries are not placed properly. It does not matter if a positive or negative pole touches the base of the handle. Be sure that a positive pole touches a negative pole or vice versa, so that electrical current will flow properly. When reassembled, the bulb should glow with a white light.
5. The lightbulb in the stainless steel blade is loose or defective. Tighten the lightbulb by turning it clockwise. It should light up if it was just loose. Unscrew and throw away a defective lightbulb. Replace it with a lightbulb of the same size. When reassembled, the bulb should glow with a white light. The newer plastic laryngoscopes use a fiberoptic bundle as the light source with no lightbulb to tighten or replace.

Besides the laryngoscope handle and blades, a number of additional items are typically needed to ensure a smooth, safe intubation procedure. These are listed in Box 12-1.

Exam Hint

Know how to troubleshoot and fix a malfunctioning laryngoscope and blade.

---

10. Intubation equipment: fiberoptic devices
a. Get the necessary equipment (WRE code: IIA7d) [Difficulty: An]

A physician may use a fiberoptic laryngoscope (Fig. 12-17) or bronchoscope (see Fig. 18-3) to visualize the larynx and trachea during a difficult intubation. Either can be used during a nasal or oral endotracheal intubation procedure.

b. Put the equipment together and make sure that it works properly (WRE code: IIA7d) [Difficulty: An]
c. Troubleshoot any problems with the equipment (WRE code: IIA7d) [Difficulty: An]

Review the discussion on bronchoscopy in Chapter 18 for the details on the equipment. The fiberoptic tube should

---

BOX 12-1 Equipment for Oral and Nasal Intubation

Pediatric and adult laryngoscope handles with batteries
Straight and curved pediatric and adult laryngoscope blades
Variety of nasal and oral endotracheal tubes
Water-soluble, sterile lubricant
Metal stylet
Magill forceps for nasal intubation
Hemostat
Tongue depressors
Oropharyngeal airways
Bite block
Nasopharyngeal airways
10-mL syringe with three-way stopcock
Manometer to measure intracuff pressure
Tape or tube restraining device
Yankauer or other oral suction device
Sterile suction catheter for tracheal suctioning
Stethoscope for listening to breath sounds

---

be lubricated so that it will easily slide through the lumen of the endotracheal tube (see Fig. 12-17). After the physician has confirmed that the distal end of the fiberoptic tube has entered the trachea, the endotracheal tube is gently pushed into the trachea. The fiberoptic tube is then withdrawn, the cuff is inflated, and the endotracheal tube is secured. If the endotracheal tube will not slide into the patient's trachea, either it is too large or not enough lubricant is on the fiberoptic tube. It may be necessary to withdraw them, correct the problem, and start over again.

11. Oral and nasal endotracheal tubes
a. Get the necessary equipment (WRE code: IIA7b) [Difficulty: An]

An endotracheal tube is the best emergency device for maintaining a secure airway. It also provides a direct suctioning route to the lungs and prevents aspiration. Mechanical ventilation can easily be provided through it. An endotracheal tube is meant to be a temporary airway; however, it can be kept in patients for weeks if necessary. Virtually all endotracheal tubes used clinically now are made of pliable plastic. Always select a tube that has a large residual volume and low pressure cuff unless a specific reason exists not to do so. For the most part, oral and nasal endotracheal tubes can be used interchangeably. The nasal endotracheal tube is longer and more curved than an oral endotracheal tube. The greater curve of the nasal tube should result in less pressure on the nasal mucosa. An anesthesiologist requests a nasal tube if he or she is going to place it by the nasal route. Oral tubes are used in the majority of patients.

The tubes come in sizes from 4-mm OD through 14-mm OD, so that patients of all ages and sizes can be

Fig. 12-17 A fiberoptic laryngoscope that is being used to insert an endotracheal tube through the nasal passage. *(From Scanlan C, Simmons K: Airway management. In Scanlan CL, Wilkins RL, Stoller JK, editors:* Egan's fundamentals of respiratory care, *ed 7, St. Louis, 1999, Mosby.)*

intubated. The OD size increments are 0.5 mm. The thickness of the outer wall of the tube varies from 0.5 to 1 mm, which results in a reduction of the inner diameter (ID) of the tube by about 1 to 2 mm. Table 12-1 lists the approximate ID of an endotracheal tube to place into a patient based on age. It is common practice to refer to the size of endotracheal tube (or tracheostomy tube) needed by its ID. Once the tube is properly placed into the patient, the excess tube, beyond 3 to 4 cm past the teeth, should be cut off. This reduces the airway resistance and mechanical dead space.

Most endotracheal tubes have the standard features shown in Fig. 12-18. A number of specialty endotracheal tubes can be found in limited use. They all share the same characteristics except for some special feature. These tubes are worth considering if available.

1. Pediatric endotracheal tubes

Pediatric endotracheal tubes come in two basic types. One type has a constant diameter. During intubation, the tube should be inserted until the black mark, about 2 cm from the tip, is at the vocal cords. The second type has a body with a relatively wide proximal part that narrows at the distal end. The design is supposed to allow the smaller diameter tip to be passed through the vocal cords but prevent the wide "shoulder" from passing into the trachea. Both types of tubes end with a single opening with a bevel cut (Fig. 12-19). It is recommended that children younger than 8 years have a tube without a cuff.

2. Armored tubes

Armored tubes have a steel spring coiled through them. An advantage of the armored tubes over regular tubes is that they do not collapse if the patient bites down.

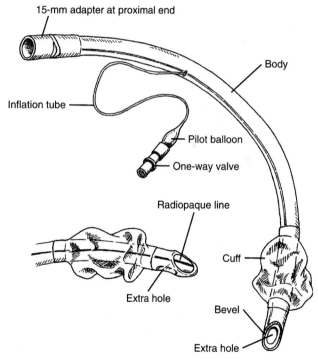

Fig. 12-18 Typical, modern endotracheal tube with its component parts. Insert shows important features found at the distal end of the tube.

Furthermore, the tube may be prebent for shape and does not kink as a plastic tube might.

3. Preformed tubes

Preformed tubes have been preshaped for better patient comfort and security. One style has a forward bend so that

Fig. 12-19 Comparison of the two different types of pediatric endotracheal tubes. The top type of tube is made by several manufacturers and has a uniform diameter. The bottom tube is made by Cole and features a narrowing of the distal tip to pass through the vocal cords. Note that neither has a cuff. (*From Burgess WR, Chernick V:* Respiratory therapy in newborn infants and children, *ed 2, New York, 1986, Thieme.*)

the tube can be taped to the chin. A pediatric tube bends back so that it may be taped to the forehead.

4. Guidable (trigger) tubes

Guidable tubes have a wire embedded within the wall of the tube (Fig. 12-20). When the ring at the proximal end is pulled, the distal tip is flexed up to shorten the radius of the curve. This allows the tube to be directed into the anterior trachea. Guidable trigger tubes make it easier to intubate a patient with an anterior larynx or to perform a blind nasal intubation.

5. Double-lumen endotracheal tubes

Double-lumen endotracheal tubes are used to allow independent lung ventilation. A double-lumen tube also is used during special procedures performed on one lung, such as bronchoscopy, bronchoalveolar lavage, lobectomy, and pneumonectomy. The other lung may be mechanically ventilated to maintain the patient's blood gas values (Fig. 12-21). An adapter can be added to join the two proximal ends of the channels together so that a single ventilator can be used to ventilate both lungs. The Carlens tube is used to preferentially intubate the left bronchus. The White tube is used to preferentially intubate the right bronchus (see Fig. 12-22 for both). Robertshaw makes tubes for either right or left bronchial intubation.

Several limitations are inherent in all double-lumen tubes. First, they can be used only on adults because the smallest size is 8-mm OD. Second, the small internal diameter of the two lumens results in a high airway resistance. Third, a much smaller than normal suction catheter must be used to remove any tracheal secretions.

6. Tubes for high-frequency jet ventilation

These special purpose tubes have a main lumen for a standard ventilator and an additional lumen to which a jet

Fig. 12-20 Guidable or "trigger"-type endotracheal tube. A wire is embedded within the wall of the tube. When the ring at the proximal end is pulled, the distal tip is flexed up to shorten the radius of the curve. This allows the tube to be directed into an anterior trachea. (*Modified from Heffner JE: Managing difficult intubation in critically ill patients.* Respir Manage *19(3):53, 1989.*)

ventilator is attached. See Chapter 15 for more discussion and an illustration.

7. Oropharyngeal suctioning tubes

In response to the concern about oropharyngeal secretions leaking around the endotracheal tube cuff causing ventilator associated pneumonia, an endotracheal tube with a built-in suctioning catheter has been invented. The catheter runs down the outer curve of the tube to just above the cuff. When vacuum is applied to the catheter, any secretions that have accumulated above the cuff are suctioned out. It functions like a standard, cuffed endotracheal tube in all other aspects.

b. Put the equipment together and make sure that it works properly (WRE code: IIA7b) [Difficulty: An]

Refer to Fig. 12-18 for these components of a standard endotracheal tube:

1. The hollow curved body is the main part of the tube through which the patient can breathe, or a suction catheter can be placed. The OD and ID size are printed on the side of the tube. Make sure that the central channel is not plugged by dried secretions, blood, or a foreign body.

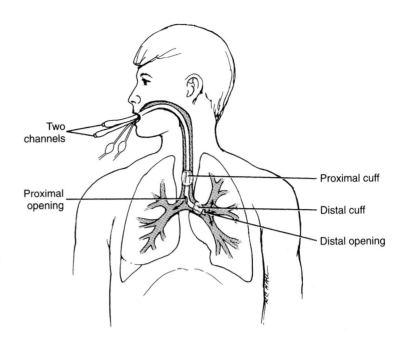

Fig. 12-21 Double-lumen endotracheal tube properly positioned in patient so that both lungs can be independently ventilated or suctioned, or have special procedures performed. *(From Eubanks DH, Bone RC: Comprehensive respiratory care, ed 2, St Louis, 1990, Mosby.)*

Fig. 12-22 Two types of double-lumen endotracheal tubes. **A,** Carlens tube; its distal tube enters left mainstem bronchus. **B,** White tube; its distal tube enters right mainstem bronchus. Note how both tubes have a cuff that seals the trachea and a cuff that seals a bronchus. Each has its own inflation tube, pilot balloon, and one-way valve. *(From Miller RD, editor: Anesthesia, New York, 1981, Churchill Livingstone.)*

Exam Hint

Know the indications, features, and any uses for the various types of endotracheal tubes.

Exam Hint

Know the proper size of endotracheal or tracheostomy tube to use with an adult (usually an 8-mm ID). A question may ask you to select the appropriate size tube.

---

2. The proximal end is left outside of the patient's nose or mouth. An adapter with a 15-mm OD equipment connector is inserted into the tube. The other end of the adapter narrows and is individually sized to fit snugly into the ID of the endotracheal tube. The adapters cannot be cross-fitted to different sizes of endotracheal tubes.

3. The distal end is inserted into the patient's trachea. The tip is cut with either a right- or left-sided bevel. The bevel cut creates an oval-shaped opening that is less likely to become plugged with secretions than is a round opening. An extra hole (the Murphy eye) is cut in the tube on the opposite side of the bevel.

4. A line of radiopaque material is imbedded in the tube from the tip back to the cuff. It is seen as a white line on the chest radiograph, showing the location of the tube tip in the trachea (see the insert in Fig. 12-18).

5. A cuff (balloon) is located a few centimeters from the tip of the tube. It is blown up with air to seal the trachea so that mechanical ventilation can be performed and aspiration is prevented. Most modern tubes have a large residual volume, low-pressure cuff.
   Note: Most tubes that are 4.0-mm ID/6.0-mm OD or greater have cuffs. However, cuffless tubes larger than this are available for pediatric patients. Neonatal tubes smaller than 4.0-mm ID/6.0-mm OD will not have a cuff.

6. A cuff filling inflation tube is connected about halfway down the tube. The proximal end is left out of the patient's mouth, and the distal end goes to

the cuff so that it can be inflated and deflated. A pilot balloon that inflates and deflates with the cuff is found in the middle of the capillary tube or connected with the one-way valve at the distal end. The one-way valve has an end that connects to any syringe. When the syringe is disconnected, the one-way valve seals to prevent the air in the cuff from escaping.

7. With a double-lumen endotracheal tube, each lumen has its own 15-mm adapter, cuff, one-way valve, pilot balloon, and inflation tube to inflate the cuff. As with traditional endotracheal tubes, both cuffs should be test-inflated. They should hold the air without a leak and then be easily deflated. One additional piece of equipment, a plastic Y, can be used with a double-lumen tube. The plastic Y can be used to connect the proximal ends of both tubes. Both 15-mm adapters are removed, and one branch of the Y is inserted into each of the proximal ends of the tubes. The open end of the Y has a 15-mm adapter so that it can be connected to a ventilator or oxygen source.

c. Troubleshoot any problems with the equipment (WRE code: IIA7b) [Difficulty: An]

The cuff(s) should be inflated, and the syringe should be disconnected from the one-way valve before the tube is placed in the patient. This ensures that the system works properly. The cuff(s) should hold the air. Do not use any tube with a leaking cuff or leaking one-way valve. Deflate the cuff before placing the tube into the patient.

MODULE B

Perform endotracheal intubation (WRE code: IIIb2) [Difficulty: An]

Oral endotracheal intubation is the recommended procedure for securing the airway during an emergency such as a cardiopulmonary resuscitation (CPR) attempt. In uncomplicated cases, the patient can be quickly intubated with an apneic period of no more than 20 seconds. This procedure is explained for a team of two respiratory therapists. It is difficult, if not impossible, for a single therapist to perform this important task without placing the patient at great risk. Usually the therapist who intubates is considered the leader, and the other therapist acts as the assistant. Therapists must feel comfortable in both roles. See Box 12-2 for a list of indications and contraindications for oral intubation and Box 12-3 for a list of complications.

Steps in an emergency oral endotracheal intubation include the following:

BOX 12-2 Indications and Contraindications for Oral Endotracheal Intubation

GENERAL INDICATIONS FOR ENDOTRACHEAL INTUBATION
Provide a secure, patent airway
Provide a route for mechanical ventilation
Prevent aspiration of stomach or mouth contents
Provide a route for suctioning the lungs
Use general anesthesia

INDICATIONS FOR ORAL INTUBATION
Fastest, easiest method to secure the airway
Simpler, less-invasive method cannot ensure an open airway

CONTRAINDICATIONS FOR ORAL INTUBATION
Cervical spine injury such that the patient's neck cannot be hyperextended
Lower facial injury
Oral surgery

BOX 12-3 Complications of Endotracheal Intubation

GENERAL COMPLICATIONS
Reflex laryngospasm
Perforation of the esophagus or pharynx
Esophageal intubation
Bronchial intubation
Reflex bradycardia
Tachycardia or other arrhythmias from hypoxemia
Hypotension
Bronchospasm
Aspiration of tooth, blood, gastric contents, laryngoscope bulb
Laceration of pharynx or larynx
Nosocomial infection
Vocal cord injury
Laryngeal or tracheal injury from the tube or the excessive cuff pressure

COMPLICATIONS OF THE ORAL ROUTE
Cervical spine injury
Tooth trauma from the blade being pulled back
Eye trauma from the handle or the operator's hand

COMPLICATIONS AFTER EXTUBATION
Reflex laryngospasm
Aspiration of stomach contents or oral secretions
Sore throat
Hoarseness
Laryngeal edema (postintubation croup)

---

1. Prepare the patient. The assistant should:
   a. Place the head and neck in the sniff position.
   b. Ventilate the patient with 100% oxygen by a face mask and manual resuscitator or demand valve.

2. The intubator should put on a surgical mask, goggles, and clean gloves on both hands, and then perform the following.
3. Prepare the endotracheal tube.
   a. Select the proper endotracheal tube (see Table 12-1 for the recommended tube sizes based on age). If time permits, the next smaller and larger tube size also should be selected.
   b. Inflate the cuff with a 10- or 20-mL syringe. Remove the syringe from the one-way valve. Make sure that it holds the air, and then deflate the cuff completely.
   c. Lubricate the last few centimeters of the endotracheal tube with a water-soluble lubricant.
   d. Lubricate a stylet with the sterile water-soluble lubricant. Place the stylet into the tube so that the natural curve of the tube is maintained. The tip of the stylet should not go past the end of the tube (Fig. 12-23). Some practitioners may prefer not to use a stylet. Many believe that the stylet offers the advantage of being able to bend the tube to match the patient's anatomy if a second attempt is needed.
4. Prepare the laryngoscope and blade.
   a. Select a laryngoscope handle.
   b. Select a laryngoscope blade. The blades come in several sizes from pediatric to adult, with two main classes of blades: straight and curved (see Fig. 12-15). The straight blades (Miller is a common brand) are designed to lift the epiglottis to expose the tracheal opening. The curved blades (MacIntosh is a common brand) are designed to fit into the vallecula (between the base of the tongue and the epiglottis). As the blade is lifted, the epiglottis is raised, and the tracheal opening can be seen. Personal experience and training leads the practitioner to select between the two styles.
   c. Attach the blade to the handle (see Fig. 12-16). Make sure that the lightbulb shines brightly.
5. The intubator should tell the assistant to stop ventilating the patient and stand clear so that an intubation can be attempted. The assistant should check his or her watch to count off 20 seconds silently. The intubator should be told when 20 seconds has passed so that the patient can be reventilated if the intubation is proving to be difficult.
6. Open the victim's mouth as widely as possible without using force. Remove any dentures or foreign material. Suction out any saliva, blood, or vomitus.
7. Grasp the laryngoscope handle in the left hand. Carefully advance the blade between the teeth or gums along the right side of the mouth. Move the tongue to the left side of the mouth to allow a clear view of the oropharynx (Fig. 12-24). Advance the blade along the base of the tongue until the epiglottis is seen.
8. With a *straight* blade:
   a. Advance the blade so that it barely passes the epiglottis.
   b. Do not advance the blade too far, or it will enter the esophagus or trachea.
   With a *curved* blade:
   a. Advance the blade tip into the vallecula.
   b. Lift the blade tip into this space.
9. With either blade, lift the laryngoscope handle and blade toward the patient's chest at a 45 degree angle (Fig. 12-25). The straight blade lifts the epiglottis. The curved blade lifts the soft tissues of the valleculae, and

Fig. 12-23 Stylet with stopper properly placed in standard endotracheal tube to maintain its curved shape. *(From Eubanks DH, Bone RC:* Comprehensive respiratory care, *ed 2, St Louis, 1990, Mosby.)*

Fig. 12-24 Proper placement of the laryngoscope blade to move the patient's tongue. **A,** Proper placement of the laryngoscope blade to the right of the patient's tongue to move it to the left. This should give a clear view of the glottis. **B,** Tongue partially obstructs the view if it is not moved to the left. *(From Shapiro BA, Kacmarek RM, Cane RD, et al, editors:* Clinical application of respiratory care, *ed 4, St Louis, 1991, Mosby.)*

Fig. 12-25 Proper use of the laryngoscope blade to expose the larynx by lifting the glottic structures. Note how the lifting is at a 45 degree angle toward the patient's chest. Never pull back on the blade against the teeth. **A**, A straight blade is used to lift the epiglottis to expose the trachea. **B**, A curved blade is used to lift soft tissues of the vallecula to expose the trachea. *(From Shapiro BA, Kacmarek RM, Cane RD, et al, editors:* Clinical application of respiratory care, *ed 4, St Louis, 1991, Mosby.)*

the epiglottis lifts with them. Do *not* pull back on the patient's upper teeth.

10. The vocal cords and glottis should be clearly seen (Fig. 12-26). If needed, tell the assistant to put gentle, downward pressure on the patient's larynx (Sellick's maneuver). This may help to bring the glottis into better view.
11. Tell the assistant to place the endotracheal tube into your right hand.
12. Place the tube into the right side of the patient's mouth, and direct it into the trachea. The assistant may feel over the larynx as the tube enters the trachea. In the adult, the proximal end of the cuff should be

placed 3 to 4 cm past the vocal cords (Fig. 12-27). In children younger than 6 months, with an uncuffed endotracheal tube, place the end of the tube about 1 cm past the vocal cords.

13. Hold the tube in place.
14. Withdraw the laryngoscope blade.
15. Tell the assistant to inflate the cuff. Place about 10 mL of air into the cuff (of an adult's tube) so that some resistance can be felt. The cuff pressure can be measured and adjusted later.
16. Pull out the stylet (if used).
17. The assistant should ventilate the patient with the manual resuscitator bag or a demand valve.

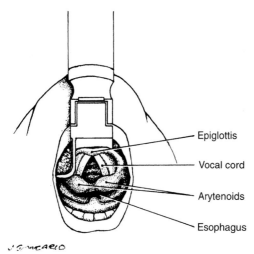

Fig. 12-26 Major anatomic features that can be seen when epiglottis is lifted. Opening to trachea can be seen between vocal cords. *(From Shapiro BA, Kacmarek RM, Cane RD, et al, editors:* Clinical application of respiratory care, *ed 4, St Louis, 1991, Mosby.)*

- Epiglottis
- Vocal cord
- Arytenoids
- Esophagus

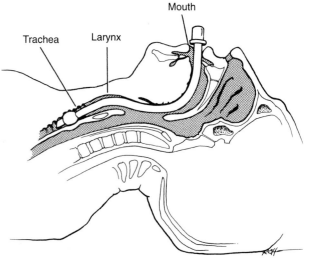

Fig. 12-27 Oral endotracheal tube properly positioned within the trachea. *(From Eubanks DH, Bone RC:* Comprehensive respiratory care, *ed 2, St Louis, 1990, Mosby.)*

Mouth

Trachea   Larynx

18. The intubator should listen to both lung fields in the upper lobes and bases. Bilateral breath sounds should be heard.

19. If the breath sounds are equal and bilateral, the assistant can secure the tube in place with tape or a tube holder. If the breath sounds are unequal or absent on one side, the tube has been placed into a bronchus (usually the right mainstem). The cuff should be deflated and the tube then withdrawn 1 to 2 cm in an adult, less in a child. The cuff should be reinflated and breath sounds listened to again. When the breath sounds are equal, the tube can be secured.

20. If no breath sounds are heard, listen over the stomach area. If air is heard bubbling into the stomach, the tube has been placed into the esophagus. Immediately remove the tube. Ventilate the patient, and prepare to attempt reintubation with a new endotracheal tube.

The practitioner should perform only those procedures for which he or she has been trained. If the patient cannot be intubated with the standard equipment and procedure, an anesthesiologist or trained physician should be called in. Be prepared to assist as necessary.

MODULE C
Ensure that the artificial airway is properly placed and maintained

1. Auscultate the patient's breath sounds and interpret any changes (WRE code: IIIE12) [Difficulty: An]

Respiratory efforts without breath sounds indicate that a complete obstruction exists in the patient's airway. Inspiratory or expiratory stridor or wheezing indicate that a partial obstruction exists in the patient's airway. Listen for stridor over the larynx and wheezing over the major airways. The restoration of the normal airway should result in the return of normal breath sounds over all areas of both lung fields (unless another, unrelated problem is present).

It is especially important to check for bilateral breath sounds after an endotracheal tube has been placed. If the tube has been inserted too far, it usually enters the right mainstem bronchus because it comes off of the trachea at a less acute angle than the left mainstem bronchus. No breath sounds are heard over the left lung field. If both lung fields cannot be auscultated, at least listen to the right apical area. This one site can be checked because the segmental bronchus to the right upper lobe comes off of the right mainstem bronchus in such a way that if the right mainstem bronchus is intubated, the upper lobe segmental bronchus will be blocked.

2. Exhaled carbon dioxide detector
a. Get the necessary equipment (WRE code: IIA7d) [Difficulty: An]

Most exhaled carbon dioxide detectors are single patient use, disposable devices that change color when exhaled carbon dioxide is sensed. The units are placed onto an endotracheal tube 15-mm adapter to monitor the proper placement of the endotracheal tube. This is often done if a patient is being transported and a possibility exists that the tube could be dislodged. Exhaled carbon dioxide detectors also are used during CPR attempts to help determine whether resuscitation attempts are being performed on a viable patient. It the patient is not producing exhaled $CO2$, no metabolic activity is present. The physician may then decide to stop CPR efforts.

Currently available disposable units include the Easy Cap, the A.C.E. STAT-Check CO_2 Indicator, and the unit produced by Resuscitation ACE, Inc. The Easy Cap end-tidal CO_2 detector (Fig. 12-28) is the original unit and is quite widely used. It comes in a neonatal/pediatric size for infants smaller than 15 kg and a standard size for larger children and adults. Its carbon dioxide indicator changes color from dark purple to yellow when CO_2 is exhaled through it. The other two disposable units also indicate the presence of exhaled CO_2 by an indicator turning purple.

Another choice is the MiniCAP III CO_2 Detector. It is a reusable item that has a mainstream type of infrared carbon dioxide detector. The unit is powered by a battery pack. Its light-emitting diode signals the presence of carbon dioxide with each exhalation. A capnograph should be selected if it is necessary to get a more accurate CO_2 reading. Its general function and the interpretation of capnography tracings were discussed in Chapter 5.

b. Put the equipment together and make sure that it works properly (WRE code: IIA7d) [Difficulty: An]

The Easy Cap comes as a single unit within a sealed foil container. Remove the unit from the container, and compare the initial purple color of the indicator with the purple color labeled CHECK on the product dome. Do *not* use an Easy

Fig. 12-28 Easy Cap ETCO$_2$ detector. This disposable device comes in adult and pediatric sizes and is able to detect exhaled carbon dioxide. Color change from dark purple to yellow indicates exhaled CO_2 to confirm tracheal placement of endotracheal tube or effective efforts at cardiopulmonary resuscitation. *(From Nellcor, Hayward, Calif.)*

Cap unit whose color is not the same as or darker than that on the product dome. Attach the Easy Cap to the patient's endotracheal tube by its 15-mm ID connector port. The Easy Cap 15-mm OD circuit end is connected to the manual resuscitator to ventilate the patient. If a heat and moisture exchanger is used, it should be placed between the patient's endotracheal tube and the Easy Cap and manual resuscitator. The Easy Cap should not be used with a heated humidifier or nebulizer because too much humidity affects its accuracy. The unit is not supposed to be used for more than 2 hours because the color change will fade away.

The MiniCAP III has a disposable adapter that connects the mainstream CO_2 detector to the patient's endotracheal tube. The adapter has a 15-mm ID end for attachment to the endotracheal tube and a 15-mm OD end to which the manual resuscitator can be attached. The assembly and operation of a capnograph are discussed in Chapter 5. Review it if necessary.

c. Troubleshoot any problems with the equipment (WRE code: IIA7d) [Difficulty: An]

Because the Easy Cap comes as a self-contained single piece unit, nothing exists to repair. The following items can contaminate the Easy Cap and cause a patchy yellow or white discoloration of the indicator: stomach contents, mucus, pulmonary edema fluid, and intratracheal epinephrine. Because of the contamination, the color does not change with the breathing cycle, and the unit should be thrown away. The 15-mm ID patient connector port fits only over the endotracheal tube adapter. The 15-mm OD circuit connector port fits only into the manual resuscitator or demand valve adapter.

The adapter is the only removable part in the MiniCAP III. It fits only in one direction into the CO_2 detection unit. The other end of the adapter fits only into a manual resuscitator outlet. Troubleshooting with a capnograph was presented in Chapter 5.

3. Review the patient's chart for information on tube placement (WRE code: IA6) [Difficulty: Ap, An]

After a patient is intubated, a chest radiograph should be taken. The chart should include information on the location of the tip of the tube and other information confirming proper tube placement within the trachea. Ideally the tip of the tube is in the middle of the trachea. In the adult, this would be several centimeters above the carina.

4. Make the recommendation for an upper airway and chest radiograph, as needed, to help determine the patient's condition, and review the chest radiograph (WRE code: IC1 and IIIE1) [Difficulty: An]

A chest radiograph should always be taken to confirm the location of a newly placed endotracheal or tracheostomy tube. The chest radiograph should be repeated after a significant change in the patient's condition or if the tube has been pulled back or pushed deeper into the trachea. A chest radiograph also confirms the presence and location of an opaque foreign body in the airway. Metallic objects, stones, and coins can be clearly seen. Less radiopaque objects can be barely seen, if at all. The chest radiograph also detects a pneumothorax related to the tracheostomy procedure or other pulmonary conditions. If needed, an upper airway radiographic examination can be performed to look for a foreign body or to check the position of the tracheostomy tube.

5. View the upper airway or chest radiograph to see the position of the endotracheal or tracheostomy tube (WRE code: IB6b) [Difficulty: An]

All modern endotracheal and tracheostomy tubes contain a strip of radiopaque material near the distal tip of the tube. This is easily noticed as the white line seen on the chest radiograph and confirms the location of the tip of the tube in the airway (see Fig. 12-18). The ideal location of the tip of the endotracheal tube is the middle third of the trachea. When the tube is positioned properly, it is less likely for the tip to be pushed into the carina when the patient bends his or her head forward or for the cuff to hit the vocal cords if the patient's head is bent back. Both endotracheal and tracheostomy tubes should be positioned midline within the trachea. They should not be twisted laterally because the tip can cause damage to the tracheal wall.

6. Identify the placement of the endotracheal tube by any available means (CSE code: IIIB4)

Review the previous discussions if needed. Often the endotracheal tube can be palpated in an infant as it is being inserted through the larynx because the laryngeal structures are so pliable. Feeling the tube being inserted through the larynx indicates that it is properly located within the trachea. If the tube cannot be palpated through the larynx, it has probably been inserted into the esophagus. It is more difficult to use this technique with confidence in adults because their laryngeal structures are stiffer.

Some limitations exist in the use of an Easy Cap carbon dioxide detector. It should not be used during mouth-to-mouth resuscitation, to detect right mainstem bronchus intubation, to detect hypercarbia, or to determine the placement of an esophageal obturator airway.

The esophageal detection device (EDD) is able to show that the endotracheal tube has been placed within an airway by pulling a small sample of gas from the patient's lungs. If the endotracheal tube has been accidentally put into the esophagus, the deflated bulb will stay collapsed (Fig. 12-29). A limitation of the EDD is that it inflates chest radiograph for positioning. If the tube is too high within the trachea, it may be pulled up through the vocal cords if the patient's head is hyperextended. An air leak may be heard at the larynx if the patient is using a mechanical ventilator. In this case, the cuff should be deflated and the tube inserted deeper into the trachea.

Conversely, if the tip of the tube is inserted too deeply into the trachea, it may be pushed into a main-stem bronchus if the patient's head is moved toward the chest. In this situation, no breath sounds would be heard in the opposite lung (usually the left). The cuff should be deflated and the tube pulled up into the middle third of the trachea. Reinflate the cuff after the tube is repositioned. A chest radiograph should be taken to confirm the tube position after it has been moved.

The endotracheal tube body has centimeter marks placed on it starting at the distal end and finishing at the proximal end. Check and record the centimeter mark present at the patient's teeth or gums. The average adult's distance from the midtrachea to the teeth is about 23 to 25 cm. The practitioner can tell if the tube has been accidentally pulled out a little or pushed further into the patient by looking at the current centimeter mark. If the tube is intentionally adjusted, the new centimeter mark should be checked and recorded.

A wide variety of handmade, as well as manufactured, devices are available to secure the endotracheal tube in the correct position. Fig. 12-30 shows one way to make a tube holder from adhesive tape. This is flexible when the

Fig. 12-29 Esophageal detection device. This squeeze bulb device is attached to proximal end of patient's endotracheal tube and air is squeezed out. **A,** Shows reinflation of bulb with air from patient's lungs when the endotracheal tube has been properly placed. **B,** Shows that the bulb fails to reinflate when the endotracheal tube has been accidentally placed into the patient's esophagus. *(From Scanlan C, Simmons K: Airway management. In Scanlan CL, Wilkins RL, Stoller JK, editors:* Egan's fundamentals of respiratory care, *ed 7, St Louis, 1999, Mosby.)*

whether the endotracheal tube is placed into the trachea or either main-stem bronchus. Remember to auscultate for bilateral breath sounds.

7. Change the position of the endotracheal or tracheostomy tube (CSE code: IIIF1g1)

As mentioned earlier, an endotracheal tube is ideally located within the middle third of the trachea. Check the

---

Exam Hint

Be prepared to determine the proper placement of the endotracheal tube by palpation of the neck, auscultation of bilateral breath sounds, detection of exhaled carbon dioxide, observation of bilateral symmetrical chest movement on inspiration, visualization of the tip of the tube on a chest radiograph, or centimeter markings on the tube.

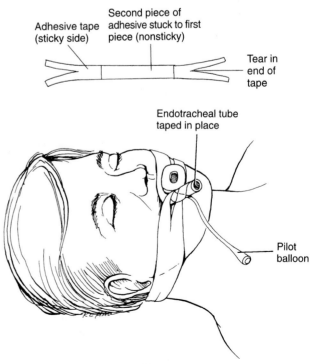

Fig. 12-30 Taping the endotracheal tube to secure it in the airway. *(From Eubanks DH, Bone RC:* Comprehensive respiratory care, *ed 2, St Louis, 1990, Mosby.)*

patient moves and is inexpensive. Tincture of benzoin can be applied to the patient's cheeks to make the tape hold more securely without tearing the skin. An oropharyngeal airway may or may not be needed.

The manufactured tube holders are made of plastic with cloth ties and usually include a built-in bite block. Make sure that it is sized properly to the patient's mouth. Too large a bite block can injure the tongue, lips, and mouth. Watch for a gag reflex. This type of holder is useful in the patient who is prone to seizures.

A tracheostomy tube should be positioned so that the flange is snug against the base of the neck and the outer cannula is within the trachea. If pulled out too far, the cuff may be seen at the stoma. An air leak may be heard or secretions may be seen to bubble out of the stoma. Correct the problem by deflating the cuff, inserting the tube so that the flange is against the base of the neck, and reinflating the cuff.

> ### Exam Hint
>
> **A**lmost always, a question deals with understanding that the lack of breath sounds over the left lung indicates that the endotracheal tube has been placed into the right main-stem bronchus. The tube must be withdrawn to the trachea.

10. Keep an endotracheal or tracheostomy tube cuff properly inflated

a. Determine tracheal tube cuff volume and pressure (WRE code: IB7k) [Difficulty: Ap]

All of the adult and larger pediatric endotracheal and tracheostomy tubes have a cuff for sealing the airway. Most brands of modern tubes have cuffs that are designed to have a relatively large reservoir volume that fills at a relatively low pressure. The soft, flexible balloon seals the airway by having a large surface area that conforms to the shape of the trachea. Two slightly different ways are known to inflate the cuff and maintain a safe cuff pressure. Both methods can be used only with patients on a positive-pressure ventilator.

1. Minimal leak

a. Connect the cuff pressure measuring device (see next discussion) to the one-way valve on the cuff inflating tube.
b. Listen with a stethoscope over the patient's larynx.
c. Inflate or deflate the cuff as necessary while listening for an air leak.
d. Stop changing the air volume when a minimal leak is heard at the peak airway pressure in the breathing cycle. The tidal volume should still be delivered, except for this minor leak.
e. Note the cuff pressure when the minimal leak was heard. Note the cuff volume, if possible.

f. Disconnect the cuff pressure measuring device.
g. It may be necessary to add more volume and pressure to the cuff if the leak gets worse when the peak airway pressure increases.

2. Minimal occluding volume

The purpose is to find the cuff pressure that results in no leak at the cuff when the patient's airway pressure is greatest. The following are the steps in the procedure:

a. Connect the cuff pressure measuring device (see next discussion) to the one-way valve on the cuff inflating tube.
b. Listen with a stethoscope over the patient's larynx.
c. Inflate or deflate the cuff as necessary while listening for an air leak.
d. Stop changing the air volume when no leak is heard at the peak airway pressure in the breathing cycle.
e. Note the cuff pressure when the seal was heard. Note the cuff volume, if possible.
f. Disconnect the cuff pressure measuring device.
g. It may be necessary to add more volume and pressure to the cuff if a leak results when the peak airway pressure increases.

This discussion relates only to those tubes that must be actively filled with air and have variable intracuff pressures. Several manufacturers have developed endotracheal and tracheostomy tubes that have built-in cuff pressure limitations. Follow the manufacturer's guidelines when inflating these cuffs. This discussion would not be complete without mentioning the recent manufacture of systems designed to increase the cuff pressure to match the peak airway pressure of a patient using a mechanical ventilator. A tube connects the inspiratory circuit to the one-way valve on the cuff inflating tube. As a positive-pressure breath is delivered, the pressure in the circuit is also applied to the patient's cuff. No loss of tidal volume should be seen. When the patient exhales and the airway pressure decreases to normal, the cuff pressure also decreases to its normal level.

b. Maintain proper tracheal tube cuff inflation (WRE code: IIIB3a) [Difficulty: An]

A cuff pressure manometer is needed to measure the air pressure within an endotracheal or tracheostomy tube cuff. When a tracheal tube is first inserted, the volume of air that is injected into the cuff should be measured and charted. The pressure within the cuff should also be noted. After that, if more air is inserted or any air is removed from the cuff, it should be measured and recorded in the chart. The resulting final cuff pressure also must be recorded. A number of manufactured units are available for measuring cuff pressure. The Cufflator is discussed here because it is widely used. This system consists of a pressure gauge calibrated in centimeters of water, a hand-pumped reservoir, internal one-way valve, pressure release valve, and adapter to fit into the one-way valve on the cuff inflating tube. A three-way stopcock can be added to the one-way valve adapter. This can be used to prepressurize the system before attaching it to the patient's one-way valve on the cuff inflating tube (Fig. 12-31). The pressure in the cuff can be measured as air is added by squeezing the hand pump or as air is removed by the pressure release valve. The volume of air added or removed cannot be measured.

A second system can be "homemade," although it is also commercially available. It consists of a 5- to 10-mL syringe, a three-way stopcock, and a pressure gauge (either millimeters of mercury or centimeters of water). The syringe and pressure gauge are attached to two of the ports on the stopcock. The third port on the stopcock is connected to the one-way valve on the cuff inflating tube. When the stopcock handle is opened to all three ports, the pressure throughout the system and the cuff are the same. Air can be added or removed with the syringe. The pressure gauge shows the system and cuff pressure as the air volume is adjusted (Fig. 12-32). One advantage of this system over the Cufflator is that the volume of air that is added or subtracted can be measured. This system also can be prepressurized so that its pressure matches the pressure anticipated in the cuff. With any of these systems, it is necessary to keep airtight connections. If the pressure decreases unexpectedly, an air leak will be noticed. Tighten the connections to create a seal so that the pressure is maintained.

c. Monitor tracheal tube cuff volume and pressure (WRE code: IIIE11) [Difficulty: An]

It is commonly recommended that the cuff pressure be monitored at least every 8 hours or whenever air is taken out of or put into the cuff.

d. Interpret the tracheal tube cuff volume and pressure (WRE code: IB10h) [Difficulty: An]

All manufacturers (except Kamen-Wilkenson) have designed cuffs that must be actively filled with air by way of a one-way valve and syringe. These cuffs have greater than atmospheric pressure within them. That pressure is placed against the wall of the trachea. The greater the pressure on the wall of the trachea, the greater the disruption of normal lymphatic and blood flow. Shapiro and colleagues stated that a patient with a normal blood pressure (120/80 mm Hg) has the following effects at these cuff pressures:

1. Lymphatic flow blockage occurs at pressures greater than 5 mm Hg (8 cm H_2O). Edema of the tracheal mucosa results.
2. Capillary blood flow blockage occurs at pressures greater than 18 mm Hg (24 cm H_2O). Venous (and lymphatic) drainage stops as a result.
3. Arterial blood flow blockage occurs at pressures greater than 30 mm Hg (42 cm H_2O). Arterial (and lymphatic and capillary) flow stops as a result.

In general, the clinical goal is to keep the cuff pressure as low as possible to make sure that the circulation through the tracheal wall is normal. Based on Shapiro and colleagues, it seems reasonable to try to keep the cuff pressure no greater than 15 mm Hg (20 cm H_2O). This holds true for all normotensive patients. Hypertensive

Fig. 12-31 Cufflator device used to measure cuff pressure with its component parts.

Fig. 12-32 Cuff measuring device made from pressure manometer, three-way stopcock, and 10-mL syringe.

patients may be able to tolerate higher cuff pressures than normotensive patients before blood flow to the tracheal tissues is stopped. Hypotensive patients have loss of blood flow to the tracheal wall at lower cuff pressures than those previously listed.

e. Inflate and deflate the cuff as indicated (WRE code: IIIF7c) [Difficulty: An]

A spontaneously breathing patient must have the cuff inflated to prevent the aspiration of oral secretions into the lungs. In general, keep the pressure at about 15 mm Hg (20 cm H_2O), as discussed earlier. It may be necessary to keep a higher cuff pressure in a mechanically ventilated patient. However, Shapiro and associates recommend that if the cuff pressure must be greater than 20 mm Hg, the endotracheal or tracheostomy tube is too small. Ideally, the tube should be replaced with a larger one. However, some patients are too unstable to tolerate reintubation of their airways and must simply have the cuff pressure increased temporarily.

It is clear that a cuff pressure greater than the patient's mucosa capillary pressure prevents the flow of blood through the area covered by the cuff. Tissue ischemia (hypoxemia) results. If the ischemia is severe enough, tissue necrosis follows. The higher the cuff pressure and the longer the high cuff pressure is maintained, the greater the likelihood of tissue necrosis. If the necrosis is circumferential (all the way around) to the trachea, tracheal stenosis may occur. Tracheal stenosis is found when the diameter of the trachea is narrowed because of scar tissue buildup after the normal mucosa and underlying tissues have died. The patient's airway is permanently narrowed and, if serious, must be surgically corrected. Another severe complication of high cuff pressures and tracheal necrosis is the development of a tracheoesophageal fistula. This is an opening between the trachea and esophagus. This is more likely when the patient also has a nasogastric tube in place. The fistula permits food to pass into the airway and lungs, causing pneumonia. Mechanical ventilation is more difficult because of the air leak from the lungs to the esophagus. Surgical repair of the fistula is required.

Exam Hint

Usually a question deals with adjusting a cuff pressure to a safe level of no more than 20 mm Hg or making a recommendation to replace a tracheal tube that is too small and requires a too high cuff pressure. A small endotracheal tube should also be replaced with a larger one if a patient cannot wean from the ventilator because of the high airway resistance created by the smaller tube.

---

1. Change the endotracheal tube (WRE code: IB7l) [Difficulty: An]

Usually only two reasons are found to replace a patient's endotracheal tube. First, the tube should be changed if it is too small and the cuff must be overfilled to seal the airway. Excessive pressure results in damage to the tracheal wall, as previously discussed.

Second, the tube should be replaced if the cuff is leaking or ruptured and the airway cannot be sealed. The patient may be reintubated by the procedure described earlier, or a tube changing stylet may be used (Fig. 12-33). The stylet is a hollow, flexible plastic tube that can be bent and holds its shape. It has a center mark and 1-cm markings counting out to each end. These are to help keep the proper depth for inserting the replacement endotracheal tube. It can be used on an endotracheal tube that is at least 7.5-mm ID. The procedure for

Fig. 12-33 Endotracheal tube changer (guide) inserted through an endotracheal tube. The JEM 400 unit can be inserted through a tube that is 7.5-mm ID or larger. The tube changer is used to aid in replacement of an esophageal obturator airway or a defective endotracheal tube with a functional endotracheal tube. See text for how to use the tube changer instead of traditional intubation equipment. *(Modified from Heffner JE: Managing difficult intubations in critically ill patients,* Respir Manage *19(3):53, 1989.)*

changing the endotracheal tube with a tube changing stylet includes the following:

a. Obtain the needed equipment: replacement endotracheal tube and one that is a size smaller, 10-mL syringe to inflate the cuff, sterile gloves, goggles, and sterile water-soluble lubricant. Make sure the cuff inflates and deflates properly.

b. Tell the patient what you are going to do. Put on the gloves and goggles.

c. Remove the patient's oxygen equipment.

d. Suction the secretions from the patient's trachea and oral pharynx.

e. Reoxygenate and ventilate the patient.

f. Place some lubricant on the outside of the stylet.

g. Remove the oxygen equipment, and pass the stylet through the endotracheal tube into the patient's trachea.

h. Insert it to about the same depth as marked on the distal end of the endotracheal tube. For example, if the distal end of the endotracheal tube is 22 cm, insert the tube changer to 22 cm.

i. Deflate the cuff on the endotracheal tube.

j. While holding the distal tip of the tube changer in place, pull the defective endotracheal tube over the tube changer and out of the patient.

k. Advance the new endotracheal tube over the stylet. Hold the distal end of the stylet, and push the new tube into the patient to the same depth mark on the stylet as the old tube had been.

l. Hold the endotracheal tube in place and remove the stylet.

m. Ensure that the tube has been placed into the trachea to the proper depth by listening for bilateral breath sounds.

n. Inflate the cuff to a safe pressure.

o. Secure the tube in place, and note the depth marking at the patient's teeth or gums.

p. Obtain a chest radiograph.

A defective one-way valve or severed cuff inflating tube may not necessarily lead to a reintubation; often it can be bypassed. This is done by slipping a small diameter needle (usually about 21 gauge) into the inflating tube, attaching a three-way stopcock to the hub of the needle, and screwing a 10-mL syringe into one of the stopcock ports (Fig. 12-34). The cuff pressure can be measured by attaching a pressure manometer to the other port on the stopcock. Air can be added by the 10-mL syringe and the pressure measured simultaneously (Fig. 12-35). A commercially available system can bypass a severed cuff inflating tube.

2. Change the tracheostomy tube (CSE code: IIIB5)

A tracheostomy tube may have to be changed because of a ruptured cuff or because of another problem. In addition, patients with a permanent tracheostomy have the tube

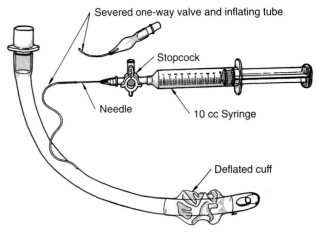

Fig. 12-34 Emergency system for inflating the cuff when the one-way valve and inflating tube are severed. *(From Sills JR: An emergency cuff inflation technique,* Respir Care *31:199–201, 1986.)*

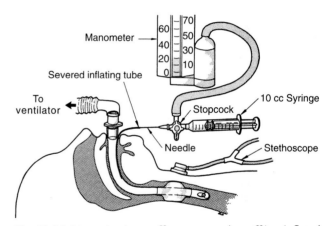

Fig. 12-35 Measuring intracuff pressure as the cuff is reinflated with an emergency system. The stethoscope is used to listen for the presence of a leak at the larynx. *(From Sills JR: An emergency cuff inflation technique,* Respir Care *31:199–201, 1986.)*

changed on a routine schedule as part of the tracheostomy care. These two different situations are discussed separately.

a. Emergency tube change

Several things can cause the clinical emergency of obstruction such as the cuff herniating over the end of the tube, a mucus plug blocking the lumen, or the end of the tube forced into the tracheal tissues. Unfortunately, these problems cannot be seen from the outside. If the patient is in acute respiratory distress and an obstruction is suspected, attempt to pass a suction catheter. Failure to pass it beyond the end of the tube confirms the obstruction. A rapid clinical decision has to be made to choose the best action. The tube should be removed if the obstruction is complete and the patient cannot breathe.

A spontaneously breathing patient can continue to breathe through the stoma. An apneic patient must be temporarily ventilated with mouth-to-stoma breaths. As rapidly and carefully as possible, another tracheostomy tube should be inserted. This usually results in a patent airway. If loose tracheal mucosa is blocking the airway, an endotracheal tube must be inserted past the tissue and deeper into the trachea. Call the physician as soon as possible to evaluate the patient's condition.

b. Routine tube change

If possible, the tube should not be changed until several days after a fresh tracheostomy procedure. This allows time for the stoma site to form granulomatous tissue as it begins to heal. The site is then less likely to bleed as the tube is changed. When the tracheostomy tube is changed, it is usually part of the tracheostomy wound care. The following are typical steps in changing the tracheostomy tube:

1. Gather the necessary equipment: a new tracheostomy tube of the same size and the next size smaller, its inner cannula, its obturator, tracheostomy tie strings to secure the tube in the patient (see Fig. 12-10), a sterile 4 × 4-in gauze pad, sterile scissors, a 10-mL syringe to inflate the cuff, sterile water-soluble lubricant, sterile gloves, and goggles. Make sure the cuff inflates and deflates properly.
2. Put on the gloves and goggles.
3. Maintaining sterile technique, make sure the obturator easily fits into and comes out of the tracheostomy tube.
4. Cut a slit into the center of the gauze pad.
5. Apply some lubricant to the tip of the tracheostomy tube.
6. Tell the patient what you are going to do.
7. Remove the oxygen or aerosol or both from the patient.
8. Suction the patient's trachea. Reoxygenate the patient.
9. Untie the tracheostomy strings.
10. Deflate the cuff.
11. Remove the 4 × 4-in gauze pad.
12. Remove the tracheostomy tube by pulling it in a curved motion toward the patient's chest.
13. Inspect the tracheostomy opening for signs of infection such as redness, pus, or swelling. Report signs of infection to the nurse or physician.
14. Carefully insert the new tracheostomy tube with obturator into the stoma. The motion should be opposite that used to remove the original tube. Make sure not to force the tube into the tissues of the trachea.
15. Remove the obturator, and insert the inner cannula. Lock it in place.

16. Give the patient oxygen or aerosol or both, as before the tube change.
17. Inflate the cuff to a safe pressure.
18. Listen for bilateral breath sounds.
19. Slide the new 4 × 4-in gauze pad around the tube so that the slit fits around it.
20. Tie the tracheostomy tie strings behind the patient's neck.

3. Perform tracheostomy care (WRE code: IIIF7d) [Difficulty: An]

Routine tracheostomy care includes these steps without the removal of the tracheostomy tube. It is done to inspect the stoma for possible signs of infection, clean the stoma site, apply a topical antibiotic, and replace the 4 × 4-inch gauze pad.

MODULE D
Extubate the patient (WRE code: IIIB4) [Difficulty: An]

Extubation should be performed only by trained personnel and under the proper conditions to ensure the patient's safety. See Box 12-4 for a list of complications that can occur after extubation.

1. Endotracheal tube

The generally recommended steps in extubation include the following:

a. Evaluate the patient's cardiopulmonary status. The reason(s) for the tube being placed should be corrected. The most recent blood gas results

---

BOX 12-4 Complications after Extubation

ENDOTRACHEAL TUBE REMOVAL
Laryngospasm
Regurgitation and aspiration of stomach contents
Aspiration of saliva
Sore throat
Dysphagia
Postintubation laryngeal edema (croup)
Hoarseness from vocal cord edema or paralysis

TRACHEOSTOMY TUBE REMOVAL
Difficult tube removal from a tight stoma
Granuloma or scar at the stoma
Unhealed, open stoma

CUFF-RELATED COMPLICATIONS
Granuloma
Tracheomalacia
Tracheal stenosis
Tracheal web formation
Tracheoesophageal fistula
Arterial fistula

should be acceptable. Tracheal secretions should be minimal and not so thick that they cannot be coughed out by the patient. Bedside spirometry results should show an acceptable tidal volume, vital capacity, and maximum inspiratory pressure.

b. Inform the patient about the removal of the tube and the follow-up care that is needed.

c. The patient's inspired oxygen percentage may be kept the same or increased before the extubation. If increased, it should be done at least 5 to 10 minutes before the tube is removed.

d. Suction the trachea until all secretions are removed.

e. Suction the oral pharynx to remove all saliva. Be prepared to suction out additional oral secretions and mucus after extubation.

f. In rapid succession:
   1. Give a deep sigh breath.
   2. Deflate the cuff. Cut the inflation tube to the cuff to ensure its collapse.
   3. Pull out the tube when the lungs are full.

   Alternatively, in rapid succession:
   1. Give a deep sigh breath.
   2. Place a suction catheter through the tube into the trachea. This works best with a self-contained catheter and sheath system.
   3. Deflate the cuff. Cut the inflation tube to the cuff to ensure its collapse.
   4. Pull out the tube when the lungs are full.
   5. Apply suction as the tube is withdrawn.

g. Have the patient cough vigorously to remove any secretions.

h. Apply a cool, bland aerosol by face mask with the previous amount of oxygen.

i. Monitor and evaluate the patient every 30 minutes for several hours. Encourage deep breathing and coughing. Check the vital signs. Measure pulse oximetry or arterial blood gases after 20 minutes. Listen to the breath sounds and larynx. Inspiratory stridor is a sign of laryngeal edema. Be prepared to nebulize racemic epinephrine (Vaponephrine) if needed. Be prepared to reintubate the patient if necessary.

2. Tracheostomy tube

a. Follow steps a through g from the previous list.

b. Depending on the physician's order, do one of the following:
   1. Apply a bland aerosol by tracheostomy mask to the stoma site with the previous amount of oxygen.
   2. Cover the stoma site with a sterile 4 × 4-in dressing. Tape it in place. Apply a bland aerosol by face mask with the previous amount of oxygen.
   3. Monitor and evaluate the patient every 30 minutes for several hours. Encourage deep breathing

and coughing. Check the vital signs and breath sounds. Measure pulse oximetry or arterial blood gases after 20 minutes. Be prepared to reintubate the patient if necessary.

4. Routine stoma care to ensure healing usually includes the following each shift:
   aa. Remove the dressing. Inspect the stoma for signs of infection such as pus, redness, and swelling.
   bb. Clean the stoma site with hydrogen peroxide on a sterile gauze pad.
   cc. Apply antibiotic ointment to the stoma site.
   dd. Reapply a sterile dressing.

MODULE E
Respiratory care plan

1. Analyze available information to determine the patient's pathophysiologic state (CSE code: IIIH1)

Be able to recognize an airway obstruction problem in a patient and recommend or place the proper airway device to correct the problem. A chest radiograph should always be taken to confirm the location of a newly placed endotracheal or tracheostomy tube. All modern endotracheal and tracheostomy tubes contain a strip of radiopaque material near the distal tip of the tube. This is easily noticed as the white line seen on the chest radiograph film and confirms the location of the tip of the tube in the airway (see Fig. 12-18). The chest radiograph examination should be repeated if a significant change has occurred in the patient's condition, or if the tube has been pulled back or pushed more deeply into the trachea. The chest radiograph would also show a pneumothorax related to the tracheostomy procedure or other pulmonary conditions.

2. Determine the appropriateness of the prescribed therapy and goals for the identified pathophysiologic state (CSE code: IIIH3)
3. Recommend changes in the therapeutic plan if supportive data exist (WRE code: IIIH2) [Difficulty: An]

The indications or uses for the various airways are listed with the information on that airway. In general, the airway should be removed when it is no longer needed. Typically, an oropharyngeal airway should be removed from a patient who has regained consciousness. A nasopharyngeal airway should be removed if the patient no longer needs it as an airway or for a suctioning route. Endotracheal and tracheostomy tubes can be removed when the patient does not need mechanical ventilation or a suctioning route, is no longer in danger of aspiration, or does not need a permanent artificial airway.

Effective communication is important for good patient care. The conscious patient with an endotracheal tube or tracheostomy is unable to speak. Alternative ways to communicate must be provided. Examples include alphabet boards and picture boards for pointing, and pencil and paper for notes. Head nods for yes and no and lip reading are often used. It is important that questions be worded so that they can be answered with a *yes* or *no*. Avoid questions that require a lengthy written answer unless the patient seems ready and willing to do so.

It is not possible to predict how a patient may react to the placement of an artificial airway or its prolonged need. Some patients react with relief and relax when the WOB is reduced. Others may become angry at the limitations imposed on them. Still others may become depressed. Be prepared to deal with these reactions or changes in the patient's emotional response to this very stressful situation.

4. Stop the treatment or procedure if the patient has an adverse reaction to it (CSE code: IIIF1)

5. Discontinue treatment based on the patient's response (WRE code: IIIG1e) [Difficulty: An]

Be prepared to stop or discontinue the use of a particular airway and initiate the use of another, as needed. The indications for each type of airway were presented earlier in the chapter.

BIBLIOGRAPHY

American Association for Respiratory Care: Clinical practice guideline: management of airway emergencies, *Respir Care* 40(7):749, 1995.

American Association for Respiratory Care: Clinical practice guideline: removal of the endotracheal tube, *Respir Care* 44(1):85, 1999.

American Heart Association, Emergency Cardiac Care Committee and Subcommittees: Guidelines for cardiopulmonary resuscitation and emergency cardiac care: adult advanced cardiac life support, *JAMA* 268(16):2199, 1992.

Durbin CG: Artificial airways. In Cairo JM, Pilbeam SP, editors: *Mosby's respiratory care equipment,* ed 7, St Louis, 2004, Mosby.

Eubanks DH, Bone RC: *Comprehensive respiratory care,* ed 2, St Louis, 1990, Mosby.

Frownfelter DL: Chest physical therapy and airway care. In Barnes TA, editor: *Core textbook of respiratory care practice,* ed 2, St Louis, 1994, Mosby.

Gorback MS: Airway management. In Dantzker DR, MacIntyre NR, Bakow ED, editors: *Comprehensive respiratory care,* Philadelphia, 1995, WB Saunders.

Heffner JE: Managing difficult intubations in critically ill patients, *Respir Manage* 19(3):53, 1989.

Hess DR, Branson RD: Airway and suction equipment. In Branson RD, Hess DR, Chatburn RL, editors: *Respiratory care equipment,* ed 2, Philadelphia, 1999, Lippincott Williams & Wilkins.

JEM 400 Endotracheal Tube Changer (Guide), product literature, Instrumentation Industries Inc, Bethel Park, Penn.

Kovac AL: Dilemmas and controversies in intubation, *Respir Manage* 21(4):77, 1991.

Levitzky MG, Cairo JM, Hall SM: *Introduction to respiratory care,* Philadelphia, 1990, WB Saunders.

Lewis RM: Airway care. In Fink JB, Hunt GE, editors: *Clinical practice in respiratory care,* Philadelphia, 1999, Lippincott-Raven.

May RA, Bortner PL: Airway management. In Hess DR, MacIntyre NR, Mishoe SC, et al, editors: *Respiratory care principles and practice,* Philadelphia, 2002, WB Saunders.

McIntyre D: Airway management. In Wyka KA, Mathews PJ, Clark WF, editors: *Foundations of respiratory care,* Albany, NY, 2002, Delmar.

Plevak DJ, Ward JJ: Airway management. In Burton GC, Hodgkin JE, Ward JJ, editors: *Respiratory care: a guide to clinical practice,* ed 4, Philadelphia, 1997, Lippincott-Raven.

PressureEasy Cuff Pressure Controller, ReviveEasy PtL Airway, and Endotracheal/Trach Tube Pilot Tube Repair Kit, product literature, Respironics, Monroeville, Penn.

Roth P: Airway care. In Aloan CA, Hill TV, editors: *Respiratory care of the newborn and child,* ed 2, Philadelphia, 1997, Lippincott-Raven.

Scanlan C, Simmons K: Airway management. In Scanlan CL, Wilkins RL, Stoller JK, editors: *Egan's fundamentals of respiratory care,* ed 7, St Louis, 1999, Mosby.

Simmons KF, Scanlan CL: Airway management. In Wilkins RL, Stoller JK, Scanlan CL, editors: *Egan's fundamentals of respiratory care,* ed 8, St Louis, 2003, Mosby.

Shapiro BA, Kacmarek RM, Cane RD, et al, editors: *Clinical application of respiratory care,* ed 4, St Louis, 1991, Mosby.

Sills JR: An emergency cuff inflation technique, *Respir Care* 31(3):199, 1986.

Whitaker K: *Comprehensive perinatal and pediatric respiratory care,* ed 2, Albany, NY, 1997, Delmar.

White GC: *Equipment theory for respiratory care,* ed 4, Albany, NY, 2005, Delmar.

SELF-STUDY QUESTIONS

1. A 59-kg (130-lb) woman must be intubated to initiate mechanical ventilation. What size tube should be used?
   A. 6.0-mm ID
   B. 7.0-mm ID
   C. 8.0-mm ID
   D. 9.0-mm ID

2. A hospitalized patient rapidly develops ventilatory failure because of an accidental overdose of morphine sulfate for pain control. The preferred way to quickly provide a safe, secure airway is to:
   A. Place an oropharyngeal airway.
   B. Hyperextend the patient's neck into the sniff position.
   C. Place a nasal endotracheal tube.
   D. Place an oral endotracheal tube.

3. After a successful CPR attempt, a patient with an oral endotracheal tube is placed on a mechanical ventilator in the Intensive Care Unit. The respiratory therapist notices that the exhaled CO_2 monitor is appropriately changing color with each breath cycle. The patient's breath sounds are present on the right side but diminished on the left side. What is the most likely cause of this situation?
   A. Left-sided pneumothorax
   B. Right bronchial intubation
   C. Malfunctioning exhaled CO_2 monitor
   D. Delivered tidal volume is too small

4. A 2-year-old child admitted with severe croup has just been extubated after 2 days with an oral endotracheal tube. The child is given oxygen and aerosolized water through a heated large volume nebulizer. Thirty minutes later, mild inspiratory stridor is heard over the child's throat area. What should be done *first*?
   A. Deliver nebulized racemic epinephrine.
   B. Reintubate the child.
   C. Perform a cricothyrotomy.
   D. Perform a tracheostomy.

5. A 55-year-old, 77-kg (170-lb) male patient has been returned from the operating room with a fresh tracheostomy. The respiratory therapist determines the cuff pressure on the 6.0-mm ID tracheostomy tube to be 35 mm Hg. The ventilator is delivering a tidal volume of 750 mL and returning a tidal volume of 650 mL, and a leak can be heard at the tracheostomy site. What should be done?
   A. Increase the tidal volume by 100 mL.
   B. Increase the cuff pressure to seal the trachea to stop the tidal volume leak.
   C. Replace the tracheostomy tube with one that is 8.5 mm ID.
   D. Deflate the cuff enough to reduce the cuff pressure to 15 mm Hg.

6. An intubated and mechanically ventilated adult patient has been returned to the long-term care unit after being transported to the Radiology Department for an abdominal radiograph examination. The respiratory therapist observes that the patient's trachea is midline. However, the patient's left chest area does not rise with inspiration as much as the right chest area. The endotracheal tube is at the 28-cm mark at the patient's teeth. What should be done now?
   A. Check the abdominal radiograph for signs of vomiting and aspiration.
   B. Pull the endotracheal tube back about 4 cm.
   C. Check the patient's end-tidal carbon dioxide level.
   D. Deliver a larger tidal volume breath to inflate the left lung better.

7. A conscious patient is recovering from Guillain-Barré syndrome and is able to breathe spontaneously off of the mechanical ventilator for several hours. She currently has a standard 7.5-mm ID tracheostomy tube. To help her weaning process but to enable her to be ventilated at night, what should be done?
   A. Remove the tracheostomy tube when she is off of the ventilator.
   B. Substitute a speaking-type tracheostomy tube.
   C. Replace the current tracheostomy tube with one that is 6.0 mm ID.
   D. Substitute a fenestrated tracheostomy tube.

8. A patient who had facial burns and smoke inhalation has recovered enough to be extubated. Although the patient is receiving 40% oxygen with a bland aerosol, significant inspiratory stridor is noticed within 15 minutes. After the inhalation of a vasoconstricting medication, the patient's breath sounds are improved. Thirty minutes later, the patient's SpO_2 is 80%, and the inspiratory stridor is more serious. The patient is very anxious and is pulling off the oxygen mask. What should the respiratory therapist recommend to best manage the patient's problem?
   A. Draw an arterial blood gas sample.
   B. Increase the patient's oxygen to 50%.
   C. Intubate the patient.
   D. Administer a sedative medication.

9. All of the following may be used to help determine the position of an endotracheal tube:
   I. End-tidal carbon dioxide monitoring
   II. An esophageal detection device (EDD)
   III. Laryngeal palpation during tube insertion
   IV. Neck and chest radiographs
   V. Observation of bilateral chest movement
      A. I, III, and IV
      B. II, IV, and IV
      C. I, II, III, and V
      D. I, II, III, IV, and V

10. A respiratory therapist replaces a patient's tracheostomy tube with another one of the same size and inflates the cuff with 5 mL of air as was done previously. Immediately, the patient has difficulty breathing, and no air can be felt coming from the tube. What could be the problem?
    A. The tip of the tube has been placed into the subcutaneous tissues.
    B. The patient has closed her epiglottis over the trachea.
    C. More air must be added to the cuff to form a seal.
    D. The tube has been placed into the esophagus by accident.

ANSWER KEY

1. **C.** Rationale: An adult woman normally has an 8.0 (or 7.5) mm ID endotracheal tube placed into her. Review Table 12-1 for the recommended sizes of endotracheal and tracheostomy tubes for patients of all sizes.

2. **D.** Rationale: In an emergency situation, it is fastest and easiest to place an oral endotracheal tube into most patients. A safe and secure airway can be assured within 20 to 30 seconds. An oropharyngeal airway only keeps the tongue from blocking the back of the throat. It does not provide a safe, secure airway. Hyperextending the patient's neck into the sniff position opens the airway but does not secure it from possible dangers such as vomiting and aspiration. Placing a nasal endotracheal tube requires an anesthesiologist and special equipment. This delay is unnecessary when oral endotracheal intubation can be done by a trained respiratory therapist.

3. **B.** Rationale: Right bronchial intubation is indicated by the presence of the patient's breath sounds on the right side but diminished on the left side. No direct evidence indicates a left-sided pneumothorax. The exhaled CO_2 monitor is functioning properly because it is supposed to change color (from dark purple to yellow when exposed to exhaled carbon dioxide) during the breathing cycle. Even a small tidal volume should deliver equal air to both lungs and result in equal breath sounds over both lungs.

4. **A.** Rationale: A mild case of stridor is first treated by nebulizing the vasoconstricting medication racemic epinephrine. This usually results in enough constriction of the throat's mucous membrane blood vessels to dilate the airway and correct the stridor. If this does not work, the patient may need to be intubated. A cricothyrotomy is done only to create an emergency airway opening if the patient's upper airway is obstructed by a foreign body or trauma. A tracheostomy is done only if a long-term surgical airway opening is needed. This patient certainly does not need either of the latter two solutions to his or her problem.

5. **C.** Rationale: Because the cuff pressure is so high on the small tracheostomy tube, it is best to replace the tube with one that is 8.5 mm ID. This is the correct size for an adult man. Increasing the tidal volume by 100 mL may deliver a larger tidal volume, or it may just increase the leak around the tracheostomy tube. The real problem is a tube that is too small for the patient's trachea. It is unsafe to increase the cuff pressure to seal the trachea to stop the tidal volume leak. Although the increased pressure overinflates the cuff to stop the leak, the circulation is cut off from the patient's tracheal mucosa, and the mucosa can die. It is unsafe to deflate the cuff enough to reduce the cuff pressure to 15 mm Hg because the patient's tidal volume leak can worsen.

6. **B.** Rationale: An adult patient usually has the proximal end of the tube at the 23- to 25-cm mark at the teeth for a midtracheal tube tip position. This, and the observation that the left side of the patient's chest is not moving as much as the right side, indicates that the tube has been pushed down into the right main-stem bronchus. The best thing to do is reposition the tube by suctioning the patient's airways and throat, deflating the cuff, withdrawing the tube about 4 cm, and reinflating the cuff. Of course, check for bilateral breath sounds, confirm a safe cuff pressure, and get a chest radiograph to complete the procedure. Nothing is to be gained by checking the abdominal radiograph because signs of vomiting and aspiration are not seen on it. Pneumonitis can be seen on a chest radiograph but not on an abdominal radiograph because an abdominal radiograph does not include the chest. Checking the patient's end-tidal carbon dioxide level demonstrates exhaled CO_2. However, this is not specific enough for this situation because the right lung can give off the gas even if the left lung is not ventilated. Delivering a larger tidal volume breath does not inflate the left lung any better because the endotracheal tube has been pushed down the right mainstem bronchus.

7. **D.** Rationale: Substituting a fenestrated tracheostomy tube for the standard tube allows her to breathe spontaneously through the upper airway when the inner cannula is removed. This allows her to talk, which can have a very positive emotional impact on the patient. It is probably going too far to remove the tracheostomy tube when she is off of the ventilator. This necessitates removing the tube, covering the stoma, and reinserting the tube later in the day. This can lead to damage to the tracheal tissue. In additional, if the patient's condition suddenly deteriorates while the tracheostomy tube is removed, no secure airway is available. Although a speaking-type tracheostomy tube allows her to speak

while on the ventilator, it does not enable her to breathe through her upper airway when she is off of the ventilator, as a fenestrated tube allows. Replacing the current 7.5-mm ID tracheostomy tube with one that is 6.0 mm ID greatly increases the patient's WOB. This can tire her and delay her recovery.

8. **C.** Rationale: The patient should be reintubated because of the serious nature of the inspiratory stridor that is unresponsive to the inhaled vasoconstricting drug (racemic epinephrine), the low SpoO$_2$ value, and the combative nature of the patient. An arterial blood gas value is not necessary because the Spo$_2$ value of 80% confirms hypoxemia. Getting the arterial blood gas sample and waiting for the results only delays the necessary intubation. Increasing the patient to 50% oxygen helps relieve the hypoxemia. However, once the patient is intubated and can breathe adequately, the Spo$_2$ value should increase to a safe level on the previous 40% oxygen. It could be very dangerous to administer a sedative medication to this patient. Sedating the patient further reduces the patient's ability to breathe through the narrowed airway.

9. **D.** Rationale: All of these may be used, along with listening for bilateral breath sounds, to confirm the location of the endotracheal tube. An end-tidal carbon dioxide monitoring system (capnograph) or disposable carbon dioxide detector such as the Easy Cap may be used to detect exhaled carbon dioxide. If the tube is placed within the esophagus, no carbon dioxide will be found. An EDD can be attached to the endotracheal tube. After the bulb has been squeezed, it inflates with air from the patient's lungs if the tube is within a major airway (see Fig. 12-29). Laryngeal palpation during tube insertion allows the tube to be felt as it passes through the larynx. Remember that these three methods differentiate only between airway and esophageal intubation. They do not detect a tube that has been inserted too deeply and has entered a mainstem bronchus (usually the right). A neck and chest radiograph shows the tube entering the larynx and its tip within the trachea (or a bronchus). Observation of bilateral chest movement is valuable because equal movement correlates with tracheal intubation and ventilation of both lungs.

10. **A.** Rationale: If the tip of the tracheostomy tube has been placed into the subcutaneous tissues, the patient will not be able to ventilate at all. The tube must be immediately withdrawn. Because the tracheotomy site is below the larynx, it does not matter if the patient has closed her epiglottis over the trachea. She still can breathe through the tracheostomy tube. It is unlikely that the new cuff requires any more air than the previous one. Even if this were the case, the patient should still be able to breathe through the tube. It should not be possible to place a tracheostomy tube into a patient's esophagus.

13 Suctioning the Airway

Note 1: The National Board for Respiratory Care (NBRC) has released the *RRT Examination Matrix* (covering the testable items on the Written Registry Exam) and the *CSE Examination Matrix* (covering the testable items on the Clinical Simulation Exam). Turn to the appendices at the back of this book for both publications in their original formats. This book is intended to cover all of the testable items in these two publications. This chapter (and all others) uses the abbreviation "WRE" for the coded items testable on the Written Registry Exam *and* Clinical Simulation Exam. The listed difficulty (R, Recall; Ap, Application; An, Analysis) relates to the question difficulty on the Written Registry Exam. The abbreviation "CSE" is used for the coded items testable on *only* the Clinical Simulation Exam. Because no question difficulty level is given for this exam, be prepared for anything.

Note 2: A review of the most recent Written Registry Examinations has shown an average of three questions (3% of the exam) that cover suctioning procedures. The Clinical Simulation Exam is comprehensive and may include everything that should be known or performed by an advanced level respiratory therapist.

MODULE A
Suctioning devices

1. **Oropharyngeal suction devices**
   a. **Get the necessary equipment for the procedure (WRE code: IIA8) [Difficulty: Ap]**

Oropharyngeal suctioning is considered a clean (not sterile) procedure. The suctioning device is packaged sterile but may be used more than once. A Yankauer suction catheter is widely used. It is made of hard plastic and has an angled catheter to reach into the back of the mouth. One large opening or several medium sized openings may be found at the tip of the catheter. The openings are large enough to permit easy suctioning of saliva, food, or vomit. Some handles include a thumb control valve so that suction can be applied to the tip only when wanted. Covering the opening with a thumb creates a vacuum at the tip for suctioning the patient's mouth (Fig. 13-1). The Yankauer

may be discarded when no longer needed or sterilized for use with another patient.

A flexible plastic or rubber catheter also can be used. It should be the largest diameter possible to reduce the chance of its becoming plugged. The opening at the catheter tip should be cut straight (perpendicular) across instead of at an angle. No side openings should be present (Fig. 13-2). The catheter is discarded when no longer needed.

   b. **Put the equipment together, make sure that it works properly, and identify any problems (WRE code: IIA8) [Difficulty: Ap]**

The catheters just mentioned are single pieces with nothing to assemble. They must be attached to a vacuum source by a length of soft rubber tubing. With clean gloves on both hands, attach the Yankauer, plastic, or rubber catheter to the vacuum tubing. The vacuum must be applied to the tip of the catheter for oral secretions to be removed. Check for a vacuum at the tip by any of the following methods:

1. Listen for the sound of air being drawn into the tip.
2. Put the tip into a container of sterile water. Close the thumb control opening. The water must be drawn up the catheter.
3. Place a clean-gloved hand over the tip if no water is available. Close the thumb control opening. The glove should be attracted to the catheter.

   c. **Fix any problems with the equipment (WRE code: IIA8) [Difficulty: Ap]**

Failure to have a vacuum at the catheter tip can mean:

1. The vacuum is not turned on. Check the following:
   a. Some centralized vacuum systems have a single dial that turns the system off and on and sets the vacuum level. Other centralized vacuum systems have an on and off switch and a dial for the vacuum level.
   b. Freestanding vacuum systems must be plugged into a working electrical outlet. The on and off switch must be turned on. The simpler systems

Fig. 13-1 Features of Yankauer suction catheter.

Fig. 13-2 Features of suction catheter with cross-cut tip.

have a preset vacuum level. Variable vacuum levels can be set with a dial in the more sophisticated systems.

2. The system is not sealed, so the vacuum is lost to the atmosphere. Check the following:
   a. Make sure that the rubber vacuum tubing fits tightly over the connectors on the catheter and on the vacuum system.
   b. Make sure that the catheter and vacuum tubing are not cracked or cut. Replace a Yankauer, plastic, or rubber catheter or vacuum tubing that is defective.

c. Close the thumb control if it has been left open.
d. Check the central or freestanding vacuum system to make sure that the secretion collection bottle is sealed properly.

3. The system is blocked, and no vacuum can get through to the tip. Check the following:
   a. Check for a pinch in the vacuum tubing or soft catheter.
   b. Check for a blockage in the catheter or vacuum tubing. Try to suction some sterile water to clear the blockage into the secretion collection bottle. Replace the catheter, or vacuum tubing, or both if the blockage cannot be cleared.
   c. Empty out a full collection bottle.

2. Suction catheters

Suctioning catheters are intended for removing secretions and foreign material from the trachea. They come sterile and individually packaged. It is highly recommended that the outer diameter (OD) of the catheter be no more than one half the inner diameter (ID) of the airway that it is passing through. This guideline is intended to minimize the obstruction to the airway so that the patient can still breathe around the catheter.

Exam Hint

Remember that the outer diameter of the suction catheter should be no more than one half the inner diameter of the endotracheal tube. This is often a test question.

See Table 13-1 for the recommended suction catheter sizes for the various endotracheal or tracheostomy tubes. The practitioner also can easily compare the relative sizes of the tube and suction catheter at the bedside before suctioning. Suction catheters are sized by the French (Fr or F) scale of their OD. Endotracheal and tracheostomy tubes are sized by ID and OD in millimeters and often by ID in French. Review Table 12-1 if necessary. The following formula and example show how to calculate the OD size of any suction catheter to find with which endotracheal or tracheostomy tube that size of suction catheter may be used. Because each French unit is about 0.33 mm, the OD in millimeters of a suction catheter can be found by multiplying the French size by 0.33. For example, calculate the OD of a 12Fr suction catheter:

$$12Fr \times 0.33 = 3.96 \text{ (about 4.0) mm OD of the catheter}$$

Therefore this size catheter could be used on an 8.0-mm ID endotracheal tube. See Fig. 13-3 for the relative sizes of this endotracheal tube and catheter.

	ID of Tube Sizes (mm)	Suction Catheter Size (Fr)
TABLE 13-1 Recommended Suction Catheter French Sizes for the various Endotracheal and Tracheostomy Tube Sizes		
Age		
NEWBORN		
1000 g	2.5	5
1000–2000 g	3.0	6
2000–3000 g	3.5	8
3000 g to 6 mo old	3.5–4.0	8
PEDIATRIC		
18 mo	4.0	8
3 yr	4.5	8
5 yr	5.0	10
6 yr	5.5	10
8 yr	6.0	10
ADULT		
16 yr	7.0	10
Normal size woman	7.5–8.0	12
Normal size man	8.0–8.5	14
Large adult	9.0–10.0	16

Note: It is recommended to use a suction catheter with an outer diameter that is no more than half of the inner diameter of the endotracheal tube.
ID, Inner diameter.

Knowing the ID of a suction catheter is helpful because it relates to the maximum particle size that can pass through it. The following formula can be used to interconvert from French to millimeters:

Fig. 13-3 Number 12Fr suction catheter inside of 8.0-mm ID endotracheal tube. The OD of the catheter should be no more than one half of the ID of the tube so that the patient can still breathe around it.

$$mm = \frac{Fr - 2}{4}$$

EXAMPLE

What is the ID in millimeters of a 12Fr suction catheter?

$$mm = \frac{12 - 2}{4}$$

$$mm = \frac{10}{4}$$

$$mm = 2.5 \ (\text{See Fig. 13-3.})$$

a. Get the necessary catheter for an open airway suctioning procedure (WRE code: IIA8) [Difficulty: Ap]

Open airway suctioning is used here to refer to the patient spontaneously breathing room air after being disconnected from the source of supplemental oxygen. This happens to the patient with a normal upper airway when the oxygen mask is removed for nasotracheal suctioning. It also happens when the patient with an endotracheal or tracheostomy tube has the aerosol T-piece (Briggs adapter) or ventilator circuit removed for suctioning purposes.

These types of catheters have been in use for many years. The two basic types are shown in Fig. 13-4. Closing the thumb control, as shown in Fig. 13-5, allows the vacuum to be selectively applied to the secretions when desired. The tips of the catheters can vary greatly. A considerable amount of effort has been spent trying to develop a catheter tip that most effectively removes secretions without damaging the tracheal mucosa. Fig. 13-6 shows some of the catheter tips that have been developed to minimize mucosal damage. Note that all feature at least one opening in the catheter that is back from the opening at the tip. Compare this with the single end opening found on the oral suction catheter (see Fig. 13-2). The side openings are designed to prevent the vacuum from being applied to the tip when it makes contact with the mucosa.

Notice in Fig. 13-4 and 13-6 that most catheters are straight throughout their length. All of these catheters tend to enter the right mainstem bronchus during deep suctioning. This is because its angle off of the trachea is less acute compared with the angle of the left mainstem bronchus. Thus it is difficult, if not impossible, for any of these catheters to suction the left main-stem bronchus. The Coudé catheter has been designed with an angled tip to better enable it to be guided into the left (or right) mainstem bronchus. See the far right example in Fig. 13-6. When these catheters are used, the direction of the thumb control valve can help determine the angle of the bent tip.

Fig. 13-4 Features of two types of suction catheters with angle-cut tips and side holes. **A,** Catheter has its own thumb control valve. **B,** Catheter must have a thumb control valve constructed from a Y connector.

Fig. 13-6 Close-up of the ends of three different suction catheters. **A,** A bevel cut of the tip with two offset side holes. **B,** A ring tip with several side holes around it. **C,** A Coudé (curved-tip) catheter, which may help in guiding it into either the left or right mainstem bronchus. *(From Rarey KP, Youtsey JW: Respiratory patient care, Englewood Cliffs, NJ, 1981, Prentice-Hall.)*

Use of these traditional types of catheters during open airway suctioning always results in some level of hypoxemia. The use of a relatively new type of suction catheter may help to alleviate this problem. The insufflating suction catheter is designed to provide alternatively oxygen through the catheter or vacuum for suctioning. The thumb control end of the catheter is modified with two male-type tubing connectors and a way to switch the lumen of the catheter between them. The thumb control is set to direct the oxygen through the catheter and into the patient as the catheter is advanced. After the catheter has been deeply placed into the trachea for suctioning, the thumb control is switched from delivering oxygen to applying suction.

Fig. 13-5 Close-up of thumb control valve showing how room air is drawn into vacuum tubing when the valve is left open. Closing valve applies vacuum to catheter tip to suction secretions.

b. Get the necessary catheter for a closed airway suctioning procedure (WRE code: IIA8) [Difficulty: Ap]

Closed airway suctioning is used here to refer to suctioning when the patient remains connected to the original source of oxygen. This may be done through a special aerosol T-piece or, more commonly, with the patient receiving mechanical ventilation. Spontaneously breathing patients are less likely to have hypoxemia with closed airway suctioning because they can continue to inhale the prescribed oxygen percentage.

In closed airway suctioning systems, a flexible, clear plastic sheath covers the catheter to maintain its sterility (Fig. 13-7). The practitioner does not need gloves. When used for patients who need frequent suctioning, the self-contained systems have a financial advantage over the traditional catheter and gloves suctioning method because they can be reused. These closed-system suction catheters come with either the traditional straight tip or the Coudé tip for selective bronchial suctioning.

Another device to create a sealed system for endotracheal tube suctioning consists of an elbow adapter that has an inner plastic sleeve or diaphragm. As the traditional catheter is inserted into the opening on the elbow adapter, the sleeve or diaphragm conforms to the catheter so that no air leak occurs (Fig. 13-8). This ensures that the ventilator delivered volumes and pressures are not lost through a leak.

c. Put the suctioning equipment together, make sure that it works properly, and identify any problems (WRE code: IIA8) [Difficulty: Ap]

Refer to Fig. 13-4 for the attachment of an open airway suction catheter to the vacuum tubing. Fig. 13-7 shows the attachment of a closed airway suction catheter to the vacuum tubing. The other end of the vacuum tubing is attached to the vacuum regulator system.

Fig. 13-7 Self-contained catheter and sheath suctioning system for closed airway suctioning. *(Based on the Kimberly-Clark/Ballard TRACH CARE® closed endotracheal suction device.)*

Fig. 13-8 Features and placement of special elbow adapter for closed airway suctioning without losing tidal volume or pressure during mechanical ventilation.

With open airway suctioning, only a hand covered by a sterile glove can be allowed to touch the area of the catheter that enters the patient's trachea. The practitioner's other hand also should be gloved. A clean glove is acceptable because it does not touch the part of the catheter that will enter the patient's trachea.

While holding the body of the catheter, the thumb control valve, and vacuum connector with the sterile-gloved hand and the vacuum tubing with the clean-gloved hand, slip the vacuum tubing over the catheter's vacuum connector. The seal should be tight so that no vacuum leak occurs. From now on, only the sterile-gloved hand may touch the part of the catheter that makes contact with the patient. The clean-gloved hand may touch only the thumb control valve and vacuum tubing. If the catheter is contaminated, it must be discarded.

The catheter can be tested for patency and vacuum at the tip by the three methods described earlier in the discussion on oropharyngeal suction devices. Note that only a *sterile* glove may be touched against the tip of the suction catheter to check for a vacuum.

The practitioner does not need gloves when a self-contained catheter is used for closed airway suctioning because the sheath covers the catheter to prevent contamination.

> **Exam Hint**
>
> **R**emember that endotracheal suctioning is a sterile procedure. Contaminated gloves or catheter must be replaced with sterile equipment.

d. Fix any problems with the equipment (WRE code: IIA8) [Difficulty: Ap]

The three common causes of an equipment failure and how to fix them are described in the earlier discussion on oropharyngeal suction devices. Remember to withdraw the closed airway suctioning catheter completely from the endotracheal tube into the sheath, or it will act as a partial obstruction.

3. Specimen collectors
a. Get the necessary equipment (WRE code: IIA8) [Difficulty: Ap]

A variety of specimen collectors (commonly called Lukens traps) exist. They are packaged as sterile so that no contamination of the sputum sample occurs with nonpatient organisms. Figs. 13-9 through 13-12 show the key features and functions of several sputum sample collectors. The sputum sample is obtained through a suction catheter or bronchoscope.

The specimen jar has volume markings and screws into either a special lid used to suction the specimen or a regular lid for shipment to the laboratory. The special lids

Fig. 13-9 Features of sputum specimen collection system with thumb control valve.

Fig. 13-10 Features of sputum specimen collection system without thumb control valve.

Specimen jar lid with suction catheter
and thumb control valve catheter

Suction
catheter

Regular specimen
jar lid

Specimen jar

Thumb control valve

Connector

Vacuum tubing

Fig. 13-11 Features of sputum specimen collection system with thumb control valve built into catheter.

used in the systems featured in Figs. 13-9 and 13-10 must be connected to a sterile catheter. Fig. 13-11 shows a system with its own catheter. The vacuum source is provided to these specimen collectors by a length of vacuum tubing as in the previously described suction catheter systems. Fig. 13-12 shows a DeLee system sometimes used in the delivery room. The physician, nurse, or practitioner uses mouth suction to remove secretions from the newborn. In all of these examples, after the sample has been collected, the special lid is unscrewed and replaced with the regular specimen jar lid.

b. Put the equipment together, make sure that it works properly, and identify any problems (WRE code: IIA8) [Difficulty: Ap]

A properly working specimen collection system provides a vacuum to the tip of the suction catheter when the thumb control valve or mouthpiece is sealed and vacuum is applied. This is tested by dipping the catheter tip into a container of sterile water or saline solution. The liquid is drawn up the catheter and deposited in the specimen jar. (The water can be emptied out of the jar by simply unscrewing the jar and discarding it.)

c. Fix any problems with the equipment (WRE code: IIA9) [Difficulty: Ap]

Failure to have a vacuum at the tip of the suction catheter may be caused by any of the previously mentioned

Suction catheter

Specimen jar
lid with suction
catheter and
mouthpiece
on catheter

Mouthpiece for suctioning

Specimen jar

Regular specimen jar lid

Fig. 13-12 Features of DeLee sputum specimen collection system with mouthpiece through which the practitioner can apply suction.

possibilities. They can be checked and corrected by the methods listed earlier. Two likely causes of an inability to suction secretions are found. One possible cause is that the jar is not screwed tightly into the special lid. This allows room air to be drawn in. Simply screw the lid in tightly. The second possible cause is that the secretion channel is plugged. Discard it and replace it with a new specimen collector.

MODULE B
Vacuum regulator systems

1. Get the necessary vacuum regulator system: vacuum pump, regulator, and collection bottle (CSE code: IIA23)

2. Put the equipment together, make sure that it works properly, and identify any problems (CSE code: IIA23)

The vacuum regulators come preassembled by the manufacturer. The two basic types are described here. Components must be added to make them fully functional.

a. Portable vacuum systems

Portable units are designed to be moved with the patient. They may be mounted on a small platform (Fig. 13-13) or mounted on a wheeled cart. The portable systems generally include an electrically powered vacuum pump with an on/off switch and a collection bottle. Some units have a control valve for adjusting the level of negative pressure. A negative-pressure gauge is used to determine how much vacuum is being applied. A length of rubber vacuum tubing is used to pass the negative pressure from the pump to the collection bottle. Another length of vacuum tubing is used to pass the vacuum through to the suction catheter. Portable systems are not as powerful as the central vacuum systems. They are not very effective at suctioning out large amounts of thick secretions.

In general, the following steps are needed to make the units operational:

Fig. 13-13 A portable suction machine. The electrically powered motor, collection bottle and cap, and connecting tubing can be seen. *(Courtesy Allied Health Care Products Inc, St Louis, Mo.)*

1. Plug the vacuum pump into a working electrical outlet. Battery-operated units should have fully charged batteries.
2. Place a clean, empty collection bottle into its holder on the cart. The bottle should be able to hold at least 500 mL of fluid.
3. Slip the rubber lid onto the open top of the collection bottle. Both vacuum tubing connectors on the lid must be patent.
4. Slip one end of a short length of vacuum tubing over the connector on the vacuum pump and the other end over one of the tubing connectors on the collection bottle lid.
5. Slip one end of a length of vacuum tubing over the other tubing connector on the collection bottle lid. The vacuum tubing should be no more than 3 feet long. The other end of the vacuum tubing is connected to the suction catheter when needed.
6. Turn on the unit, and determine the negative pressure by:
   a. Pinching closed the long vacuum tubing
   b. Turning on the vacuum pump
   c. Observing the pressure on the negative-pressure gauge
7. If the unit has a fixed vacuum level, the observed negative pressure should match that listed by the manufacturer.
8. If the unit has a variable vacuum level, adjust the vacuum control knob to the desired level.

b. Central vacuum systems

Central (wall) vacuum systems are usually available at each patient's bedside in all special care units. Each of the wall outlets is connected through a hospital-wide piping system to a large electrically powered vacuum pump. It is capable of generating a negative pressure far greater than what is needed in most patient care situations. A regulator is used to reduce the vacuum to the desired clinical level (Fig. 13-14). Either a Quick Connect or Diameter Index Safety System (DISS) connector is used to attach the regulator to the central vacuum system.

Most regulators have a selector knob that allows the user to turn the vacuum off (Off setting) or switch between full vacuum (Full setting) and a regulated level of vacuum (Reg setting). The Full setting opens the unit to the maximum level of vacuum available from the central pump. The Reg setting allows the user to adjust the vacuum level through a wide range.

In general, the following steps are needed to make the units operational:
1. Connect the regulator into a working suction outlet.
2. Screw a clean, empty collection bottle onto its connector on the regulator. The bottle must be able to hold at least 500 mL of fluid.

Fig. 13-14 Features of Ohmeda central vacuum regulator with three-position selector knob. *(Courtesy of Ohmeda Medical, Columbia, Md.)*

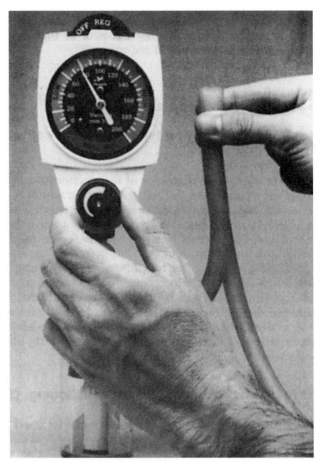

Fig. 13-15 Setting the level of negative pressure on Ohmeda central vacuum regulator by pinching vacuum tubing and adjusting vacuum control knob. Vacuum pressure is seen on pressure gauge. *(Courtesy of Ohmeda Medical, Columbia, Md.)*

3. Slip one end of a length of vacuum tubing over the tubing connector on the collection bottle. The vacuum tubing should be no more than 3 feet long. The other end of the vacuum tubing is connected to the suction catheter when needed.
4. Determine the negative pressure by:
   a. Pinching closed the vacuum tubing (Fig. 13-15).
   b. Turning the selector knob to Reg.
   c. Observing the pressure on the negative-pressure gauge.
5. Adjust the vacuum control knob to the desired level. If the secretions are too thick to be drawn up the suction catheter, the negative pressure must be increased.

3. Fix any problems with the equipment (CSE code: IIA23)

With a *portable* vacuum system, check the following when trying to determine the cause of a loss of vacuum:
   a. The vacuum pump is plugged into a working electrical outlet.
   b. The vacuum pump is turned on.
   c. The vacuum control valve is set at the desired negative pressure.
   d. The lid to the collection bottle is tightly sealed.
   e. The vacuum tubing tightly connects the pump to the collection bottle and the collection bottle to the suction catheter.
   f. No knots or obstructions are in the vacuum tubing or catheter.
   g. The collection bottle is not filled above its maximum level.

Correct any potential problems. Do not use a portable vacuum system that will not generate the negative pressure that it is supposed to.

With a *central* vacuum system, check the following when trying to determine the cause of a loss of vacuum:
   a. The regulator is plugged into a working vacuum outlet.
   b. The vacuum control valve is set at the desired negative pressure.
   c. The collection bottle is tightly screwed onto the suction-regulator outlet.

d. The vacuum tubing tightly connects the collection bottle to the suction catheter.

e. No knots or obstructions are present in the vacuum tubing or catheter.

f. The collection bottle is not filled above its maximum level.

Correct any potential problems. Do not use a central vacuum system outlet that will not generate the negative pressure that it should. Occasionally, less negative pressure is found than expected when the central vacuum system is being heavily used. No problem exists with the regulator or tubing, and the vacuum pressure will increase when fewer people are using it.

MODULE C

Initiate suctioning procedures to remove tracheal and oral secretions (WRE code: IIIF7b) [Difficulty: An]

Tracheal or oral secretions must be actively removed by suctioning whenever the patient cannot clear them out and there is a risk of airway obstruction. Suctioning may be needed in patients who are unconscious and lack swallowing or coughing reflexes, or in patients who may be too weak to cough effectively to remove tracheal secretions. Often the physician writes a standing order to suction the patient on a regular basis or as needed. However, in many institutions, a protocol exists to suction any patient who is at risk of obstructing his or her airway. For example, the comatose patient who vomits should have the mouth suctioned out even though no specific physician's order is written.

Suctioning secretions from a patient's trachea, by any method, places the patient at risk. The following two factors must be understood, identified when they occur, and prevented or corrected.

1. Prevent hypoxemia during the suctioning procedure (WRE code: IIID6) [Difficulty: An]

Suctioning the trachea removes air (including oxygen), as well as secretions, from the lungs. Hypoxemia, however, can be minimized by hyperoxygenating the patient for 1 to 2 minutes before suctioning. It is generally recommended that the patient receive 100% oxygen, if possible. Infants younger than 6 months should be given a fractional concentration of inspired oxygen (FIO_2) only 10% to 20% greater than their base level. This is because of the risk of retinopathy of prematurity (ROP), also known as retrolental fibroplasia.

Check the patient's arterial blood gas results or SpO_2 value to see whether the patient is hypoxic before beginning the procedure. SpO_2 values also can be monitored throughout the suctioning procedure to see how low the saturation decreases. After suctioning, give the patient supplemental oxygen until SpO_2 reaches at least 90%. The patient's chart also should be checked for any history of cardiac problems. Sudden hypoxemia from suctioning can result in life-threatening dysrhythmias such as premature ventricular contractions (PVCs). Check the patient's pulse rate and rhythm before and after suctioning. If the patient is using a cardiac monitor, it should be watched for rate and rhythm changes that are related to the suctioning procedure. Tachycardia is frequently seen with hypoxemia. Check the blood pressure of any patient who has suctioning-related dysrhythmias. The patient's vital signs should return to normal when oxygenation is restored.

Any modern mechanical ventilator can be set to deliver 100% oxygen. The most current ventilators have a 100% oxygen button designed just for this purpose. Pushing it results in the patient receiving pure oxygen for 1 to 2 minutes (depending on the manufacturer). Several sigh breaths also can be delivered. A closed airway suction catheter can be used with the ventilator, as discussed earlier, to minimize hypoxemia.

A spontaneously breathing patient can have a nonrebreathing mask placed and set to deliver close to 100% oxygen. If a nonrebreathing mask is not available, turn up the oxygen flow or percentage on whatever appliance the patient is using. A spontaneously breathing patient with an endotracheal or tracheostomy tube can have 100% oxygen delivered through a Brigg adapter/aerosol T-piece. A manual resuscitation bag also can be used to give the patient several sigh breaths.

All patients must be reoxygenated before another attempt at suctioning is made. Giving 100% oxygen after the suctioning episode helps the patient to reoxygenate faster. Giving several sigh breaths also helps reoxygenation to occur faster than normal tidal volume breathing does.

Vagus or vagal nerve stimulation. Vagal nerve endings are found in the hypopharynx and trachea. When they are mechanically stimulated by a suction catheter, any of the following may be seen:

a. The patient may have an induced bronchospasm.

b. The patient may become bradycardic.

c. The patient's blood pressure may decrease because of the bradycardia.

Listen to the patient's breath sounds before and after suctioning to determine whether an increase in wheezing is present, which shows bronchospasm. Check the patient's heart rate and rhythm by palpation or cardiac monitor to determine whether he or she is becoming bradycardic. The blood pressure also can be measured to check for hypotension.

Further suctioning should be delayed, if possible, until the patient's wheezing and vital signs have returned to normal. It may be necessary to modify the suctioning procedure by not going as deeply and striking the carina, not twisting the catheter, or not suctioning for as long to reduce the risk of vagal stimulation. A local anesthetic such as lidocaine (Xylocaine) can be nebulized (with a physician's order) to reduce the local reaction to the catheter.

Exam Hint

Understand the importance of hyperoxygenating a patient before and after a suctioning procedure. Hypoxemia and vagal stimulation can result in unstable vital signs and bronchospasm. Be prepared to stop suctioning, give extra oxygen, or get help.

---

2. Perform endotracheal or tracheostomy tube suctioning on the patient (WRE code: IIIC2) [Difficulty: An]

The procedure for endotracheal or tracheostomy tube suctioning is the same for both tubes, except to note that the catheter does not need to be inserted as far into the tracheostomy tube before hitting the carina.

The generally accepted steps in the procedure follow:

a. Check the chart for specific orders, an order to suction as needed, or any special patient considerations.

b. Gather the needed equipment:
   1. Suction catheter no larger than one half the ID of the patient's endotracheal or tracheostomy tube
   2. Two sterile gloves or one sterile glove and one clean glove (this may be skipped if a closed airway, self-contained system is used)
   3. Specimen collector if ordered
   4. Vacuum system
   5. Sterile water or normal saline in a sterile basin

c. Tell the patient what to expect during the procedure.

d. If possible, place the patient in semi-Fowler and sniff positions.

e. Give the patient 100% O_2 for at least 30 seconds before suctioning and for at least 1 minute afterward until the patient is no longer hypoxemic. (The infant who is younger than 6 months can have the F_{IO_2} increased by 10% to 20%.)

f. Get help if necessary.

g. Wash hands. (This may be skipped if a self-contained system is used or in an emergency.)

h. With sterile technique, put on the gloves, get the catheter out of its packaging, and connect the vacuum tubing to the catheter.

i. The American Association for Respiratory Care (AARC) Clinical Practice Guidelines suggest that the vacuum be set at the lowest possible level that still effectively removes secretions. A number of authors suggest the following ranges for vacuum:
   1. Adults: −100 to −120 mm Hg
   2. Children: −80 to −100 mm Hg
   3. Neonates: −60 to −80 mm Hg

j. Test that the vacuum is reaching the tip of the catheter.

k. Disconnect the ventilator circuit or O_2 appliance from the tube (except with a self-contained system).

l. Suction the tube:
   1. Without any vacuum, quickly and gently pass the catheter down the tube until an obstruction is felt. Withdraw the catheter 2 cm.
   2. In the adult, the entire procedure of disconnection of the O_2, suctioning, to reconnection of the O_2 and normal breathing should take no longer than 10 to 15 seconds. In the infant, the entire procedure should take no longer than 10 seconds.
   3. Withdraw the catheter with a twisting motion while suctioning intermittently. Suction to clear out any secretions. Typically, in the adult, suctioning may be applied for between 5 and 10 seconds. In the infant, suctioning may be applied for no more than 5 seconds.
   4. Turning the patient's head to the right might help direct the catheter down the left main-stem bronchus. The catheter tends to enter the right main-stem bronchus if the head is in a neutral position or twisted to the left.

m. Reoxygenate the patient for at least 1 minute before suctioning again. Giving 100% O_2 (or 10% to 20% more than the base level in the infant) and several sigh breaths helps this happen faster.

n. Monitor the patient's vital signs, O_2 level, and breath sounds before suctioning again. Suction again, if needed, when the patient is stable.

o. Normal saline solution may be instilled into the tube if the secretions are too thick to be suctioned out easily. The saline solution may help to loosen the secretions. The patient also is likely to cough vigorously. The amount of saline solution to be instilled varies with the size of the patient and the thickness of the secretions. The following are general guidelines for the instillation of normal saline solution:
   1. Neonates may be given a few drops to 0.33 mL at a time.
   2. Adults may be given 5 to 10 mL at a time or in divided doses.
   3. A physician's order may be needed to instill saline solution.

p. Dispose of the catheter and glove by pulling the glove inside out over the catheter. Self-contained systems may be left in place for up to 24 hours.

q. Rinse the vacuum tubing clear of secretions.

r. Turn off the suction unit.

Refer to Box 13-1 for hazards and complications of endotracheal suctioning.

BOX 13-1   Hazards and Complications of Endotracheal Suctioning

Cardiac arrest
Respiratory arrest
Hypoxemia
Cardiac dysrhythmias
Bronchospasm
Increased intracranial pressure
Hypertension
Hypotension
Apnea from interruption of mechanical ventilation
Pulmonary hemorrhage
Mechanical trauma to tracheal and bronchial mucosa
Infection to and/or from patient and respiratory care
    practitioner
Atelectasis

---

3. Perform nasotracheal suctioning on the patient (WRE code: IIIC1b) [Difficulty: An]

The generally accepted steps in the procedure follow:

a. Check the chart for specific orders, an order to suction as needed, or any special patient considerations.

b. Gather the needed equipment:
   1. Suction catheter no larger than one half the diameter of the patient's nostril
   2. Appropriate size and type of nasopharyngeal airway to minimize nasal mucosal damage
   3. Sterile, water-soluble lubricant jelly
   4. Sterile 4 × 4-inch gauze pad

c. Tell the patient what to expect during the procedure.

d. If possible, place the patient in semi-Fowler and sniff positions.

e. Give the patient 100% O_2 for at least 30 seconds before suctioning and for at least 1 minute afterward until the patient is no longer hypoxemic. (The infant younger than 6 months can have the F_{IO_2} increased by 10% to 20%.)

f. Get help if necessary.

g. Wash hands. (This may be skipped in an emergency.)

h. With sterile technique, put on the gloves, get the catheter out of its packaging, apply lubricant jelly to the catheter tip, and connect the vacuum tubing to the catheter.

i. The AARC Clinical Practice Guidelines suggest that the vacuum be set at the lowest possible level that still effectively removes secretions. A number of authors suggest the following ranges for vacuum:
   1. Adults: −100 to −120 mm Hg
   2. Children: −80 to −100 mm Hg
   3. Neonates: −60 to −80 mm Hg

j. Test that the vacuum is reaching the tip of the catheter.

k. Remove the O_2 appliance from the patient so that the nose may be reached. Directing the end of the O_2 tubing or nasal cannula prongs toward the patient's mouth may help to prevent hypoxemia.

l. Suction the trachea:
   1. Without any vacuum, advance the catheter into the nasopharyngeal airway. If no nasopharyngeal airway is available, advance the catheter into the most open nasal passage without any vacuum. The catheter should be advanced parallel to the turbinates to minimize tissue trauma. Never force the catheter. (The most patent nasal passage can be determined by checking the chart for a history of deviated septum, asking the patient if one side feels more open, or feeling which nostril has more airflow through it.)
   2. Have the cooperative patient stick out his or her tongue. The practitioner or assistant can grasp the uncooperative patient's tongue with a 4 × 4-inch gauze pad or gloved hand.
   3. Advance the catheter as the patient inspires. The epiglottis and vocal cords are open at this time, and it is easiest to slip the catheter into the trachea. The cooperative patient should be told to inhale slowly and deeply. Some practitioners find it helpful to disconnect the catheter from the vacuum tubing and listen to the end of the catheter for the sound of air movement. The patient will cough vigorously when the catheter is in the trachea (Fig. 13-16).
   4. Advance the catheter until an obstruction is felt. Then pull the catheter back about 2 cm.
   5. Withdraw the catheter with a twisting motion while suctioning intermittently. Suction to clear out any secretions. Typically, in the adult, suctioning may be applied for between 5 and 10 seconds. Suctioning in the infant should be applied for no more than 5 seconds. If the secretions are cleared, the catheter is pulled out. Practitioners disagree on whether the catheter should be withdrawn or left in place if the patient still has secretions. Some prefer to withdraw the catheter, let the patient rest and reoxygenate, and reinsert the catheter for more suctioning. Others prefer to leave the catheter in place to minimize tissue trauma from a reinsertion, let the patient rest and reoxygenate, and then suction again.
   6. The entire procedure usually takes longer than 20 seconds, so the O_2 tubing must be kept directed toward the patient's mouth.
   7. Turning the patient's head to the right might help direct the catheter down the left main-stem bronchus. The catheter will tend to enter the

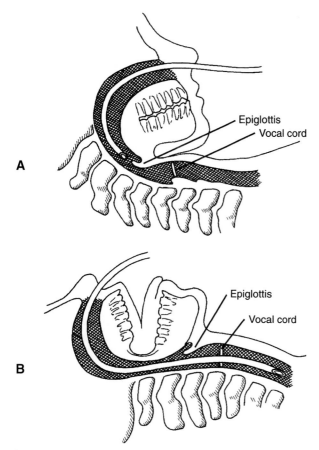

Fig. 13-16 Cross section through airway showing nasotracheal suctioning. **A,** With the patient's head in the sniff position, the catheter is advanced through a nostril to the level of the vocal cords. **B,** During an inspiration, the catheter is advanced into the trachea. The patient will cough, and secretions can be suctioned out.

BOX 13-2   Contraindications and Hazards and Complications of Nasotracheal Suctioning

CONTRAINDICATIONS
Absolute:
  Epiglottitis
  Laryngotracheobronchitis (croup)
Relative:
  Blocked nasal passages
  Nasal bleeding
  Acute facial, neck, or head injury
  Bleeding disorder
  Upper respiratory tract infection
  Irritable airway
  Laryngospasm

HAZARDS AND COMPLICATIONS
  Cardiac arrest
  Respiratory arrest
  Hypoxemia
  Cardiac dysrhythmias
  Bronchospasm
  Increased intracranial pressure
  Hypertension
  Hypotension
  Pulmonary hemorrhage
  Infection to and/or from patient and respiratory therapist
  Atelectasis
  Pain
  Catheter misdirected into esophagus
  Gagging and/or vomiting
  Uncontrolled coughing
  Mechanical trauma: nasal turbinates, perforation of pharynx, nasal bleeding, bleeding of the tracheal and bronchial mucosa

---

right mainstem bronchus if the head is in a neutral position or twisted to the left.

m. Reoxygenate the patient for at least 1 minute before suctioning again. Giving 100% O_2 (or 10% to 20% more than the base level in the infant) helps this happen faster.

n. Monitor the patient's vital signs, O_2 level, and breath sounds before suctioning again. Suction again, if needed, when the patient is stable.

o. Normal saline solution may be instilled down the suction catheter by pulling off the vacuum tubing, inserting the tip of the syringe (not needle) into the end of the catheter, covering the thumb control valve, and squirting the saline solution into the catheter. The other considerations listed earlier would apply here.

p. Dispose of the catheter and glove by pulling the glove inside out over the catheter.

q. Rinse the vacuum tubing clear of secretions.

r. Turn off the suction unit.

Refer to Box 13-2 for contraindications and hazards and complications of nasotracheal suctioning.

4. Perform orotracheal suctioning on the patient (WRE code: IIIC1b) [Difficulty: An]

Orotracheal suctioning is a more difficult procedure than nasotracheal suctioning and is not performed as often.

The generally accepted steps in the procedure follow:

a. Check the chart for specific orders, an order to suction as needed, or any special patient considerations.

b. Gather the needed equipment:

1. Suction catheter no larger than one half the diameter of the patient's nostril. Even though the catheter is going through the mouth, the critical diameter is the trachea. This guideline helps prevent too large a catheter being forced into the trachea.

2. The nasopharyngeal airway is not needed.

3. The sterile, water-soluble lubricant jelly and 4 × 4-inch gauze pad may not be needed if the patient's mouth is moist. Some may always prefer to lubricate the catheter tip.

4. Use sterile water or normal saline solution and sterile basin. Pour some water or saline into the basin.

c. Tell the patient what to expect during the procedure.

d. If possible, place the patient in semi-Fowler and sniff positions.

e. Give the patient 100% O_2 for at least 30 seconds before suctioning and for at least 1 minute afterward until the patient is no longer hypoxemic. (The infant younger than 6 months can have the F_{IO_2} increased by 10% to 20%.)

f. Get help if necessary.

g. Wash hands. (This may be skipped in an emergency.)

h. With sterile technique, put on the gloves, get the catheter out of its packaging, and connect the vacuum tubing to the catheter. Add the following steps if necessary:
   1. With the clean gloved hand, squeeze some of the lubricant jelly on the 4 × 4-inch gauze pad.
   2. Lubricate the tip and first few centimeters of the catheter.

i. The AARC Clinical Practice Guidelines suggest that the vacuum be set at the lowest possible level that still effectively removes secretions. A number of authors suggest the following ranges for vacuum:
   1. Adults: −100 to −120 mm Hg
   2. Children: −80 to −100 mm Hg
   3. Neonates: −60 to −80 mm Hg

j. Test that the vacuum is reaching the tip of the catheter.

k. Remove the O_2 appliance from the patient so that the mouth may be reached. A nasal cannula may be placed on the patient to give supplemental O_2. An assistant may be able to direct the end of the O_2 tubing toward the patient's mouth to help prevent hypoxemia.

l. Suction the trachea:
   1. Without any vacuum, advance the catheter into the oral pharynx.
   2. Have the cooperative patient stick out his or her tongue. The practitioner or assistant can grasp the uncooperative patient's tongue with a 4 × 4-inch gauze pad or gloved hand.
   3. Advance the catheter as the patient inspires. The epiglottis and vocal cords are open at this time, and it is easiest to slip the catheter into the trachea. The cooperative patient should be told to inhale slowly and deeply. Try to avoid stimulating the patient's gag reflex by not striking the oropharynx with the tip of the catheter. The patient will cough vigorously when the catheter is in the trachea.
   4. Advance the catheter until an obstruction is felt. Then pull the catheter back about 2 cm.
   5. Withdraw the catheter with a twisting motion while suctioning intermittently. Suction to clear out any secretions. Typically, in the adult, suctioning may be applied for between 5 and 10 seconds. Suctioning in the infant may be applied for no more than 5 seconds. If the secretions are cleared, the catheter is pulled out. Practitioners disagree on whether the catheter should be withdrawn or left in place if the patient still has secretions. Some prefer to withdraw the catheter, let the patient rest and reoxygenate, and reinsert the catheter for more suctioning. Others prefer to leave the catheter in place to minimize tissue trauma from a reinsertion, let the patient rest and reoxygenate, and then suction again.
   6. The entire procedure usually takes longer than 20 seconds, so the O_2 tubing must be kept directed toward the patient's mouth.
   7. Turning the patient's head to the right might help direct the catheter down the left main-stem bronchus. The catheter will tend to enter the right main-stem bronchus if the head is in a neutral position or twisted to the left.

m. Reoxygenate the patient for at least 1 minute before suctioning again. Giving 100% O_2 (or 10% to 20% more than the base level in the infant) helps this happen faster.

n. Monitor the patient's vital signs, O_2 level, and breath sounds before suctioning again. Suction again, if needed, when the patient is stable.

o. Normal saline solution may be instilled down the suction catheter by pulling off the vacuum tubing, inserting the tip of the syringe (not needle) into the end of the catheter, covering the thumb control valve, and squirting the saline into the catheter. The other considerations listed earlier would apply here.

p. Dispose of the catheter and glove by pulling the glove inside out over the catheter.

q. Rinse the vacuum tubing clear of secretions.

r. Turn off the suction unit.

MODULE D
Respiratory care plan

1. Analyze available information to determine the patient's pathophysiologic state (CSE code: IIIH1)

Hearing coarse, intermittent expiratory sounds (crackles, or rhonchi) indicates that secretions are in the airway. Tracheal suctioning should clear these secretions and result in the return of normal breath sounds (or at least an improvement). Pneumonia and bronchitis result in chest radiograph changes that show areas of infiltrate. Disease involvement of right or left lung (or both), individual lobes, and segments can be determined. As the patient's condition improves, the chest radiograph should show clearing of infiltrates.

2. Determine the appropriateness of the prescribed therapy and goals for the identified pathophysiologic state (CSE code: IIIH3)

The standard physician's order for suctioning states that suctioning should be done as needed (PRN). The respiratory therapist or nurse or both should be able to evaluate the patient and perform suctioning when it is justified. It is inappropriate for the physician to suction the patient on a set schedule (for example, every hour). This could result in the patient being suctioned when it is not needed. Additionally, the therapist and nurse could not suction the patient more often. The respiratory care plan should allow the therapist to make the following changes.

a. Make a change in the size and type of suction catheter (WRE code: IIIF8b) [Difficulty: An]

As discussed earlier, the OD of the suction catheter should be no more than half the ID of the patient's endotracheal tube. If the secretions are easy to suction out, a smaller catheter may be used. The spontaneously breathing patient is less likely to become hypoxic if the tube is less obstructed.

A catheter with a Coudé tip should be used if the catheter must be directed into one or the other main-stem bronchus (usually the left). Closed airway catheters such as those made by Ballard Medical Products offer two advantages over single-use catheters. First, they are more economical if the patient needs frequent suctioning. Second, a patient using a mechanical ventilator continues to be ventilated and oxygenated and have positive end-expiratory pressure (PEEP) maintained during the suctioning episode. The newer catheters that offer intermittent or continuous insufflation of oxygen may reduce the hypoxemia that many patients experience during the suctioning procedure. However, they can be difficult to use and costly.

b. Change the level of vacuum used when suctioning (WRE code: IIIF8c) [Difficulty: Ap, An]

In general, the lowest possible vacuum level should be used that adequately removes secretions. Several authors have listed recommended maximum vacuum levels to be applied to adults, children, and neonates. However, the AARC Clinical Practice Guidelines on suctioning state that there is a lack of experimental data to support these or any other written maximum pressures.

c. Instill an irrigating solution into the trachea (WRE code: IIIF8d) [Difficulty: An]

Sterile normal saline solution (0.9%) is widely accepted as useful to instill into the trachea to dilute and mobilize pulmonary secretions. It should be used whenever secretions are difficult to suction out. Because the secretions are easier to remove, the respiratory therapist also can use a lower vacuum level. In adults, about 5 to 10 mL is instilled into the trachea and then suctioned out with any secretions. Less is used with children, but no universal guidelines are available. Neonates have been reportedly given a few drops to 0.33 mL.

d. Change the frequency of suctioning (WRE code: IIIF8a) [Difficulty: An]

Secretions obstruct the airways and should be removed if possible. Often this requires more than one suctioning episode. No harm is found in repeatedly suctioning the patient as long as he or she is reoxygenated between each session. Watch for any complications as listed in Boxes 13-1 and 13-2. Listen to the patient's breath sounds for rhonchi, or palpate the chest for secretions in between suctioning efforts. Stop suctioning when it is no longer needed.

e. Change the duration of the suctioning procedure (WRE code: IIIF8a) [Difficulty: An]

Suctioning generally takes between 5 and 10 seconds; the entire procedure should take between 10 and 15 seconds. Some patients may not be able to tolerate this. Be prepared to suction for a shorter period. Suction repeatedly rather than increasing the suctioning time.

As listed in Boxes 13-1 and 13-2, stop the procedure if the patient becomes hypoxic or has tachycardia, bradycardia, dysrhythmias, hypotension, or bronchospasm. Bloody secretions may indicate mucosal damage and justify stopping the procedure. Hypoxemia, tachycardia, bradycardia, dysrhythmias, hypotension, bronchospasm, pneumothorax, or pulmonary hemorrhage that place the patient's life in danger indicate the cancellation of the suctioning order. Once the underlying problem has been corrected and safe suctioning can be performed, the order may be resumed.

f. Stop the treatment or procedure if the patient has an adverse reaction to it (CSE code: IIIF1)

As listed in Boxes 13-1 and 13-2, stop the procedure if the patient becomes hypoxic or has tachycardia, bradycardia, arrhythmias, hypotension, or bronchospasm. Bloody secretions indicate possible mucosal damage and justify stopping the procedure. A conscious patient should be able to communicate how he or she feels after sections have been suctioned. It is hoped that the feeling of dyspnea will improve. Hypoxemia and vagal stimulation can cause unstable vital signs and bronchospasm. Be prepared to stop suctioning, give extra oxygen, or get help.

A conscious patient should be able to communicate with you about how he or she feels after suctioning of secretions. Hopefully, the feeling of dyspnea is improved. Inform the patient's nurse or physician and the supervising therapist if any serious question or problem occurs with the patient. Routine communication should occur as needed between these people and any other caregiver.

g. Discontinue treatment based on the patient's response (WRE code: IIIG1e) [Difficulty: An]

Hypoxemia, tachycardia, bradycardia, arrhythmias, hypotension, bronchospasm, pneumothorax, or pulmonary hemorrhage that places the patient's life in danger justifies the cancellation of the suctioning order. Once the underlying problem has been corrected and safe suctioning can be performed, the order may be resumed.

MODULE E

Record in conventional terminology any treatment(s) or procedure(s) performed, including the date, time, frequency of therapy, medication, and ventilatory data

1. Record and evaluate the patient's response to the treatment(s) or procedure(s), including the following:

a. Record and interpret the following: heart rate and rhythm, respiratory rate, blood pressure, body temperature, and pain level (WRE code: IIIA1b, IIIA1c) [Difficulty: An]

See the discussion on these topics in Chapter 1 or earlier in this chapter.

b. Record and interpret the patient's breath sounds (WRE code: IIIA1a) [Difficulty: An]

If suctioning is effective, the patient's breath sounds will improve. The rhonchi (crackles) that were heard before suctioning should now be absent. Normal breath sounds should be heard.

c. Record and interpret the type of cough the patient has and the nature of the sputum (WRE code: IIIA1a) [Difficulty: An]

The amount and consistency of sputum that a patient produces depends on the lung problem and whether it is worsening or improving. For example, if pneumonia or bronchitis is worsening, secretion production is increased. If the patient is dehydrated, the sputum contains less water than normal. The patient may complain that the secretions are "thicker" and harder to cough out. Airway suction may be needed to remove the secretions. As the patient's condition improves, a return to normal sputum consistency should occur, and less should be produced. The patient should be able to cough it out effectively.

BIBLIOGRAPHY

AARC Clinical Practice Guideline: Endotracheal suctioning of mechanically ventilated adults and children with artificial airways, *Respir Care* 38:500, 1993.

American Association for Respiratory Care: Clinical Practice Guideline: nasotracheal suctioning: 2004 revision and update, *Respir Care* 49(9):1080, 2004.

AARC: Clinical Practice Guideline: nasotracheal suctioning, *Respir Care* 37:898, 1992.

Burton GG: Patient assessment procedures. In Barnes TA, editor: *Respiratory care practice,* St Louis, 1998, Mosby.

Caldwell SL, Sullivan KN: Suctioning protocol. In Burton GG, Hodgkin JE, editors: *Respiratory care,* ed 2, Philadelphia, 1984, Lippincott.

Durbin CG: Airway management. In Cairo JM, Pilbeam SP, editors: *Mosby's respiratory care equipment,* ed 7, St. Louis, 2004, Mosby.

Eubanks DH, Bone RC: *Comprehensive respiratory care,* ed 2, St Louis, 1990, Mosby.

Fink JB, Hess DR: Secretion clearance techniques. In Hess DR, MacIntyre NR, Mishoe SC, et al, editors: *Respiratory care principles and practice,* Philadelphia, 2002, WB Saunders.

Guidelines for the prevention of nosocomial infections, *AARTimes* 7(9):x, 1983.

Hess DR, Branson RD: Airway and suctioning equipment. In Branson RD, Hess DR, Chatburn RL, editors: *Respiratory care equipment,* ed 2, Philadelphia, 1999, Lippincott Williams & Wilkins.

Lewis RM: Airway care. In Fink JB, Hunt GE, editors: *Clinical practice in respiratory care,* Philadelphia, 1999, Lippincott Williams & Wilkins.

McIntyre D: Airway management. In Wyka KA, Mathews PJ, Clark WF: *Foundations of respiratory care,* Albany, NY, 2002, Delmar.

Pettignano MM, Pettignano R: Airway management. In Barnhart SL, Czervinske MP, editors: *Perinatal and pediatric respiratory care,* Philadelphia, 1995, WB Saunders.

Plevak DJ, Ward JJ: Airway management. In Burton GG, Hodgkin JE, Ward JJ, editors: *Respiratory care,* ed 4, Philadelphia, 1997, Lippincott-Raven.

Rarey KP, Youtsey JW: *Respiratory patient care,* Englewood Cliffs, NJ, 1981, Prentice-Hall.

Roth P: Airway care. In Aloan CA, Hill TV, editors: *Respiratory care of the newborn and child,* ed 2, Philadelphia, 1997, Lippincott.

Scott AA, Koff PB: Airway care and chest physiotherapy. In Koff PB, Eitzmann DV, Neu J, editors: *Neonatal and pediatric respiratory care,* ed 2, St Louis, 1993, Mosby.

Shapiro BA, Kacmarek RM, Cane RD, et al: *Clinical application of respiratory care,* ed 4, St Louis, 1991, Mosby.

Simmons KF, Scanlan CL: Airway management. In Wilkins RL, Stoller JK, Scanlan CL, editors: *Egan's fundamentals of respiratory care,* ed 8 St Louis, 2003, Mosby.

Wilkins RL: Physical examination of the patient with cardiopulmonary disease. In Wilkins RL, Krider SJ, Sheldon RL, editors: *Clinical assessment in respiratory care,* ed 3, St Louis, 1995, Mosby.

Wilkins RL, Hodgkin, JE, Lopez B: *Lung sounds, a practical guide,* St Louis, 1988, Mosby.

Wojciechowski WV: Incentive spirometers, and secretion evacuation devices, and inspiratory muscle training devices. In Barnes TA, editor: *Core textbook of respiratory care practice,* ed 2, St Louis, 1994, Mosby.

SELF-STUDY QUESTIONS

1. Your patient is being mechanically ventilated with 60% oxygen and 8 cm of PEEP. Twice she has had her Spo$_2$ value and blood pressure decrease when she was removed from the ventilator for suctioning. What should be recommended to prevent this from happening again?
   A. Switch to a smaller suction catheter.
   B. Switch to a larger suction catheter.
   C. Increase her PEEP to 10 cm water before and after the suctioning.
   D. Use a closed-system suction catheter.

2. It is difficult to remove the tracheal secretions from your adult patient when using 60 mm Hg of vacuum pressure. What should be done?
   A. Suction for 20 seconds.
   B. Suction more frequently.
   C. Increase the vacuum pressure to 80 mm Hg.
   D. Change from the central vacuum system to a portable one.

3. When selecting a catheter OD for suctioning through an endotracheal tube, it is important that it be:
   A. No more than one fourth the ID of the tube
   B. No less than one half the ID of the tube
   C. No less than three fourths the ID of the tube
   D. No more than one half the ID of the tube

4. Your 40-year-old patient has pneumonia in her left lower lobe with a large amount of secretions. What would you recommend to be able to suction her better?
   A. Use the largest diameter suction catheter that is available.
   B. Use a suction catheter with a Coudé tip.
   C. Use the longest suction catheter that is available.
   D. Increase the length of time that you apply suction.

5. Your patient is receiving mechanical ventilation and has an 8.0-mm oral endotracheal tube in place. Over the course of the shift, it is noticed that the patient has more tracheal secretions. What is the best course of action?
   A. Suction more often.
   B. Suction for longer periods.
   C. Change to a closed airway suction catheter.
   D. Administer nebulized atropine.

6. A conscious patient requires nasotracheal suctioning. During the suctioning procedure, the patient's blood pressure decreases to 100/60 mm Hg, and heart rate decreases from 110 to 60 beats/min. What should be done?
   A. Change to a catheter with a larger diameter.
   B. Shorten the suctioning time.
   C. Insert an oropharyngeal airway before suctioning.
   D. Squirt 5 mL of saline down the suction catheter into the patient's trachea.

7. The respiratory therapist is called to set up a suctioning system for a new patient in the intensive care unit. To measure the vacuum pressure, what should be done?
   A. Check the manometer while occluding the catheter tip.
   B. Set the vacuum control to maximum.
   C. Close the thumb control valve on the catheter.
   D. Check the manometer while pinching off the connecting tubing.

8. A 16-year-old female patient is intubated with a 7.0-mm endotracheal tube and is receiving mechanical ventilation. After suctioning with a 14Fr catheter, it is noticed on the electrocardiogram monitor that the patient is bradycardic. What should be recommended?
   A. Administer 10 cm PEEP.
   B. Limit suctioning to twice a shift.
   C. Change to a 10Fr catheter.
   D. Use a catheter with a Coudé tip.

9. An intubated patient with pneumonia must have a sputum sample sent to the laboratory for culture and sensitivity testing. What is the most appropriate way to get a sample?
   A. Place a Lukens trap between the suction catheter and the vacuum tubing.
   B. Suction the oropharynx with a sterile Yankauer suction catheter.
   C. Place a Lukens trap between the vacuum tubing and the collection bottle.
   D. Suction the patient, and place the catheter inside the Lukens trap.

ANSWER KEY

1. **D.** Rationale: A closed-system suction catheter allows the patient to be ventilated and keep the PEEP level while suctioning is being performed. This should help to prevent hypoxemia. Changing to a smaller or larger diameter open airway suction catheter will not significantly improve the patient's situation. When the patient is taken off of the ventilator and suctioned, she will become hypoxemic. Additional PEEP will not prevent hypoxemia when the patient is taken off of the ventilator.

2. **C.** Rationale: Increasing the vacuum pressure from 60 to 80 mm Hg will result in the secretions being removed more quickly. The whole suctioning procedure is usually limited to 15 seconds. Suctioning for

20 seconds will remove more secretions but is also likely to cause hypoxemia. Suctioning more frequently will not prove effective if the suctioning level is too low at 60 mm Hg. A hospital's central vacuum system is more powerful than a portable one and will suction more effectively.

3. **D.** Rationale: It is commonly accepted practice to limit the OD of a suction catheter to no more than one half the ID of the endotracheal or tracheostomy tube. This allows the patient to breathe spontaneously around the catheter during the procedure, as shown in Fig. 13-3. See Table 13-1 for recommendations on tube size and suction catheter. A smaller catheter may be used but will not remove as many secretions with each suctioning effort. This may result in the need to suction more frequently. Too frequent suctioning can result in greater risk of trauma to the mucous membrane, hypoxemia, and vagal stimulation. A larger suction catheter prevents the patient from being able to breathe around it.

4. **B.** Rationale: A suction catheter with a Coudé tip may enable you to guide the catheter to either the left or right mainstem bronchus. A straight catheter has a tendency to go down the right mainstem bronchus of an adult. This is because it comes off of the trachea at the carina at a more acute angle than the left mainstem bronchus. (A newborn patient does not have a significant difference in the angle of the main-stem bronchi from the trachea.) As discussed in question 3, the diameter of the catheter should not be more the one half the ID of the endotracheal tube. Any adult size suction catheter is long enough to suction adequately. Increasing the time of suctioning puts the patient at risk for hypoxemia.

5. **A.** Rationale: More frequent suctioning is called for if the patient has more secretions. Suctioning for longer periods puts the patient at risk for hypoxemia. No indication exists that a closed airway suction catheter is needed (hypoxemia or therapeutic PEEP) or will be more effective than a standard catheter. Nebulized atropine in a large enough dose decreases secretion production. However, a dose large enough to do this is also likely to cause tachycardia. Atropine is rarely given to control secretions outside of the operating room. A physician's order is needed to give this medication.

6. **B.** Rationale: Because the patient is having an adverse reaction to the suctioning procedure, the suctioning time should be shortened. Changing to a catheter with a larger diameter increases the risk of trauma to the mucous membrane of the patient's nasal passage. Inserting an oropharyngeal airway before suctioning may stimulate the conscious patient's gag reflex. In addition, the airway may block the suction catheter from passing through the patient's oropharynx to the larynx and trachea. Squirting 5 mL of saline down the suction catheter into the patient's trachea will probably trigger coughing. This could worsen the patient's distress with the whole procedure.

7. **D.** Rationale: To seal the system and determine the set vacuum pressure, check the manometer while pinching off the connecting tubing. The system is not sealed off if the therapist just occludes the catheter tip; the thumb control valve is still open. Setting the vacuum control to maximum without sealing off the system allows an air leak. Therefore the pressure cannot be measured. The system is not sealed off if the therapist just closes the thumb control valve on the catheter; the catheter tip opening is still open.

8. **C.** Rationale: Change to a 10Fr catheter because the 14Fr catheter is too large for the endotracheal tube. See Table 13-1 for the catheter and tube combinations that should be used. A physician's order is needed to administer 10 cm PEEP. There is no indication that the patient is having any difficulties other than bradycardia during the suctioning procedure. Suctioning should be done as often as needed and not limited to twice per shift. The patient experiences bradycardia whenever she is suctioned because the catheter is too large. No indication is found that a catheter with a Coudé tip is needed to guide the catheter down the left (or right) mainstem bronchus.

9. **A.** Rationale: The only way to get an uncontaminated sputum sample is to place a Lukens trap between the suction catheter and the vacuum tubing. This way, the patient's secretions are collected within the Lukens trap after they have passed through the sterile suction catheter. Suctioning the patient's oropharynx with a sterile Yankauer suction catheter provides an oral sample, not a tracheal sample. It is likely that the patient's mouth contains additional microorganisms besides the ones causing the pneumonia. Placing a Lukens trap between the vacuum tubing and the collection bottle will provide a contaminated sample. This is because the vacuum tubing is not sterile as is a suction catheter. The Lukens trap is designed to hold secretions and keep them from becoming contaminated. It is not designed to hold a suction catheter.

14 Intermittent Positive-Pressure Breathing

Note 1: The National Board for Respiratory Care (NBRC) has released the *RRT Examination Matrix* (covering the testable items on the Written Registry Exam) and the *CSE Examination Matrix* (covering the testable items on the Clinical Simulation Exam). Turn to the appendices at the back of this book for both publications in their original formats. This book is intended to cover all of the testable items in these two publications. This chapter (and all others) uses the abbreviation "WRE" for the coded items testable on the Written Registry Exam *and* Clinical Simulation Exam. The listed difficulty (R, Recall; Ap, Application; An, Analysis) relates to the question difficulty on the Written Registry Exam. The abbreviation "CSE" is used for the coded items testable on *only* the Clinical Simulation Exam. Because no question difficulty level is given for this exam, be prepared for anything.

Note 2: *A review of the most recent Written Registry Examinations has shown an average of two questions (2% of the exam) that cover IPPB therapy. The Clinical Simulation Exam is comprehensive and may include everything that should be known or performed by an advanced level respiratory therapist.*

MODULE A

Initiate and adjust intermittent positive-pressure breathing therapy to achieve adequate spontaneous ventilation and oxygenation (WRE Code: IIID2a) [Difficulty: An]

1. Indications

The following indications and guidelines are listed in the American Association for Respiratory Care (AARC) Clinical Practice Guideline on intermittent positive-pressure breathing (IPPB).

To treat atelectasis when other deep breathing methods are ineffective. Patients who are uncooperative, unconscious, or physically incapable of being coached in deep breathing and coughing techniques or in performing incentive spirometry may be helped by IPPB. The patient who cannot generate an inspiratory capacity (IC) of greater than 12 mL/kg, a vital capacity (VC) of greater than 15 mL/kg, or who has a postoperative IC less than 33% of the preoperative value can benefit from IPPB rather than incentive spirometry. An inspiratory pause at the end of the IPPB breath helps to distribute the gas better to open areas of atelectasis.

The AARC Guideline lists the following poor pulmonary function values as supporting the need for IPPB. This guideline suggests that the patient would have an ineffective cough: VC less than 70% of predicted or less than 10 mL/kg, forced expiratory volume in 1 second (FEV_1) less than 65% of predicted, or maximum voluntary ventilation (MVV) less than 50% of predicted.

To deliver aerosolized medications more effectively. If the patient cannot coordinate his or her breathing pattern to make use of a metered dose inhaler or hand-held nebulizer, IPPB may be used. Examples of when IPPB is preferable include any situation in which the patient is unconscious, uncooperative, or physically incapable. These patients are physically unable to make effective use of simpler methods of lung inflation (incentive spirometry) or to take an aerosolized medication (metered dose inhaler or hand-held nebulizer). Examples of these types of patients include the elderly, the chronically debilitated, patients with neuromuscular diseases, and patients with kyphoscoliosis. It also may be used to provide temporary support to home care patients.

To enhance the patient's cough effort and sputum clearance. The combination of aerosolized saline, with or without a bronchodilator or mucolytic, and deeper tidal volumes may help the patient to cough more productively. The practitioner must stop the treatment periodically to coach the patient's cough effort.

The following additional indications were listed in Guidelines for the Use of Intermittent Positive-Pressure Breathing:

To treat impending ventilatory failure as seen by an increased arterial carbon dioxide pressure ($PaCO_2$ more effectively). It may be possible to delay or avoid intubation and mechanical ventilation in the deteriorating chronic obstructive pulmonary disease (COPD) patient. The patient is able to relax and reduce the work of breathing (WOB) during a passive IPPB treatment. It may be necessary to give IPPB for 5 to 10 minutes as often as every one half to 1 hour. The treatment also should be given with the intention of helping the patient's cough and sputum clearance.

To help manage the patient with acute pulmonary edema. IPPB can help in the management by temporarily reducing the venous return to the heart. The IPPB procedure does not correct the underlying cardiac problem, which must be treated by other means.

To induce a sputum sample for culture and sensitivity or other diagnostic studies. Inducing a sputum sample by IPPB is indicated only if simpler methods have failed.

To deliver medications for special purposes when simpler methods do not work. IPPB should be used to deliver medication when simpler methods fail (for example, using a small volume nebulizer to deliver a local anesthetic such as lidocaine [Xylocaine] before a bronchoscopy procedure).

2. Contraindications

Untreated pneumothorax is listed by all authors and the AARC Guideline as an absolute contraindication. An increased intrathoracic pressure converts a simple pneumothorax into a tension pneumothorax. The consequences can be fatal. Once a chest tube has been inserted into the pleural space and a pleural drainage system set up, IPPB can be administered. An increase in the air leak may occur, but it should not be life threatening.

The AARC Guideline lists the following as relative contraindications. Any patient with one of the following contraindications should be evaluated carefully before a decision about the clinical use of IPPB is made:

a. Active hemoptysis. Coughing up blood indicates that a tear has occurred in the airway or lung tissues. The IPPB treatment should be stopped if a large amount of hemoptysis is present. Certainly massive hemoptysis (defined as >600 mL of blood coughed out in a 16-hour period) contraindicates IPPB.

b. Hemodynamic instability

c. Intracranial pressure greater than 15 mm Hg

d. Chest radiograph that shows a bleb

e. Tracheoesophageal fistula

f. Recent surgery on the esophagus, skull, face, or mouth

g. Untreated, active tuberculosis (hazard to the practitioner)

h. Nausea, air swallowing, or hiccups (singultation)

3. Hazards and precautions

The AARC Guideline lists the following hazards and precautions for IPPB therapy:

a. Pneumothorax

b. Barotrauma

c. Increased airway resistance from a bronchospastic reaction to the positive pressure or an adverse reaction to a medication. This can result in alveolar overdistention and air trapping.

d. Hyperoxia when 100% oxygen is delivered to the patient. Some COPD patients who are hypercarbic and breathing on hypoxic drive may hypoventilate as a result.

e. Secretions that may become impacted when the inhaled gas is not humidified adequately

f. Nosocomial infection

g. Decreased venous return

h. Increased ventilation-to-perfusion mismatch. This may worsen any hypoxemia.

i. Hyperventilation

j. Psychological dependence. This may be seen in the long-term home care patient who does not want to switch to another method of taking inhaled medications.

k. Hypocarbia

l. Hemoptysis

m. Gastric distention

n. Air trapping, auto-PEEP, or overdistended alveoli

4. Initiation of therapy
a. Steps in the basic procedure

1. Check for a complete and proper order specifying the patient, oxygen percentage, frequency of treatment, medication, and any special considerations.

2. Gather the necessary equipment, medication, and so on.

3. Set up the equipment outside of the patient's room.

4. Introduce yourself, the department, and your purpose to the patient.

5. Confirm the patient's identity.

6. Have the patient sit up in bed or in a chair; an obese patient may stand.

7. Interview the patient.

8. Assess the patient's vital signs.

9. Assess the patient's breath sounds.

10. Prepare the IPPB unit for operation:
    a. If the unit is electrical, plug into a working outlet.
    b. If the unit is pneumatic, plug into either a compressed air or oxygen outlet, as ordered.
    c. Set the following controls:
       i. Set sensitivity at -1 cm H_2O pressure.
       ii. Set nebulizer to run on inspiration only.
       iii. Adjust the flow as necessary.
       iv. Set the peak pressure at about 10 to 15 cm H_2O.

d. Test the nebulizer by turning on the machine.

e. Cover the mouthpiece with a clean tissue to ensure that it cycles off at the preset pressure.

11. Instruct the patient to sip on the mouthpiece like a straw to turn the machine on. Have the patient relax and let the machine fill his or her lungs with air. The patient should hold his or her breath in for 2 to 3 seconds and exhale slowly.

b. Giving a passive treatment

Most authors describe the patient taking a passive treatment. In a passive treatment, the patient relaxes and lets the machine fill the lungs until the preset pressure is reached. As mentioned earlier, the patient is then told to hold in his or her breath before exhaling passively. This treatment is given with the intent of minimizing the patient's work of breathing (WOB). As slow a flow rate as possible is used so that any nebulized medication is deposited deeply into the small airways and lungs.

c. Giving an active treatment

Several authors advocate having the patient take an active treatment in which he or she interacts with the IPPB machine to get as deep a breath as possible.

Welch and colleagues found that the patient's post-treatment IC is greatest when the practitioner (1) uses as high a peak pressure as the patient can tolerate, and (2) coaches the patient to inhale as deeply as possible with the IPPB machine. They and others believe that this is the best way to treat or prevent atelectasis.

5. Initial settings on the Bird Mark 7

The older version of the Mark 7 is used as the model respirator of the Bird series. The current Mark 8 has similar features. Other Bird units have slightly different controls and features. Refer to Fig. 14-1 for the following:

a. Adjust the *air mix* knob to the desired gas mix.

b. Sensitivity should be set so that the patient has to generate about -1 cm H_2O pressure to cycle the unit on. Set the *sensitivity* control (on the left-hand side of the unit when facing it) to the reference number 15. This is at approximately the 2 o'clock position. Turning the control lever counterclockwise makes the unit more sensitive. Push in the hand-timer rod to note that the unit cycles on easily.

c. Flow should be set so that the patient feels comfortable with the inspiratory time. Set the *flow rate* knob so that the reference number 15 is at the 12 o'clock position; the *off* sign will be at the 8 o'clock position. Turning the *flow rate* knob counterclockwise increases the flow.

d. Peak pressure should be set at about 10 to 15 cm H_2O pressure. Set the *pressure* control (on the right-hand side of the unit when facing it) to the reference number 15. This is at approximately the 10 o'clock position. Turning the control lever more clockwise increases the peak pressure. Hold a clean tissue against the patient's mouthpiece to see that the unit cycles off at the desired peak pressure.

6. Initial settings on the Bennett PR-2

The PR-2 is used as the model respirator of the Bennett series. (Although the PR-2 is no longer being produced, many are still in clinical use.) Other Bennett units have slightly different controls and features. Refer to Figs. 14-2 and 14-3 for the following:

a. Adjust the *air dilution* knob to the desired gas mix.

b. Sensitivity should be set so that the patient has to generate about -1 cm H_2O pressure to cycle the unit on. Turning the control lever counterclockwise makes the unit more sensitive. Push up on the Bennett valve strut to note that the unit cycles on easily.

c. Flow should be set so that the patient feels comfortable with the inspiratory time. The Bennett valve is designed to automatically open and close itself to allow the patient as much flow as desired. Set the *peak flow* control knob as counterclockwise as possible so that it is at the maximum setting. Turning the *peak flow* knob more clockwise will decrease the patient's peak flow.

d. Peak pressure should be set at about 10 to 15 cm H_2O pressure. Dial the *pressure* control clockwise until the *control pressure* gauge shows the desired peak pressure. Hold a clean tissue against the patient's mouthpiece to see that when the unit cycles off, the *system pressure* gauge reads the same as the *control pressure* gauge.

e. Turn the *inspiration nebulization* control counterclockwise for medication to be nebulized only during an inspiration. Some practitioners believe that the *expiration nebulization* control should be turned on slightly so that the mouthpiece and circuit dead space are filled with medication before the next breath. Others are opposed to this because it wastes medication when the patient stops the treatment.

f. A small leak in the circuit, mouthpiece, or face mask can be overcome by adding some additional flow by turning on the *terminal flow* control. It is normally left off. Turn the control counterclockwise to add as much additional flow as necessary to overcome the leak.

Details on the design and control specifications for the various Bird and Bennett models can be found in the manufacturers' literature and books on respiratory therapy equipment.

Fig. 14-1 Controls and features of the Bird Mark 7 intermittent positive-pressure breathing unit.

MODULE B

Independently adjust IPPB therapy based on the patient's response

1. Change the patient machine interface (WRE code: IIIF1) [Difficulty: An]

a. Mouthpiece

A conscious, cooperative patient can take a treatment with a mouthpiece. He or she must be instructed to place the mouthpiece between the teeth (or gums) and seal the lips around it so that no leak occurs. Instruct the patient to sip gently on it to turn on the IPPB machine. As long as the lips are sealed and no other leaks occur, the positive-pressure breath will stop when the preset pressure is reached. Nose clips are often helpful to prevent a leak through the nose as the patient is learning how to take the treatment. The nose clips can be removed after the patient has learned how to seal the nasopharynx with the soft palate.

A variety of mouthpieces are available. All share the common features of a raised edge so that the teeth do not

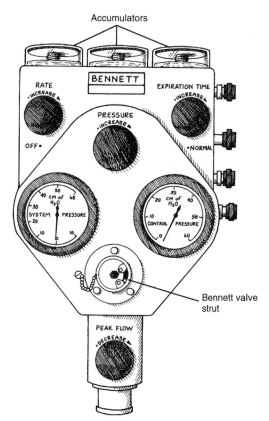

Fig. 14-2 Front controls and features of the Bennett PR-2 intermittent positive-pressure breathing unit.

slip off and a 22-mm outer diameter (OD) connector end to insert into the IPPB circuit (Fig. 14-4).

b. Mouth seal (Bennett seal)

An unconscious, uncooperative, or aged patient who cannot seal his or her lips can be aided by placing a soft rubber seal around the mouthpiece. The practitioner gently holds the seal around the patient's lips to seal the airway so that the patient can trigger the breath and cycle the machine off (Fig. 14-5). Nose clips also are commonly needed.

c. Face mask

The face mask can be used if the mouth seal does not provide an airtight seal. This might be because of the patient's facial structure or lack of teeth. Mouth trauma, surgery, or lip sores are other reasons to use a face mask.

The mask should be clear and properly sized to fit comfortably over the patient's nose and mouth. The practitioner should be able to get a seal with a minimum amount of hand pressure (Fig. 14-6). The equipment connection opening in the mask has a 22-mm inner diameter (ID) so that it connects directly to the IPPB circuit. A 22-mm OD male adapter and short length of aerosol tubing can be added for flexibility and patient comfort. The clear mask is important so that the practitioner can see whether the patient has vomited or has a large amount of secretions or saliva in his or her mouth. The mask should never be strapped to the patient's face so that the practitioner can attend to another patient.

Fig. 14-3 Right side controls and features of the Bennett PR-2 intermittent positive-pressure breathing unit.

Fig. 14-4 Universal intermittent positive-pressure breathing mouthpiece with a tapered 22- to 18-mm machine connector.

Fig. 14-6 Giving an intermittent positive-pressure breathing treatment with the use of a face mask.

Fig. 14-5 *Top,* Bennett or mouth flange seal. *Bottom,* Intermittent positive-pressure breathing mouthpiece inserted into the seal.

Fig. 14-7 Giving an intermittent positive-pressure breathing (IPPB) treatment with the use of a tracheostomy/endotracheal tube adapter.

This is the least effective patient attachment device if the therapeutic goal is to deliver an aerosolized medication. Much of the medication rains out on the patient's face or in the nasal passages if he or she is a nose breather.

d. Tracheostomy/endotracheal tube (elbow) adapter

The elbow adapter is designed to connect the patient's tracheostomy or endotracheal tube to the IPPB circuit (or other respiratory care equipment). The IPPB end has a 22-mm ID connector. The tracheostomy/endotracheal tube end has a 15-mm ID connector (Fig. 14-7). If the

patient has had the cuff deflated, it must be reinflated to seal the airway. An unsealed cuff results in an air leak, and the gas flow will not turn off.

2. Adjust the sensitivity (WRE code: IIIG3a) [Difficulty: An]

The sensitivity of the IPPB unit refers to how much effort or work the patient must perform to turn the unit on for a breath. Commonly, the sensitivity is set so that the patient has to generate a negative pressure of only about −1 cm H_2O pressure to begin an inspiration. This can be seen by looking at the needle deflecting into the negative range on the pressure manometer. Ask the patient whether the machine can be easily turned on to get a breath. The IPPB unit should not be set at a level so sensitive that it self-cycles.

The sensitivity range on the Bird series is −0.01 to −5 cm H_2O. Turning the *sensitivity/starting effort* adjustment lever counterclockwise toward the smaller reference numbers makes the unit more sensitive. The sensitivity range on the Bennett series is −0.5 to −1 cm H_2O. Turning the *sensitivity* control counterclockwise makes the unit easier to turn on.

3. Adjust the fractional concentration of inspired oxygen (WRE code: IIIF1) [Difficulty: An]

Compressed air or oxygen can power both the Bird and Bennett units. The patient's condition determines the oxygen percentage administered. The physician may include the oxygen percentage in the treatment order. Some departments have oxygen protocols in their treatment procedure. Generally, compressed air (21% oxygen) should be used whenever the patient does not need supplemental oxygen.

A patient with COPD who is retaining carbon dioxide and breathing on hypoxic drive should also be given room air via the IPPB unit. The patient may be allowed to keep wearing a nasal cannula with oxygen during the treatment so that the blood oxygen level is kept normal. The unavailability of piped-in compressed air should not be an excuse to give a patient a high oxygen percentage when it may be harmful. IPPB can be given through a gas-powered unit powered by a compressed air cylinder or an electrically powered unit.

Supplemental oxygen is given if either unit is powered by oxygen and the *air mix/air dilution* knobs are set to dilute the source gas with room air. This is appropriate for patients who require supplemental oxygen and are not at risk of stopping their spontaneous ventilation. Most practitioners use this method of giving IPPB because piped oxygen is usually available in all patients' rooms.

Pure oxygen should be given to the patient who is severely hypoxemic. Examples include acute pulmonary edema, respiratory failure, and carbon monoxide poisoning. The *air mix/air dilution* knobs must be set so that only the source gas (oxygen) is delivered to the patient.

For varying oxygen percentages on the Mark 7, note the following guidelines:

a. Pushing the *air mix* knob into the center body results in pure source gas. This can be either air or oxygen.
b. Pulling the *air mix* knob out of the center body results in a dilution of the source gas with room air. If oxygen

is the source gas, the room air will dilute the delivered gas to between 60% and 90% (or more) oxygen.

For varying oxygen percentage on the PR-2, note the following guidelines:

a. Pulling the *air dilution* knob out of the body results in pure source gas. This can be either air or oxygen.
b. Pushing the *air dilution* knob into the body results in a dilution of the source gas with room air. If oxygen is the source gas, the room air will dilute the delivered gas to between 40% and 80% oxygen.
c. Turning on the *terminal flow* control results in the dilution of source gas with room air. This dilutes the final percentage if the source gas is oxygen.

4. Adjust the flow (WRE code: IIIF1) [Difficulty: An]

The patient should initially feel comfortable with the flow rate and the inspiratory time. Ideally, the flow should result in a smooth, steady increase in the pressure up to the pre-set maximum pressure. Reduce the flow if the pressure increases too quickly. Increase the flow if the pressure wavers higher and lower; this indicates the patient is breathing in faster than the gas is being delivered. Ask the patient a simple question, such as, "Is the breath coming too fast or too slowly?" He or she can give you a short answer or even a hand gesture in response. As the treatment progresses, the practitioner may be able to adjust the flow to modify the patient's breathing pattern to better achieve the therapeutic goal, for example:

a. Anxious patients may initially need a fast flow. As they are coached to relax and get used to the treatment, the practitioner should try to reduce the flow.
b. Slower flows result in medications being deposited deeper into the lungs. This is important if the patient is having a bronchodilator, mucolytic, or antibiotic nebulized.
c. Faster flows result in the deposition of medications in the upper airways. This is important if the patient is receiving racemic epinephrine for laryngeal edema or lidocaine for a local anesthetic of the upper airway before bronchoscopy.

Turning the *inspiratory time/flow rate* control counterclockwise increases the flow rate on the Bird series. Pulling the *air mix* knob out from the center body increases the total flow by allowing room air to be entrained along with the source gas. Flow rate in the PR-2 is determined by the patient's inspiratory effort and how open the Bennett valve is. Flow can be decreased somewhat by turning the *peak flow* control clockwise. Flow is not affected by the position of the *air dilution* knob.

5. Adjust the volume, pressure, or both (WRE code: IIIF1) [Difficulty: An]

A review of the current respiratory care textbooks reveals that all authors agree that the basic goal of IPPB is to increase how deeply the patient inspires. Unfortunately, considerable differences are found about what inspiratory volume is being measured or by how much that breath should be increased for therapeutic goals to be achieved. The AARC has released the following on the subject:

a. The AARC Clinical Practice Guideline (1993) on IPPB: The tidal volume delivered during an IPPB-assisted breath should be at least 25% greater than the patient's spontaneous breaths.

b. The AARC Clinical Practice Guideline (1991) on incentive spirometry: IPPB is indicated to treat atelectasis rather than incentive spirometry if (i) the patient's IC is less than 33% of the preoperative value, or (ii) the patient's VC is less than 10 mL/kg of ideal body weight.

If the therapeutic goal is to prevent or treat atelectasis, having the patient inspire a deeper than spontaneous tidal volume breath should help. It seems reasonable to follow the AARC guidelines both as indications and as clinical goals. They can be used as guidelines if an increased tidal volume is used as a substitute for the VC. Based on this assumption, an IPPB delivered tidal volume goal of at least 10 mL/kg of ideal body weight seems reasonable. Because all of the current IPPB units are pressure cycled, the only way to increase the inspired volume during a passive treatment is to increase the peak pressure. Coaching the patient during an active treatment results in a larger volume without the need for as great a peak pressure. Decrease the peak pressure if the patient complains of discomfort or cannot hold that much pressure without losing the lip seal.

6. Eliminate auto-PEEP by adjusting the expiratory retard (WRE code: IIIG3k1) [Difficulty: An]

Expiratory retard is indicated in patients who have small airway disease and are air trapping on exhalation. Over the course of an IPPB treatment, this can lead to an increased functional residual capacity (FRC), which is seen as auto-PEEP. This lung overinflation increases the risk of pulmonary barotrauma. Adding expiratory retard to the treatment has the same effect as pursed-lips breathing. The increased backpressure on the smallest airways keeps them open longer so that the more distal air can be exhaled.

It is important to measure the exhaled volumes during the treatment and monitor the patient's response to know how much retard is needed. Too little retard results in some air trapping and an incompletely exhaled tidal volume. Too much retard results in an uncomfortably long expiratory time and an increased mean intrathoracic pressure. The proper amount of expiratory retard should result in the patient feeling comfortable with the breathing cycle and being able to exhale the tidal volume completely. Listening to the patient's breath sounds also is

helpful. If wheezing is present, it can be minimized when the proper amount of retard is added. This is because the backpressure is properly adjusted to minimize the small airway collapse.

Bird makes a retard cap that fits over the exhalation valve port on their permanent circuit. The cap has a series of different size holes through which the exhaled gas can pass (Fig. 14-8). By rotating the cap progressively from the largest to the smallest opening and evaluating the patient at each setting, the proper size opening and amount of retard can be found.

Bennett makes a retard exhalation valve that can be substituted for the regular exhalation valve on their permanent circuit (Fig. 14-9). The valve consists of a spring attached to a nut and a diaphragm. As the nut is turned counterclockwise, the spring pushes the diaphragm closer to the exhalation valve opening. This

Fig. 14-8 Bird retard cap for providing adjustable expiratory resistance. *(From McPherson SP: Respiratory therapy equipment, ed 5, St Louis, 1995, Mosby.)*

Fig. 14-9 Bennett retard exhalation valve for providing adjustable expiratory resistance. *(From McPherson SP: Respiratory therapy equipment, ed 5, St Louis, 1995, Mosby.)*

causes resistance to the exhalation of the tidal volume, and a backpressure is created against the airways. If too much pressure is placed against the exhalation valve opening, the patient will not be able to exhale back to atmospheric pressure. This should not be done without an order from the physician.

Be sure to ask the patient's opinion about the use of expiratory retard. The conscious, cooperative patient can tell you if he or she feels as if more air is getting out by the use of the retard or if the lungs feel more full because too much retard is being used. Too much retard may also make the expiratory time uncomfortably long.

Exam Hint

Commonly a question deals with adjusting the equipment settings to increase the tidal volume (increase the pressure) or needing to give a faster breath (increase the flow).

MODULE C
IPPB equipment

1. Get the proper IPPB circuit for the patient's treatment (WRE code: IIA10b) [Difficulty: Ap, An]

The two most widely used IPPB machines are the Bird Mark 7/8 (or a variation on it found in the series) and the Bennett PR-2. Both are pneumatically powered and found in most hospitals. Each unit requires a circuit that is designed specifically for it. See Fig. 14-10 for a drawing of a permanent (reusable after cleaning) and disposable circuit for a Bird machine. See Fig. 14-11 for a drawing of a permanent (reusable after cleaning) and disposable circuit for a Bennett machine.

2. Put the IPPB circuit together, make sure that it works properly, and identify any problems (WRE code: IIA10b) [Difficulty: Ap, An]

See Fig. 14-10 for the Bird setup and Fig. 14-11 for the Bennett setup.

a. General setup procedures

1. Check for plentiful source gas. Make sure that the oxygen or air tank has the proper regulator. Check the pressure in the gas cylinder.

Fig. 14-10 Features of permanent and disposable Bird intermittent positive-pressure breathing circuits.

Fig. 14-11 Features of permanent and disposable Bennett intermittent positive-pressure breathing circuits.

2. Attach the high-pressure hose to the source gas and the IPPB unit at the gas inlet. Make sure that the connections are tight.

3. Bacteria filters are optional. They are inserted between the IPPB unit gas outlets and the mainstream and nebulizer hoses.

4. A cascade-type humidifier is optional. Some practitioners prefer to warm and humidify the mainstream gas before it reaches the patient.

5. Check to see that the IPPB circuit is put together properly and that all of the connections are tight.

6. Set the initial treatment parameters for sensitivity, flow, and peak pressure. Manually cycle the unit on. Cover the mouthpiece to see that the unit cycles off at the preset pressure.

7. Add any medication to the nebulizer. Check to see that the nebulizer is producing a mist.

b. Bird setup

1. One end of the mainstream (large bore) hose is connected to the mainstream breathing hose connector on the right side of the unit. The other end is connected to the nebulizer.

2. One end of the nebulizer (small bore) hose is connected to the small nipple on the right-hand side of the unit. The other end is connected to a T-piece at the nebulizer.

3. A piece of small bore hose is used to connect one limb of the T-piece and the exhalation valve. Gas flowing through this hose powers both the nebulizer and the exhalation valve.

c. Bennett setup

1. One end of the mainstream (large bore) hose is connected to the mainstream breathing hose connector on the underside of the unit. The other end is connected to the nebulizer.

2. One end of the nebulizer (medium bore) hose is connected to the larger of two nipples on the underside of the unit. The other end is connected to the nebulizer nipple.

3. One end of the exhalation (small bore) hose is connected to the smaller of two nipples on the underside of the unit. The other end is connected to the exhalation valve nipple.

3. Fix any problems with the equipment (WRE code: IIA10b) [Difficulty: Ap, An]

Fixing a problem is possible only after the problem has been identified. The practitioner should be familiar with both permanent and disposable types of Bird and Bennett circuits. Leaks of any sort in the circuit prevent the unit from cycling off so that the patient can exhale. Tighten any friction fit or screw-type connections to stop the leak. A leak at the source gas connection or high-pressure hose gas inlet connection results in a rather loud hissing sound. When connections are tightened properly, the hissing and leak will stop.

Debris such as mucus or blood can plug the nebulizer capillary tube and prevent any mist from being formed. Disassemble the nebulizer, and rinse it under running water to try to clear the capillary tube. Replace the nebulizer if necessary.

Exam Hint

Commonly a question covers the reason(s) that an IPPB machine may fail to cycle off. Know to seal off an air leak around the patient's mouthpiece, within the circuit, or to inflate the cuff on a tracheostomy tube.

MODULE D
Respiratory care plan

1. Analyze available information to determine the patient's pathophysiologic state (CSE code: IIIH1)

Atelectasis is determined by characteristic chest radiograph findings and decreased or absent breath sounds over the affected area. Wheezing breath sounds is a finding indicating bronchospasm. Pulmonary edema has characteristic chest radiograph findings and cardiovascular indicators. Review discussion on these conditions and their findings in Chapters 1 and 5. IPPB has been used in the management of patients with these conditions if other methods are not effective.

2. Determine the appropriateness of the prescribed therapy and goals for the identified pathophysiologic state (CSE code: IIIH3)
   a. **Review the interdisciplinary patient and family care plan (WRE code: IIIH1b) [Difficulty: An]**
   b. **Review the planned therapy to establish the therapeutic plan (WRE code: IIIH1a) [Difficulty: An]**
   c. **Recommend changes in the therapeutic plan if supportive data exist (WRE code: IIIH2) [Difficulty: An]**

For the patient to receive the best care possible, the respiratory therapist must know the indications, contraindications, complications, and hazards of the respiratory care procedures the patient will receive. The patient must be assessed before, during, and after the treatment or procedure to determine whether it was effective. The key goal of an appropriate care plan is that the patient's condition be treated in the best way possible. Modifications to the care plan must be made, as needed, as the patient's condition changes.

The respiratory therapist should be a member of the patient care team of the physician, nurse, and others in deciding how best to care for the patient. The following steps are necessary in developing the respiratory care plan for any patient:

1. Determine an expected outcome or goal(s).
2. Develop a plan to achieve success.
3. Decide how to measure whether the goal(s) have been achieved.
4. Plan a timeline to measure the patient's progress.
5. Document the patient's response to care and the final outcome.

The patient should be fully cooperative to make the best use of IPPB. It may be counterproductive to try to force an IPPB treatment on a combative or uncooperative patient. A patient who has a neuromuscular deficit may need assistance in holding the IPPB circuit or keeping a good mouth seal. A mouth seal or face mask treatment may have to be given. Be prepared to make a recommendation to have a patient use either incentive spirometry, positive end-expiratory pressure therapy, or IPPB for hyperinflation therapy. Also be prepared to make a recommendation for a patient to use either a metered dose inhaler, small volume nebulizer, or IPPB for the delivery of an aerosolized medication.

d. Stop the treatment or procedure if the patient has an adverse reaction to it (CSE code: IIIF1)

Patient safety should always be an important consideration during the treatment or procedure. The respiratory therapist should know the complications and hazards of any patient care activity that is performed. Be prepared to stop the treatment or procedure if the patient has an adverse reaction to it. In addition, be prepared to recommend to the physician that the treatment or procedure be discontinued if it is likely to result in additional adverse reactions.

As previously mentioned, the general treatment length is 15 to 20 minutes. The patient may not be able to tolerate that length of time because of fatigue. This is often seen in aged or debilitated patients. Stop the treatment if the patient has a pulse change of 20 beats/min or more. It is most common to see the pulse increase because of a nebulized bronchodilator drug. A decreased venous return to the heart may be shown by an increased heart rate or decrease in blood pressure.

e. Discontinue treatment based on the patient's response (WRE code: IIIG1e) [Difficulty: An]

The contraindications, hazards, and precautions to IPPB were discussed earlier. The treatment should be canceled if the patient has an untreated pneumothorax or massive hemoptysis. Other serious problems also justify the cancellation of the order.

3. Respiratory care protocols

a. Develop the outcomes of respiratory care protocols (WRE code: IIIH4b) [Difficulty: An]

b. Apply respiratory care protocols to patient care situations (WRE code: IIIH6) [Difficulty: Ap]

c. Explain planned therapy and goals to the patient in understandable (nonmedical) terms to achieve the best results from the treatment or procedure (WRE code: IIIA6) [Difficulty: An]

d. Monitor the outcomes of respiratory care protocols (WRE code: IIIH5) [Difficulty: An]

The goal of all protocols is to restore the patient's condition to as close to normal as possible. When it is not possible to restore normal conditions, acceptable conditions must be listed as the target for care. The patient must be evaluated before, during, and after a protocol is used to determine whether improvement has occurred. Based on the results of the patient assessment, the care can be upregulated (increased) or downregulated (decreased).

IPPB should be used for hyperinflation therapy only when less expensive options (such as incentive spirometry) are not practical. Bedside spirometry should confirm that IPPB is indicated and that the patient's IPPB breath is at least 25% greater than spontaneous breath. Breath sounds should be heard more clearly to the bases of the lungs. One of the goals of IPPB is to give the patient larger tidal volumes than normal. More secretions may be heard in the airways if the larger tidal volumes result in their mobilization. However, if the deeper breaths enable the patient to cough more effectively, more secretions should be coughed out. Wheezing should be diminished if a bronchodilator medication is nebulized to a patient with bronchospasm.

4. Communicate the outcomes of therapy and change the therapy based on the protocol (WRE code: IIIA5) [Difficulty: An]

Inform the patient's nurse or physician and the supervising therapist if any serious question or problem occurs with the patient. Routine communication should occur as needed between these people and any other caregiver.

5. Record and evaluate the patient's response to the treatment(s) or procedure(s), including the following:

a. Record and interpret the following: heart rate and rhythm, respiratory rate, blood pressure, body temperature, and pain level (WRE code: IIIA1b, IIIA1c) [Difficulty: An]

Ask about the patient's feelings toward the treatment, and write them in the chart. Note any significant comments made by the patient. Note the patient's preferred flow and pressure or volume settings.

b. Record and interpret the patient's breath sounds (WRE code: IIIA1a) [Difficulty: An]

If atelectatic areas have been opened up, normal breath sounds should be heard there.

c. Record and interpret the type of cough the patient has and the nature of the sputum (WRE code: IIIA1a) [Difficulty: An]

If IPPB helps to deliver a larger tidal volume to the patient, the cough may be more effective. If IPPB has been used to deliver a nebulized mucolytic drug, the patient's sputum may be easier to cough out.

d. Recheck any math work and make note of incorrect data (WRE code: IIIA2) [Difficulty: An]

Make sure that the patient's IPPB tidal volume goal is properly calculated.

6. Communicate information relevant to coordinating patient care and discharge planning (e.g. scheduling, avoiding conflicts, and sequencing of therapies) (WRE code: IIIA3) [Difficulty: An]

Common scheduling problems include eating times and when the patient must go to another department such as radiology or physical therapy. Some procedures, such as giving an IPPB treatment with aerosolized medications and performing chest physiotherapy, should be performed before eating.

BIBLIOGRAPHY

AARC Clinical Practice Guideline: Incentive spirometry, *Respir Care* 30:1402, 1991.

AARC Clinical Practice Guideline: Intermittent positive pressure ventilation, *Respir Care* 38:1189, 1993.

AARC Clinical Practice Guideline: Intermittent positive pressure ventilation: 2003 revision and update, *Respir Care* 48:540, 2003.

Branson RD, Hess DR, Chatburn RL, editors: *Respiratory care equipment*, ed 2, Philadelphia, 1999, Lippincott Williams & Wilkins.

Cairo JM: Lung expansion devices. In Cairo JM, Pilbeam SP, editors: *Mosby's respiratory care equipment,* ed 7, St Louis, 2004, Mosby.

Eubanks DH, Bone RC: *Comprehensive respiratory care,* ed 2, St Louis, 1990, Mosby.

Fink JB: Volume expansion therapy. In Burton GG, Hodgkin JE, Ward JJ, editors: *Respiratory care,* ed 4, Philadelphia, 1997, Lippincott.

Fink JB: Bronchial hygiene and lung expansion. In Fink JB, Hunt GE, editors: *Clinical practice in respiratory care,* Philadelphia, 1999, Lippincott Williams & Wilkins.

Fink JB: Volume expansion therapy. In Burton GG, Hodgkin JE, Ward JJ, editors: *Respiratory care,* ed 4, Philadelphia, 1997, Lippincott.

Fink JB, Hess DR: Secretion clearance techniques. In Hess DR, MacIntyre NR, Mishoe SC, editors: *Respiratory care principles and practices,* Philadelphia, 2002, WB Saunders.

Fluck RJ Jr: Intermittent positive-pressure breathing devices and transport ventilators. In Barnes TA, editor: *Respiratory care practice,* ed 2, St Louis, 1994, Mosby.

McPherson SP: *Respiratory care equipment,* ed 5, St Louis, 1995, Mosby.

Miller WF: Intermittent positive pressure breathing (IPPB). In Kacmarek RM, Stoller JK, editors: *Current respiratory care,* Philadelphia, 1988, BC Decker.

Respiratory Care Committee of the American Thoracic Society: Guidelines for the use of intermittent positive pressure breathing (IPPB), *Respir Care* 25:365, 1980.

Shapiro BA, Kacmarek RM, Cne RD, et al: *Clinical application of respiratory care,* ed 4, St Louis, 1991, Mosby.

Weizalis CP: Intermittent positive-pressure breathing. In Barnes TA, editor: *Respiratory care practice,* ed 2, St Louis, 1994, Mosby.

Welch MA Jr, Shapiro BJ, Mercurio P, Wagner W, Hirayama G: Methods of intermittent positive pressure breathing, *Chest* 78:463, 1980.

White GC: *Equipment theory for respiratory care,* ed 3, Albany, NY, 1999, Delmar.

Wilkins RL, Scanlan CL: Lung expansion therapy. In Wilkins RL, Stoller CL, Scanlan CL, editors: *Egan's fundamentals of respiratory care,* ed 8, St Louis, 2003, Mosby.

SELF-STUDY QUESTIONS

1. In the emergency department, you are giving an IPPB treatment with metaproterenol sulfate (Alupent) to an asthmatic patient. During a break in the treatment, the patient complains that his lungs feel too full, and he does not feel as if all the IPPB volume is getting out. What would you recommend?
   A. Increase the flow.
   B. Add expiratory retard.
   C. Increase the system pressure.
   D. Change to 100% oxygen.

2. While giving an IPPB, a hissing sound is heard, and the patient complains that the inspiratory time is too long. What is the most likely problem?
   A. The nebulizer hose is attached to the exhalation valve.
   B. The nebulizer medication jar is loose.
   C. The bacteria filter is missing.
   D. The inspiratory and expiratory hoses are reversed.

3. You are delivering an IPPB treatment to an elderly patient without teeth or dentures. He has difficulty keeping his lips tight around the mouthpiece, and pressure fails to increase enough to cycle off the breath. What should be done?
   A. Switch the mouthpiece to a mask.
   B. Increase the inspiratory flow.
   C. Place nose clips on the patient.
   D. Change from IPPB to incentive spirometry.

4. You are about to give an asthmatic 16-year-old patient her second IPPB treatment with a bronchodilator medication. When checking the equipment, you notice that it is set with a rather fast inspiratory flow. Her chart had a note that she was very anxious when first admitted. She seems calmer now. How would you start the treatment?
   A. Increase the pressure setting to deliver a larger breath.

   B. Keep the flow the same to deliver a larger breath.
   C. Make the machine as sensitive as possible to trigger it easily.
   D. Decrease the flow on the machine.

5. Your patient with atelectasis has a spontaneous tidal volume of 600 mL and weighs 82 kg (180 lb). Based on this information, what should his IPPB tidal volume be?
   A. 500 mL
   B. 600 mL
   C. 700 mL
   D. 900 mL

6. Atelectasis has been diagnosed by chest radiograph in a patient whom you are treating with IPPB. To evaluate the effectiveness of the treatment, which of the following would you evaluate?
   I. Repeat the chest radiograph after the treatments have been given for 2 days
   II. Complete blood count
   III. Percussion sound for the positions of the hemidiaphragms
   IV. Breath sounds
   V. MVV after the treatments have been given for 2 days
      A. I, III, IV
      B. I, II
      C. III, V
      D. III, IV, V

7. Your patient with COPD has been receiving IPPB treatments on a Bird Mark 7 for 5 days. Expiratory retard was added 4 days ago. Because the retard has not been evaluated since then, the physician asks you to do so. You proceeded to make the following adjustments in the retard cap settings and make the following observations:

Retard cap setting	Exhaled tidal volume (mL)	Wheezing	Patient's impression
1 (smallest)	850	None	Exhalation too long
2	825	Some in bases	Exhalation too long
3	800	Some in bases	Comfortable
4	700	All lobes	Lungs feel full

Based on this information, which retard cap setting would you recommend?
A. 1
B. 2
C. 3
D. 4

8. A 13-year-old patient with cystic fibrosis is receiving IPPB to deliver an aerosolized bronchodilator and mucolytic. You notice that the pressure gauge needle is bouncing higher and lower as she takes a breath. What should you do?
  A. Increase the target pressure.
  B. Increase the sensitivity setting.
  C. Increase the flow.
  D. Tell the patient to inhale more quickly.
9. Your patient has an IPPB tidal volume goal of 900 mL but is only exhaling 700 mL. What would you do to deliver a larger volume?
  A. Increase the delivered pressure.
  B. Decrease the flow.
  C. Add expiratory retard.
  D. Have the patient inhale more forcefully.

ANSWER KEY

1. **B.** Rationale: Adding expiratory retard adds some back-pressure to the patient's airways and allow a more complete exhalation. Increasing inspiratory flow increases turbulence, and increasing system pressure increases tidal volume. Neither of these will help the patient's problem of air trapping. There is no indication that the patient is hypoxic and needs 100% oxygen.
2. **B.** Rationale: A loose nebulizer medication jar would result in a hissing sound from the leaking air and a prolonged inspiratory time. If any of the hoses is misconnected, the IPPB machine will fail to function properly, but the described problems will not be found. A missing bacteria filter does not cause any hissing sound or prolong the inspiratory time.
3. **A.** Rationale: The patient has a leak at the mouthpiece; correct it by switching to a face mask. Increasing the inspiratory flow will not correct the leak at the patient's mouth. Nose clips will not fix the patient's leak around the mouthpiece. There is no listed reason to switch the patient from IPPB to incentive spirometry.
4. **D.** Rationale: Because the patient is calmer now, it is best to reduce the flow from the IPPB machine. This allows the delivered tidal volume and medication to be more equally delivered to all areas of the lungs. No need exists at this time to deliver a larger tidal volume. The goal is to deliver medication effectively to the lungs. Machine sensitivity is not a problem at this time.
5. **D.** Rationale: The AARC Clinical Practice Guideline states that an IPPB-assisted breath should be at least 25% greater than the patient's spontaneous tidal volume. This would result in an IPPB breath goal of at least 750 mL. Therefore the best answer is 900 mL.
6. **A.** Rationale: The chest radiograph should be repeated to determine whether the lungs are more inflated in areas that earlier showed atelectasis. If atelectasis were decreased or gone, the patient's lung percussion note

would reveal lowered hemidiaphragms indicating larger lung volumes. If atelectasis were decreased or absent, the patient's breath sounds would be normal in the former problem areas. No specific marker is noted in the complete blood count for atelectasis or its correction. The MVV test is not specific for atelectasis.
7. **C.** Rationale: Expiratory retard cap setting 3 is best because the patient's tidal volume is adequate, wheezing is found only in the bases, and the patient is comfortable with the breath. The smaller settings (1 and 2) resulted in too long an exhalation for patient comfort. With the largest setting (4), the patient's tidal volume decreased, wheezing was heard in all lobes, and the patient said that the lungs feel full.
8. **C.** Rationale. Increasing the flow of gas to the patient will result in a smoother delivery of tidal volume to the patient. This will be seen as a gradual, steady increase in the pressure. Increasing the target pressure will only deliver a larger tidal volume. It will not meet the patient's need for a faster breath. Increasing the sensitivity setting lets the patient start a breath more easily but does not deliver a faster breath. If the patient inhales more quickly, she will increase her work of breathing even more. If her breathing pattern is to be coached, she should be told to inhale more slowly.
9. **A.** Rationale: The best way to deliver a larger tidal volume is to deliver more pressure to the lungs. Decreasing the flow will only deliver the gas more slowly to the preset pressure. Less flow will not increase the tidal volume. Expiratory retard is added only if the patient has a problem with air trapping on exhalation. It will help with the exhalation of the delivered tidal volume but will not increase the size of the delivered tidal volume. If the patient inhales more forcefully, he or she will only increase the work of breathing because the flow will be inadequate.

15 Mechanical Ventilation of the Adult

Note 1: The National Board for Respiratory Care (NBRC) has released the *RRT Examination Matrix* (detailing the testable items on the Written Registry Exam) and the *CSE Examination Matrix* (detailing the testable items on the Clinical Simulation Exam). Turn to the appendices at the back of this book for both publications in their original formats. This book is intended to cover all of the testable items in these two publications. This chapter (and all others) uses the abbreviation "WRE" for the coded items testable on the Written Registry Exam *and* Clinical Simulation Exam. The listed difficulty (R, Recall; Ap, Application; An, Analysis) relates to the question difficulty on the Written Registry Exam. The abbreviation "CSE" is used for the coded items testable on *only* the Clinical Simulation Exam. Because no question difficulty level is given for this exam, be prepared for anything.

Note 2: A review of the most recent Written Registry Examinations has shown an average of 23 questions (23% of the exam) that cover mechanical ventilation of the adult. Mechanical ventilation of the adult patient is the most heavily tested area on the examination. The Clinical Simulation Exam is comprehensive and may include everything that should be known or performed by an advanced level respiratory therapist. Expect several of the scenarios tested on the Clinical Simulation Examination to deal with mechanical ventilation of the adult patient.

MODULE A

Review the patient's chart for the following data and recommend and perform the following diagnostic procedures

1. Work of breathing

a. Review the patient's chart for information on work of breathing (WRE code: IA7c) [Difficulty: An]

Work of breathing (WOB) normally refers to how much energy the patient has to expend to inhale. Patients with stiff lungs or high airway resistance or both have an increased WOB. Exhalation is normally passive and requires no work. However, some patients with high airway resistance have to work to exhale. Look in the patient's chart for information on patient complaints of shortness of breath and easy tiring as signs of increased WOB.

A patient who has been intubated and placed on a modern mechanical ventilator with a microprocessor and graphics software can have WOB measured. See Fig. 15-1 for a pressure/volume loop tracing that shows a patient's WOB. WOB is minimized when the ventilator is set to minimize the negative pressure and inspiratory flow the patient has to generate.

b. Recommend that work of breathing be evaluated to get additional information (WRE code: IC2) [Difficulty: An]

If the breathing of an intubated and ventilated patient appears to be unsynchronized with the ventilator, his or her WOB should be evaluated. Ask the conscious patient simple questions to try to determine what the problem is. If the ventilator is capable, program it to perform a pressure/volume loop of the patient's WOB. Be prepared to adjust parameters such as the machine's sensitivity and inspiratory flow to minimize the patient's workload.

2. Ventilator flow, volume, and pressure waveforms

a. Review the patient's chart for information on airway graphics (WRE code: IA7b) [Difficulty: An]

A patient who has been intubated and placed on a modern mechanical ventilator with a microprocessor and graphics software can have ventilator flow, volume, and pressure waveforms visualized on the monitor, stored in memory, or printed out. Look for this information and compare it with the patient's current situation.

b. Perform the procedure to measure ventilator pressure/volume and flow/volume loops (WRE code: IB7h) [Difficulty: An]

Follow the ventilator manufacturer's steps to direct the unit to create flow, volume, and pressure waveforms. The patient can be instructed, based on the breathing test, either to perform a breathing maneuver actively or to lie passively as the ventilator delivers a breath.

Baseline = 0 cm H$_2$O
Relative pressure range = 60 cm H$_2$O
Inspiratory area = 0.031

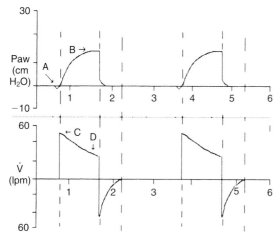

Fig. 15-1 Two graphic tracings of pressure support ventilation. **Top graphic** shows pressure/volume loop of a patient triggering a breath. *A,* Amount of work patient has to provide. *Shaded area* on right side indicates how much work was provided by ventilator. **Bottom graphic** shows pressure (Paw) versus time and flow ($\dot{V}$) versus time tracings. *A,* Where patient initiated a breath. *B,* Where ventilator cycled off when pressure support level of 15 cm water was reached. *C,* High peak flow at start of the breath. *D,* How flow rate decreases as pressure support level is reached. *(Reprinted by permission of Nellcor Puritan Bennett Inc., Pleasanton, Calif.)*

c. Interpret ventilator pressure/volume and flow/volume loops (WRE code: IB8j) [Difficulty: An]

A number of flow, volume, and pressure waveforms have been included in this chapter for practice. In addition, review Figs. 4-1 and 4-10 for examples of pulmonary function test waveform tracings. The examples in this chapter include common clinical situations and have explanations to help with interpretation. For example, Fig. 15-2

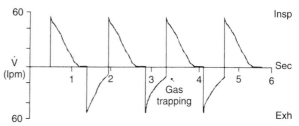

Fig. 15-2 Two graphic tracings of expiratory air trapping. **Top,** Volume versus time. *A* shows that the exhaled tidal volume tracing does not reach the baseline. Inspiratory tidal volume is greater than expiratory tidal volume, indicating air trapping. **Bottom,** Flow versus time. Inspiratory flow is the tracing above the horizontal baseline of zero flow. Expiratory flow is the tracing below the horizontal baseline. The patient's expiratory flow does not return to zero; this indicates air trapping. The higher the flow rate, the more air trapping. Air trapping leads to auto–positive end-expiratory pressure. It can be minimized by increasing expiratory time, giving an aerosolized bronchodilator to treat bronchospasm, or suctioning out any secretions. *(Reprinted by permission of Nellcor Puritan Bennett Inc., Pleasanton, Calif.)*

demonstrates two ways that air trapping on exhalation can be identified as auto–positive end-expiratory pressure (PEEP).

3. Airway resistance
a. Review the patient's chart for information on airway resistance (WRE code: IA7c) [Difficulty: An]

Airway resistance may have been measured earlier in either the pulmonary function laboratory or on the ventilator. Compare any earlier values with new measurements. This is important for understanding the patient's trends toward an improving or worsening pulmonary condition.

Airway resistance is measured in units of centimeters of water per liter per second at a standard flow rate of 0.5 L/sec (30 L/min). The normal spontaneously breathing adult's airway resistance (R_{AW}) is 0.6 to 2.4 cm water/L/sec; the normal 3-kg infant's R_{AW} is 30 cm water/L/sec. Do not forget that this procedure is being performed on a patient with an intubated airway on a ventilator. The endotracheal tube adds to the patient's total R_{AW}. The smaller the tube, the greater the resistance it offers to gas flowing through it. Altering inspiratory flow has an influence on the peak pressure measured for the calculation. As flow is reduced, gas turbulence is reduced, and peak pressure is reduced. Conversely, a higher flow creates more turbulence, and a higher peak pressure is seen.

> **Exam Hint**
>
> **E**xpect to see at least one examination question that either describes a waveform or shows a waveform that must be analyzed.

b. Recommend the measurement of the patient's airway resistance (WRE code: IC2) [Difficulty: An]

This calculation is important because it provides valuable information on the patient's pulmonary condition. The Raw value indicates how difficult it is to move the tidal volume through the patient's airways and whether aerosolized bronchodilating medications are effective.

It is reasonable to recommend an airway resistance measurement on any patient who has an increased airway resistance problem such as chronic obstructive pulmonary disease (COPD), asthma, bronchospasm, or wheezing breath sounds. It also is reasonable to measure airway resistance before and after a bronchodilator medication is given to determine whether it had any benefit.

c. Determine the patient's airway resistance (WRE code: IB7g) [Difficulty: An]

Most of the microprocessor ventilators offer software for calculating all of these values. However, in other situations, they must be calculated manually.

Procedure for calculating airway resistance.

1. Cycle a tidal volume. The patient should be breathing passively; fighting the breath will result in an erroneously high peak pressure, and assisting with the breath will result in an erroneously low peak pressure.
2. Note the peak airway pressure on the manometer.
3. Briefly prevent the tidal volume from being exhaled. No air should be moving. Note that the pressure manometer shows a peak pressure and then a static or plateau pressure that is stable as long as the tidal volume is held in the lungs. Record the plateau pressure.
4. Calculate the flow in liters per second by taking the flow in liters per minute and dividing it by 60 seconds.
5. Place the peak airway pressure, plateau pressure, and flow into the following formula and solve for airway resistance:

$$Raw = \frac{\text{peak airway pressure} - \text{plateau pressure}}{\text{flow in L/sec}}$$

EXAMPLE

A mechanically ventilated patient has a peak airway pressure of 30 cm water and plateau pressure of 20 cm water. The peak flow is set at 60 L/min.

Calculate peak flow in liters per second:

$$\frac{60 \text{ L/min}}{60 \text{ sec}} = 1 \text{ L/sec}$$

Calculate airway resistance:

$$Raw = \frac{\text{peak airway pressure} - \text{plateau pressure}}{\text{flow in L/sec}}$$

$$Raw = \frac{30 \text{ cm H}_2\text{O} - 20 \text{ cm H}_2\text{O}}{1 \text{ L/sec}} = 10 \text{ cm H}_2\text{O/L/sec}$$

This value is greater than normal for a patient breathing spontaneously. However, remember that the patient's airway is intubated. This results in a smaller airway diameter and more resistance. Some practitioners use the calculated airway resistance as the basis for setting the pressure support ventilation (PSV) level (discussed later). An increased airway resistance may indicate bronchospasm or secretions in the airways. Delivering an aerosolized bronchodilator or suctioning should result in the resistance returning to the original level.

> **Exam Hint**
>
> **A**ll past examinations have had questions that deal with identifying when the patient has an increased airway resistance and how it can be managed.

4. Auto-PEEP detection

a. Perform the procedure to detect auto-PEEP (WRE code: IB7n) [Difficulty: R, Ap, An]

Auto-PEEP is end-expiratory pressure in the lungs that cannot be seen on the ventilator's pressure manometer. (The terms *inadvertent PEEP* and *intrinsic PEEP* also are used). Auto-PEEP is caused by air trapping because of an inadequate expiratory time. It becomes more likely when the inspiratory time is increased or the expiratory time is decreased, or in patients with long time constants of ventilation. Simply put, the next breath is delivered before the patient has exhaled completely. This problem is frequently seen in a patient with status asthmaticus or COPD because of early small airway closure. In patients with acute respiratory distress syndrome (ARDS) receiving pressure controlled inverse ratio ventilation (PCIRV), the long inspiratory times used increase the risk of expiratory air trapping. Auto-PEEP is more likely to be found when the I:E ratio becomes 2:1 or greater.

The level of auto-PEEP can be determined in different ways, depending on the type of ventilator being used. It can be measured on the pressure manometer of most ventilators. The trapped expiratory gas also can be seen on the graphic display of microprocessor ventilators such as the Servo *i*, Nellcor Puritan Bennett 7200, Hamilton Veolar, and Drager Evita 4. The following procedure can be followed for determining the presence or level of auto-PEEP:

1. Note the delivery of a tidal volume.
2. Watch the pressure gauge as it decreases to zero (or the level of therapeutic PEEP) at the end of exhalation. Make sure that the patient is exhaling passively to get an accurate reading.
3. Reduce the rate control to delay the next breath.
4. Occlude the expiratory tubing (or push the expiratory-hold button or add inflation hold on

other ventilators) to prevent any further exhalation for about 3 to 5 seconds.

5. If the pressure gauge is being monitored, note any pressure increase above the baseline pressure, or if the ventilator has a graphics monitor, noting the failure of the exhaled tidal volume or expiratory flow to return to baseline confirms the presence and amount of auto-PEEP (see Fig. 15-2).

6. Listen to the patient's breath sounds during a standard breath and during the prolonged exhalation. It is likely that during the standard breath, the expiratory sounds will be heard until the inspiratory sounds begin. During the prolonged exhalation, the expiratory sounds continue for a longer time and then end with silence. This silent pause time indicates that no more expiratory airflow is occurring.

It is important to add any auto-PEEP to the amount of therapeutic PEEP the patient has. This should be recorded as the total PEEP. For example, the patient has 5 cm of therapeutic PEEP and 2 cm of auto-PEEP for 7 cm of total PEEP. It may be thought that the total PEEP level places the patient at risk for volutrauma or decreased venous return and lowered cardiac output. The amount of auto-PEEP can be reduced by decreasing the inspiratory time, increasing the expiratory time, or decreasing the tidal volume. Lack of auto-PEEP can be confirmed by this procedure. If the auto-PEEP cannot be eliminated, therapeutic PEEP can be added to match it. By increasing the baseline pressure, the patient can more easily trigger an assisted or synchronous intermittent mandatory ventilation (SIMV) breath. It is especially important to decrease the auto-PEEP and therapeutic PEEP levels as the patient's lung compliance improves and airway resistance returns to normal.

b. Interpret ventilator graphics to detect auto-PEEP (WRE code: IB8k) [Difficulty: An]

Fig. 15-2 demonstrates two ways that air trapping on exhalation can be identified as auto-PEEP (unintended positive end-expiratory pressure). Note in Fig. 15-2, *bottom*, that the patient's expiratory flow does not reach the baseline pressure before another breath is delivered. This proves that air trapping has occurred. The larger the gap between the pressure at the end of expiration and the baseline, the greater the air trapping.

5. Determine the patient's plateau pressure (WRE code: IB7g) [Difficulty: An]

The plateau pressure on the ventilator is determined to evaluate the patient's lung compliance (C_{LT}). A change in the patient's lung compliance will correlate with changes in the patient's lung condition. The following two areas of discussion cover lung compliance, performing the lung compliance procedure, and interpreting the results.

There are two ways to determine the plateau pressure. First, have the patient lie passively and set the ventilator to prevent a delivered tidal volume from being exhaled (inflation hold). Second, have the patient lie passively, and manually cover the end of the expiratory tubing to prevent a delivered tidal volume from being exhaled.

The hold should be held for about 2 seconds so that the pressure manometer value is stable. Note the pressure as the plateau pressure. After the plateau pressure has been determined, the patient must exhale completely. It may be necessary to delay the next timed ventilator tidal volume breath not to "stack" a new breath when the first has not yet been exhaled. It is recommended that the plateau-pressure procedure be repeated to be sure that the measured pressure is accurate.

6. Lung compliance

a. Review the patient's chart for information on lung compliance (WRE code: IA7c) [Difficulty: An]

This value may have been measured earlier in either the pulmonary function laboratory or on the ventilator. Compare any earlier values with new values. This is important for understanding the patient's trends toward an improving or worsening pulmonary condition.

The compliance values indicate how easily the tidal volume can be delivered into the lungs. Static compliance (Cst) is the measurement of work required to overcome the elastic resistance to ventilation. It is a measurement of the compliance of the lungs and thorax (C_{LT}). Static compliance is measured in units of milliliters per centimeters of water pressure. The normal adult's static compliance is 100 mL/cm water; the normal 3-kg infant's static compliance is 5 mL/cm water.

Dynamic compliance (Cdyn), sometimes called *dynamic characteristic*, is the measurement of the combination of the patient's static compliance and airway resistance. As discussed previously, airway resistance is the pressure required to move a tidal volume through the airways. It also is known as *nonelastic resistance to ventilation*.

b. Recommend the measurement of the patient's lung compliance (WRE code: IC2) [Difficulty: An]

It is reasonable to recommend that lung compliance be measured on any patient who has clinical evidence of a significant change in lung compliance. This may occur in conditions such as ARDS, pneumonia, pulmonary edema, or pulmonary fibrosis. Compliance can be measured to document the worsening of the patient's condition as well as to determine whether the compliance is improving with treatment.

c. Determine the patient's lung compliance (WRE code: IB7g) [Difficulty: An]

Most of the microprocessor ventilators offer software for calculating all of these values. However, in other situations, they must be calculated manually.

1. Procedure for calculating the compliance factor

Before the actual calculation of the patient's static and dynamic compliance can be performed, the static compliance of the breathing circuit should be determined. In most older ventilators, some of the set tidal volume never reaches the patient because it is "lost" in the circuit. For highest accuracy in the calculation of static and dynamic compliance and the calculation of actual tidal and sigh volumes, this lost volume must be subtracted from the exhaled tidal volume. The term "compressed volume" is commonly used to describe this lost volume.

1. Remove the patient from the ventilator and manually ventilate him or her during this procedure.
2. Set the pressure limit as high as possible.
3. Block the breathing circuit at the patient connector.
4. Cycle a tidal volume.
5. Perform either of the following: (a) note the peak pressure developed in the circuit as the tidal volume stretches out the circuit; or (b) if the ventilator's peak pressure hits the pressure limit, note the delivered tidal volume and the pressure limit.
   Note: If the patient is receiving PEEP therapy, subtract the PEEP level from the measured peak pressure to find the true peak pressure.
6. The compliance factor is found by dividing the measured tidal volume by the peak pressure.

EXAMPLE

The patient has a set tidal volume of 600 mL. By using step 5b, the peak pressure is found to be 80 cm water, and the measured tidal volume is found to be 320 mL.

$$\text{Compliance factor} = \frac{320 \text{ mL}}{80 \text{ cm}} = 4 \text{ mL/cm water}$$

The compressed volume is found by multiplying the compliance factor by either the peak or the plateau pressure. The compressed volume is then subtracted from the exhaled tidal volume to determine the patient's actual tidal volume.

Exam Hint

Commonly, examinations have had a question requiring the calculation of static compliance or dynamic compliance or both. Be able to perform the following calculations.

---

2. Procedure for calculating static compliance

1. Determine the compliance factor of the breathing circuit (as described previously).
2. Reattach the patient to the ventilator. Reset all controls to their ordered or preset positions.

3. Cycle a tidal volume. The patient should be breathing passively; fighting the breath will result in an erroneously high peak pressure, and assisting with the breath will result in an erroneously low peak pressure.
4. Briefly prevent the tidal volume from being exhaled. No air should be moving. Note that the pressure manometer shows a peak pressure and then a static or plateau pressure that is stable as long as the tidal volume is held in the lungs. Note the *plateau* pressure.
5. Calculate the Cst by using this formula:

$$\text{Cst} = \frac{\text{Exhaled tidal volume} - \text{Compressed volume}}{\text{plateau pressure} - \text{PEEP}}$$

in which compressed volume is the compliance factor × plateau pressure.

3. Procedure for calculating dynamic compliance

1. Determine the compliance factor of the breathing circuit (as described previously).
2. Reattach the patient to the ventilator. Reset all controls to their ordered or preset positions.
3. Cycle a tidal volume. The patient should be breathing passively; fighting the breath will result in an erroneously high peak pressure and assisting with the breath will result in an erroneously low peak pressure.
4. Note the *peak pressure* on the manometer. If the pressure at the end of inspiration is less than the peak pressure, the pressure at the end of inspiration should be used in the calculation.
5. Calculate the dynamic compliance (Cdyn) by using this formula:

$$\text{Cdyn} = \frac{\text{Exhaled tidal volume} - \text{Compressed volume}}{\text{peak pressure} - \text{PEEP}}$$

in which compressed volume is the compliance factor × peak pressure.

EXAMPLE

Calculate the static and dynamic compliance on a ventilated patient *without PEEP* therapy.

The patient has an exhaled tidal volume of 600 mL. The peak pressure is 30 cm water, and the static or plateau pressure is 20 cm water. The compliance factor has been determined to be 4 mL/cm water. The compressed volume at the plateau pressure is determined to be 80 mL (4 mL/cm compliance factor × 20 cm). The compressed volume at the peak pressure is determined to be 120 mL (4 mL/cm compliance factor × 30 cm).

$$\begin{aligned} \text{Cst} &= \frac{600 \text{ mL} - 80 \text{ mL}}{20 \text{ cm} - 0} \\ &= \frac{520 \text{ mL}}{20 \text{ cm}} \\ &= 26 \text{ mL/cm water} \end{aligned}$$

$$Cdyn = \frac{600 \text{ mL} - 120 \text{ mL}}{30 \text{ cm} - 0}$$
$$= \frac{480 \text{ mL}}{30 \text{ cm}}$$
$$= 16 \text{ mL/cm water}$$

EXAMPLE

Calculate the static and dynamic compliance on a ventilated patient *with PEEP* therapy.

The same patient has an exhaled tidal volume of 600 mL. Because of refractory hypoxemia, 10 cm of PEEP therapy is started. The peak pressure is now 36 cm water, and the static or plateau pressure is now 25 cm water. The compliance factor has been determined to be 4 mL/cm water. The compressed volume at the plateau pressure is determined to be 60 mL [4 mL/cm compliance factor × 15 cm (25 cm − 10 cm PEEP)]. The compressed volume at the peak pressure is determined to be 104 mL [4 mL/cm compliance factor × 26 cm (36 cm − 10 cm PEEP)].

$$Cst = \frac{600 \text{ mL} - 60 \text{ mL}}{25 \text{ cm} - 10 \text{ cm}}$$
$$= \frac{540 \text{ mL}}{15 \text{ cm}}$$
$$= 36 \text{ mL/cm water}$$
$$Cdyn = \frac{600 \text{ mL} - 104 \text{ mL}}{36 \text{ cm} - 10 \text{ cm}}$$
$$= \frac{496 \text{ mL}}{26 \text{ cm}}$$
$$= 19 \text{ mL/cm water}$$

7. Interpret the patient's plateau pressure, airway resistance, dynamic lung compliance, and static lung compliance values on the ventilator (WRE code: IB8f) [Difficulty: An]

> **Exam Hint**
>
> Every examination has had questions that deal with the interpretation of increasing or decreasing peak pressure, plateau pressure, airway resistance, or lung compliance. Be able to identify a clinical change, possible causes of the change, and corrective actions.

Any increase in airway resistance or decrease in lung compliance or both creates an increase in the patient's WOB. Examples of conditions or situations in which an increased airway resistance is found include bronchospasm, secretions, mucosal edema, airway tumor, placement of a small endotracheal tube, and biting or kinking of the endotracheal tube. Lung compliance is decreased by pneumonia, pulmonary edema, ARDS, pulmonary fibrosis, atelectasis, consolidation, hemothorax, pleural effusion, air trapping, pneumomediastinum, and pneumothorax. Examples of chest wall and abdominal conditions that reduce compliance include the various chest wall deformities,

circumferential chest or abdominal burns, enlarged liver, pneumoperitoneum, peritonitis, abdominal bleeding, herniation, and advanced pregnancy. Correction of the problem should return the patient's ventilator pressure(s) to baseline and normalize the patient's WOB.

Six possible combinations of increasing or decreasing static and dynamic lung compliance exist. Each has its own possible causes and is covered in turn. The patient must be passive on the ventilator for the measured values to be accurate. Check two or three breaths for increased accuracy. Let the patient have a normal breath or two between each of the peak and plateau pressure measurement breaths.

a. Decreased dynamic compliance with stable static compliance

Decreased dynamic compliance with stable static compliance is noticed as an *increase* in the peak pressure with an unchanged plateau pressure (Fig. 15-3). It is caused by an increased airway resistance (bronchospasm, etc.). Correcting the underlying problem results in the peak pressure returning to the original level.

Note that the inspiratory resistance has doubled from the original 10 to 20 cm while the plateau pressure has not changed. This confirms that the problem originates in the airway or breathing circuit. The patient's lung compliance has not changed.

b. Increased dynamic compliance with stable static compliance

Increased dynamic compliance with stable static compliance is noticed as a *decrease* in the peak pressure with an

Fig. 15-3 Decreased dynamic compliance (Cdyn) with a stable static compliance (Cst). **A,** Original pressure manometer reading and pressure/volume curve. **B,** Altered pressure manometer reading and pressure/volume curve.

Fig. 15-4 Increased dynamic compliance (Cdyn) with a stable static compliance (Cst). **A,** Original pressure manometer reading and pressure/volume curve. **B,** Altered pressure manometer reading and pressure/volume curve.

Fig. 15-5 False decreased dynamic compliance (Cdyn) with true decreased static compliance (Cst). **A,** Original pressure manometer reading and pressure/volume curve. **B,** Altered pressure manometer reading and pressure/volume curve.

unchanged plateau pressure (Fig. 15-4). This represents an improvement in the patient's airway resistance from the original condition. Secretions can be diminished, mucus plugs cleared, bronchospasm corrected, and so on.

Note that the inspiratory resistance has decreased from the original level of 20 to just 5 cm. This confirms that the patient's airway resistance has decreased. The patient's lung compliance has not changed.

c. False decreased dynamic compliance with true decreased static compliance

False decreased dynamic compliance with true decreased static compliance is noticed as an *increase* in *both* the peak and plateau pressures (Fig. 15-5). This is seen when the patient's lung/thoracic compliance worsens. The plateau pressure is elevated, and the static compliance is decreased.

As an artifact of the stiffer lungs, the peak pressure also is elevated, and the dynamic compliance is decreased. However, the difference between the peak and plateau pressures remains the same. This demonstrates that no real increase in the patient's airway resistance has occurred.

d. True decreased dynamic compliance with true decreased static compliance

True decreased dynamic compliance with true decreased static compliance also is noticed as an *increase* in *both* the peak and plateau pressures (Fig. 15-6). This is seen with the combination of a decreased lung compliance and an increased airway resistance. Causes of both of these problems were discussed earlier.

e. False increased dynamic compliance with true increased static compliance

False increased dynamic compliance with true increased static compliance is noticed as a *decrease* in *both* the peak and plateau pressures (Fig. 15-7). This is seen when the patient's lung/thoracic compliance improves. The plateau

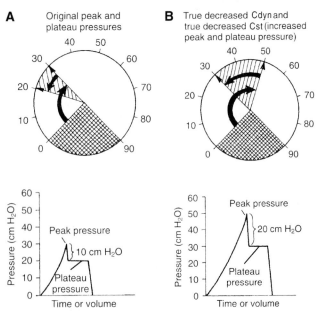

Fig. 15-6 True decreased dynamic compliance (Cdyn) with true decreased static compliance (Cst). **A,** Original pressure manometer reading and pressure/volume curve. **B,** Altered pressure manometer reading and pressure/volume curve.

Fig. 15-7 False increased dynamic compliance (Cdyn) with true increased static compliance (Cst). **A**, Original pressure manometer reading and pressure/volume curve. **B**, Altered pressure manometer reading and pressure/volume curve.

Fig. 15-8 True increased dynamic compliance (Cdyn) with true increased static compliance (Cst). **A**, Original pressure manometer reading and pressure/volume curve. **B**, Altered pressure manometer reading and pressure/volume curve.

pressure decreases, and as an artifact, the peak pressure also decreases. Notice that the difference between the peak and plateau pressures remains the same. This indicates that the patient's airway resistance is unchanged.

f. True increased dynamic compliance with true increased static compliance

True increased dynamic compliance with true increased static compliance also is noticed as a *decrease* in *both* the peak and plateau pressures (Fig. 15-8). This is seen when both the patient's airway resistance and his or her lung/thoracic compliance improve. Notice that the plateau pressure has decreased, thus indicating more compliant lungs. Also notice that the difference between the peak and plateau pressures has decreased. This demonstrates that the airway resistance also has decreased.

All six examples of increasing or decreasing static or dynamic lung compliance or both make use of a single tidal volume that is analyzed for peak and plateau pressures. Some practitioners advocate using several different tidal volumes (for example 8, 10, and 12 mL/kg of ideal body weight) when measuring dynamic and static pressures. The measured values are plotted on a graph to find the patient's optimal tidal volume that results in the highest static compliance value. Fig. 15-9 shows a series of these graphs. The curves for diseased lungs and airways are quite different from those of a normal person or a patient with a pulmonary embolism. Because of this, a pulmonary embolism should be considered if the patient's condition deteriorates rapidly and no change in the dynamic or static compliance values is observed.

MODULE B

Provide mechanical ventilation to adequately oxygenate and ventilate the patient

A number of physiologic criteria have been compiled to help the clinician determine when a patient is in respiratory or ventilatory failure (Box 15-1). Remember that the patient may not fail each and every criterion; however, the patient will often fail one or more criteria in each category.

1. Perform the following procedures to make sure that the patient is adequately oxygenated

a. Minimize hypoxemia by positioning the patient properly (WRE code: IIID7) [Difficulty: Ap, An]

This was discussed in Chapter 6. Review as necessary.

b. Administer oxygen, as needed, to prevent hypoxemia (WRE code: IIID4b) [Difficulty: An]

Oxygen administration and adjustment were discussed in Chapter 6. In brief, the goal of oxygen administration is to keep the PaO_2 level of most patients between 60 and 90 torr and the SpO_2 level greater than 90%. Exceptions are the COPD patient who is breathing on hypoxic drive and the patient who is in a cardiac arrest situation. The following formula can be used to help guide the use of supplemental oxygen in most stable patients:

$$\text{Desired } FIO_2 = \frac{\text{desired } PaO_2 \times \text{current } FIO_2}{\text{current } PaO_2}$$

Normal

Pulmonary emboli

Mucus plugging bronchospasm

Tension pneumothorax, atelectasis, pulmonary edema, pneumonia, bronchial intubation

Fig. 15-9 Pressure/volume curves for normal airways and lungs, pulmonary embolism (no change in airway resistance or lung compliance), increased airway resistance, and decreased lung compliance. *(From Pilbeam SP: Mechanical ventilation: physiological and clinical applications, St Louis, 1986, Mosby.)*

EXAMPLE

Your patient has a Pa_{O_2} level of 55 mm Hg on 30% oxygen. The clinical goal is a Pa_{O_2} level of 90 mm Hg. What oxygen percentage should the patient have?

$$\text{Desired } F_{IO_2} = \frac{\text{desired } Pa_{O_2} \times \text{current } F_{IO_2}}{\text{current } Pa_{O_2}}$$

$$\text{Desired } F_{IO_2} = \frac{90 \text{ mm Hg} \times 0.3}{55 \text{ mm Hg}}$$

$$\text{Desired } F_{IO_2} = \frac{27}{55}$$

$$\text{Desired } F_{IO_2} = 0.49 \text{ or } 49\% \text{ oxygen}$$

Those patients who have refractory hypoxemia (e.g., ARDS) will not respond with a normal increase in Pa_{O_2} level as the oxygen percentage is increased. In the short term, use whatever oxygen percentage is needed to achieve the clinical goal. The risk of oxygen toxicity increases when the F_{IO_2} is greater than 0.5 for periods of more than 48 hours. Always recheck the patient's arterial oxygen level after a change has been made in the F_{IO_2}.

Either of the following formulas can be used in the special situation of determining the flows of air and oxygen into a "bleed in" type of intermittent mandatory ventilation (IMV) or continuous positive airway pressure (CPAP) system to obtain an ordered F_{IO_2}. Either version can also be used for determining the gas flows, total flow, and oxygen/air ratio through an air entrainment (Venturi) mask.

The first formula follows:

$$(\text{L/min air} \times F_{IO_2} \text{ of air}) + (\text{L/min } O_2 \times F_{IO_2} \text{ pure } O_2) = \text{Total flow} \times \text{unknown } F_{IO_2}$$

The second formula follows:

$$F_1 C_1 + F_2 C_2 = F_T C_T$$

in which F_1 is the flow of first gas (oxygen), C_1 is the concentration of oxygen in the first gas (1.0 for pure oxygen), F_2 is the flow of second gas (air), C_2 is the concentration of oxygen in the second gas (0.21 for air), F_T is the total flow of both gases, and C_T is the concentration of oxygen in the mix of both gases. Use algebraic manipulation to solve for the unknown.

EXAMPLE

Determine the oxygen percentage through a bleed-in system that has an oxygen flow of 10 L/min and an airflow of 15 L/min. Determine the total flow through the system. Determine the ratio of oxygen to air.

VENTILATION
Apnea
$Paco_2 \geq 55$ torr in a patient who is not ordinarily hypercapneic
Dead space: tidal volume (V_D/V_T ratio) of $> 0.55-0.6$ (55%–60%)

OXYGENATION
$Pao_2 < 80$ torr on 50% oxygen or more
$P(A-a)o_2 < 300-350$ torr on 100% oxygen
Intrapulmonary shunt $> 15\%-20\%$

PULMONARY MECHANICS
Spontaneous tidal volume 3–4 mL/lb or 7–9 mL/kg of ideal body weight
Vital capacity $< 10-15$ mL/kg
Maximum inspiratory pressure (MIP) < -20 to -25 cm water pressure
Forced expiratory volume in one second (FEV_1) < 10 mL/kg
Respiratory rate < 12 breaths/min or > 35 breaths/min in an adult
Rapid, shallow breathing index (breaths/minute divided by tidal volume in liters) > 105

MISCELLANEOUS
Unconscious patient
Unstable and unacceptable vital signs
Unstable cardiac rhythm caused by hypoxemia and/or acidosis
Worsening cardiopulmonary or other major organ system

$$(\text{L/min air} \times Fio_2 \text{ of air}) +$$
$$(\text{L/min } O_2 \times Fio_2 \text{ pure } O_2) = \text{total flow} \times \text{unknown } Fio_2$$
$$(15 \times 0.21) + (10 \times 1.0) = (15 + 10) \times \text{unknown } Fio_2$$
$$(3.15) + (10) = (25) \times \text{unknown } Fio_2$$
$$13.15 = 25 \, Fio_2$$
$$(\text{Divide both sides by 25.})$$
$$0.526 \text{ or } 52.6\% = Fio_2$$
$$\text{Total flow} = 15 + 10 = 25 \text{ L/min}$$
$$\text{Ratio} = \frac{10 \text{ L/min oxygen}}{15 \text{ L/min air}}$$

c. Adequately oxygenate the patient to prevent accidental hypoxemia before and after suctioning, changing the ventilator circuit, or performing other procedures in which the patient is disconnected from the ventilator (WRE code: IIID6) [Difficulty: An]

Ensuring adequate oxygenation when suctioning is discussed in Chapter 13. In brief, remember to give the adult patient 100% oxygen for at least 30 seconds before suctioning. Perform the task as quickly and safely as possible to minimize time off the ventilator. Leave the patient on 100% oxygen for at least 1 minute after the procedure or until he or she returns to a stable condition as before the procedure. Children younger than 6 months can have the Fio_2 increased by 10% for the procedure.

In an adult, it is acceptable to increase the inspired oxygen up to 100% before and after a procedure that requires disconnection from the ventilator. The goal is to prevent hypoxemia. The patient should be manually ventilated with a resuscitation bag if indicated. Always remember to return the patient to the original oxygen percentage when clinically indicated.

2. Initiate and adjust continuous mechanical ventilation modes (WRE code: IIID2b) [Difficulty: An]

The following modes of ventilation are delivered through most types of electrically powered, volume cycled ventilators such as the Servo *i*, Puritan-Bennett 840, and Drager Evita 2 Dura.

a. Control

Control (C) is the simplest method of providing ventilatory support and is used on an apneic patient. The ventilator is set with a mandatory respiratory rate and tidal volume. The machine is incapable of allowing any patient interaction. For example, the ventilator might be set to deliver a tidal volume of 700 mL at a rate of 14 times/min. Because of this limitation, it is rarely, if ever, used in modern medicine except when the patient must be kept sedated or pharmacologically paralyzed (Fig. 15-10, *A*, shows the pressure/time curve).

b. Assist/control

The assist/control (A/C) mode has a set backup respiratory rate but allows the patient to trigger additional machine delivered breaths. A sensitivity control is adjusted to allow the patient to start a breath easily as needed. All tidal volumes are the same (Fig. 15-10, *B*, shows the pressure/time curve).

c. Intermittent mandatory ventilation

IMV has a set backup respiratory rate and tidal volume that is delivered to the patient. In addition, in between the mandatory breaths, the patient can breathe spontaneously as frequently as desired. The patient also can take in as large a spontaneous tidal volume as needed. The sensitivity control is set so that the patient cannot trigger any extra ventilator tidal volumes. For example, the ventilator might be set to deliver a 700-mL tidal volume 8 times/min. Let us say that the patient breathes spontaneously 10 more times and has an average tidal volume of 400 mL. The total rate is counted at 18. The total minute volume is the combination of the machine's volume and the patient's volume (Fig. 15-10, *C*, shows the pressure/time curve).

Fig. 15-10 Pressure versus time waveforms for various modes of mechanical ventilation. **A,** Control (C) mode shows no patient effort and consistent inspiration/expiration ratios. **B,** Assist/control (A/C) mode shows that patient's initial effort triggers machine tidal volume breath. **C,** Intermittent mandatory ventilation (IMV) mode shows spontaneous tidal volume breaths occurring between predetermined machine tidal volume breaths. Note "stacked" breaths that happen when patient takes in a breath that is then supplemented by a machine breath. **D,** Synchronous intermittent mandatory ventilation (SIMV) mode shows that a patient effort within a time window results in delivery of machine tidal volume. Any other patient efforts within the time window result in a spontaneous tidal volume. If no patient efforts occur within the time window, machine tidal volume will be automatically delivered. **E,** Pressure support ventilation (PSV) mode shows how patient must initiate all breaths that are then supported to the predetermined airway pressure. Stable tidal volumes are seen if the patient inhales passively. Variably larger tidal volumes result if the patient inhales more actively. **F,** Positive end-expiratory pressure (PEEP) therapy can be added to A/C mode (as shown) or any other mode. The elevated baseline pressure prevents alveolar collapse. The sensitivity control must be set at −1 to −2 cm water so that the patient is able to trigger a breath without undue effort. **G,** Continuous positive airway pressure (CPAP) shows that the patient takes spontaneous tidal volumes while exhaling against an elevated baseline pressure.

d. Synchronous intermittent mandatory ventilation

SIMV is similar to IMV except that the sensitivity control is functional. The patient can trigger a machine delivered tidal volume during a preset time interval. The timing of the backup rate is such that the patient can get only as many ventilator breaths as are set. Spontaneous tidal volumes vary with the patient's efforts. The total respiratory rate and total minute volume would be calculated as discussed previously (Fig. 15-10, *D*, shows the pressure/time curve).

e. Pressure support ventilation

PSV is similar to intermittent positive-pressure ventilation (IPPB) in that when the patient initiates a ventilator

breath, a preset pressure is delivered to the airway. The patient has the flexibility to determine the respiratory rate. The physician orders a PSV level that is enough either to overcome the patient's calculated airway resistance or to deliver a minimum tidal volume, depending on the clinical goal. The tidal volume will be stable if the patient passively takes the PSV breath, or it can be larger if the patient interacts actively with the pressure that is delivered (Figs. 15-1 and 15-10, *E*, show the pressure/time curve).

f. Pressure control ventilation

Pressure control ventilation (PCV) involves the delivery of tidal volume breaths that are pressure limited and time cycled. A set ventilator rate can be set and the patient also can trigger additional breaths. Because the pressure is limited, the tidal volumes may vary. This must be monitored closely in patients with frequently changing lung compliance and airway resistance. As the inspiratory time is increased, it can become longer than the expiratory time. This results in pressure control inverse ratio ventilation (PCIRV). Fig. 15-11 shows the volume, flow, and pressure tracings.

g. Airway pressure release ventilation

Currently only the Drager ventilator series offers the airway pressure release ventilation (APRV) mode (as well as other modes). These ventilators are microprocessor controlled and include a monitor for patient data and graphics. The APRV mode has been used with success in ARDS patients who have not responded well to constant volume ventilation. APRV can be described simply as a mode in which the patient can breathe spontaneously at two different levels of CPAP. A difference from conventional CPAP is that the two levels are held for set periods. The ventilator options for this mode are quite simple. The practitioner sets the low pressure (P_{low}), high pressure (P_{high}), and times that the patient will be at those pressure levels. The low pressure is sometimes referred to as CPAP and high pressure as *release pressure*. The timing changes from low pressure to high pressure and back to low

pressure effectively deliver a tidal volume. (See Fig. 15-12 for a pressure/time tracing.)

When comparing APRV with other modes of ventilation, there appear to be several similarities between it and PCIRV with PEEP and bilevel ventilation. All have an elevated baseline pressure that allows the patient to breathe spontaneously. All have variable inspiratory times for the higher pressure level. None delivers a set tidal volume to the patient. The only real difference seems to be that the patient can breathe spontaneously at the higher pressure level only with APRV. If the patient does not make any respiratory efforts, APRV functions like PCV or bilevel ventilation.

A set of blood gases, vital signs, pulmonary artery catheter values, and so forth should be obtained on the current constant volume ventilator settings as a baseline before starting APRV. The following suggestions for initiating APRV are similar to those listed earlier for starting PCIRV:

1. Set the high pressure (release pressure) at the patient's optimal PEEP/CPAP level. Often this is in a range between the patient's static lung compliance pressure and peak pressure (see Fig. 15-30). The clinical goal is safely to maximize the patient's functional residual capacity (FRC).
2. Set the low pressure (CPAP) at the level of PEEP that was used on the constant volume ventilator.

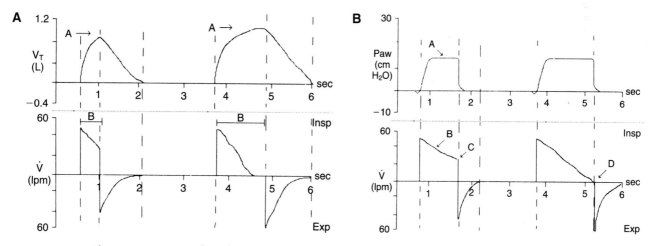

Fig. 15-11 Two sets of graphic tracings of pressure control ventilation. **A,** Two tracings show volume (V_T) versus time and flow (V) versus time. *A* shows tidal volume; *B* shows inspiratory flow. Note how tidal volume increases as inspiratory time is increased. However, as shown in lower right tracing, as flow decreases to zero, no more volume is delivered. **B,** Two tracings show pressure versus time and flow versus time. *A* shows the pressure control level being reached with an inspiratory plateau or "square wave" appearance. *B* shows declining inspiratory flow. *C* shows final flow when inspiration is time cycled off and exhalation begins. This graphic can be used to help adjust a longer inspiratory time. If pressure control inverse ratio ventilation (PCIRV) were being optimally adjusted, the inspiration time could be increased until inspiratory flow reached zero (indicated by *D*). *(Reprinted by permission of Nellcor Puritan Bennett Inc., Pleasanton, Calif.)*

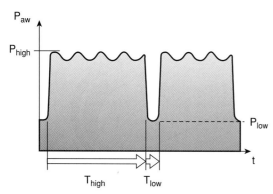

Fig. 15-12 APRV—Airway Pressure Release Ventilation. Spontaneous breathing under continuous positive airway pressure with brief pressure release. The patient breathes spontaneously at a high pressure level (P_{high}) for an adjustable length of time (T_{high}). For very short expiratory times (T_{low}), the EvitaXL switches to a low pressure level (P_{low}). The normal lung areas are emptied, but the "slow" lung areas only change volume to a lesser extent.* In this way, the ventilation/perfusion ratio can be improved for patients with a poor gas exchange. The steepness of the increase from the lower pressure level to the upper pressure level is controlled by the rise time setting (slope). The effective time for the increase in pressure cannot become greater than the set time (T_{high}).

> This is to maintain the patient's FRC. See point *A* of Fig. 15-30.
>
> 3. Set the inspired oxygen the same as before. Some may prefer to set it at 100%, as with PCIRV, until blood gas results show that it can be lowered.
>
> 4. Set the timing of the high pressure and low pressure values so that more time is spent at the high pressure than at the low pressure. Often the low pressure time is limited to 1 to 1.5 seconds. Keep the same respiratory rate as before. Even if the patient is apneic, as the ventilator switches from high pressure to low pressure, the patient exhales a tidal volume to blow off carbon dioxide.

Monitor the patient's ventilator delivered and spontaneous tidal volumes and rates. Check vital signs. Get an arterial blood gas (ABG) sample in about 15 minutes.

If the patient's initial blood gas results on APRV show hypoxemia, the following options are available: (1) increase the inspired oxygen percentage if it is not already at 100%, (2) increase the low pressure level, (3) increase the high pressure level, or (4) increase the time the patient is kept at the high pressure level. Reducing any or all of these options will decrease the patient's PaO_2 if it is too high.

If the blood gas results show hypoventilation, the following options are available: (1) increase the high pressure level, or (2) decrease the time at the high pressure level to increase the respiratory rate. Do the opposite to increase the $PaCO_2$ if the patient is being hyperventilated.

As with the previous ventilator modalities, the patient should be closely monitored and have an ABG drawn to evaluate every change.

Exam Hint

The National Board of Respiratory Care (NBRC) examinations have used a variety of terms and phrases to describe modes or modifications of modes of ventilation, including the following.

Terms related to delivering a set tidal volume include volume ventilation; volume cycled mechanical ventilation; volume controlled ventilation; volume preset ventilation; volume controlled, flow limited ventilation; volume controlled, pressure limited ventilation; volume controlled with SIMV, A/C, or C; and volume controlled with continuous flow IMV circuit added.

Terms related to *not* delivering a set tidal volume include pressure cycled ventilation; pressure control; pressure-controlled, pressure-limited, time cycled ventilation; pressure-controlled with constant inspiratory time; pressure-limited; and any previous term with inverse ratio ventilation.

---

h. Initiate high frequency ventilation and select appropriate settings

High frequency ventilation (HFV) is needed whenever the patient's condition calls for a higher respiratory rate or smaller tidal volume than usually delivered on a conventional volume cycled ventilator. A high frequency ventilator can deliver a respiratory rate far higher than the limit of 150/min set by the Food and Drug Administration (FDA) on all conventional adult and neonatal/pediatric ventilators.

The FDA has approved HFV for use on adults during bronchoscopy and laryngoscopy procedures and when a patient with a bronchopleural fistula cannot be managed on a conventional ventilator. Although patients with ARDS have not been officially approved for HFV, the procedure has been used when a patient is hypoxic despite maximum settings on a conventional ventilator. (Box 16-5 lists clinical uses for HFV with infants and children.)

Currently three different ways exist to deliver HFV. The first involves the use of a conventional ventilator set at a rate of up to the FDA maximum of 150/minute. This method is called high frequency positive-pressure ventilation (HFPPV). With it, the set tidal volume is decreased to something less than standard (less than 10 mL/kg). The second involves the use of a high frequency jet ventilation (HFJV) and a special endotracheal tube with a standard lumen and an additional small diameter air entrainment lumen (see Fig. 15-22). The HFJV unit is connected to the air entrainment lumen. Gas from the HFJV unit entrains other gas through the main lumen to create the patient's tidal volume. HFJV units can deliver a small tidal volume several hundred times per minute. The third method involves a high frequency oscillation (HFO) ventilator. HFO makes use of a conventional endotracheal tube (as does HFPPV). However, the delivered tidal volume is the smallest, and the respiratory rate can be the fastest of all three methods. Table 16-2 has a comparison of all three methods. The equipment used for HFJV and HFO is described later in this chapter. Table 15-1 lists considerations for the initial settings and adjustment of HFV delivered to infants and adults by either a jet ventilator or an oscillator ventilator.

Current clinical experience is recommended with any HFV method. Although adult patients have been successfully treated with HFV, far greater use of these techniques has occurred with infants and children. Therefore, Chapter 16 has further discussion.

i. Independent (differential) lung ventilation

Independent lung ventilation (ILV) involves the use of a separate mechanical ventilator for each lung. A double-lumen endotracheal tube must be placed into the patient to allow this procedure. (See Figs. 12-21 and 12-22 and the related discussion.) Box 15-2 lists indications for double-lumen endotracheal tubes and ILV. In all cases, the patient has one normal lung and one abnormal lung. The overriding concerns with ILV are to ventilate the patient adequately through the normal lung and to allow the injured lung to heal.

A common initial approach is to select two identical ventilators that allow synchronization of the patient's respiratory rate. The Servo 900C and the Drager Evita 1 and Evita 4 ventilators are suited for this. They allow one unit to be designated the "primary" ventilator to set the respiratory rate for it and the "secondary" unit. Each unit can then also have the same mode and I:E ratio. This synchronized ILV method still allows the independent setting of tidal volume, oxygen percentage, and PEEP for each lung.

For example, an 80-kg adult man normally receives an initial tidal volume of about 800 mL (10 mL × 80 kg). If both lungs functioned normally, each would receive 400 mL. However, with unilateral lung disease, the bad lung receives little tidal volume, and the normal lung receives too much and becomes overdistended. It is therefore important to set the initial tidal volume to the good lung at *half* the normal volume for both lungs. With this patient example, the normal lung's initial tidal volume should be set at 400 mL (5 mL × 80 kg). To avoid changing too many parameters at once, the same oxygen percentage and PEEP level are kept as originally set. The abnormal lung is ventilated based on its pathologic condition or may be left unventilated.

After 15 minutes, check the patient's ABG values. Depending on the results, adjust the ventilator settings for the good lung as would typically be done to remove carbon dioxide and maintain oxygenation. The ventilator settings for the diseased lung must be carefully adjusted

to allow healing and prevent complications such as atelectasis and pneumonia.

When the patient has a bronchopulmonary fistula, the air leak through the bad lung can be so great that an HFV must be used rather than a conventional ventilator. In this situation, no synchronization of rate or any other parameters can be set. The good lung is conventionally ventilated to maintain the patient's blood gas values. The HFV is set to provide some support with a small tidal volume and low ventilating pressures. The clinical goal is to prevent excessive lung pressure so that the lung tear heals.

The patient can be converted back to breathing through one conventional ventilator when normal functioning returns to the injured lung. This can be done when the peak pressure, plateau pressure, and mean airway pressure for both lungs are about the same. When these values match, or are close, they indicate similar lung compliance and airway resistance values. The first step in converting from ILV to conventional ventilation involves combining the proximal ends of the double-lumen endotracheal tube with a Y adapter. By doing this, one ventilator can deliver tidal volume breaths to each lung. It is suggested that the PC mode be used so that excessive pressure is not applied to the healing lung. Set the peak pressure at or just below the previous peak pressure used with the healing lung. Set the PEEP level at the previous pressure used with the healing lung. Check the patient's ABG values after 15 minutes. Be prepared to adjust the conventional ventilator as needed to get the desired blood gas values. Watch for problems with the healing lung, and be prepared to go back to independent lung ventilation if necessary. When it appears certain that the patient is tolerating conventional ventilation, the double-lumen endotracheal tube should be removed and replaced with an appropriate single-lumen tube. This allows better suctioning and results in less airway resistance through the tube. Wean and extubate the patient when appropriate.

j. External negative-pressure ventilation

These ventilators have proven useful in patients with the following characteristics: (1) normal, intact upper airway, (2) ability to swallow, (3) normal airway resistance, (4) normal lung/thoracic compliance, and (5) ability to ventilate until respiratory muscle fatigue becomes too great.

Patients with the following disease conditions have been successfully ventilated by a negative-pressure ventilator: (1) neuromuscular defects such as poliomyelitis, postpolio syndrome, muscular dystrophy, and high spinal cord injury; (2) kyphoscoliosis with resulting restrictive lung disease; and (3) COPD during an acute worsening.

Negative-pressure ventilators work by creating a negative pressure either around the patient's whole body or over the anterior chest and abdomen. The negative pressure expands the thorax, and a tidal volume is inhaled.

TABLE 15-1 High Frequency Ventilation Operational Considerations

	Infant Jets	Adult Jets	Infant Oscillators	Adult Oscillators
Initial recommended frequency	7 Hz (IMV background rate of 2)	5 Hz	15 Hz	3–5 Hz
Initial tidal volume parameters	Jet-drive pressure to produce 90% of CMV peak pressure; I time = 0.02 sec	Jet-drive pressure of 25–35 psi; I:E = 1:2–1:1	Amplitude to create chest vibration visually; I:E = 1:1	Amplitude to create chest vibration visually; I:E = 1:2–1:1
To change effective V_A	Alter drive pressure*; alter inspiratory time†; alter frequency‡	Alter drive pressure*; alter inspiratory time†; alter frequency‡	Alter pressure amplitudes*; alter inspiratory time†; alter frequency‡	Alter pressure amplitudes*; alter inspiratory time†; alter frequency‡
To change mean $\overline{Paw}$ (for $\dot{V}/\dot{Q}$ effects on PaO_2)	Alter applied PEEP; alter inspiratory time†	Alter applied PEEP (if available); alter inspiratory time†	Alter bias flow pressures; alter inspiratory time†	Alter bias flow pressures; alter inspiratory time†

*↑ Pressure = ↑ tidal volume = ↑ V_A.

†↑ Inspiratory time = ↑ tidal volume = ↑ V_A *unless* air trapping develops, in which case, tidal volume may ↓.

‡Frequency response may be variable: ↑ frequency may increase total ventilation *but* ↑ frequency can ↓ tidal volume through shorter inspiratory time and pulse attenuation through narrow endotracheal tubes.

CMV, Continuous mandatory ventilation; I, inspiratory; I:E, inspiratory/expiratory; IMV, intermittent mandatory ventilation; PaO_2, arterial oxygen pressure; $\overline{Paw}$, airway pressure; PEEP, positive end-expiratory pressure; V_A, alveolar ventilation; $\dot{V}/\dot{Q}$, ventilation–perfusion. In MacIntyre NR: High-frequency ventilation. In MacIntyre NR, Branson RD: *Mechanical ventilation*, Philadelphia, 2001, WB Saunders.

BOX 15-2   Indications for Double-lumen Endotracheal Tubes and Independent Lung Ventilation

Thoracic surgery
    Pneumonectomy
    Some lobectomies
    Thoracic aortic surgery
    Thoracoscopy
    Some esophageal surgery
Selective airway protection
    Secretions (tuberculosis, bronchiectasis, or abscess)
    Whole-lung lavage
    Massive hemoptysis
Bronchopleural fistula
Unilateral lung disease
    Unilateral parenchymal injury
        Aspiration
        Pulmonary contusion
        Pneumonia
        Massive pulmonary embolism
        Reperfusion edema
        Asymmetrical ARDS
        Asymmetrical pulmonary edema
    Atelectasis
Unilateral airflow obstruction
    Single-lung transplant for chronic airflow obstruction
    Unilateral bronchospasm
Severe bilateral lung disease
    ARDS
    Aspiration
    Pneumonia

ARDS, Acute respiratory distress syndrome.
From Tuxen D: Independent lung ventilation. In Tobin MJ, editor: *Principles and practice of mechanical ventilation,* New York, 1994, McGraw-Hill, pp 571–588.

If the patient needs supplemental oxygen, it must be given by nasal cannula or face mask. Three basic types of external negative-pressure ventilators are available: Drinker body respirator (so-called "iron lung"), body wrap, and chest curaisse (Fig. 15-13).

The following steps are used to initiate ventilation:

1. Select a ventilator rate that meets the patient's needs. This can be about 5 to 10 breaths less than the patient's own in a patient with some breathing ability. In an apneic patient, the rate can be varied between 14 and 24 per minute.
2. Gradually increase the negative pressure until the patient cannot speak during the inspiratory phase. A pressure of −7 to −15 cm water is enough for most patients. A maximum pressure of −35 cm water can often be achieved. It is possible to create a positive pressure during exhalation, if needed, by closing a valve. This is usually limited to times when an assisted cough is called for.

Fig. 15-13 Patient in chest curaisse (LifeCare). Note control box on right that contains vacuum motor. Hose connects vacuum motor to patient inside chest shell. *(From Hill NS: Clinical application of body ventilators,* Chest 90(6):897, 1986.)

3. Use a hand-held spirometer to measure the patient's tidal volume.
4. After a few minutes, ask the patient, "Does the breath feel deep enough, too deep, or not enough? Do you have tingling fingers or feel dizzy (signs of hyperventilation)?"
5. Adjust the negativity or rate or both to meet the patient's needs.
6. Draw an ABG sample after about 15 minutes. Speed is important because the unit must be opened to collect the sample. Interpret the ABG results as usual.
7. If the carbon dioxide level is higher than desired, increase the rate or set a more negative pressure to increase the minute volume. Do the opposite if the patient is being hyperventilated. If the patient is hypoxic, provide supplemental oxygen by nasal cannula or face mask.

Exam Hint

Recent exams have focused on mechanical ventilation being delivered with conventional modes or combinations of modes (see later). Typically only one or two questions deal with rarely used modes such as high frequency ventilation, independent lung ventilation, or negative-pressure ventilation.

---

3. Begin and modify combinations of ventilatory techniques to oxygenate the patient adequately: synchronous intermittent mandatory ventilation, pressure support ventilation, pressure control ventilation, and positive end-expiratory pressure (WRE code: IIID2e) [Difficulty: An]

The current generation of mechanical ventilators offers the physician and practitioner a number of options for how best to tailor ventilatory support to meet the patient's needs. The following should be considered when deciding what modes to use and combine.

a. Increased work of breathing

Patients who show increased WOB may have a very high airway resistance, as in status asthmaticus, or may have a very low lung/thoracic compliance, as in ARDS. Some practitioners believe that the C or A/C modes, when properly applied to a sedated patient, are best for these problems because the patient's breathing efforts are almost eliminated. Other practitioners believe that IMV and SIMV are physiologically superior modes of ventilation. More recently, PSV has been shown to be beneficial to patients with increased efforts at breathing from the high airway resistance caused by a small diameter endotracheal tube.

b. Hypercapnia

A patient may have hypercapnia (a high carbon dioxide level) because of sedation from a morphine or heroin overdose or may have COPD with worsening of the chronic hypercapnia. In either case, the patient becomes progressively more hypoxemic (unless given supplemental oxygen) as the carbon dioxide level increases. Control or A/C modes are best for setting a minimum minute volume to determine the maximum carbon dioxide level. As the patient recovers, IMV/SIMV or PSV allows the gradual reduction of ventilatory support. See Box 15-3 for indications of IMV/SIMV tolerance.

BOX 15-3   Indications of Intermittent Mandatory Ventilation (IMV)/Synchronous Intermittent Mandatory Ventilation (SIMV) Tolerance

INDICATIONS THAT IMV/SIMV IS BEING WELL TOLERATED
Stable spontaneous respiratory rate
Stable heart rate
Stable spontaneous tidal volume
Stable vital capacity, minimal inspiratory pressure (MIP), and/or FEV_1
No use or stable use of accessory muscles of ventilation
Patient indicates he or she is comfortable
Stable blood gases

INDICATIONS THAT IMV/SIMV IS NOT BEING WELL TOLERATED
Increased spontaneous respiratory rate
Tachycardia or dysrhythmias such as premature ventricular contractions
A decrease in the spontaneous tidal volume
A decrease in the vital capacity, MIP, and/or FEV_1
Beginning or increased use of accessory muscles of ventilation
Patient complains of dyspnea
Deterioration of blood gases as seen by a falling Pao_2 or Spo_2 and a rapidly falling or rising $Paco_2$

Mandatory minute ventilation (MMV) also has shown success at setting a minute volume that limits the increase in carbon dioxide as the patient is weaning. MMV is a relatively new variation on the IMV/SIMV mode. With MMV, the patient is assured of a preset minute volume regardless of his or her spontaneous breathing. It has been proposed as an effective way to ventilate and wean patients who can spontaneously breathe but who have an unreliable respiratory drive and unstable tidal volume. Examples include patients who have received narcotic, sedative, anesthetic, or neuromuscular blocking medications. Patient conditions for which MMV is indicated include encephalopathy and cerebral disorders such as stroke. In addition, MMV may be used during the recovery period of a neuromuscular disease. Ventilators that include the MMV mode are all controlled by a microprocessor and include the Drager series and the Hamilton Veolar. The following parameters have been recommended for the initiation of MMV:

1. Set the ventilator tidal volume according to established guidelines (10 to 15 mL/kg of ideal body weight).
2. The spontaneous breaths may be taken through a demand valve or may be pressure supported.
3. Determine the minimum minute volume according to the patient's preexisting condition and the clinical goals:

The patient who has been on IMV/SIMV should have the MMV set at 90% of the IMV-delivered minute volume. For example, the patient has an IMV/SIMV rate of 5 breaths/min and tidal volume of 800 mL. Therefore the ventilator is delivering 4 L of minute volume (5 × 800 mL), and the MMV would be set at 3600 mL (90% of 4 L).

The patient who has been on A/C should have the mandatory minute volume set at 80% of the A/C-delivered minute volume. For example, the patient has an A/C rate of 10 breaths/min and tidal volume of 1000 mL. Therefore the ventilator is delivering 10 L of minute volume (10 × 1000 mL), and the MMV would be set at 8 L (80% of 10 L).

1. Set the inspired oxygen percentage, inspiratory flow, and so forth as the patient's clinical condition requires

Ideally MMV establishes a minimum safe volume of ventilation. If the patient inhales less than this volume, the ventilator delivers as many breaths as necessary at the preestablished tidal volume to make up the difference. Be aware that a patient breathing rapidly with a small tidal volume may move enough gas to exceed the minimum minute volume. Because of this risk, it is important to set a low tidal volume alarm or a high respiratory rate alarm or both to give warning. Do not let the programming of an MMV create a false sense of security with these patients.

c. Hypoxemia

If hypoxemia is secondary to a decreased FRC, as in ARDS or atelectasis, the treatment of choice for hypoxemia is CPAP on a freestanding system or PEEP on a conventional volume cycled ventilator. If the problem is from an increased intrapulmonary shunt, the patient may need PEEP or CPAP as well as up to 100% oxygen. See Box 15-4 for patient monitoring during PEEP and CPAP. PCIRV and HFJV have been used with success in hypoxemic patients with a pulmonary air leak for whom conventional volume ventilation has failed. All the following were discussed earlier as individual modes of ventilation. When a patient has more than one problem, more than one solution may be needed. The following are combinations of modes from which to choose.

d. Pressure control/pressure control inverse ratio ventilation, synchronous intermittent mandatory ventilation, and positive end-expiratory pressure

PCV or, if necessary, PCIRV has been used with success in patients with low compliance and a pulmonary air leak. By limiting the peak pressure, less air seems to leak out and the tissues are more likely to heal. Therapeutic PEEP is applied to increase the patient's FRC to correct hypoxemia. The SIMV feature is added to let the patient breathe spontaneously if desired and stay more synchronized with the ventilator. With lung healing, the PEEP level is decreased and the inspiratory time is shortened. SIMV with a constant tidal volume may be used during the weaning phase. Fig. 15-11 shows pressure and flow tracings during PCV.

e. Intermittent mandatory ventilation/synchronous intermittent mandatory ventilation with pressure support ventilation and positive end-expiratory pressure

IMV/SIMV is used to give the patient a controlled number of deep tidal volume breaths. The patient can breathe as often as desired between the mandatory breaths. The patient's total minute volume can be determined by adding the combination of IMV/SIMV and pressure supported breaths. A maximum acceptable $PaCO_2$ can be established with the proper combination of IMV/SIMV breaths and pressure support (PS) level. A PS level of more than 10 cm water may be needed. In addition, the PS ensures that the airway resistance of the endotracheal tube is overcome. (See the airway resistance calculation earlier in the chapter.) PEEP therapy is applied to the level necessary to obtain a clinically safe PaO_2 at the lowest possible FIO_2. Fig. 15-14, *A*, shows the pressure/time curve.

Patients who have both a ventilation and an oxygenation problem benefit from these modes of ventilation. They have the desire to breathe on their own but a very limited ability to do so. All three modes can be independently adjusted for more or less support, as indicated by the patient's clinical condition and blood gas results.

f. Intermittent mandatory ventilation/synchronous intermittent mandatory ventilation with positive end-expiratory pressure

IMV/SIMV and PEEP therapy are applied as indicated. Pressure support is not needed if the patient is strong enough to overcome the airway resistance of the endotracheal tube and breathe with a clinically acceptable tidal volume. Fig. 15-14, *B*, shows the pressure/time curve.

g. Intermittent mandatory ventilation/synchronous intermittent mandatory ventilation with pressure support ventilation

IMV/SIMV and PS levels are increased or decreased based on the factors discussed earlier. This patient has the ability to provide some, but not all, of his or her own ventilation. The PaO_2 is clinically acceptable at an oxygen percentage probably no higher than 40%.

A fairly common clinical situation is seen in which the recovering patient does well on a gradually decreasing

---

BOX 15-4 Patient Monitoring during Positive End-expiratory Pressure (PEEP) or Continuous Positive Airway Pressure (CPAP) Therapy

GOOD TOLERANCE OF CPAP/PEEP THERAPY

Increased PaO_2
Increased static lung compliance
Stable cardiac output as shown by the following:
  Stable heart rate without rhythm disturbances
  Stable blood pressure
  The following can be measured only through a pulmonary artery/Swan-Ganz catheter:
    Stable or increased $P\bar{v}O_2$ (mixed venous oxygen)
    Stable cardiac output
    Decreased pulmonary vascular resistance
    Decreased intrapulmonary shunt

POOR TOLERANCE OF CPAP/PEEP THERAPY

Increased PaO_2 (This can be deceiving if this is the only information observed)
Decreased static lung compliance
Decreased cardiac output as shown by the following:
  Increased heart rate or rhythm disturbances
  Decreased blood pressure
  The following can be measured only through a pulmonary artery/Swan-Ganz catheter:
    Decreased $P\bar{v}O_2$ (mixed venous oxygen)
    Decreased cardiac output
    Increased pulmonary vascular resistance
    Increased intrapulmonary shunt

Fig. 15-14 Modification of combinations of intermittent mandatory ventilation (IMV)/synchronous intermittent mandatory ventilation (SIMV), pressure support ventilation (PSV), and positive end-expiratory pressure (PEEP). **A**, IMV/SIMV with PSV and PEEP. **B**, IMV/SIMV with PEEP. **C**, IMV/SIMV with PSV. **D**, PSV with PEEP. See text for descriptions of various combinations and their clinical application.

number of IMV/SIMV breaths until he or she can go no lower. The barrier seems to be the airway resistance of the endotracheal tube. (See the airway resistance calculation earlier in this chapter.) The addition of some PS overcomes that resistance so that the IMV/SIMV level can be further reduced. When the IMV/SIMV frequency is down to four or less, the patient is providing almost all of his or her minute volume. The greatest barrier to breathing is likely to be the resistance of the endotracheal tube. The decision can then be made to extubate the patient. Fig. 15-14, *C*, shows the pressure/time curve.

h. Pressure support ventilation with positive end-expiratory pressure

PSV and PEEP are applied as discussed earlier. This patient has the drive to breathe on his or her own; however, he or she has some limitation in the ability to overcome the resistance of the endotracheal tube or generate a consistently large enough tidal volume. (See the airway resistance calculation earlier in the chapter.) In addition, the patient has a significant oxygenation problem and needs some PEEP therapy. With recovery, both PS and PEEP can be

reduced. They may be reduced individually or simultaneously as the patient's strength and/or oxygenation improve. Fig. 15-14, *D*, shows the pressure/time curve.

The following subjects are not specifically listed as testable on the Written Registry Examination. However, an analysis of the most recent examinations finds questions related to modifying the following ventilator settings.

Sensitivity. Sensitivity is the term used to describe the amount of work or effort the patient must perform to trigger the ventilator to deliver a tidal volume breath. Many ventilators require the patient to generate a *negative pressure* to trigger the unit. With these machines, the sensitivity is usually set at about −1 to −2 cm water pressure.

Several of the newer ventilators also have an option in which the patient generates an *inspiratory flow* to trigger a ventilator tidal volume breath. The Puritan-Bennett 7200 ventilator is an example of such a ventilator. The term "flow-by" is used to describe this sensitivity option on the ventilator. With a ventilator using flow sensitivity, the patient triggers a tidal volume when his or her inspiratory flow is about 2 L/min (33 mL/sec) less than the set baseline flow through the circuit.

Flow. Flow is adjusted to set the inspiratory time and inspiratory/expiratory (I:E) ratio to meet the patient's needs. Inspiratory flow should be great enough to meet the patient's needs and minimize the WOB. Increase flow if the patient has signs of greater demand, such as using accessory muscles of inspiration, lack of synchrony with the ventilator, or the pressure manometer deflects greatly below the baseline pressure or shows a low initial increase in inspiratory pressure.

In addition, most current generation ventilators offer more than one inspiratory flow pattern (Fig. 15-15). The sine wave is the most physiologically like a normal, spontaneous inspiration. The other wave forms can be compared with the sine wave to determine which one best meets the patient's needs. Ideally, the best flow pattern is one in which the patient's peak and mean airway pressures are lowest, exhalation is complete, breath sounds are improved bilaterally, heart rate and blood pressure are stable, and the patient feels most comfortable.

I:E ratio. The I:E ratio is adjusted to ensure that the patient can inhale in as physiologically appropriate a manner as possible and completely exhale the inspired tidal volume. Typically, the I:E ratio should be 1:2 or

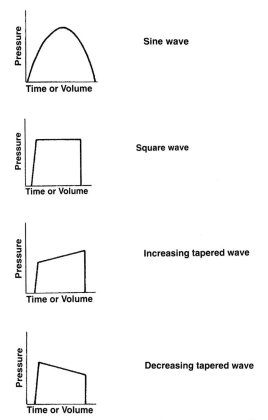

Sine wave

Square wave

Increasing tapered wave

Decreasing tapered wave

Fig. 15-15 Graphic tracings of typical inspiratory waveforms that are available on current mechanical ventilators.

more. Incomplete exhalation will cause air trapping and auto-PEEP (see Fig. 15-2).

Usually two questions are related to modifying the inspiratory flow to meet the patient's need for a faster breath or modifying the I:E ratio. Remember that if the patient has auto-PEEP, the expiratory time must be increased to allow a more complete exhalation.

Alarms. Alarm systems are different for each type of ventilator. Generally speaking, they are set with a safety margin of ±10% from the patient's normal ventilator settings. A variation of greater than 10% results in an audible or visual alarm condition. Most ventilators alarm if the I:E ratio is 1:1 or less.

Gas temperature. The goal for most patients is to minimize their humidity deficit by giving gas that is humidified and warmed to near body temperature. This can be accomplished by either a cascade- or a wick-type humidifier or a heat-moisture exchanger (HME). It is common to see the gas warmed to 90°F to 95°F (31°C to 35°C). This decreases the patient's humidity deficit to a miniscule level and reduces the "rain out" of water vapor condensing in the ventilator circuit. A temperature probe should be placed in the inspiratory tubing as close to the patient as possible to monitor the inspired gas temperature.

i. Choose and adjust the tidal volume for mechanical ventilation

A spontaneously breathing 70-kg (154-lb) adult with normal lungs and metabolism needs a tidal volume at 7 to 9 mL/kg (3 to 4 mL/lb) of ideal body weight to remove carbon dioxide adequately. Splitting the differences, a spontaneous tidal volume of about 500 mL is considered normal. The Radford nomogram can be used for predicting normal spontaneous tidal volumes and rates based on body weights. It can be used to establish an initial tidal volume for most patients (Fig. 15-16).

Most authors recommend a *set* ventilator tidal volume of *10 to 15 mL/kg* of ideal body weight. These are the values used by the NBRC in most patient situations. For example, the 70-kg (154-lb) adult with normal lungs needs a *set* mechanical ventilator tidal volume in the following range:

$$10 \text{ mL} \times 70 \text{ kg} = 700 \text{ mL}$$
$$15 \text{ mL} \times 70 \text{ kg} = 1050 \text{ mL}$$

This volume is higher than spontaneous for two reasons. First, some of the set volume is lost to the patient because of gas compression and tubing stretch/compliance (discussed previously). Second, some patients need larger-than-normal tidal volumes because their lungs are not functioning normally. Exceptions are patients with severe chronic restrictive lung disease, pneumonectomy patients, or patients with COPD. The tidal volume for these patients should be set at about 5 to 10 mL/kg of ideal body weight to avoid excessive ventilating pressure. In addition, giving a COPD patient a ventilator delivered tidal volume in the normal range may result in blowing off too much carbon dioxide and causing a respiratory alkalosis.

It is common practice to get a set of ABG values after the patient is stable on the ventilator. The tidal volume can be adjusted within the range depending on whether the patient's arterial CO_2 pressure (Pa_{CO_2}) value is too high or low for the therapeutic goal. The most direct way to change alveolar ventilation is to modify the delivered tidal volume. If everything else remains the same, a larger tidal volume results in a lower Pa_{CO_2} value. Conversely, while everything else remains the same, a smaller tidal volume results in a higher Pa_{CO_2} value.

The following formula can be used to help predict what *tidal volume* produces a *desired* Pa_{CO_2} value:

$$(V_T - [V_{D_{anat}} + V_{D_{mech}}]) \times f \times Pa_{CO_2} =$$
$$(V_T' - [V_{D_{anat}} + V_{D_{mech}}]) \times f \times Pa_{CO_2}'$$

in which

V_T = current tidal volume

$V_{D_{anat}}$ = anatomic dead space (This is calculated at 1 mL/lb or 2.2 mL/kg of ideal body weight)

$V_{D_{mech}}$ = added mechanical dead space

f = respiratory (ventilator) rate

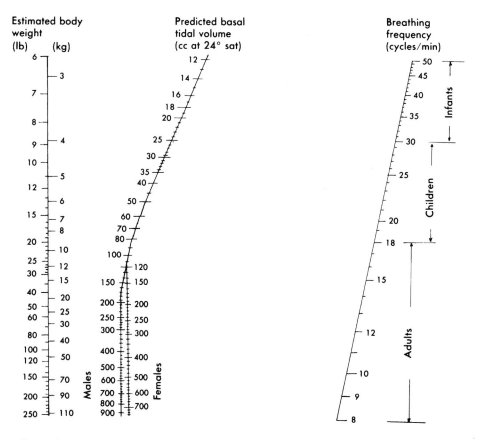

Estimated body weight (lb) (kg)

Predicted basal tidal volume (cc at 24° sat)

Breathing frequency (cycles/min)

Corrections of predicted basal tidal volumes.
    For patients not in coma: add 10%
    Fever: add 5% for each °F above 99 (rectal)
            add 9% for each °C above 37 (rectal)
    Altitude: add 5% for each 2000 feet above sea level
            add 8% for each 1000 meters above sea level
    Intubation: subtract volume equal to one-half body weight in pounds
            subtract 1 cc/kg of body weight
    Dead space: add equipment dead space

Fig. 15-16 Radford nomogram. To use the nomogram, place the left edge of a ruler on the patient's estimated body weight and move the right edge to the patient's breathing frequency. The predicted basal tidal volume can now be found. For example, a 150-pound male breathing 12 times per minute will have a predicted tidal volume of 500 cc (mL). *(From Radford EP Jr: Ventilation standards for use in artificial respiration.* J Appl Physiol *7:451–460, 1955.)*

Pa_{CO_2} = actual patient Pa_{CO_2} value

V_T' = *desired tidal volume*

Pa_{CO_2}' = desired patient Pa_{CO_2} value

Note that other, simpler formulas are available for calculating a change in minute volume or tidal volume. This one is presented because it takes into account more factors and can be used to calculate a change in tidal volume, rate, or mechanical dead space.

EXAMPLE

The patient is a 70-kg (154-lb) man who is being ventilated on the control mode (he is apneic). His ventilator settings are a tidal volume of 1000 mL, rate of 12 times/min, fractional inspired oxygen concentration (F_{IO_2}) of 0.3, and no added mechanical dead space. His ABG values are an arterial oxygen pressure (Pa_{O_2}) of 90 torr, Pa_{CO_2} of 30 torr, pH of 7.48, Sa_{O_2} of 95%, and a base excess (BE) of 0. The clinical goal is to adjust the patient's tidal volume as needed to produce a Pa_{CO_2} value of 40 torr. In summary:

V_T = 1000 mL current tidal volume

$V_{D_{anat}}$ = 154 mL of anatomic dead space (This is calculated at 1 mL/lb or 2.2 mL/kg of ideal body weight.)

$V_{D_{mech}}$ = no added mechanical dead space

f = 12 times/min for the ventilator rate

Pa_{CO_2} = 30 torr actual patient Pa_{CO_2} value

V_T' = *desired tidal volume*

Pa_{CO_2}' = 40 torr desired patient Pa_{CO_2} value

Placing the data and goal into the formula results in the following:

$$(V_T - [VD_{anat} + VD_{mech}]) \times f \times Paco_2 =$$
$$(V_T' - [VD_{anat} + VD_{mech}]) \times f \times Paco_2'$$
$$(1000 - [154 + 0]) \times 12 \times 30 = (V_T' - [154 + 0]) \times 12 \times 40$$

Simplifying produces the following:

$$(846) \times 12 \times 30 = (V_T' - 154) \times 480$$
$$304,560 = 480\, V_T' - 73,920$$
$$378,480 = 480\, V_T'$$
$$788\ mL = V_T'$$

The solution is to reduce the patient's tidal volume from 1000 to 788 mL.

Exam Hint

Every available NBRC examination has had several problems that require the test taker to determine an original ventilator tidal volume or a new tidal volume to correct for overventilating (low carbon dioxide level) or underventilating (high carbon dioxide level) a patient. Typically, start with a tidal volume of 10 mL/kg of body weight. Increase or decrease the tidal volume as needed from this starting point.

---

j. Choose and adjust the rate for mechanical ventilation

See Table 1-11 for a listing of the normal resting respiratory frequencies based on age. If the patient is apneic and has a normal temperature and an appropriately set tidal volume, the respiratory rates in the indicated ranges will produce a normal Paco2 level. This must be confirmed by ABG measurements. If the tidal volume cannot be changed, adjusting the respiratory rate will modify alveolar ventilation. A higher respiratory rate, while everything else remains the same, will result in a lower Paco2 level. Conversely, a lower respiratory rate, while everything else remains the same, will result in a higher Paco2 level.

See Fig. 15-16 for the Radford nomogram for predicting a normal respiratory rate and tidal volume based on weight. It can be used to establish an initial rate for most patients. As mentioned earlier, chronically hypercapneic patients must be ventilated with some caution. To give this type of patient a higher ventilator delivered rate and larger tidal volume may result in blowing off too much carbon dioxide and cause a respiratory alkalosis. Adult patients with severe chronic restrictive lung disease or those who have had a pneumonectomy may need respiratory rates of 20 to 30 per minute or greater to meet their minute volume needs. This is because their delivered tidal volume must be smaller than normal because of their condition.

The same formula that was used to predict a tidal volume change can be used to help predict what *respiratory rate* will produce a desired Paco2 value:

$$(V_T - [VD_{anat} + VD_{mech}]) \times f \times Paco_2 =$$
$$(V_T - [VD_{anat} + VD_{mech}]) \times f' \times Paco_2'$$

EXAMPLE

The patient is the same 70-kg (154-lb) man who is being ventilated on the control mode (he is apneic). His ventilator settings are a tidal volume of 1000 mL, rate of 12 times/min, FIO_2 of 0.3, and no added mechanical dead space. His ABG values are an arterial oxygen pressure (Pao_2) of 90 torr, $Paco_2$ of 30 torr, pH of 7.48, Sao_2 of 95%, and a base excess (BE) of 0. The clinical goal is to adjust the patient's rate as needed to produce a $Paco_2$ value of 40 torr. In summary:

V_T = 1000 mL current tidal volume

VD_{anat} = 154 mL of anatomic dead space (This is calculated at 1 mL/lb or 2.2 mL/kg of ideal body weight.)

VD_{mech} = no added mechanical dead space

f = 12 times/min for the ventilator rate

f' = desired ventilator rate

$Paco_2$ = 30 torr actual patient $Paco_2$ value

$Paco_2'$ = 40 torr desired patient $Paco_2$ value

Placing the data and goal into the formula results in the following:

$$(V_T - [VD_{anat} + VD_{mech}]) \times f \times Paco_2 =$$
$$(V_T - [VD_{anat} + VD_{mech}]) \times f' \times Paco_2'$$
$$(1000 - [154 + 0]) \times 12 \times 30 = (1000 - [154 + 0]) \times f' \times 40$$
$$[846] \times 12 \times 30 = [846] \times f' \times 40$$
$$304,560 = 33,840\, f'$$
$$9 = f'$$

The solution is to reduce the patient's respiratory rate from 12 to 9 breaths/min.

Exam Hint

Every available NBRC examination has had several problems that require the test taker to determine an original ventilator respiratory rate or a new respiratory rate to correct for overventilating (low carbon dioxide level) or underventilating (high carbon dioxide level) a patient. Typically start with a respiratory rate of 10 to 14 in an adult. Increase or decrease the rate needed from this starting point.

---

k. Choose and adjust the minute ventilation for mechanical ventilation

The subjects of minute ventilation and alveolar minute ventilation were covered in Chapter 4. Review the calculations as needed. Blood gases must always be evaluated for the $PaCO_2$ level to tell whether the patient's minute ventilation is adequate. A high carbon dioxide level indicates a need to increase the tidal volume, respiratory rate, or both. A low carbon dioxide level indicates a need to decrease the tidal volume, respiratory rate, or both. In both cases, the key to modifying the carbon dioxide level is to modify the alveolar ventilation. That is best accomplished by changing the tidal volume rather than the rate. The following formula can be used to calculate a change in the minute volume:

$$\dot{V}_E' = \frac{PaCO_2 \times \dot{V}_E}{PaCO_2'}$$

in which:

$\dot{V}_E'$ = *desired minute volume*
$\dot{V}_E$ = current minute volume
$PaCO_2$ = current carbon dioxide level
$PaCO_2'$ = *desired* carbon dioxide level

EXAMPLE

The patient is the same 70-kg (154-lb) man who is being ventilated on the control mode (he is apneic). His ventilator settings are a tidal volume of 1000 mL, rate of 12 times/min, FIO_2 of 0.3, and no added mechanical dead space. His ABG values are a PaO_2 of 90 torr, $PaCO_2$ of 30 torr, pH of 7.48, SaO_2 of 95%, and a BE of 0. The clinical goal is to adjust the patient's minute volume as needed to produce a $PaCO_2$ value of 40 torr. Placing the data and goal into the formula results in the following:

$$\dot{V}_E' = \frac{PaCO_2 \times V_E}{PaCO_2}$$
$$\dot{V}_E' = \frac{30 \times 12,000}{40 \, \dot{V}_E'}$$
$$\dot{V}_E' = \frac{360,000}{40 \, \dot{V}_E'}$$
$$\dot{V}_E' = 9000 \text{ mL}$$

The goal can be accomplished by reducing the minute volume from 12,000 to 9000 mL. As mentioned earlier, this is best done by reducing the tidal volume. Remember that the tidal volume must be kept at no less than 10 mL/kg of ideal body weight to avoid the development of atelectasis. The respiratory rate may be decreased, if necessary, to provide this reduced minute volume.

4. Begin and modify positive end-expiratory pressure therapy (WRE code: IIID2d) [Difficulty: An]

PEEP is a residual pressure above atmospheric pressure maintained at the airway opening at the end of expiration. PEEP is administered through a mechanical ventilator and is not a mode by itself. Rather, it is used in conjunction with any of the previously mentioned modes. PEEP is set to prevent the patient from exhaling back to ambient (atmospheric) pressure. The higher the level of PEEP, the more progressively the patient's FRC is increased. The therapeutic goal of this is to increase the patient's arterial oxygen pressure (PaO_2). (Fig. 15-10, *F*, shows the pressure/time curve.)

PEEP is generally indicated in any bilateral, generalized pulmonary condition in which the FRC is decreased. Examples include generalized atelectasis, pulmonary edema, ARDS, and infant respiratory distress syndrome (RDS). All of these patients show a decreased lung compliance as measured by their static compliance (Cst). Specific indications for PEEP include:

a. Intrapulmonary shunt greater than 15%
b. Refractory hypoxemia (PaO_2 less than 60 mm Hg despite an FIO_2 of up to 0.8 to 1.0)
c. The patient has had an FIO_2 of greater than 0.5 for 48 to 72 hours and shows no indication of a rapidly improving PaO_2. PEEP is added so that the FIO_2 can be lowered to a safer level.

Before PEEP is begun, the patient should be carefully monitored to establish the baseline condition. The same parameters should be monitored after each change in the PEEP level to determine how the patient is tolerating it. The best or optimal level of PEEP is the level that results in the best delivery of oxygen to the tissues (not necessarily the arterial blood). Often, a secondary goal is to reduce the inspired oxygen to a safe level. The patient is at risk of oxygen toxicity if more than 50% oxygen is inhaled for more than 48 to 72 hours. See Box 15-4 for recommendations on what to monitor during the application of PEEP and how to evaluate the data.

The application of PEEP has risks. Clinically, these risks must be weighed against the potential benefit to the patient. In the profoundly hypoxic patient, PEEP can be lifesaving. Some clinicians use low levels of PEEP (up to 5 cm water) in patients with normal lungs or overly compliant lungs (emphysema) to maintain the baseline level of FRC. Hazards of PEEP include:

Pulmonary barotrauma: pneumothorax, tension pneumothorax, mediastinal emphysema, pulmonary interstitial emphysema (PIE) in the neonate, subcutaneous emphysema

Decreased venous return to the heart, causing a decreased cardiac output and tachycardia, decreased blood pressure, decreased tissue perfusion as measured by a decreased mixed venous oxygen ($P\bar{v}O_2$) level, decreased urine output

PEEP therapy is usually begun at initial levels of 2 to 5 cm water. After the patient's response is determined, 2 to 5 cm more PEEP may be applied. The patient is reevaluated. This process goes on until the best or optimal level of PEEP is determined. See Fig. 15-17 for a number of physiologic parameters that can be measured and evaluated.

Different approaches to the application of PEEP are used to find the best level. One approach could be called

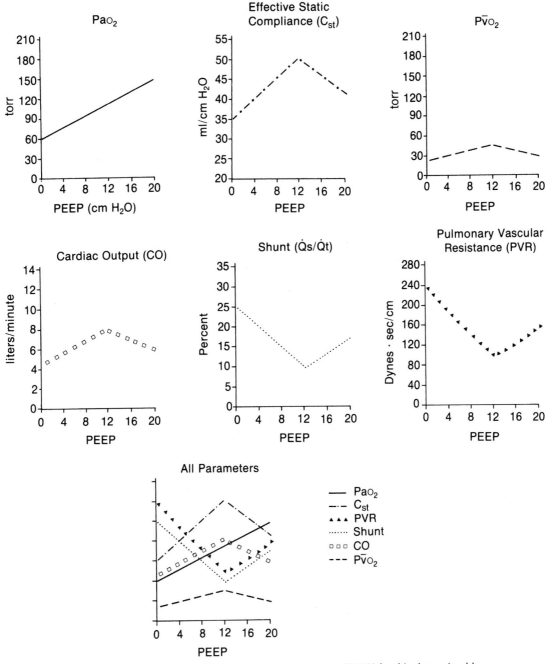

Fig. 15-17 Optimal or best positive end-expiratory pressure (PEEP) level is determined by monitoring some or all of the following parameters: Pao_2, effective static compliance (Cst), pressure of mixed venous oxygen ($P\bar{v}o_2$), cardiac output (CO), shunt ($\dot{Q}s/\dot{Q}t$), and pulmonary vascular resistance (PVR). Ideally, as functional residual capacity (FRC) is increased by PEEP, lung compliance is improved, and ventilation and perfusion are better matched. Cardiac output should remain stable. It can be measured by use of pulmonary artery (Swan-Ganz) catheter or indirectly followed by monitoring patient's heart rate and blood pressure. As can be seen, the optimal PEEP is found at 12-cm water pressure. Excessive PEEP is seen by the resulting decrease in static compliance and cardiac output.

minimum PEEP. It involves the application of PEEP to the minimum level that allows the inspired oxygen percentage to be lowered to a safer level. A clinical goal is to minimize the risk of oxygen toxicity. In this approach, PEEP is raised until the Pao_2 is greater than 60 torr or the

Spo_2 is greater than 90% on 60% oxygen or less. Usually no more than 10 to 15 cm water of PEEP is needed.

Another approach could be called maximum or optimal PEEP. This approach has the clinical goal of reducing the patient's shunt fraction to less than 15%. Often this requires more pressure than the minimal PEEP approach. Because this higher pressure level is more likely to cause hemodynamic problems, the patient should have a pulmonary artery catheter inserted. With it, the patient's cardiac output, mixed venous oxygen level, pulmonary capillary wedge pressure, and pulmonary vascular resistance can be measured. In addition, the patient may need increased intravenous fluids, dopamine (Intropin), and digitalis (Digoxin) for cardiovascular support. The higher PEEP levels increase the risk of pulmonary barotrauma. Therefore the patient must be watched closely for signs of a pneumothorax.

As the patient begins to recover, the PEEP level may be reduced in steps of 2 to 5 cm water. Again, the patient is evaluated after every change in the PEEP level. If the patient's cardiovascular status is normal, the following are recommendations for how to decrease PEEP and oxygen levels:

Decrease PEEP first if the Pa_{O_2} level is greater than 60 torr and the F_{IO_2} is less than 0.5.

Decrease oxygen first if the Pa_{O_2} level is greater than 60 torr and the F_{IO_2} is greater than 0.5.

If the patient is showing an adverse reaction to the PEEP level, such as decreased cardiac output or barotrauma, the PEEP level should be decreased before the oxygen percentage. Clinical judgment must be used to decide whether a high oxygen percentage or a high PEEP level is a greater danger to the patient. Minimize or remove the element that puts the patient at greater risk.

Exam Hint

Typically, several questions deal with the clinical application and modification of PEEP. Know to increase PEEP if the patient is hypoxic, is receiving a high oxygen percentage, and is hemodynamically stable. Know to decrease PEEP if the patient is well oxygenated and receiving a moderate oxygen percentage, is not hemodynamically stable, or has a PEEP-related complication. A decrease in the patient's cardiac output is a key indicator of excessive PEEP causing hemodynamic problems.

---

5. Begin and modify continuous positive airway pressure (WRE code: IIID2d) [Difficulty: An]

CPAP is a pressure above atmospheric maintained at the airway opening throughout the respiratory cycle during spontaneous breathing. CPAP is similar to PEEP in purpose and effect. It is different from the previously mentioned modes in that the patient does not receive any ventilator delivered tidal volume breaths. The patient must be capable of providing all of the minute ventilation for carbon dioxide removal. CPAP can be delivered through some mechanical ventilators when the rate is turned off or through a freestanding system (Fig. 15-10, G, shows the pressure/time curve).

CPAP has the same indications, hazards, and patient evaluation processes discussed earlier in PEEP therapy. One possible physiologic benefit of CPAP over PEEP is that less reduction occurs in the venous return to the heart. This is because with CPAP, the patient is breathing spontaneously. Therefore patients treated with CPAP may be able to tolerate higher pressure levels than those patients being ventilated with PEEP therapy.

CPAP is usually increased and decreased in steps of 2 to 5 cm water. As with PEEP, the patient is evaluated before CPAP is begun and again after every pressure change. See Box 15-4 for recommendations on what to monitor during the application of CPAP and how to evaluate the data.

Before a patient receives CPAP therapy, the practitioner and physician must be assured that the patient has the ability to breathe adequately to eliminate carbon dioxide. CPAP is contraindicated in an apneic patient or in one who may become apneic. (This patient must be fully supported on the ventilator.) The patient must have an adequate respiratory rate, tidal volume, and minute volume. The heart rate and blood pressure should be stable. Maximum inspiratory pressure and vital capacity values may be acceptable or low. Blood gas analysis typically shows refractory hypoxemia but a normal or low Pa_{CO_2} level. This shows that the patient would benefit from an elevated baseline pressure to increase the FRC but is quite capable of ventilating.

The patient must be carefully monitored for fatigue because the patient is providing all of the minute ventilation. Signs of fatigue include increasing respiratory rate, decreasing tidal volume or vital capacity, decreasing maximum inspiratory pressure, and tachycardia. Blood gas measurement may show a stable or decreasing Pa_{O_2} value. An increasing Pa_{CO_2} level is a definite sign of fatigue. The patient may complain of dyspnea. The practitioner may notice the patient is working harder than normal to breathe, as shown by the increased use of the accessory muscles of ventilation and heavy perspiration. When these signs occur, CPAP therapy should be discontinued and mechanical ventilation instituted in a mode that best fits the patient's needs.

Exam Hint

Know that CPAP can be used and increased if the patient's carbon dioxide level is normal and hypoxemia is present. Increase or decrease CPAP by following the same parameters used to evaluate a change in PEEP. Know to switch to mechanical ventilation when the maximum level of CPAP is being used and the patient is still hypoxemic.

6. Noninvasive positive-pressure ventilation
a. Begin nasal/mask noninvasive positive-pressure ventilation (WRE code: IIID2b) [Difficulty: An]

Noninvasive positive-pressure ventilation (NPPV) is indicated in stable, unintubated, spontaneously breathing patients with any of the following clinical situations: elevated carbon dioxide level, hypoxemia despite supplemental oxygen, chronic ventilatory muscle dysfunction, or sleep apnea from upper airway obstruction. Most of the time, these patients are ventilated with the aid of a nasal mask similar to that used to deliver mask CPAP. A full face mask is needed if the patient leaks through the mouth with a nasal mask. If the patient is critically ill, unstable, must be intubated to secure the airway for secretion removal, needs a high level of therapeutic PEEP to maintain the FRC, or a combination of these, he or she should be placed on a standard volume cycled ventilator.

Often patients receiving NPPV are ventilated with two different levels of positive pressure. This is referred to as *bilevel ventilation*. The baseline pressure is greater than zero (CPAP or PEEP), and the peak pressure is set to deliver a desired tidal volume (similar to PS ventilation). Both levels can be independently adjusted. If only the baseline pressure is elevated, the patient is receiving CPAP. If only the peak pressure is elevated, the patient is receiving PS ventilation. Respironics has developed two devices for bilevel ventilation that can be used in the hospital or home for noninvasive mask ventilation. They are the BiPAP S-D and the newer BiPAP S/T-D Ventilatory Support System. Supplemental oxygen is not available through the machines; however, it can be added though a side port on the nasal mask to meet clinical goals.

The patient must have a properly fitting nasal or face mask to receive noninvasive ventilation. These ventilation masks are similar to CPAP masks and are referred to as such. CPAP masks come in different sizes for children older than 3 years and for adults. Nasal masks are designed to cover only the nose. They allow the patient to eat, drink, speak, and use the mouth as a second airway for breathing in case a malfunction of the CPAP system occurs. The mouth also acts as a pressure relief route if the CPAP pressure should become too great. Pressures of up to 10 to 15 cm water can usually be maintained (Fig. 15-18). Usually the mask is made of a transparent plastic. Face masks are designed to cover the nose and mouth. They are similar in design to the masks used during bag/mask ventilation and also are made of a transparent plastic. The face mask must be used if the patient has persistent mouth breathing and cannot use a nose mask. With a good seal, pressures of greater than 15 cm water can be maintained.

Both types of CPAP mask have a soft, very compliant seal to fit closely the contours of the face. Straps are needed to hold the mask in place (Fig. 15-19). Too large a mask will not seal and will allow gas to leak and pressure to decrease. The patient may show increased snoring or airway obstruction with periods of apnea. A mask that is too small or misfitting can cause an uneven distribution of pressure on the face. This can lead to abrasions or pressure sores and ulcers on the face.

The BiPAP S/T-D system can be used for bilevel ventilation or in the CPAP mode. It makes use of a relatively simple smooth interior circuit and does not have a humidifier, alarm system, or the other attachments seen in a volume cycled ventilator. A bacteria filter should be inserted between the BiPAP unit and the patient circuit. If a humidifier is desired, it must be a cascade- or wick-type humidifier. An HME cannot be used because it creates too much resistance.

b. Adjust nasal/mask noninvasive ventilation (WRE code: IIID2b) [Difficulty: An]

The bilevel settings must be determined at the bedside by asking for the patient's subjective opinion, listening to breath sounds, checking vital signs, and evaluating ABG values. If supplemental oxygen is needed, it can be added at a port on the patient's mask, at the humidifier, or at the outlet from the BiPAP unit. Up to 15 L/min can be added without affecting the performance of the BiPAP system. It is not possible to know the delivered oxygen percentage until after the bilevel ventilation settings are determined. The oxygen flow should then be gradually increased while the patient's Spo_2 value increases to the desired saturation level.

Only the function of the BiPAP S/T-D system is reviewed because it is newer and has more features. The operator can choose among the following five modes of operation:

1. Expiratory positive airway pressure (EPAP) from 2 to 20 cm water. This is functionally similar to CPAP.
2. Inspiratory positive airway pressure (IPAP) from 2 to 25 cm water. This is functionally similar to setting the peak pressure on a pressure cycled ventilator. The patient must trigger each IPAP-assisted breath.
3. Spontaneous (S) functions like the PS mode in which the patient must initiate each assisted breath. The therapist can set IPAP and EPAP levels. This delivers bilevel ventilation.
4. Spontaneous/timed (S/T) delivers between 6 and 30 ventilator breaths per minute when the patient's respiratory rate decreases below the set number. Otherwise, it functions like the spontaneous mode and delivers bilevel ventilation.
5. Times (T) varies the percentage of each cycle in IPAP from 10% to 90%. This allows the therapist to set an I:E ratio. All of the first four functions are maintained, except that the patient cannot trigger an IPAP breath.

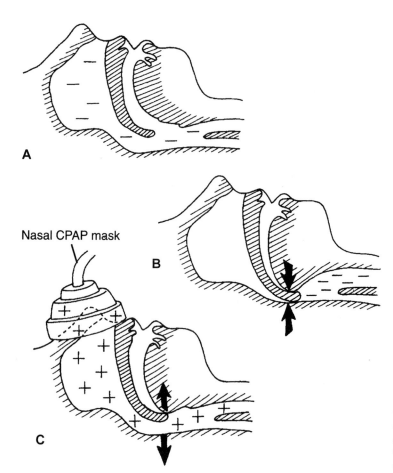

Fig. 15-18 Effect of nasal continuous positive airway pressure (CPAP) mask. **A,** Normal upper airway remains patent during sleep. **B,** Abnormal upper airway of patient with obstructive apnea collapses on inspiration during sleep. **C,** Pressure from nasal CPAP mask keeps abnormal upper airway patent during sleep. *(Modified from Scanlan CL. In Scanlan CL, Spearman CB, Sheldon RL, editors:* Egan's fundamentals of respiratory care, *ed 5, St Louis, 1990, Mosby.)*

With the BiPAP units, the difference between IPAP and EPAP is called *pressure boost* and delivers the tidal volume. It is important to remember that the delivered tidal volume varies depending on changes in the patient's airway resistance and lung/thoracic compliance as well as the machine settings.

MODULE C
Mechanical ventilation equipment

Note: The literature produced by the manufacturers and the descriptions used in many standard texts break down the various ventilators into more categories than used by the NBRC. To avoid confusion, this text uses the NBRC more simplified terminology. A *pneumatically powered ventilator* is defined here as a ventilator powered by compressed gas and without any electrically powered control systems (electrically powered alarm systems may or may not be added). An *electrically powered ventilator* is defined here as a ventilator that is either electrically powered or controlled. Most volume cycled ventilators fall into this category. *Microprocessor ventilators* are electrically powered but controlled by one or more microprocessors (computers). Many of the most current volume cycled ventilators have microprocessors to control their functions. *Fluidic ventilators* typically make use of electrical circuits with flip-flops to respond to changes in gas flow and pressure through the system. Fluidic ventilators are powered by compressed gas. *Noninvasive positive-pressure ventilators* are designed for home use or short-term hospital use and are electrically powered and controlled. They have fewer controls and alarms than hospital-based critical care ventilators. A nasal or full face mask, rather than an endotracheal tube, is used to attach the ventilator to the patient. *High-frequency ventilators* are used in a limited population of critically ill patients who are doing poorly despite all attempts at conventional mechanical ventilation. These units are designed to deliver very rapid respiratory rates and very small tidal volumes.

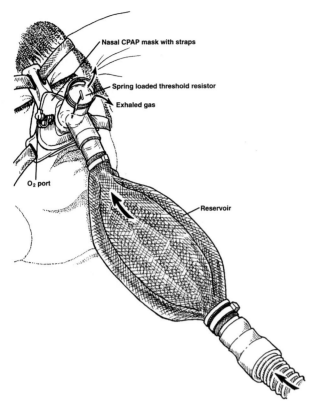

Fig. 15-19 Nasal continuous positive airway pressure (CPAP) mask in place on adult patient. Note straps to hold mask in place to create a seal around the patient's nose. If patient needs supplemental oxygen, small bore tubing can be connected to the oxygen port.

1. Pneumatically powered ventilators
a. Get the necessary equipment for the procedure (WRE code: IIA6a) [Difficulty: An]

The only commonly used pneumatically powered ventilators are the Bird series and the Bennett PR-2. A control or backup rate can be set on these units in case the patient is apneic. All other controls and functions are the same as discussed in Chapter 14. The following equipment and procedures are necessary:

1. Bennett PR-2 or Bird ventilator with an air/oxygen blender and hoses
2. Bennett or Bird breathing circuit
3. Bacteria filters
4. Proper humidification system: either a passover- or cascade-type humidifier or an HME, (discussed later). Put sterile, distilled water in the passover- or cascade-type humidifier.
5. One or two water traps for condensation from the circuit
6. Add an alarm system(s) such as a low volume bellows spirometer or a low-pressure/disconnection alarm

7. If a low volume bellows spirometer alarm is used, a length of large bore tubing is needed to connect the exhalation valve to the bellows

b. Put the equipment together and make sure that it works properly (WRE code: IIA6a) [Difficulty: An]

Refer to Figs. 14-10 and 14-11 in Chapter 14 for the IPPB circuits. The ventilator and circuits are similar to those used in IPPB therapy with the following exceptions:

1. Set the ordered oxygen percentage on the blender; set the Bird *air mix* and Bennett *air dilution* selection controls to pure source gas from the blender. Analyze the F_{IO_2} through a port in the inspiratory limb of the circuit.
2. If a passover or cascade humidifier is used, a short length of large bore tubing is connected between the outlet of the mainstream in-line bacteria filter and the inlet of the humidifier. The inspiratory limb of the circuit is connected to the outlet of the humidifier. If an HME is used, it is added between the circuit and the tracheostomy/endotracheal tube adapter (Fig. 15-20).

Fig. 15-20 Heat-moisture exchanger inserted into a patient's breathing circuit. Any extra tubing placed between the Y of the circuit and the endotracheal tube acts as mechanical dead space.

3. A tracheostomy/endotracheal tube adapter is always used to connect the circuit to the patient (see Fig. 15-20).

4. Add at least one disconnection alarm to the circuit. It could be a low volume bellows spirometer alarm (e.g., on the Puritan-Bennett MA-1 ventilator) on the expiratory limb or a low pressure or disconnection alarm added into the inspiratory limb of the circuit with a Briggs adapter/T-piece.

5. Water traps are placed in the lowest part of the inspiratory and expiratory limbs of the circuit to hold any condensed water vapor.

Fig. 15-21 shows a complete circuit to a volume cycled ventilator. It is essentially the same circuit as used on a pressure cycled ventilator.

c. Troubleshoot any problems with the equipment (WRE code: IIA6a) [Difficulty: An]

Both of these types of ventilators send gas through the circuit during an inspiration and do not cycle off until the preset pressure is reached. Test the tightness of the circuit, backup rate, and delivered tidal volume by placing a test lung on the patient connection of the circuit. Set the controls to deliver the prescribed order. Be prepared to make final adjustments once either unit has been placed on the patient. The patient's airway resistance and lung compliance greatly affect the functioning of both units.

Troubleshooting problems with these units were discussed in Chapter 14. Make sure that all connections are tight; more exist now with the addition of the humidification system and expiratory limb to the spirometer.

A defective exhalation valve or one in which the small bore tubing has popped off sends gas through the circuit and not to the patient. If a bellows spirometer is being used, you will notice that it fills during inspiration instead of during expiration as normal.

2. Electrically powered ventilators
a. Get the necessary equipment for the procedure (WRE code: IIA6a) [Difficulty: An]

The majority of mechanical ventilators are electrically powered or controlled. They function primarily as volume cycled units, meaning that a preset volume is delivered from the ventilator with each breath regardless of the

Fig. 15-21 The basic components of a patient breathing circuit for continuous mechanical ventilation.

patient's condition. Each ventilator is unique in its abilities, modes, and so forth. It is beyond the scope of this book to discuss each and every volume cycled ventilator. They are presented in a generic manner. The learner should become familiar with the function of the Servo *i* and other widely used machines.

b. Put the equipment together and make sure that it works properly (WRE code: IIA6a) [Difficulty: An]

c. Troubleshoot any problems with the equipment (WRE code: IIA6a) [Difficulty: An]

Each ventilator must be learned for its specifics. Generally speaking, the following steps should be taken to ensure that the ventilator is functioning properly:

1. Select the proper ventilator for the physician's orders and patient's needs.
2. Attach the circuit properly, and make sure that all connections are tight (see Fig. 15-21).
3. Select the appropriate humidification device: a passover type, cascade type, or HME. Put sterile, distilled water in the passover or cascade unit.
4. Preset all of the physician-ordered parameters and any other settings that are needed to make the ventilator fully functional.
5. Place a test lung on the circuit at the patient connection.
6. Make sure that the ventilator delivers the preset rate, volume, oxygen percentage, I:E ratio, and so forth.

A low volume can be caused by a leak; check all connections, and tighten them as needed. The volume can be measured directly as it leaves the ventilator and at the exhalation valve to help determine the source of the wrong volume. If the unit shows a volume entering the exhalation valve and spirometer instead of the test lung during inspiration, the exhalation valve is broken. All alarms must be working properly. Batteries must be replaced when discharged.

3. Microprocessor ventilators

a. Get the necessary equipment for the procedure (WRE code: IIA6a) [Difficulty: An]

The microprocessor ventilators (e.g., Servo *i*, Hamilton Veolar, Drager Evita 4) are the most advanced generation of mechanical ventilators. They are electrically powered but controlled by one or more microprocessors (computers). They offer all commonly found modes of ventilation. In addition, many of these machines offer computer software for measuring bedside spirometry for weaning, WOB, and other parameters that give the clinician much valuable information. Airway resistance and static and dynamic lung compliance can be automatically calculated. Flow, volume, and pressure tracings are graphically displayed on the computer screen. Auto-PEEP can be documented and

measured. These units offer the greatest amount of patient data and clinical flexibility of all currently available ventilators. The most challenging patients can probably be best cared for on one of these machines.

b. Put the equipment together and make sure that it works properly (WRE code: IIA6a) [Difficulty: An]

c. Troubleshoot any problems with the equipment (WRE code: IIA6a) [Difficulty: An]

All of the previous general discussion on electrically powered ventilators applies to the microprocessor ventilators as well. An additional advantage to these units is that they self-diagnose most problems and display the problem for you. If a microprocessor should fail, the unit should be removed from the patient. The biomedical department or manufacturer has to replace the computer chip.

4. Fluidic ventilators

a. Get the necessary equipment for the procedure (WRE code: IIA6a) [Difficulty: An]

Examples of commonly available fluidic ventilators include the Sechrist IV-100B and Bio-Med MVP-10. Both are neonatal/pediatric units.

b. Put the equipment together and make sure that it works properly (WRE code: IIA6a) [Difficulty: An]

Make sure that high pressure gas hoses between the unit and wall outlets are tightly connected to prevent leaks. The patient circuit and humidification system must be properly installed and operating.

c. Troubleshoot any problems with the equipment (WRE code: IIA6a) [Difficulty: An]

Typically, fluidic ventilators are pneumatically powered and have fluidic controls. Make sure that the oxygen and air sources are up to the required pressure (usually 50 psig). Fluidic controls are very sensitive to any obstruction and to changes of other settings. Make sure that gas inlet and outlet filters are kept clear of obstructions.

5. Bilevel/noninvasive positive-pressure ventilators

a. Get the necessary equipment for the procedure (WRE code: IIA6b) [Difficulty: An]

A bilevel or NPPV is intended for an adult patient who is capable of breathing spontaneously for a limited period. The unit is typically used for a short period with a patient who is having breathing difficulty but does not require intubation and full ventilatory support. Current ventilators include the Respironics BiPAP S/T-D series, Respironics

BiPAP Vision, Nellcor Puritan-Bennett KnightStar 320, and Healthdyne Quantum PSV.

b. Put the equipment together and make sure that it works properly (WRE code: IIA6b) [Difficulty: An]

c. Troubleshoot any problems with the equipment (WRE code: IIA6b) [Difficulty: An]

Follow the manufacturer's guidelines for putting the circuit on the unit and adding a cascade- or passover-type humidifier. A proper size nasal or full face mask is needed to attach the circuit to the patient. Check carefully for any leakage between the mask and the patient's face.

6. High frequency ventilators
a. High frequency jet ventilators
1. Get the necessary equipment for the procedure (WRE code: IIA6c) [Difficulty: R, Ap, An]

Examples of freestanding jet ventilators include the Instrument Development Corporation Model VS600, Bunnell Life Pulse, and APT 1010. Bear Medical Systems developed the BEAR Jet, which must be used with a volume cycled ventilator that is placed in the CPAP or IMV mode during use of the jet.

In addition, a special endotracheal tube must be placed into the patient before HFJV can be initiated. Ideally, the patient must be intubated with a HiLo Jet tube from Mallinckrodt (Fig. 15-22) or the similar APT Ultracheal tube. These tubes are designed with a catheter through which the jetted gas is sent to the main lumen. Based on the physical principles that govern jets, additional gas is entrained through the main lumen. This entrained gas should be humidified if the jet gas is dry. All exhaled gas passes out through this main lumen. If the jet ventilator is used with a conventional volume cycled ventilator, the exhaled tidal volume can be measured through the ventilator's spirometry system. The ventilator's alarm systems also can be used, and IMV breaths and PEEP can be added if needed. If the patient is too unstable to be extubated and reintubated, a special endotracheal tube adapter can be added (Fig. 15-23). Jet gas enters through the cannula, and additional inspiratory and all expiratory gas goes through the main lumen of the adapter.

2. Put the equipment together and make sure that it works properly (WRE code: IIA6c) [Difficulty: R, Ap, An]

3. Troubleshoot any problems with the equipment (WRE code: IIA6c) [Difficulty: R, Ap, An]

Fig. 15-24 shows a schematic drawing of an HFJV. Although the currently available ventilators have basic

Fig. 15-22 A HiLo Jet endotracheal tube from Mallinckrodt. This special purpose endotracheal tube features four lumens. **A,** Pilot line to the cuff. **B,** Jet catheter used for delivering small bursts of tidal volume gas from a high frequency jet ventilator. It opens within the endotracheal tube above the cuff. **C,** Catheter for measuring proximal airway pressure within endotracheal tube near its tip. The main lumen of the endotracheal tube is used for suctioning and adding entrained, humidified gas from a conventional volume cycled ventilator. *(From McPherson SR: Respiratory therapy equipment, ed 4, St Louis, 1990, Mosby.)*

differences in how they are designed, they share these common features:

1. 50 psig source gas(es) of oxygen or oxygen and air are needed to generate a driving pressure.
2. A patient circuit specifically suited to the jet ventilator.
3. A drive pressure control lets the operator set the peak pressure of the jet.
4. An inspiratory time control sets the I:E ratio.

Fig. 15-23 Schematic drawing of tracheostomy/endotracheal tube adapter that has been modified for use with high frequency jet ventilator. Jet injector cannula has been added to tracheostomy/endotracheal tube adapter. A needle has been pushed through endotracheal tube adapter to drip saline into it for humidity. This system would be used if patient could not be intubated with HiLo Jet endotracheal tube. *(From Carlon GC, Miodownik S, Ray C Jr, Kahn RC: Technical aspects and clinical implications of high frequency jet ventilation with a solenoid valve. Crit Care Med 9:45, 1981.)*

Fig. 15-24 Schematic diagram of a high-frequency jet ventilator concept. *(From MacIntyre NR: Jet ventilation in the adult with breathing rates up to 150 bpm, Riverside, Calif, 1985, Bear Medical Systems. Courtesy of Viasys Respiratory Care, Inc.)*

5. Rate can be varied within the limits set by the unit.
6. The inspired oxygen percentage can be dialed either on the unit itself or on an external air/oxygen blender before going into the unit.
7. Humidification must be provided by either a dedicated cascade system or one joined to a volume cycled ventilator. The BEAR Jet does not have a humidification system of its own. It is used with a conventional volume ventilator, and the entrained gas is humidified through the cascade-type humidifier on it.

As with any ventilator, make sure that all connections are tight. Leaks are a particular problem because of the high pressures leaving the unit and the small tidal volumes that are delivered.

b. High frequency oscillator ventilators
1. Get the necessary equipment for the procedure (WRE code: IIA6c) [Difficulty: R, Ap, An]

The Percussionaire VDR 4 and the SensorMedics 3100B high-frequency oscillatory ventilators (HFOVs) are available for adults. Both units require a special circuit.

2. Put the equipment together and make sure that it works properly (WRE code: IIA6c) [Difficulty: R, Ap, An]
3. Troubleshoot any problems with the equipment (WRE code: IIA6c) [Difficulty: R, Ap, An]

Experience with the equipment is recommended to assemble the circuit as needed. The SensorMedics 3100B circuit is designed to combine two separate flows of gas for the patient's tidal volume. As with any circuit, make sure

that all connections are tight. The SensorMedics 3100B ventilator is controlled by a microprocessor that can help to diagnose any problems with the equipment.

7. Continuous mechanical ventilation and noninvasive ventilation breathing circuits
a. Get the necessary equipment for the procedure (WRE code: IIA10a and IIA10b) [Difficulty: Ap, An]

Either a permanent or a disposable circuit may be selected, based on the type of ventilator on which it must be placed. A circuit with an external exhalation valve must be used with older ventilators such as the Bennett MA-1 and Bear 1 and 2. The Drager Evita 2 Dura, Servo *i*, and other newer ventilators feature internal exhalation valves and do not need a circuit. If the patient must receive aerosolized medications, the circuit should either include a nebulizer or be able to accept one. If not included, the nebulizer or metered dose inhaler adapter must be added into the inspiratory limb of the circuit.

Also consider whether it is better to use an unheated or heated circuit. Usually the circuit is unheated. With these, a cascade-type humidifier or HME is used to warm and humidify the inspired gas. However, some practitioners prefer to use a heated circuit for the care of neonates. These circuits either have heated wires loosely running through the lumen of the tubing or have a wire embedded within the tubing itself. A heated-wire circuit offers finer control over the temperature of the inspired gas and minimizes condensation. Follow the manufacturer's guidelines to make sure that the system can adequately humidify the minute volume that is being used.

Noninvasive ventilators, such as the Respironics series, have specific circuits designed only for the unit. Traditional ventilator circuits cannot be placed on a non-invasive ventilator.

b. Put the equipment together and make sure that it works properly (WRE code: IIA10a and IIA10b) [Difficulty: Ap, An]

Assemble the circuit with the features needed to manage the patient. Common, but not universal, features of the inspiratory limb of the circuit include a water trap, a humidification system, a nebulizer, a thermometer or temperature probe, a pressure monitoring port, and an oxygen monitoring port. Common, but not universal, features of the expiratory limb of the circuit include an exhalation valve and a water trap.

The heated-wire circuits must be used only with the humidifier with which they are specifically designed to work. The humidifier has a thermostat that regulates warming the humidifier water and heated wires to the same temperature. Never cover a heated-wire circuit with a patient's sheets or blanket or any other material. Do not rest the circuit on anything such as the bed rail, patient's body, or medical equipment. These circuits should always be supported on a boom arm or tube-tree.

Noninvasive ventilator circuits must be set up as specified for the ventilator. Typically, an HME is added to humidify the patient's tidal volume gas. This is because of the high airway resistance of a wick- or bubble-type humidifier. These ventilators are not powerful enough to provide a stable tidal volume when airway resistance is high.

All circuits use a Y-connector to tie the inspiratory and expiratory limbs together and attach the circuit to the patient. See Fig. 15-21 for a generic ventilator circuit. Make sure that the water level is properly maintained in the humidifier.

c. Troubleshoot any problems with the continuous ventilation circuit (WRE code: IIA10a and IIA10b) [Difficulty: Ap, An]

Check the circuit and connections for leaks if the volume returned from the patient is less than what was set or delivered. The set volume should be measured with a hand-held spirometer as it exits the ventilator, at connection points through the circuit, and at the exhalation valve or ventilator spirometer or both. The volume control or ventilator spirometer may be out of calibration. If the unit shows a volume entering the spirometer instead of the test lung during inspiration, the exhalation valve is broken. Replace a circuit with a leak or a defective exhalation valve that cannot be fixed.

d. Change the patient's ventilator circuit as needed (CSE code: IIIF2i9)

A circuit must be replaced if it is damaged in a way that prevents the patient from being ventilated. This is most commonly seen in circuits with external exhalation valves. If the valve is damaged and will not close, the circuit should be replaced.

Routine circuit changes are done for infection control purposes. A circuit that is not clean in appearance (mucus or blood contamination) should be changed. The American Association for Respiratory Care (AARC) Clinical Practice Guideline on ventilator circuit changes includes the following recommendations:

1. The circuit should be changed every 24 hours if a nebulizer is used for humidification.
2. The circuit may be used for up to 5 days if a cascade- or wick-type humidifier is used for humidification.
3. If an HME is used, it should be changed every 24 hours.

8. Ventilator breathing circuits: PEEP valve assembly

a. Get the necessary equipment for the procedure (WRE code: IIA10c) [Difficulty: Ap, An]

A variety of PEEP systems can be added to a ventilator or CPAP circuit. Consult an equipment book for the details of their operation. A number of newer ventilators such as the Servo i and Hamilton Veolar have internal exhalation valves and PEEP-generating venturi systems with nothing to assemble at the bedside. Failure to generate PEEP indicates that the exhalation valve or PEEP-generating venturi system has failed in some manner.

Most older ventilators (Bennett MA-1 and Bear 1 and 2) use a balloon-like exhalation valve. A direct relation exists between the volume of gas that is kept in the balloon, the pressure and resistance that it creates, and the PEEP level that is generated (see Fig. 15-21).

b. Put the equipment together and make sure that it works properly (WRE code: IIA10c) [Difficulty: Ap, An]

The key thing to check with any PEEP-generating system is that the proper level of PEEP is generated and maintained. Once the ordered PEEP level is set, it should be seen as stable on the pressure manometer throughout the respiratory cycle. Sensitivity should be set at no more than −1 to −2 cm water. That way, the PEEP level is maintained at close to the ordered level even during an assisted breath. For example, PEEP is set at 10 cm, and the sensitivity is set at −1 cm. When the patient triggers a breath, it will occur at 9 cm PEEP.

c. Troubleshoot any problems with the equipment (WRE code: IIA10c) [Difficulty: Ap, An]

Malfunctioning internal exhalation valves or PEEP-generation venturi systems cannot be easily repaired at the bedside. The ventilator must be replaced. Balloon-type exhalation valves (see Fig. 15-21) are prone to the following two problems:

1. The small bore tube carrying gas from the ventilator to the balloon valve is pulled off. Reconnect the tubing to either the ventilator nipple connection or exhalation valve nipple connection.
2. The balloon is torn, and the gas leaks out. This can be confirmed by disassembling the exhalation valve assembly. Replace the balloon, and reassemble the exhalation valve.

Both of these problems are exhibited when the inspiratory tidal volume flows past the patient and directly into the exhaled tidal volume spirometer. Little or no airway pressure is generated. The patient is poorly ventilated, if at all. This problem must be corrected immediately while the patient is manually ventilated.

9. Continuous positive airway pressure systems: breathing circuits

a. Get the necessary equipment for the procedure (WRE code: IIA10c) [Difficulty: Ap, An]

Most current generation ventilators have a built-in CPAP mode. No additional circuitry is needed. After switching to the CPAP mode, set the desired level by adjusting the PEEP/CPAP dial and watching the reading on the pressure manometer.

Several manufacturers make CPAP systems for home use in the treatment of obstructive sleep apnea patients. These CPAP systems typically include an air pump to generate flow to the patient, CPAP generating device, circuit designed to work with the system, patient mask(s), and alarm system.

Freestanding CPAP breathing circuits used in hospitals vary considerably. No manufacturer has developed a system that dominates the marketplace. Most commonly, each respiratory care department develops its own breathing circuit to meet its own needs.

b. Put the equipment together and make sure that it works properly (WRE code: IIA10c) [Difficulty: Ap, An]

Fig. 15-25 shows the typical components used in a CPAP breathing circuit. The components include

1. Air/oxygen blender
2. Pediatric or adult flowmeter on the blender
3. Cascade-type humidifier
4. Inspiratory circuit of large bore or aerosol tubing with the following additions: water trap, one-way valve, and thermometer
5. Y-connector to connect the inspiratory and expiratory limbs of the circuit
6. Patient connector (elbow adapter) to endotracheal or tracheostomy tube, CPAP prongs, or CPAP mask
7. Expiratory circuit of large bore or aerosol tubing with the following additions: water trap, high pressure pop-off valve (not shown), pressure manometer for measuring the CPAP level, low pressure or disconnection audible alarm, anesthesia bag as a reservoir, variable resistance clamp on the tail of the anesthesia bag, Briggs adapters/T-pieces for connecting the various features, emergency pop-in valve in case gas flow is stopped, and CPAP device.

The CPAP level is adjusted by means of a variety of devices collectively called *threshold resistors,* which include the following:

1. A column of water with a length of expiratory tubing inserted the needed depth below the surface (so-called "bubble CPAP").
2. A vertically mounted ball bearing. It creates a resistance as gas flows up past it. These ball-bearing resistors come in weights of 2.5, 5, and 10 cm water.
3. A spring-loaded resistor that is adjusted to apply the desired CPAP level against the airway.
4. A freestanding venturi PEEP system. Gas from the venturi jet creates backpressure against the escaping patient tidal volume.

Air exits through each of these devices when it is working properly. All CPAP systems must be adjusted by checking the pressure level on the manometer. Set the low pressure or disconnection audible alarm to sound at a few centimeters below the CPAP level. For example, if 10 cm CPAP is ordered, set the alarm to sound if the pressure drops below 8 cm of CPAP.

c. Fix any problems with the equipment (WRE code: IIA10c) [Difficulty: Ap, An]

Flow through the CPAP breathing circuit must be sufficient to meet the patient's needs. Adjust the flowmeter setting, and clamp on the anesthesia bag so that it is somewhat inflated, with excess air escaping out past the clamp. With all of the devices, gas escapes through the path of least resistance. All or some may escape through the anesthesia bag, the CPAP device, or both. The bag should collapse somewhat during the patient's inspiration and expand somewhat during the expiration. The CPAP level should not decrease more than 1 or 2 cm from the baseline during an inspiration.

Make sure that the water level is properly maintained in the humidifier. Fill it with sterile, distilled water as often as necessary.

A sudden decrease in the CPAP level to zero indicates a disconnection at the patient or somewhere in the breathing circuit. Check all connections, and reassemble the break. The patient may need to be manually ventilated while the problem is corrected.

If the CPAP level decreases more than 2 cm water during an inspiration, the flow is inadequate and should be increased. Flow also is inadequate if the patient shows an increased use of accessory muscles of respiration or complains of increased WOB. Too high a flow is seen by an inadvertently high level of CPAP or the patient complaining of difficulty exhaling.

Fig. 15-25 Patient breathing circuit for continuous positive airway pressure (CPAP).

Water-column systems must be frequently monitored because of water loss caused by evaporation. The actual CPAP level is progressively less than desired as the water is gradually lost. This system must regularly have water added to it or have the expiratory tubing inserted deeper to keep the desired CPAP level.

The ball-bearing resistor system must be mounted vertically for gravity to keep the desired weight against the circuit. If it falls over and is horizontal, the CPAP pressure will be lost.

10. CPAP systems: masks, nasal, and bilevel

a. Get the necessary equipment for the procedure (WRE code: IIA2) [Difficulty: An]

A CPAP mask and breathing circuit are used primarily for patients who have obstructive sleep apnea. CPAP, by means of the mask, forces the soft tissues open to the point that the airway is never obstructed (see Fig. 15-18). The patient is now able to sleep normally and remain oxygenated. The patient should have the CPAP mask, breathing circuit, and proper CPAP level determined by a sleep study in the hospital. The patient can use the system at home once it is set up properly and he or she has been trained in its use.

In recent years, a CPAP mask has been used with a non-invasive mechanical ventilator to assist temporarily in the breathing of a patient with respiratory distress. The hope is to support the patient's breathing long enough to treat the underlying problem(s). If this is successful, the patient does not need to be intubated. These patients require careful assessment and monitoring.

The two main categories of CPAP masks come in different sizes for children older than 3 years to adults. See Fig. 15-26 for examples. Nasal mask and pillow systems are designed to cover only the nose. These allow the patient to speak and offer the mouth as a second airway for breathing in case a malfunction of the CPAP system occurs. The mouth also acts as a pressure relief route if the CPAP pressure should become too great. Pressures of up to 15 cm water can usually be maintained in an adult.

Fig. 15-26 Types of masks used to deliver continuous positive airway pressure or noninvasive positive-pressure ventilation. **A,** Nasal mask designed to cover the entire nose. **B,** Full face mask (oronasal mask) designed to cover the nose and mouth. **C,** Nasal pillows that fit into the nostrils. **D,** Total face mask that covers the entire facial area. The key elements to consider in deciding which mask to use are patient fit without leaks and comfort. (**A, C, D,** From Hess DR, Kacmarek RM: Essentials of mechanical ventilation, *ed 2, New York, 2002, McGraw-Hill.* **B,** From Hill NS: Complications of noninvasive positive pressure ventilation, Respir Care *42:432–442, 1997.*)

Pressures of up to 10 cm water can usually be maintained in a child.

Full face mask and total face mask systems are designed to cover the nose and mouth. These are transparent and similar to the mask used during bag/mask ventilation. The face mask must be used if the patient has persistent mouth breathing and cannot use a nose mask. With a good seal, pressures of greater than 15 cm water can be maintained.

All types of CPAP masks have a soft, very compliant seal to closely fit the contours of the face. Straps are needed to hold the mask in place. It is imperative that the mask properly fit the patient's face.

b. Put the equipment together and make sure that it works properly (WRE code: IIA2) [Difficulty: An]

Several companies manufacture mask CPAP systems for home care. These are relatively simple circuits and do not have a humidification system or the other attachments seen in the hospital. Check the manufacturer's literature for specific directions on their application to the patient. As shown in Figures 15-19 and 15-26, the straps must be tight enough to seal the mask to the face but not so tight as to cut off circulation to the skin. Any mask CPAP system must be able to generate enough flow to meet the patient's minute volume and peak flow needs. The CPAP level must be stable throughout the breathing cycle.

c. Troubleshoot any problems with the equipment (WRE code: IIA2) [Difficulty: An]

Too large a mask does not seal and allows gas to leak out. This is seen as a decreased CPAP pressure on the manometer. The patient may show increased snoring or airway obstruction with periods of apnea. A mask that is too small or misfitting can cause an uneven distribution of pressure on the face. This can lead to abrasions or pressure sores and ulcers on the face.

A sudden decrease in the CPAP level to zero indicates a disconnection at the patient or somewhere in the breathing circuit. Check all connections, and reassemble the break. If the CPAP level decreases more than 2 cm water during an inspiration, the flow is inadequate and should be increased. Flow also is inadequate if the patient shows an increased use of accessory muscles of respiration or complains of increased WOB. Too high a flow is seen by an inadvertently high level of CPAP or by the patient complaining difficulty exhaling.

Exam Hint

Two questions usually relate to troubleshooting equipment problems. Expect a question that involves a leak with the loss of delivered tidal volume. If the source of the leak is a loose CPAP or NPPV mask, it must be adjusted or replaced. Also be prepared to troubleshoot problems with a leak in the circuit tubing or the exhalation valve.

---

11. Humidifiers: passover and cascade type

a. Get the necessary equipment for the procedure (WRE code: IIA3) [Difficulty: An]

A cascade-type humidifier is indicated in these situations:

1. The patient has thick or copious secretions. An increase in the amount or thickness of secretions or a change from white to yellow or green justifies the switch to a cascade-type humidifier.
2. The patient will probably require mechanical ventilation for more than 96 hours.
3. The patient cannot have mechanical dead space added to the breathing circuit. If the patient's (especially a child's) tidal volume is smaller than the HME dead space, it should not be used. IMV systems typically are set up without mechanical dead space, so an HME should not be used.
4. An HME should not be used for a patient receiving very large tidal volumes. This is because the filter's ability to hold moisture is exceeded, and the patient will breathe in some dry air. Check the manufacturer's literature for the maximum recommended tidal volume.

5. If the patient has a large air leak, as seen with a deflated cuff or bronchopleural fistula, an HME should not be used. With a large air leak, more air is inspired than expired, and the exchanger will not be able to fully humidify the inspired tidal volume.

b. Put the equipment together and make sure that it works properly (WRE code: IIA3) [Difficulty: An]

The general discussion of this equipment was presented in Chapter 8. See Figs. 15-21 and 15-25 for setups in ventilator and CPAP breathing circuits. Both types are capable of providing 100% relative humidity. Passover-type systems are preferred with neonates.

The humidifier's temperature is usually maintained between 31°C and 35°C. Normally, the temperature should never be greater than 37°C at the patient's airway. An exception to this rule is the hypothermic patient. Inhaled gas that is warmed a few degrees above normal body temperature speeds the rewarming process.

Typically, a temperature probe is added into the inspiratory limb of the circuit near the Y. If a heated-wire circuit is being used with an infant, the temperature probe should be outside of the incubator and away from a radiant warmer's direct heat. The humidifier should provide at least 30 mg/L of water vapor.

Make sure that the water level is kept in the recommended range to humidify the gas properly. Avoid being sprayed with any circuit water during disconnections from the patient. It is considered contaminated and should be disposed of like any other contaminated fluid from the patient.

An AARC Clinical Practice Guideline recommends that a cascade- or wick-type humidifier and patient circuit be changed at least every 5 days for infection control purposes. The guideline also recommends that a nebulizer used for humidification purposes and the patient circuit be changed every 24 hours for infection control purposes.

c. Troubleshoot any problems with the equipment (WRE code: IIA3) [Difficulty: An]

A loose connection at the humidifier (or anywhere else in the circuit) results in a loss of volume or pressure or both to the patient. Check the entire circuit. When the leak is fixed the volume and pressure are restored. The humidifier should warm to the desired temperature. Do not use a humidifier that does not warm properly.

12. Humidifiers: heat and moisture exchangers

a. Get the necessary equipment for the procedure (WRE code: IIA3) [Difficulty: An]

HMEs are designed to be warmed by the patient's exhaled breath and absorb the water vapor from the gas. The next inspired volume is then warmed and humidified by evaporation. The key element in the exchanger is a hygroscopic filter medium. Under ideal conditions, the units can achieve up to 70% to 90% body humidity. They should minimally provide 30 mg/L of water at 30°C. The general discussion of this equipment was presented in Chapter 8. See Fig. 15-21 for a setup in a ventilator breathing circuit.

An HME is indicated in the following situations:
1. The patient has few, if any, secretions.
2. The patient will probably be weaned from the ventilator within 96 hours.
3. The patient is being transported on mechanical ventilation.

An HME is contraindicated in the following situations:
1. The patient has thick, bloody, or large amounts of secretions.
2. The patient has a large air leak such that the exhaled volume is less than 70% of the inhaled tidal volume. This results in a relatively dry hygroscopic filter. (Patients with uncuffed or torn cuffs on their endotracheal tubes or large bronchopleurocutaneous fistulas have large tidal volume leaks.)
3. The patient's temperature is less than 32°C.
4. The patient's spontaneous minute volume is greater than 10 L/min.
5. Always remove the HME when delivering nebulized medications through the circuit.

Consider the following when selecting an HME:
1. Select a unit with the smallest possible dead space volume. Watch for an increase in the patient's $Paco_2$ if the HME adds too much dead space or the patient's tidal volume is too small.
2. Pick the unit that provides the greatest percentage of body humidity. Do not use one that cannot meet these minimum standards.
3. If the patient has a known pulmonary infection, select an HME that is also a bacteria filter.
4. Should the unit be disposable or reusable? Staffing, infection control, and equipment processing considerations make a difference in choosing which unit to use.

b. Put the equipment together and make sure that it works properly (WRE code: IIA3) [Difficulty: An]

Most of these units are preassembled by the manufacturer, with nothing to add. It may be necessary to attach a length of large bore or aerosol tubing or an elbow adapter to make the unit fit onto the Y or endotracheal tube. All come with standard 15- or 22-mm connector ends. Air should flow easily through them with little resistance (see Fig. 15-20).

An AARC Clinical Practice Guideline states that HMEs can be used for up to 4 days if the patient does not have a major secretion problem. Each individual HME can be used for at least 24 hours unless it is obviously fouled. The whole patient circuit should be changed at least every 5 days for infection control purposes.

c. Troubleshoot any problems with the equipment (WRE code: IIA3) [Difficulty: An]

Any disconnections can be easily noticed and reconnected. Replace any unit that has a mucus plug or other debris obstructing the channel. This might be demonstrated by the patient's peak airway pressure suddenly increasing. Typically, HME units are replaced every 24 hours.

When secretions are coughed into an HME, it becomes obstructed. This is seen as a rapid increase in the peak pressure during an inspiration. Remove the obstructed HME. Either replace it or change to a cascade-type humidifier.

13. Perform quality control procedures on mechanical ventilators (WRE code: IIC4) [Difficulty: Ap, An]

Follow the manufacturer's guidelines for quality control procedures on a mechanical ventilator. The microprocessor ventilators usually have a software package that performs self-diagnostic tests on the unit. Obviously, the ventilator should deliver the volume, flow, and pressure that is set on the controls. Do not use a unit that fails a quality control check.

MODULE D
Evaluate and monitor the patient's response to mechanical ventilation

1. Observe the patient for signs of patient/ventilator dysynchrony (WRE code: IIIE6) [Difficulty: An]

Because a patient with an intubated airway cannot speak, it is necessary to communicate by asking simple questions that can be answered in a *yes* nod or *no* shake of the head. Other methods of communication are a pad of paper and pencil or picture boards.

It is not possible to predict how a patient will react to the initiation of mechanical ventilation or its prolonged need. Some patients react with relief and relax when the WOB is reduced. Others may become angry at the limitations imposed on them. Still others may become depressed. The issue of a patient's emotional reaction to illness is discussed in detail in Chapter 1.

2. Measure the patient's lung compliance and airway resistance (WRE code: IB7g) [Difficulty: An]

These measurements and their interpretation are presented earlier in this chapter.

3. Interpret the patient's plateau pressure, lung compliance, and airway resistance (WRE code: IB8f) [Difficulty: An]

Review and interpret the various waveforms presented in the chapter and the flow/volume loops in Chapter 4.

4. Monitor the tidal volume (WRE code: IIIE9) [Difficulty: An]

The patient's exhaled tidal volume is usually measured and recorded in his or her chart. Many of the newer ventilators also display an inhaled and exhaled tidal volume. If possible, compare the two volumes. If they do not match closely, check for a leak or other reason for the difference. The patient on an IMV, SIMV, or PSV mode should have both the machine delivered and spontaneous tidal volumes measured and recorded.

The weaning patient must have his or her spontaneous tidal volume measured along with the vital capacity. These and other parameters are used to judge weanability (discussed later; see Box 15-5 for more information).

5. Monitor the respiratory rate (WRE code: IIIE9) [Difficulty: An]

Count and record the machine delivered respiratory rate. If the patient is on an IMV, SIMV, or PSV, count and record both the machine and spontaneous rates. The weaning patient should have his or her spontaneous rate counted and recorded.

BOX 15-5   Indications That the Patient Can Probably Be Weaned from the Ventilator

OXYGENATION
$Pao_2 \geq 80$ torr or $Spo_2 > 90\%$ on 50% oxygen or less
$P(A-a)o_2 < 300-350$ torr on 100% oxygen
Intrapulmonary shunt of < 15%

VENTILATION
$Paco_2 < 55$ torr in a patient who is not ordinarily hypercapneic
Dead space/tidal volume ($V_D:V_T$) ratio < 0.55-0.6 (55%-60%)
Rapid, shallow breathing index (breaths/minute divided by tidal volume in liters) < 105

PULMONARY MECHANICS
Spontaneous tidal volume of 3-4 mL/lb or 7-9 mL/kg of ideal body weight
Vital capacity of $\geq 10-15$ mL/kg
Maximum inspiratory pressure (MIP) more than -20 to -25 cm water pressure
Forced expiratory volume in one second (FEV_1) > 10 mL/kg
Respiratory rate of 12-35/min (adult)

MISCELLANEOUS
Conscious and cooperative patient who wants to breathe spontaneously
Stable and acceptable normal blood pressure and temperature
Stable cardiac rhythm; heart rate should not increase by > 15% to 20%
Corrected underlying problem that led to ventilatory support
Normal fluid balance and electrolyte values
Proper nutritional status

6. Monitor the inspiratory/expiratory ratio (WRE code: IIIE9) [Difficulty: An]

The I:E ratio should be calculated and recorded. Some newer ventilators display it. Others show inspiratory time and expiratory time. The I:E ratio can then be calculated, as shown in Table 15-2.

7. Monitor airway pressures (WRE code: IIIE9) [Difficulty: An]

a. Peak pressure (or P_{peak}): The peak pressure reached during the delivery of a tidal volume is the pressure required to push the gas through the circuit, endotracheal tube, and the patient's airways, and to expand the lungs. The sigh volume requires a greater pressure because it is a larger volume. These pressures should be recorded regularly whenever the patient and machine are checked. The importance of peak pressure in calculating dynamic compliance was discussed earlier in the chapter.

b. Plateau pressure (or P_{plat}): The plateau pressure is found when the tidal volume has been delivered to the lungs and is temporarily held within them. The importance of plateau pressure in calculating static compliance was discussed earlier in the chapter.

c. Baseline pressure: The baseline pressure is the pressure measured at the end of exhalation. Normally it is seen as zero on the ventilator's pressure manometer. (Remember that in this case, zero is actually local barometric pressure.) If the patient has therapeutic PEEP or CPAP, the baseline pressure will be greater than zero.

8. Monitor mean airway pressure (WRE code: IIIE9) [Difficulty: An]

Mean airway pressure ($\overline{Paw}$) is the average pressure over an entire breathing cycle. Most of the newer ventilators display a mean airway pressure. This pressure results from changes in the patient's peak and baseline pressures plus the I:E ratio.

9. Measure the patient's inspired oxygen percentage (WRE code: IIIE10) [Difficulty: Ap, An]

Most ventilators have very accurate oxygen delivery systems. However, standard practice requires the use on a calibrated, external oxygen analyzer to confirm the oxygen percentage. If the patient is receiving IMV with an added flow system, it too must be analyzed. Make sure that the ventilator and the IMV gas have the same, ordered oxygen percentage.

10. Monitor the ventilator alarm systems and adjust them as needed (WRE code: IIIE9 and IIIF9a) [Difficulty: An]

All alarm systems must function properly. Test all audible and visual alarms. The practitioner should be familiar with the most widely used adult and infant ventilators and their alarm systems. It is common practice to set most alarms at ±10% of the set value. For example:

1. The tidal volume is 1000 mL. Set the low volume alarm at 900 mL and the high volume alarm at 1100 mL.
2. The minute volume is 10,000 mL. Set the high volume alarm at 11,000 mL and the low volume alarm at 9000 mL.
3. The oxygen percentage is set at 40%. Set the high percentage alarm at 45% and the low percentage alarm at 35%.

TABLE 15-2	Time Variables in Mechanical Ventilation		
	Term	Symbol	Formula for Calculation
	Frequency (rate)	f	Count breaths/min or $\dfrac{60}{t_I + t_E}$
	Cycle time	$t_I + t_E$	Add $t_I + t_E$ or $\dfrac{60}{f}$
	Inspiratory time	t_I (I)	$t_I = \dfrac{60}{f} - t_E$ or $t_I = \%t_I \times (t_I + t_E)$
	Expiratory time	t_E (E)	$t_E = \dfrac{60}{f} - t_I$
	Inspiratory/expiratory ratio	I:E or t_I/t_E	$I:E = \dfrac{t_I}{t_E}$, usually numerator
	Percentage inspiratory time	$\%t_I$	$\%t_I = \dfrac{t_I}{t_I + t_E} \times 100$

From Scanlan CL: Physics and physiology or ventilatory support. In Scanlan CL, Spearman CB, Sheldon RL, editors: *Egan's fundamentals of respiratory care,* ed 5, St Louis, 1990, Mosby.

4. The low pressure or disconnection alarm is set to sound if the ventilator delivered pressure is about 5 cm water below the peak pressure. For example, if the peak pressure has been about the 40 cm water, the low pressure or disconnection alarm should be set at 35 cm water. If a leak or disconnection occurs, the alarm sounds when the peak pressure does not reach 35 cm water. If the patient is on a CPAP system, the low pressure or disconnection alarm should be set to sound if the pressure decreases about 2 to 3 cm water below the set level. For example, if the patient is on 10 cm water CPAP, the alarm should be set at 8 cm water.

Many types of alarms have a timer that can be set to delay when the alarm sounds. If the alarm is on a ventilator, the delay should be set for about 3 to 5 seconds longer than the cycling time. For example, if the patient has a backup rate of 10 times/min, the cycling time between mandatory breaths is 6 seconds. Set the timer to delay the alarm sounding for about 10 seconds. If the patient is disconnected from the ventilator and the peak pressure does not reach 35 cm water, the alarm will sound in 10 seconds. If the patient is on a CPAP system, the timer may be set for no delay or a short delay. Adjust all the alarms to fit the clinical setting and the patient's condition. Some may need tighter limits, and others may need wider limits than those just discussed.

> ### Exam Hint
>
> **B**e able to troubleshoot an alarm situation, correct the problem, and reset the alarms settings as needed. For example, the high pressure alarm will go off if the peak pressure hits the alarm setting because of an increase in airway resistance or a decrease in lung compliance.

11. Monitor the cuff pressure to the patient's endotracheal or tracheostomy tube (WRE code: IIIE11) [Difficulty: An]

This was presented in Chapter 12. Review it if necessary.

12. Auscultate the patient's chest, and interpret the breath sounds (WRE code: IB3a) [Difficulty: An]

This was presented in Chapter 1. Review it if necessary.

13. Interpret arterial blood gas results (WRE code: IIIE4) [Difficulty: R, Ap]

An ABG sample should be obtained after every significant change in the ventilator settings. This includes a change in the inspired oxygen percentage, rate, tidal volume, or PEEP level. The interpretation of the ABG results will give vital information to guide further ventilator changes.

> ### Exam Hint
>
> **E**xpect to see many ABG values incorporated into questions about adjusting the ventilator. Hypoxemia should be treated by increasing the oxygen percentage or increasing the PEEP level. As the patient improves, they can be reduced. If the patient's carbon dioxide level is too high, increase either the rate or the tidal volume. If too much carbon dioxide is being blown off, decrease either the rate or the tidal volume.

MODULE E
Recommend modifications in mechanical ventilation based on the patient's response

1. Recommend a change in the type of mechanical ventilator (WRE code: IIIG3i) [Difficulty: An]

Selecting the type of mechanical ventilator was discussed earlier in this chapter. In brief, a pressure cycled unit can be used with a patient without cardiopulmonary disease. Most patients with conditions that cause abnormal Raw or C_{LT} should be placed on electrically powered, volume cycled units. The microprocessor ventilators offer more ventilating options and monitoring of clinical information; they are best for the most critical patients. Noninvasive ventilation and negative-pressure ventilation are used with patients who do not need intubation and have some ability to breathe for themselves.

Be prepared to change from one type of ventilator to another as the patient's condition warrants. A malfunctioning ventilator should be replaced with one that is capable of providing the same level of ventilatory support.

2. Recommend a change in the ventilator breathing circuit (WRE code: IIIG3i) [Difficulty: An]

Changing circuits was discussed earlier in this chapter. In brief, change a circuit that has a leak or is contaminated. Routine changes are performed for infection control purposes.

3. Change the type of humidification equipment (WRE code: IIIF7a) [Difficulty: An]

An HME is indicated in the following situations:
  a. The patient has few, if any, secretions.
  b. The patient will probably be weaned from the ventilator within 96 hours.
  c. The patient is being transported on mechanical ventilation.

An HME is contraindicated in the following situations:

a. The patient has thick, bloody, or copious secretions.

b. The patient has a large air leak such that the exhaled volume is less than 70% of the inhaled V_T. This causes a relatively dry hygroscopic filter. (Patients with uncuffed or torn cuffs on their endotracheal tubes or large bronchopleural fistulas would have large V_T leaks.)

c. The patient's temperature is less than 32°C.

d. The patient's spontaneous $\dot{V}_E$ is greater than 10 L/min.

c. Always remove the HME when delivering nebulized medications through the circuit

A cascade-type bubble humidifier is indicated in these situations:

a. The patient has thick or copious secretions. An increase in the amount or thickness of secretions or a change from white to yellow or green justifies the switch to a cascade-type humidifier.

b. The patient will probably require mechanical ventilation for more than 96 hours.

c. The patient cannot have mechanical dead space added to the breathing circuit. If the patient's V_T (especially a child's) is smaller than the HME dead space, it should not be used. IMV systems typically are set up without mechanical dead space, so an HME should not be used.

d. An HME should not be used with a patient receiving very large V_Ts because the filter's ability to hold moisture will be exceeded, and the patient will breathe in some dry air. Check the manufacturer's literature for the maximum recommended V_T.

e. If the patient has a large air leak, as seen with a deflated cuff or bronchopleural fistula, an HME should not be used. With a large air leak, more air is inspired than expired, and the exchanger cannot fully humidify the inspired V_T.

4. Enhance oxygenation
a. Make a recommendation to change the oxygen percentage (WRE code: IIIG3b) [Difficulty: An]
b. Change the oxygen percentage (WRE code: IIIF4a) [Difficulty: An]

As discussed earlier, the goal of O_2 administration is to keep the PaO_2 level of most patients between 60 and 90 torr and the SpO_2 level greater than 90%. Exceptions are patients who are breathing on hypoxic drive and who are in a cardiac arrest situation. The COPD patient who has a chronically low PaO_2 level and chronically high $PaCO_2$ level may be allowed to have a PaO_2 value as low as 50 to 55 torr and an SpO_2 value as low as 85%.

The patient who is extremely hypoxic must be given up to 100% O_2. Those patients who have refractory hypoxemia (e.g., ARDS) do not respond with a normal increase in the PaO_2 level as the O_2 percentage is increased.

5. Make a recommendation to change ventilator settings based on ventilator graphics (WRE code: IIIG3h) [Difficulty: An]

See the previous discussion and example figures.

6. Improve alveolar ventilation (WRE code: IIIG3c) [Difficulty: An]
a. Tidal volume

The specific V_T to select was discussed earlier in this chapter. Conditions in which the V_T should be increased include atelectasis, consolidation, and when the present V_T is at the small end of the normal range and the patient has an elevated CO_2 level. The NBRC uses the upper level for a set V_T in an adult as 15 mL/kg of ideal body weight. Conditions in which the V_T should be decreased include air trapping, hyperinflated lungs as seen on the chest radiograph film by wide intercostal margins or flattened hemidiaphragms, and when the present V_T is at the large end of the normal range and the patient has a decreased CO_2 level. The NBRC uses the lower level for a set V_T in an adult as 10 mL/kg of ideal body weight.

An additional consideration is whether to give the patient a sigh breath, which is a volume larger than the normal V_T. People normally sigh every few minutes. It serves the purpose of opening up atelectatic alveoli and reorienting the surfactant in the alveoli so that they are stable. A sigh breath is usually given to a patient only in A/C mode.

Most patients being ventilated in the A/C mode receive a ventilator sigh volume just as they do a V_T. A sigh volume is typically 1.5 to 2 times the V_T if the V_T is in the low to middle range of normal. If the patient has a problem of atelectasis or consolidation, a larger sigh volume may be indicated. The patient may not need a sigh volume if the set V_T is at the 15 mL/kg upper limit. A patient with bullous emphysema, pneumothorax, or cardiac status that is sensitive to high peak pressures may be contraindicated for a sigh volume. The patient with air trapping of the V_T should have a smaller (possibly no) sigh volume. Compare the inspired and expired volumes to ensure that no air trapping exists. Most current ventilators allow the clinician to tailor the sigh frequency to best meet the patient's clinical needs. The sigh frequency should be increased in patients with atelectasis or consolidation. The sigh frequency may need to be decreased or eliminated in patients who are air trapping the V_T or sigh volume. Sighs are usually not given when the patient is on the IMV/SIMV mode.

b. Respiratory rate

Respiratory rate was discussed earlier in this section. Increase the backup rate on the ventilator if the patient has an elevated CO_2 level and the V_T is at the high end of the normal range. Decrease the backup rate on the ventilator if the patient has a decreased CO_2 level and the V_T is at the low end of the normal range.

7. Make a recommendation to change inspiratory effort (sensitivity) to improve patient synchrony (WRE code: IIIG3a) [Difficulty: An]

Sensitivity was discussed earlier in this chapter. If the patient seems to be working too hard to trigger a ventilator breath, make a recommendation to increase the sensitivity. Be careful not to make the ventilator so sensitive that it self-cycles.

8. Monitor and adjust the alarm settings (WRE code: IIIG3a) [Difficulty: R, Ap]

Alarm settings were discussed earlier in this chapter. Be prepared to adjust the alarm settings based on the patient's clinical situation.

9. Mechanical dead space
a. Make a recommendation to change the mechanical dead space (WRE code: IIIG3j) [Difficulty: Ap, An]
b. Change the mechanical dead space (WRE code: IIIF9b) [Difficulty: R, Ap, An]

Mechanical dead space is added to increase the patient's $PaCO_2$ level. This is done by having the patient rebreathe gas from his or her anatomic dead space. This high CO_2 gas is then inhaled back to the alveolar level and increases the patient's $PaCO_2$ level. The more dead space tubing there is, the more carbon dioxide is retained. It is important to realize that this same rebreathed volume of gas is lower in oxygen because of its diffusion into the patient's pulmonary circulation. If a large amount of mechanical dead space is added, it will be necessary to increase the FIO_2 to keep the ordered level. Measure the oxygen percentage between the dead space and the endotracheal or tracheostomy tube adapter.

Mechanical dead space is used only in the C and A/C modes. It should not be used in IMV/SIMV, pressure support, or CPAP modes. Typically, a length of large bore or aerosol tubing is added into the breathing circuit between the Y and the patient's endotracheal or tracheostomy tube (see Fig. 15-20). The following formula can be used to predict what amount of *mechanical dead space* (VD_{mech}') produces a desired $PaCO_2$ level:

$$([V_T - VD_{anat}] - VD_{mech}) \times f \times PaCO_2 = ([V_T - VD_{anat}] - VD_{mech}') \times f \times PaCO_2'$$

In which:

V_T = current tidal volume

VD_{anat} = anatomic dead space. This is calculated at 1 mL/lb or 2.2 mL/kg of ideal body weight.

VD_{mech} = current mechanical dead space

f = ventilator rate

$PaCO_2$ = actual patient $PaCO_2$ value

VD_{mech}' = *desired mechanical dead space*

$PaCO_2'$ = desired patient $PaCO_2$ value

EXAMPLE

Your patient is a 70-kg (154-lb) man who is being ventilated on the Control mode (he is apneic). His ventilator settings are tidal volume of 1000 mL, rate of 12/min, FIO_2 of 0.3, no added mechanical dead space. His ABGs are PaO_2 of 90 torr, $PaCO_2$ of 30 torr, pH of 7.48, SaO_2 of 95%, BE of 0. The clinical goal is to adjust the patient's mechanical dead space as needed to produce a $PaCO_2$ of 40 torr. In summary:

V_T = 1000 mL current tidal volume

VD_{anat} = 154 mL anatomic dead space. This is calculated at 1 mL/lb or 2.2 mL/kg of ideal body weight.

VD_{mech} = no added mechanical dead space

f = 12 for ventilator rate

$PaCO_2$ = 30 torr actual patient $PaCO_2$ value

VD_{mech}' = *the desired amount of mechanical dead space*

$PaCO_2'$ = 40 torr desired patient $PaCO_2$ value

Placing the data and goal into the formula results in the following equation:

$$([V_T - VD_{anat}] - VD_{mech}) \times f \times PaCO_2 = ([V_T - VD_{anat}] - VD_{mech}') \times f \times PaCO_2'$$

$$([1000 - 154] - 0) \times 12 \times 30 = ([1000 - 154] - VD_{mech}') \times 12 \times 40$$

Simplifying produces the following equation:

$$(846) \times 12 \times 30 = (846 - VD_{mech}') \times 480$$
$$304{,}560 = (846 \times 480) - (VD_{mech}' \times 480)$$
$$304{,}560 = 406{,}080 - 480\, VD_{mech}'$$
$$-101{,}520 = -480\, VD_{mech}'$$
$$211.5 \text{ mL} = VD_{mech}'$$

The solution is to increase the patient's mechanical dead space from 0 to 212 mL.

Exam Hint

Usually one question deals with recommending the addition of mechanical dead space when ABG results show that the patient is being hyperventilated.

10. Make a recommendation to change the mode of ventilation to improve patient synchrony (WRE code: IIIG3a) [Difficulty: An]

Changing the mode of ventilation was discussed earlier in this chapter. Be prepared to change the mode as the patient's condition varies. A patient who is apneic can be placed on the A/C mode. A patient with an acceptable spontaneous tidal volume can be placed on the SIMV mode. Pressure support can be added to any mode to reduce the patient's WOB.

> ### Exam Hint
>
> Usually one question requires changing the mode of ventilation, depending on the patient's condition. This could involve a patient who can breathe spontaneously being changed from the A/C mode to the SIMV mode, or it could involve a patient receiving volume cycled ventilation being changed to pressure cycled ventilation because of a very high plateau pressure.

11. Make a recommendation to change the level of positive end-expiratory pressure therapy to improve oxygenation (WRE code: IIIG3b) [Difficulty: An]

PEEP therapy was discussed earlier in this chapter. Remember that therapeutic PEEP is indicated for situations in which the patient has bilaterally small lungs with a reduced FRC. This causes hypoxemia. The proper level of PEEP restores the FRC and improves oxygenation. Watch for side effects of barotrauma or decreased cardiac output from too much pressure. The patient should be carefully monitored with blood gas analysis and vital sign checks before starting PEEP and after each change.

12. Make a recommendation to change continuous positive airway pressure therapy to improve oxygenation (WRE code: IIIG3b) [Difficulty: An]

CPAP therapy was discussed earlier. In brief, all of the considerations for PEEP apply to CPAP except that the patient must be able to breathe adequately to maintain a normal CO_2 level.

13. Recommend a change in the pressure support level (WRE code: IIIG3e) [Difficulty: An]

When the PSV level is adjusted to deliver a V_T, it is called maximum PSV (PSV_{max}). The clinical guidelines for PSV_{max} are

1. Use enough pressure to deliver a V_T of 10 to 12 mL/kg of ideal body weight.
2. The patient should not have to assist the ventilator at a rate greater than 20 times/min to achieve acceptable ABG values.

PSV_{max} has been used in patients with resolving acute respiratory failure. Usually these patients have been maintained on the A/C mode for several days to minimize their WOB while undergoing treatment for their condition. PSV_{max} is considered ideal for reconditioning the diaphragm and other respiratory muscles. Reconditioning occurs when the assist or "trigger" pressure for the breath is kept as low as possible (−1 to −2 cm H_2O pressure) and the V_T is kept large. This pattern results in a low respiratory muscle workload. As the patient continues to improve, the PSV level is reduced. The patient's V_T is stable as long as the patient passively takes in the PSV-supported breath; the V_T can be larger if the patient interacts actively with the delivered pressure. See Fig. 15-1 for a pressure/flow curve, and Fig. 15-10, E, for a pressure/time curve.

The PSV level also has been used to overcome the R_{AW} caused by the patient's endotracheal tube. (See the example calculated earlier in the chapter.) Too small an endotracheal tube may prevent some patients from successfully weaning by the IMV/SIMV mode. The addition of enough PSV to overcome the additional WOB caused by the tube enables the patient to wean successfully and the airway to be extubated.

The PSV level is reduced, as tolerated, when the patient's C_{LT} or R_{AW} improves. As both return to normal, the only barrier to extubation is the resistance offered by the endotracheal tube. Some practitioners advocate extubation when the PSV level is 10 cm H_2O or less, which is probably the pressure level needed to overcome the tube's resistance. Thus the patient should tolerate extubation without any increase in the WOB.

14. Recommend a change in the pressure control ventilation level (WRE code: IIIG3e) [Difficulty: An]

PCV involves the delivery of V_T breaths that are pressure limited and time cycled. It has been advocated for patients with bilateral low-compliance conditions (e.g., ARDS).

The PCV level is set as low as possible to achieve an adequate V_T for gas exchange. The exhaled volume must be monitored continuously because the V_T will decrease if the patient's C_{LT} or R_{AW} worsens. If either or both improve, the V_T will increase. The patient with a pulmonary air leak loses variable amounts of V_T from the chest tube depending on changes in compliance and resistance. An ABG sample must be evaluated with a change in the PCV level or V_T. The PCV mode is well tolerated by many patients because of the freedom they have to set the rate, inspiratory flow through the demand valve, and $\dot{V}_E$. PCV also may be combined with SIMV and PSV as the clinical situation indicates. The following are some suggestions for initial PCV settings:

a. Set the PEEP to the same level used on the constant volume ventilator to maintain the patient's FRC.
b. Set the PCV level at the patient's static lung compliance pressure. Be prepared to increase this pressure.

The clinical goal is to give a V_T close to that delivered previously.

c. Set the rate the same as before.

d. Set the inspired O_2 the same as before. Some may prefer to set it at 100% until blood gas results show that it can be lowered.

e. Set the inspiratory time under pressure control so that the I:E ratio is the same as before.

Check the patient's vital signs for tolerance, and get an ABG sample in about 15 minutes. If the R_{AW} or C_{LT} worsens, the PCV level must be increased to maintain or increase the V_T. Obviously, as the patient's R_{AW} and C_{LT} improve (or pulmonary air leak decreases), the PCV level must be decreased to maintain the desired V_T.

15. Recommend a change in the ventilator to reduce the inspiratory plateau pressure (WRE code: IIIG3k2) [Difficulty: An]

Inspiratory hold (also known as *inflation hold*) is a technique whereby the patient is temporarily prevented from exhaling the ventilator delivered V_T. Fig. 15-27 shows the pressure/time waveform. The pressure found during the inspiratory-hold period is called the *inspiratory plateau*. Inspiratory hold is added therapeutically to improve the distribution of the V_T. Patients with ARDS and pulmonary edema can benefit from it. Oxygenation should improve in direct proportion to the duration of the inspiratory plateau. The duration of inspiratory plateau is measured in different ways, depending on the ventilator. For example, the Bear 1000 and Puritan-Bennett 7200 can have it added in steps of 0.1 second up to several seconds total. The Servo 900C can have it added as a variable percentage of the total duration of the breathing cycle.

The inspiratory plateau must be reduced as the patient's ventilation and C_{LT} improve. Patients with normal ventilation and compliance should not receive any inspiratory plateau.

Notice that the use of an inspiratory plateau increases the inspiratory phase of the breathing cycle, which causes a shorter expiratory time if the rate is kept the same (or the rate must be reduced to keep the same I:E ratio). Again, as discussed earlier, make sure that the V_T is completely exhaled. The patient's condition should be monitored closely to determine if the level of inspiratory plateau is appropriate.

Nontherapeutic inspiratory plateau is added temporarily to determine the plateau pressure on the ventilator. This is considered to be the pressure needed to deliver the V_T. With this information, the patient's effective Cst can be calculated. Its calculation and interpretation were discussed earlier in this chapter. An inspiratory plateau of 1.0 second is usually long enough to find the plateau pressure. Remember to turn off the inspiratory plateau afterward.

Expiratory retard also is shown in the Fig. 15-27 pressure/time waveform. Some ventilators have a control that adjusts both inspiratory hold and expiratory retard, so care must be taken when a change is made in either. As discussed in Chapter 14, expiratory retard is indicated in any patient who is air trapping and not exhaling completely. It functions like pursed-lip breathing in the spontaneously breathing patient. The backpressure prevents the collapse of the smallest airways (see Fig. 15-27 for the pressure/time waveform). Expiratory retard may be indicated in a patient with asthma, emphysema, or bronchitis. It is important with these types of patients to

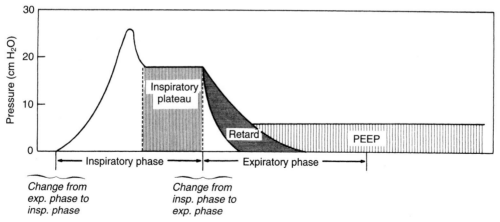

Fig. 15-27 Pressure/time waveform showing how exhalation can be modified. Inspiratory plateau (inflation hold) is seen when the tidal volume is held within the lungs for a period of time. With expiratory retard, the gas is more slowly exhaled than during a passive breath. These two modifications of exhalation may or may not be combined with positive end-expiratory pressure. *(From Kirby RR, Smith RA, Desautels DA: Modes of mechanical ventilation. In Burton GG, Hodgkin JE, editors:* Respiratory care: a guide to clinical practice, *ed 2, Philadelphia, 1984, Lippincott.)*

measure the inspiratory and expiratory V_T. Air trapping is confirmed by the expiratory volume being less than the inspiratory volume. When listening to the patient's breath sounds, it will be noted that no pause occurs at the end of exhalation before the next inspiration is started. In extreme cases, the pressure manometer does not return to the baseline level. These patients should be checked for the presence and level of auto-PEEP. The proper level of expiratory retard is determined by trial and error. The following parameters should be monitored to find the proper amount:

a. The inspiratory and expiratory V_Ts should be the same.
b. The patient's breath sounds should reveal wheezing to be absent or minimal and a silent pause at the end of exhalation before the next V_T is delivered.
c. Auto-PEEP should not occur.
d. The patient should subjectively feel that he or she has exhaled completely before the next breath is given.

The patient must be monitored frequently when expiratory retard is being used. As the patient is treated with bronchodilating medications, the bronchospasm should diminish. Expiratory retard should not be necessary when the airway resistance has returned to normal.

16. Inspiratory to expiratory ratio
   a. Recommend a change in the inspiratory/expiratory ratio (WRE code: IIIG3d) [Difficulty: An]
   b. Change the inspiratory/expiratory ratio to enhance oxygenation (WRE code: IIIG3b) [Difficulty: An]

The general discussion of I:E ratio was presented earlier. Increasing expiratory time to eliminate auto-PEEP is discussed in the next section. This discussion will focus on the need to increase the inspiratory time. This is done to improve oxygenation by holding the tidal volume in the lungs for longer than normal. When the inspiratory time is longer than the expiratory time (for example, 2:1) the patient is said to have an *inverse I:E ratio* and *inverse ratio ventilation* (IRV). This technique has been successfully used in low lung compliance adult patients who do not respond to PCV. Increased inspiratory time and decreased expiratory time should be used in any condition in which the patient has a small time constant of ventilation (T_C). ($T_C = C_{LT} \times R_{AW}$.) This would be observed clinically as a normal R_{AW} but a low C_{LT} in such conditions as ARDS, pulmonary edema, pneumonia, or an enlarged abdomen. Increasing the inspiratory time to create an inverse I:E ratio keeps the alveoli inflated longer to provide more time for O_2 to diffuse, prevent atelectasis, and maintain the FRC. Typically patients being considered for IRV are already being ventilated in the PC mode. Therefore the

merging of the two modes is called *pressure controlled inverse ratio ventilation* (PCIRV). The following have been recommended as initial PCIRV settings:

a. If the patient is being switched from volume cycled ventilation to PCIRV, set the PCV level at the patient's static lung compliance pressure. However, if the patient was already on PCV at a higher pressure, keep this higher pressure.
b. Set the O_2 at 100%.
c. Keep the current respiratory rate.
d. Keep the I:E ratio at 1:1 for now.
e. PEEP should be removed if it is currently less than 8 cm H_2O. Cut the PEEP level in half if it is currently more than 8 cm H_2O. As the I:E ratio is made inverse, air trapping increases the patient's FRC.

Draw a set of ABGs after 15 min on PCIRV, and check the patient's vital signs. Monitor the exhaled V_T for a decrease. If the ventilator gives a real-time graph of pressure, volume, and flow, these should be monitored for air trapping (auto-PEEP). See Fig. 15-2 for an auto-PEEP flow/time tracing.

If the initial set of blood gases on PCIRV does not show adequate oxygenation, the inspiratory time will have to be increased. The inspiratory time must be progressively increased and expiratory time decreased if the patient's C_{LT} worsens. It is also possible to alternate a 2- to 3-cm H_2O increase in the PCV level with small increases in the inspiratory time. Blood gases must be analyzed with each increase in inspiratory time, decrease in expiratory time, or increase in PCV. Once an acceptable PaO_2 is established, it is usually not necessary to make further increases in the inspiratory time if the patient's pulmonary condition does not worsen. Look for an increase in $PaCO_2$ or end-tidal CO_2 as a sign of inadequate V_T. It may be necessary to increase the PCV level to increase the V_T. Also monitor the patient's vital signs and cardiac output, if possible, to look for a decrease in cardiac output. PCIRV ratios as inverse as 3:1 or 4:1 have been reported. When this happens, the pressure/volume curve takes on a characteristic "square wave" shape, as shown in Fig. 15-11, *B*. The I:E ratio must be returned to normal as the patient's C_{LT} improves by gradually decreasing the inspiratory time or increasing the expiratory time. The patient's blood gas result should be evaluated with each step to be sure that oxygenation is maintained at a safe level.

17. Recommend a modification in the ventilator settings to eliminate auto-PEEP (WRE code: IIIG3k1) [Difficulty: An]

If a patient has auto-PEEP (see Fig. 15-2), every attempt should be made to determine why the patient is air trapping. Although the basic problem is an expiratory time that is too short for full exhalation of the tidal volume, a more specific reason should be found, and then a solution can be found. The following are possible reasons for air trapping and auto-PEEP and solutions:

Problem	Solution(s)
a. Bronchospasm causing slow expiratory flow.	Administer a bronchodilator medication. Increase expiratory time. Add expiratory retard.
b. Secretions causing slow expiratory flow.	Suction the patient's airway.
c. Large tidal volume that is not fully exhaled.	Reduce the tidal volume. Increase the expiratory time.

Not every possible solution can be used. The patient's situation must be considered. For example, increasing the expiratory time will reduce the inspiratory time if the same rate is to be kept. Increasing the expiratory time and keeping the same inspiratory time will reduce the patient's respiratory rate. This will reduce the minute volume and increase the patient's carbon dioxide level. Additionally, reducing the tidal volume will reduce the minute volume and increase the patient's carbon dioxide level.

18. Recommend a change in noninvasive positive-pressure ventilation (WRE code: IIIG3f) [Difficulty: An]

NPPV was discussed earlier in this chapter. In brief, if the patient's V_T needs to be increased, the level of positive pressure must be increased. Lowering the level of positive pressure decreases the V_T. Blood gases and vital signs should always be monitored after any change is made.

19. Monitor the mean airway pressure to determine the patient's response to respiratory care (WRE code: IIIE9) [Difficulty: An]

Mean airway pressure (P$\overline{aw}$ or MAP) is the average pressure over an entire breathing cycle. A number of current neonatal and adult ventilators are able to calculate the value (Fig. 15-28). MAP is influenced by the patient's lung/thoracic compliance (C_{LT}), airway resistance (Raw), and ventilator settings. If a volume cycled ventilator is being used, a decrease in compliance or an increase in resistance results in an increase in the MAP. This is because it takes more pressure to deliver the tidal volume; a higher peak pressure is seen. Conversely, if the patient's compliance increases or the resistance decreases, the MAP decreases. It is important to evaluate further the patient when a change in MAP is noticed. This is because the new pressure, by itself, does not clarify whether a change in compliance, resistance, or both has occurred. Any treatments that improve lung

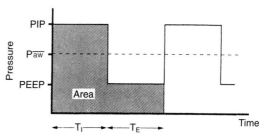

Fig. 15-28 Pressure/time tracing showing mean airway pressure (P$\overline{aw}$). PEEP, positive end-expiratory pressure; PIP, Peak inspiratory pressure; T_E, expiratory time; T_I, inspiratory time. *(From Chatburn RL: Classification of mechanical ventilators, Respir Care 36:569, 1991.)*

compliance and reduce airway resistance are shown by a reduced MAP. It is important to calculate both dynamic and static compliance (discussed earlier) when trying to determine how the patient's condition has changed.

In general, an increase in MAP increases the patient's oxygenation. This is because the alveoli are kept open longer, allowing more time for diffusion and preventing alveolar collapse. (Fig. 16-9 shows how several ventilator adjustments can change the mean airway pressure.) If alveolar ventilation is improved, the $PaCO_2$ also may be reduced. If the MAP is too high, there is an increased risk of pulmonary barotrauma and decreased cardiac output. This is especially true if PEEP is increased to raise the MAP. Watch the patient closely whenever a ventilator change is made that increases the MAP. A sudden deterioration in cardiopulmonary function may be caused by a pneumothorax. A reduction in urine output, an increased heart rate, and decreased blood pressure are often seen when the cardiac output is reduced. The MAP should be reduced if any of these situations is seen. To prevent these complications, it is necessary to reduce the MAP whenever the patient's pulmonary condition improves. As the compliance increases toward normal, it is not necessary to use as high an MAP to maintain acceptable blood gases.

20. Recommend the use of sedatives or muscle relaxants (paralyzing agents) as needed (WRE code: IIIG1b) [Difficulty: An]

An adult who is attempting to inhale or exhale out of sequence with the ventilator is considered to be "bucking" or "fighting" the ventilator. This problem is most commonly seen in the control and A/C modes. If the asynchrony between the patient's efforts and the ventilator is too great, an increased risk of hypoxemia, air trapping, and pneumothorax exists. Carefully evaluate the patient to determine whether he or she is breathing rapidly because of pain, anxiety, or improper adjustment of the ventilator. Make sure that the settings (inspiratory flow, respiratory rate, pressure limit, etc.) are correctly set for the patient's condition. Sedation or paralysis should be considered only after all other causes of asynchrony have been ruled out. The following patient conditions must be considered before making a medication choice for controlling the patient's breathing efforts:

Is the patient in pain? If so, an opiate analgesic such as morphine sulfate is commonly administered intravenously for fast onset. Morphine has the additional effects of reducing anxiety and inducing sleep. Because all opiates are central nervous system depressants, make sure that the ventilator alarm systems are functioning properly in case the patient becomes disconnected.

Is the patient agitated? Asynchrony with the ventilator for no known physical reason can often be attributed to anxiety or fear. Benzodiazepines, including diazepam (Valium) and midazolam (Versed), are the drugs of choice for treatment of agitation. They have a sedating effect within minutes when given intravenously.

Does the patient need to be paralyzed? If total muscular relaxation along with apnea is necessary, a skeletal muscle paralyzing agent should be used. Usually a short-term, depolarizing neuromuscular blocker such as succinylcholine (Anectine) is used during a difficult intubation. A single intravenous dose paralyzes a combative patient for about 10 minutes. For paralysis during mechanical ventilation, one of the following long-term, nondepolarizing neuromuscular-blocking agents is commonly used: pancuronium (Pavulon), atracurium (Tracrium), or vecuronium (Norcuron). These are given intravenously and cause paralysis lasting 2 to 4 hours.

Remember that these paralyzing agents have no effect on the patient's ability to feel pain or fear of what is happening. Pain medications such as morphine must be given as necessary. A sedating agent such as Valium is always given to counteract the emotional stress of being awake but unable to move.

Exam Hint

Expect to see one question requiring the therapist to recommend a medication for sedating an agitated patient receiving mechanical ventilation.

---

21. Wean the patient from the ventilator

a. Recommend procedures for weaning the patient (WRE code: IIIG1d) [Difficulty: An]

Indications that the patient can tolerate weaning should include some, if not all, of the criteria listed in Box 15-5. The patient need not pass each and every criterion. However, the more the patient can attain, the more likely he or she is to wean successfully. Individual physicians

and practitioners may favor some of these conditions over others and may include other factors not listed.

Some patients do not wean successfully even though objective criteria indicate that they should. Conversely, some patients wean successfully even when objective criteria indicate otherwise. Keep in mind that each patient must be evaluated individually. Look at the objective criteria and how the patient actually performs during weaning.

b. Initiate and modify weaning procedures (CSE code: IIID5)

Indications that the patient will tolerate weaning should include some, if not all, of the criteria listed in Box 15-5. It is not necessary that the patient pass each and every criterion. However, the more the patient can attain, the more likely he or she is to wean successfully. Individual physicians and practitioners may favor some of these conditions over others and may include other factors not listed.

Some patients will not wean successfully even though objective criteria indicated that they should. Conversely, some patients can wean successfully even when objective criteria indicate that the patient will not succeed. The key point to keep in mind is that each patient must be evaluated individually. Look at the objective criteria, as well as how the patient actually performs during weaning.

Each of the five methods presented here has its advocates and a body of clinical evidence to show that it is a valid weaning technique. The practitioner must evaluate the patient before recommending any particular weaning method. The patient also must be evaluated during the weaning trial to determine whether the method chosen is meeting his or her needs. The practitioner must be prepared to discontinue weaning if the patient is failing and be ready to try another weaning approach to help ensure success.

Ventilator discontinuance. Ventilator discontinuance is widely used with patients who have been ventilated for a short period and are now fully prepared to breathe on their own (Fig. 15-29, *A*). When the patient is stable, awake, and alert and meets the criteria listed in Box 15-5, he or she can be prepared for weaning. The patient should be instructed about the weaning, suctioned, and put in Fowler or semi-Fowler position if possible. The ventilator circuit is disconnected, and an aerosol and oxygen mix is breathed in through a T-piece (Briggs adapter). The oxygen percentage should be the same as originally inspired or up to 10% higher, depending on the patient's Pa_{O_2} level on the ventilator.

Ventilator discontinuance and weaning begin at the same moment. The patient goes from having the ventilator provide 100% of the minute volume needs to providing none of it. The patient should be watched continuously because he or she is now breathing totally

Part of minute volume provided by:

▨ = Ventilator   ☐ = Patient

Fig. 15-29 A–E, Options for weaning a patient from mechanical ventilator. PSV, pressure support ventilation; SIMV, synchronous intermittent mandatory ventilation.

than successful. The patient is started on a schedule of intermittent weaning periods and rest periods on the ventilator (Fig. 15-29, *B*). The method shown has a cycle of lengthening weaning periods and shortening rest periods. This goes on until the patient is weaning for an extended period, as discussed earlier. Another method involves a cycle of set rest periods (commonly 0.5 to 1 hour) and lengthening weaning periods as the patient becomes stronger. Again, blood gas values should be monitored after about 20 minutes of weaning. The weaning period can be extended as long as the patient is stable or until extubated.

Regular steps in SIMV weaning. As discussed earlier, IMV/SIMV was originally developed as a ventilating mode and has since become a widely used weaning mode. It allows the patient a more gradual transition toward totally providing all of the WOB. SIMV seems to work especially well in weaning patients who have been ventilator dependent for an extended period. By gradually taking over more of the WOB, the patient reconditions respiratory muscles that may have atrophied through lack of use. The patient also is gaining self-confidence that complete weaning will occur. An additional benefit is that all ventilator alarm systems are functional, and the patient does not need to be directly watched as closely as in the two previously mentioned weaning methods.

This particular SIMV weaning pattern can be applied to a patient who is stable and making rapid progress (Fig. 15-29, *C*). The weaning pattern might involve the IMV rate being reduced in increments of about 2 per minute on a set time schedule. About 20 minutes after reducing the SIMV rate, blood gas values should be monitored. The patient's respiratory mechanics are monitored closely. It is important to calculate the patient's spontaneous minute volume (rate × tidal volume). It should be approximately the same volume as was subtracted from the ventilator delivered minute volume. The process continues as long as the patient tolerates each decrease in the SIMV rate. The stable, strong patient can be rather quickly weaned down to an SIMV rate of two to four times/min. The decision is often made at this point either to use a T-piece, as discussed earlier, or to extubate the airway.

Irregular steps in SIMV weaning. This method is applied when the regular SIMV method is unsuccessful. Often the patient starts out on a cycle of regular reductions in the SIMV rate. This goes on until a point is reached at which the patient has a setback and cannot tolerate any further reductions in the SIMV rate. The rate may be kept at that level for an extended period until the patient is ready for a further decrease (Fig. 15-29, *D*). Further decreases in the IMV rate proceed as the patient tolerates them. No attempt is made to set up a regular pattern of reducing the rate.

independently. Vital signs and respiratory mechanics should be measured every 5 to 10 minutes throughout the procedure. If the patient deteriorates, ventilator therapy is reestablished. After a rest period, intermittent ventilator discontinuance or another mode of weaning might be tried. If the patient is stable, an ABG sample should be taken after about 20 minutes. Alternatively, pulse oximetry and end-tidal carbon dioxide can be monitored. If the blood gas results are acceptable and the patient appears stable, the weaning is continued, or the patient can be extubated. Approximately 75% of patients who tolerate this procedure can be extubated.

Intermittent ventilator discontinuance. This method is used after the previously mentioned method proves less

It may be necessary to increase the rate to higher previous levels if the patient has a serious setback. One possible cause that may prevent the SIMV rate from decreasing is the resistance to breathing through the demand valve and breathing circuit. A trial on a T-piece (which offers no resistance) may prove to be the final step in weaning. If this fails for the patient, the reason is probably the resistance caused by the endotracheal tube. The pressure support weaning method should then be tried on the patient.

Weaning by pressure support ventilation. The PSV mode is available on most modern electrically powered and microprocessor ventilators. It can be used as the newest weaning method (Fig. 15-29, *E*). When used as a weaning method, the pressure support level is gradually reduced. Decreasing pressure support steps of 2 to 5 cm water are commonly made. The patient has to increase the WOB gradually to inspire a tidal volume. Blood gas values and respiratory mechanics should be evaluated after each decrease in the pressure support level. A modest pressure support level of 2 to 5 cm water is maintained to overcome any resistance of the endotracheal tube. If the patient does well during an extended trial of minimum pressure support, extubation is performed unless the endotracheal tube is needed for other reasons.

The criteria listed in Box 15-5 can be used in evaluating any patient being weaned by any of these methods. General signs that the patient is not tolerating weaning include anxiety, agitation, a large increase or decrease in the respiratory rate, angina, tachycardia, an increase in premature ventricular contractions or other serious dysrhythmias, bradycardia, hypertension, hypotension, cyanosis, hypoxemia, and hypercarbia with acidemia. The patient probably will not exhibit all of these signs. Some tend to be seen together because they relate to the patient's WOB. Others appear to give conflicting signals of success or failure. It is the practitioner's responsibility to evaluate the patient's condition to determine whether weaning should be continued or ventilatory support resumed.

Make a recommendation to extubate the patient. Extubation can usually be safely accomplished when the patient has met the criteria listed in Box 15-5, has demonstrated the ability to breathe effectively for a clinically significant period as measured by the listed criteria, has acceptable blood gas results, is alert enough to protect his or her airway, and can effectively cough out any secretions. It may be found that some patients need the endotracheal tube even though they no longer need ventilatory support. The tube provides a suctioning route if the patient is unable to cough out large amounts of secretions. The tube also protects the airway from the risk of aspiration in a comatose patient who may vomit.

Exam Hint

Expect to see at least one question that relates to evaluating a weaning patient and recommending extubation if the patient is meeting weaning and extubation criteria or the resumption of mechanical ventilation if the patient has failed weaning and extubation criteria.

MODULE F
Respiratory care plan

1. **Analyze available information to determine the patient's pathophysiologic state (CSE code: IIIH1)**
2. **Determine the appropriateness of the prescribed therapy and goals for the identified pathophysiologic state (CSE code: IIIH3)**

Be prepared to make recommendations on changing ventilator parameters based on the patient's pathologic condition, blood gas values, chest radiograph findings, breath sounds, and vital signs. Common recommendations follow.

Exam Hint

Past Written Registry Examinations have had questions about the management of patients with specific conditions such as increased intracranial pressure (ICP), COPD, congestive heart failure (CHF), ARDS, and pneumothorax. In addition, the Clinical Simulation Examination has at least one adult scenario on each of the following: a patient with COPD, a patient with trauma, a patient with cardiovascular disease, and a patient with neuromuscular or neurologic diseases. The management of these patients is briefly discussed next.

Increased intracranial pressure

ICP is the pressure within the cranium (skull) and is normally less than 10 mm Hg. It is measured by a catheter placed into the subarachnoid space, subdural space, or ventricular space. The most common cause of an increased ICP is an acute head injury in which the brain is shaken. Other causes of increased ICP include craniotomy for brain tumor resection and stroke (cerebral vascular accident [CVA]). Any significant increase in the pressure within the skull will further injure the brain. Clinical experience has shown that when the ICP exceeds 20 mm Hg, the patient's outcome significantly worsens.

The A/C mode is usually selected with constant volume ventilation so that the patient is assured of a set minute volume if apnea occurs. It has been demonstrated that hyperventilating the patient to a $Paco_2$ between 25 and 30 torr reduces the increased ICP. This is the result of the lowered carbon dioxide pressure causing cerebral vasoconstriction. Because the cerebral blood flow is decreased by hyperventilation, it is important to maintain the patient's Pao_2 in the 90 to 110 torr range.

Chronic obstructive lung disease

Patients with COPD are usually well known because of previous hospitalizations for acute exacerbations related to problems such as a lung infection or heart failure. When the patient must be ventilated, it is important to maintain baseline "normal" blood gas values. This usually means accepting moderate hypoxemia and hypercarbia with a compensated respiratory acidosis. Ventilating the patient to provide textbook normal ABGs must be avoided. This is because the COPD patient cannot maintain this level of breathing efficiency when ready to come off of the ventilator.

The A/C or SIMV mode may be used with either a constant volume set or PC used to set the tidal volume. A COPD patient must have the ventilator adjusted, including the addition of mechanical dead space, to maintain the patient's normally elevated $Paco_2$ level. A Pao_2 of 60 to 70 torr is usually adequate. Keep the plateau pressure (alveolar pressure) less than 30 cm water to avoid overdistention of the patient's compliant lungs and resulting volutrauma.

If the patient has air trapping and auto-PEEP, a small amount of therapeutic PEEP may be added to help the patient exhale and to trigger the ventilator. Increase the therapeutic PEEP in 1-cm water steps until the patient is synchronized with the ventilator. Many COPD patients need 5 cm water of PEEP or more. When the condition that caused the sudden deterioration is corrected, the patient should be weaned off of the ventilator as soon as possible to prevent atrophy of the ventilatory muscles.

Congestive heart failure

Patients with CHF usually also have a pulmonary edema problem. This results in hypoxemia and low lung compliance. Mechanical ventilation with the A/C or SIMV mode with constant volume ventilation is needed to reduce the patient's WOB, deliver supplemental oxygen, and add therapeutic PEEP. Usually a pulmonary artery catheter is placed to measure pulmonary artery pressure (PAP), pulmonary capillary wedge pressure (PCWP), and cardiac output (CO). If the PEEP level is increased and the patient's cardiac output decreases, the PEEP should be reduced to its previous level. The patient must be given a diuretic such as furosemide (Lasix) to increase urine output. The patient's heart function is improved by giving digitalis (Lanoxin). Closely follow the patient's cardiovascular val-

ues to monitor improvement after the administration of a diuretic and digitalis. Reduce the PEEP and inspired oxygen as the pulmonary edema problem is corrected.

Acute respiratory distress syndrome

ARDS is caused by a variety of pulmonary and circulatory conditions that result in nonhomogeneous damage to alveolar capillary membranes throughout the lungs. This results in noncardiac pulmonary edema with decreased pulmonary compliance and hypoxemia. Like the patient with CHF, the patient with ARDS needs mechanical ventilation to reduce the WOB, provide supplemental oxygen, and provide therapeutic PEEP. A pulmonary artery catheter is also needed to follow the patient's cardiovascular status. Also shunt ($\dot{Q}s$) studies may be performed.

Unlike the patient with CHF, the patient with ARDS does not respond as favorably to diuretic and digitalis medications. The continued problem of low compliance and resulting high ventilating pressures has been linked to volutrauma. Recent research has led to the following lung protective strategies.

Small tidal volume ventilation. Initially, most ARDS patients are started on the A/C or SIMV mode with constant volume ventilation. Unfortunately, many severe ARDS patients cannot be managed in this manner. The stiff lungs result in a very high plateau pressure and risk of pulmonary volutrauma. Recent studies have shown that the plateau pressure found in the alveoli (P_{plat}) must be kept 35 cm water or less to avoid this serious complication. To lower a dangerously high alveolar pressure, the tidal volume must be reduced. Many clinicians recommend that the patient be switched from constant volume ventilation to PCV to do this. Recent evidence has shown a higher survival rate in ARDS patients when the tidal volume was lowered from 12 mL/kg to 6 mL/kg of ideal body weight.

If the initial set of blood gases on PC with a small tidal volume does not show adequate oxygenation, the inspiratory time must be increased. Some ARDS patients need an increased inspiratory time such that the I:E ratio is inverse. This results in PCIRV. The advantages of PCIRV over conventional volume ventilation are the lowered peak airway pressure and the longer inspiratory time. The lowered peak pressure is thought to reduce the risk of volutrauma. The longer inspiratory time allows alveoli with long time constants of ventilation to fill and areas of atelectasis to reopen.

Permissive hypercapnia. The small tidal volumes used with PCIRV can result in failure to blow off carbon dioxide to a normal level. At times, this must be clinically accepted. Permissive hypercapnia involves allowing a $Paco_2$ of 50 torr up to 100 to 150 torr. It is very important to prevent the carbon dioxide level from increasing too rapidly because it causes cerebral vasodilation and increases the patient's ICP. To minimize this risk, the Pa_{CO_2} should not be allowed to increase faster than 10 torr/hour to a maximum of 80 torr. If the Pa_{CO_2} must be allowed to increase to more than 80 torr, the rate of increase must be slower than 10 torr/hour. The high Pa_{CO_2} also results in a respiratory acidosis. Keep the patient's arterial pH at 7.25 or more to avoid problems related to the acidosis. It may be necessary to administer intravenous bicarbonate to correct the respiratory acidosis. When the patient recovers, the Pa_{CO_2} can be gradually lowered. If permissive hypercapnia was used for less than 24 hours, the Pa_{CO_2} can probably be lowered by 10 to 20 torr/hr. If permissive hypercapnia was used for more than 24 hours or bicarbonate was given to buffer the pH, the Pa_{CO_2} must be lowered more slowly. It is important to monitor the patient's arterial pH throughout this process to prevent too rapid an increase.

Lung inflection points. An optimal PEEP study is justified to find the PEEP level needed to correct the low lung compliance, severe hypoxemia, and large shunt problems these patients have. If possible, the lungs low and high inflection points should be determined. They relate to the lung compliance points at FRC and near total lung capacity. (Review Fig. 15-17 if needed.) A modern microprocessor ventilator with graphics software and a monitor should be used to evaluate these conditions. Set the unit to display a pressure/volume loop as shown in Fig. 15-30. Point *A* on the figure shows the low inflection point. This identifies the pressure needed to open up alveoli and

establish the patient's FRC. When the therapeutic PEEP level is set at or above the lungs' low inflection point, they will be most effectively ventilated. This PEEP will likely need to be maintained for several days until the patient begins to recover. Point *B* on the figure shows the high inflection point. This identifies the highest lung volume and highest lung pressure that should be allowed. Further pressure does not greatly increase tidal volume and can result in volutrauma to any overstretched alveoli. Many clinicians use the high inflection point as the maximum pressure allowed with PCV to deliver a tidal volume.

Auto-PEEP recognition. With ARDS, as the lungs become more compliant, the PCIRV inspiratory time must be reduced toward normal to prevent the pressure from compressing the heart. Full exhalation of the tidal volume must be assured. This is not usually a problem because the stiff lungs rapidly recoil to the resting level (FRC).

Pneumothorax. Recognize the signs of a pneumothorax on a mechanically ventilated patient (suddenly increasing peak and plateau pressures, hypoxemia, mediastinal shift to the side opposite the pneumothorax, hyper-resonant percussion note over the pneumothorax, and asymmetrical chest movement on inspiration) and be prepared to recommend the insertion of a pleural chest tube or to treat a tension pneumothorax (discussed later in this chapter and in Chapter 18). Common causes of the pneumothorax include lung puncture during the insertion of a CVP line via the subclavian vein, overinflated lungs from too large a tidal volume on the ventilator, punctured lung from a sharp broken rib, and thoracentesis.

Remember to get an ABG after every ventilator change that could result in a different Pa_{O_2} (pulse oximetry or transcutaneous oxygen may be substituted) or Pa_{CO_2} (end-tidal CO_2 or transcutaneous carbon dioxide may be substituted). Mixed venous blood gas values should also be obtained when possible.

Physical responses to mechanical ventilation, as measured by the vital signs, can vary considerably. A patient who is anxious, angry, or in pain will have an increase in the vital signs. A patient who is relaxed has reduced WOB, and a patient whose blood gas values are now normal will have a return to normal vital signs. Watch carefully for the patient whose decrease in blood pressure coincides with a tachycardia. This patient may be having decreased venous return to the heart from an increased intrathoracic pressure.

Because an intubated patient cannot speak, it is necessary to communicate by asking simple questions that can be answered in a *yes* nod or *no* shake of the head. Other methods of communication are a pad of paper and pencil or picture boards. It is not possible to predict how a patient will react to the initiation of mechanical ventilation or its prolonged need. Some patients react with relief and relax when the WOB is reduced. Others may become

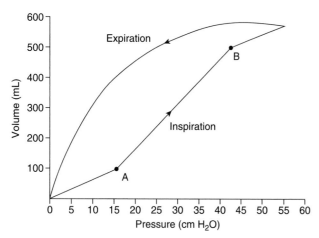

Fig. 15-30 Pressure/volume loop showing lower and upper inflection points in an acute respiratory distress syndrome patient. *A,* Lower inflection point indicating opening pressure of alveoli. This is minimum positive end-expiratory pressure level needed to maintain patient's functional residual capacity. *B,* Upper inflection point indicating that lungs are being overstretched. This should be upper limit of peak airway pressure to avoid overdistention and volutrauma. Flattening of pressure/volume loop to right of point *B* shows that little volume is delivered despite increased pressure.

Exam Hint

Be prepared to make recommendations on changing ventilator parameters based on the patient's condition, blood gas values, chest radiograph films, breath sounds, and vital signs. This information can be found in this chapter and throughout this text.

Exam Hint

Usually one question deals with recognizing that a patient is losing tidal volume through a pleural chest tube or that a pneumothorax has developed. Know the signs and symptoms of a pneumothorax.

angry at the limitations imposed on them or become depressed.

3. Treat a tension pneumothorax (WRE code: III I2) [Difficulty: Ap, An]

A chest radiograph and physical examination of the patient will reveal whether air (or fluid) is abnormally found around the lung(s) or heart. If a patient has a tension pneumothorax, a pleural chest tube must be inserted on the affected side to remove the air and relieve the pressure within the chest. In an emergency, a large-gauge needle may be placed between the second and third ribs (second intercostal space) in the midclavicular line. These and related subjects are discussed in detail in Chapter 18. A nontension pneumothorax of greater than 10% is often also treated by inserting a pleural chest tube. In addition, a pleural chest tube is placed to remove blood or other fluid from the pleural space.

A pneumomediastinum, pneumopericardium, or pneumoperitoneum that puts the patient at risk also must be treated. A chest tube is then inserted into the area where the abnormal air is found. The same chest tube would also remove any abnormal collection of fluid. A pericardial chest tube is usually placed behind the heart to remove any blood that may leak out after open heart surgery.

If the patient is being ventilated on a constant volume ventilator, the amount of air that is lost through the pleural chest tube can be calculated. This is done by subtracting the measured exhaled volume from the measured inhaled volume (the set tidal volume). The following equation demonstrates:

Inspired tidal volume = 500 mL
Exhaled tidal volume = −400 mL

100 mL of tidal volume is lost through the pleural chest tube.

It is not always possible to measure a consistent tidal volume when PCV or a similar mode is used. In a case like this, it is possible to make only a qualitative judgment on pleural air leak. In other words, if air is seen to bubble out through the pleural drainage system, an air leak is present. When the air stops bubbling, the pleural tear has healed. See Chapter 18 for a complete discussion on pleural drainage systems.

4. Stop the treatment or procedure if the patient has an adverse reaction to it (CSE code: IIIF1)

5. Discontinue treatment based on the patient's response (WRE code: IIIG1e) [Difficulty: An]

Be prepared to stop a treatment or procedure related to mechanical ventilation if the patient has an adverse reaction to it.

BIBLIOGRAPHY

Aloan CA, Hill TV, editors: *Respiratory care of the newborn and child,* ed 2, Philadelphia, 1997, Lippincott-Raven.

American Association for Respiratory Care: Clinical Practice Guideline: humidification during mechanical ventilation, *Respir Care* 37(8):887, 1992.

American Association for Respiratory Care: Clinical Practice Guideline: patient-ventilator system checks, *Respir Care* 37(8):882, 1992.

American Association for Respiratory Care: Clinical Practice Guideline: endotracheal suctioning of mechanically ventilated adults and children with artificial airways, *Respir Care* 38(5):500, 1993.

American Association for Respiratory Care: Clinical Practice Guideline: application of continuous positive airway pressure in neonates via nasal prongs or nasopharyngeal tube, *Respir Care* 39(8):817, 1994.

American Association for Respiratory Care: Clinical Practice Guideline: neonatal time-triggered, pressure-limited, time-cycled mechanical ventilation, *Respir Care* 39(8):808, 1994.

American Association for Respiratory Care: Clinical Practice Guideline: ventilator circuit changes, *Respir Care* 39(8):797, 1994.

American Association for Respiratory Care: Clinical Practice Guideline: long-term invasive mechanical ventilation in the home, *Respir Care* 40(12):1313, 1995.

American Association for Respiratory Care: Clinical Practice Guideline: capnography/capnometry during mechanical ventilation, *Respir Care* 40(12):1321, 1995.

American Association for Respiratory Care: Clinical Practice Guideline: capnography/capnometry during mechanical ventilation: 2003 revision and update, *Respir Care* 48(3):534, 2003.

American Association for Respiratory Care: Clinical Practice Guideline: removal of the endotracheal tube, *Respir Care* 44(1):85, 1999.

American Association for Respiratory Care: Clinical Practice Guideline: selection of device, administration of bronchodilator, and evaluation of responses to therapy in mechanically ventilated patients, *Respir Care* 44(1):105, 1999.

American Association for Respiratory Care: Consensus statement on the essentials of mechanical ventilation, *Respir Care* 37(9):1000, 1992.

American Association for Respiratory Care: Clinical Practice Guideline: in-hospital transport of the mechanically ventilated patient: 2002 revision and update, *Respir Care* 47 (6):721–723, 2002.

AARC Evidence-Based Clinical Practice Guidelines: Care of the ventilator circuit and its relation to ventilator-associated pneumonia, *Respir Care* 48(9):869–879, 2003.

Banner MJ, Lampotang S: Clinical use of inspiratory and expiratory waveforms. In Kacmarek RM, Stoller JK, editors: *Current respiratory care,* Philadelphia, 1988, BC Decker.

Barnes TA, editor: *Core textbook of respiratory care practice,* ed 2, St Louis, 1994, Mosby.

Bone RC: Pressure-volume measurements in detection of bronchospasm and mucous plugging in acute respiratory failure, *Respir Care* 21(7):620, 1976.

Boysen PG, McGough E: Pressure-control and pressure-support ventilation: flow patterns, inspiratory time, and gas distribution, *Respir Care* 33(2):620, 1988.

Branson RD, Campbell RS, Davis K Jr, et al: Altering flowrate during maximum pressure support ventilation (PSV_{max}): effects on cardiorespiratory function, *Respir Care* 35(11):1056, 1990.

Branson RD, Chatburn RL: Technical description and classification of modes of ventilator operation, *Respir Care* 37(9):1026, 1992.

Branson RD, Hess DR, Chatburn RL, editors: *Respiratory care equipment,* ed 2, Philadelphia, 1999, Lippincott Williams & Wilkins.

Branson RD, Hurst JM: Laboratory evaluation of moisture output of seven airway heat and moisture exchangers, *Respir Care* 32(9):741, 1987.

Burton GC, Hodgkin JE, Ward JJ, editors: *Respiratory care: a guide to clinical practice,* ed 4, Philadelphia, 1997, Lippincott-Raven.

Cairo JM, Pilbeam SP: *Mosby's respiratory care equipment,* ed 7, St Louis, 2004, Mosby.

Campbell RS, Davis BR: Pressure-controlled versus volume-controlled ventilation: does it matter? *Respir Care* 47(4):416–426, 2002.

Chang DW: *Clinical application of mechanical ventilation,* ed 2, Albany, NY, 2001, Delmar.

Chatburn RL: A new system for understanding mechanical ventilation, *Respir Care* 36(10):1123, 1991.

Chatburn RL: Classification of mechanical ventilators, *Respir Care* 37(9):1009, 1992.

Dantzker DR, MacIntyre NR, Bakow ED, editors: *Comprehensive respiratory care,* Philadelphia, 1995, WB Saunders.

Dhand R: Ventilator graphics and respiratory mechanics in the patient with obstructive lung disease, *Respir Care* 50(2):246–261, 2005.

Drinker PA, McKhann CF III: Landmark perspective: the iron lung: first practical means of respiratory support, *JAMA* 256(11):1476, 1986.

Epstein SK: Extubation, *Respir Care* 47(4):483–495, 2002.

Epstein SK: Weaning from mechanical ventilation, *Respir Care* 47(4):454–468, 2002.

Evidence-based guidelines for weaning and discontinuing ventilator support, *Respir Care* 47(1):69–90, 2002.

Felix WR Jr, MacDonnell KF, Jacobs L: Resuscitation from drowning in cold water, *N Engl J Med* 304(14):843, 1981.

Fink JB, Hunt GE, editors: *Clinical practice in respiratory care,* Philadelphia, 1999, Lippincott-Raven.

Fink JB, Tobin MJ, Dhand R: Bronchodilator therapy in mechanically ventilated patients, *Respir Care* 44:53, 1999.

Greer K: Hypothermia: a quiet killer, *Adv Respir Ther* Jan 15, 1990.

Gregg BL: Invasive mechanical ventilation. In Wyka KA, Mathews PJ, Clark WF, editors: *Foundations of respiratory care,* Albany, NY, 2002, Delmar.

Gurevitch MJ: Selection of the inspiratory:expiratory ratio. In Kacmarek RM, Stoller JK, editors: *Current respiratory care,* Philadelphia, 1988, BC Decker.

Hess DR: Mechanical ventilation of the adult patient: initiation, management, and weaning. In Burton GG, Hodgkin JE, Ward JJ, editors: *Respiratory care: a guide to clinical practice,* ed 4, Philadelphia, 1997, Lippincott-Raven.

Hess DR, Branson RD: Mechanical ventilation. In Hess DR, MacIntyre NR, Mishoe SC, et al, editors: *Respiratory care principles and practice,* Philadelphia, 2002, WB Saunders.

Hess DR, Kacmarek RM: *Essentials of mechanical ventilation,* ed 2, New York, 2002, McGraw-Hill.

Hess DR, McCurdy S, Simmons M: Compression volume in adult ventilator circuits: a comparison of five disposable circuits and a nondisposable circuit, *Respir Care* 36(10): 1113, 1991.

Hill NS: Clinical application of body ventilators, *Chest* 90(6):897, 1986.

Hill NS, Eveloff SE, Carlisle CC, et al: Efficacy of nocturnal nasal ventilation in patients with restrictive thoracic disease, *Am Rev Respir Dis* 145(2):365, 1992.

Hirsch C, Kacmarek RM, Stanek K: Work of breathing during CPAP and PSV imposed by the new generation mechanical ventilators: a lung model study, *Respir Care* 36(8):815, 1991.

International Consensus Conferences in Intensive Care Medicine: Ventilator-associated lung injury in ARDS, *Am J Respir Crit Care Med* 160:2118–2124, 1999.

Kacmarek RM: The role of pressure support ventilation in reducing work of breathing, *Respir Care* 33(2):99, 1988.

Kacmarek RM, Foley K, Cheever P: Determination of ventilatory reserve in mechanically ventilated patients: a comparison of techniques, *Respir Care* 36(10):1085, 1991.

Kacmarek RM, Hess D: Pressure-controlled inverse-ratio ventilation: panacea or auto-PEEP? *Respir Care* 35(10):945, 1990.

Kirby RR: Modes of mechanical ventilation. In Kacmarek RM, Stoller JK, editors: *Current respiratory care,* Philadelphia, 1988, BC Decker.

Kuhlen R, Rossaint R: The role of spontaneous breathing during mechanical ventilation, *Respir Care* 47(3):296–307, 2002.

MacIntyre NR: Setting the frequency-tidal volume pattern, *Respir Care* 47(3):266–278, 2002.

MacIntyre NR: Pressure support: inspiratory assist. In Kacmarek RM, Stoller JK, editors: *Current respiratory care,* Philadelphia, 1988, BC Decker.

MacIntyre NR: Weaning from mechanical ventilatory support: volume-assisting intermittent breaths versus pressure-supporting every breath, *Respir Care* 33(2):121, 1988.

MacIntyre NR, Branson RD: *Mechanical ventilation,* Philadelphia, 2001, WB Saunders.

Martz KV, Joiner JW, Rodger MS: *Management of the patient-ventilator system: a team approach,* ed 2, St Louis, 1984, Mosby.

Nilsestuen JO, Hargett KD: Using ventilator graphics to identify patient-ventilator asynchrony, *Respir Care* 50(2):202-234, 2005.

Pennock BE, Kaplan PD, Carlin BW, et al: Pressure support ventilation with a simplified ventilatory support system administered with a nasal mask in patients with respiratory failure, *Chest* 100(5):1371, 1991.

Pierson DJ: Indications for mechanical ventilation in adults with acute respiratory failure, *Respir Care* 47(3):249-265, 2002.

Pilbeam SP: *Mechanical ventilation: physiological and clinical applications,* ed 3, St Louis, 1998, Mosby.

Quan SF, Parides GC, Knoper SR: Mandatory minute volume (MVV) ventilation: an overview, *Respir Care* 35(9):898, 1990.

Radford EP Jr: Ventilation standards for use in artificial respiration, *J Appl Phys* 7:451, 1955.

Respironics: Guidelines for invasive applications with BiPAP systems, Monroeville, Penn.

Respironics: Product literature on the suggested protocol for initiation of the BiPAP S/T or BiPAP S/T-D ventilatory support system, Monroeville, Penn.

Saura P, Blanch L: How to set positive end-expiratory pressure. *Respir Care* 47(3):279-295, 2002.

Scanlan CL, Wilkins RL, Stoller JK, editors: *Egan's fundamentals of respiratory care,* ed 8, St Louis, 2003, Mosby.

Shapiro BA, Kacmarek RM, Cane RD, et al, editors: *Clinical application of respiratory care,* ed 4, St Louis, 1991, Mosby.

Shelledy DC, Mikles SP: Newer modes of mechanical ventilation, I: pressure support, *Respir Manage* July/Aug,14-20, 1988.

Shelledy DC, Mikles SP: Newer modes of mechanical ventilation, II: mandatory minute volume ventilation, *Respir Manage* July/Aug 21, 1988.

Stoller JK: Establishing clinical unweanability, *Respir Care* 36(3):186, 1991.

Strumpf DA, Carlisle CC, Millman RP, et al: An evaluation of the Respironics BiPAP Bi-Level CPAP device for delivery of assisted ventilation, *Respir Care* 35(5):415, 1990.

The Acute Respiratory Distress Syndrome Network: Ventilation with lower tidal volumes as compared with traditional tidal volumes for acute lung injury and the acute respiratory distress syndrome. May 2000. http://www.nejm.org/content/browser/1.asp.

Tobin MJ: Monitoring of pressure, flow, and volume during mechanical ventilation, *Respir Care* 37(9):1081, 1992.

Tobin MJ, Lodato RF: PEEP, auto-PEEP, and waterfalls, *Chest* 96(3):449, 1989.

Waldhorn RE: Nocturnal nasal intermittent positive pressure ventilation with bi-level positive airway pressure (BiPAP) in respiratory failure, *Chest* 101(2):516, 1992.

Waugh JB, Deshpande VM, Harwood RJ: *Rapid interpretation of ventilator waveforms,* Upper Saddle River, NJ, 1999, Prentice-Hall.

Whitaker K: *Comprehensive perinatal and pediatric respiratory care,* ed 2, Albany, NY, 1997, Delmar.

White GC: *Equipment theory for respiratory care,* ed 3, Albany, NY, 1999, Delmar.

Wright J, Gong H: "Auto-PEEP": incidence, magnitude, and contributing factors, *Heart Lung* 19(4):352, 1990.

SELF-STUDY QUESTIONS

1. PCIRV is indicated in which following condition?
   A. Asthma
   B. Chronic bronchitis
   C. Pulmonary contusion
   D. ARDS

2. Mean airway pressure is defined as:
   A. P_{peak} minus the plateau pressure
   B. P_{peak} divided by inspiratory time
   C. The average pressure throughout the breathing cycle
   D. Tidal volume divided by peak pressure

3. Clinical factors causing decreased lung compliance include:
   I. Pulmonary edema
   II. Pulmonary fibrosis
   III. Emphysema
   IV. ARDS
      A. I and II
      B. II and III
      C. I, II, and IV
      D. I, II, III, and IV

4. MMV ventilation is:
   I. Similar to A/C ventilation.
   II. Indicated when weaning a patient with an unstable respiratory drive.
   III. Designed to make sure that at least a minimum minute volume is delivered.
   IV. A substitute for CPAP.
      A. II and III
      B. I
      C. III
      D. I and IV

5. The Food and Drug Administration has approved high frequency ventilation for management of all of the following situations *except:*
   A. Laryngoscopy
   B. Near drowning
   C. Bronchopleural fistula
   D. Bronchoscopy

6. Weaning should be terminated when:
   I. The patient's rapid, shallow breathing index is 120.
   II. Cardiac dysrhythmias occur.

III. The patient's $Paco_2$ is 60 torr.

IV. The patient's Pao_2 is 70 torr on 40% oxygen.
    A. I and III
    B. II and IV
    C. II, III, and IV
    D. I, II, and III

7. If a patient has just returned from surgery for a left pneumonectomy, the ventilator delivered tidal volume should be:
    A. Less than normal based on ideal body weight.
    B. The same as normal based on ideal body weight.
    C. Larger than normal based on ideal body weight.
    D. The same volume as delivered before surgery.

8. A negative-pressure ventilator is indicated for all the following types of patients *except:*
    A. ARDS
    B. Neuromuscular defects
    C. Kyphoscoliosis
    D. COPD in acute failure

9. The parameters found with an ideal optimal PEEP study are:
    I. Pulmonary compliance improves
    II. Pao_2 increases
    III. Percentage shunt decreases
    IV. Pulmonary vascular resistance increases
    V. Pulmonary vascular resistance decreases
    VI. Blood pressure decreases and heart rate increases
    A. II, IV, and VI
    B. I, II, III, and V
    C. II, III, V, and VI
    D. I, II, III, and IV

10. What would be a patient's static compliance (Cst) if the corrected tidal volume is 600 mL, the ventilator's peak pressure is 65 cm water, the plateau pressure is 48 cm water, and there is 12 cm water of PEEP?
    A. 9 mL/cm water
    B. 11 mL/cm water
    C. 13 mL/cm water
    D. 17 mL/cm water

Use the following information for questions 11 and 12: Your ventilated patient has an exhaled tidal volume of 700 mL. Because of refractory hypoxemia, 6 cm of PEEP therapy is started. The peak pressure is 35 cm water, and the static or plateau pressure is 25 cm water. The compliance factor has been determined to be 4 mL/cm water.

11. Calculate the static compliance (Cst) for this patient.
    A. 19 mL/cm water
    B. 24 mL/cm water
    C. 28 mL/cm water
    D. 32 mL/cm water

12. Calculate the dynamic compliance (Cdyn) for this patient.
    A. 16 mL/cm water
    B. 19 mL/cm water

    C. 24 mL/cm water
    D. 32 mL/cm water

13. When preparing to ventilate a patient with HFJV, it is necessary to have all of the following *except:*
    A. Spirometer to measure tidal volume
    B. Jet injector line
    C. High pressure oxygen source
    D. Humidifier

14. Over the course of an 8-hour shift, the respiratory therapist notices that a patient receiving constant volume ventilation has had an increase in the peak pressure from 25 to 40 cm water. What could have caused this change?
    I. Airway resistance decreased
    II. Lung compliance increased
    III. Airway resistance increased
    IV. Lung compliance decreased
    A. III
    B. IV
    C. III and IV
    D. I and II

15. A 45-year-old patient has developed ARDS. The physician asks the respiratory therapist for the best ventilator adjustment to reduce the patient's intrapulmonary shunting. The therapist should recommend:
    A. Increasing the inspiratory time
    B. Increasing the sigh volume
    C. Decreasing the respiratory rate
    D. Increasing the PEEP

16. A trauma patient has a pleural chest tube to the left lung. A volume cycled ventilator is delivering an inspiratory tidal volume of 800 mL. The expiratory tidal volume is shown to be 600 mL. What could best explain the volume difference?
    A. Air leak through the chest tube
    B. Deflated endotracheal tube cuff
    C. Miscalibrated spirometer
    D. Bronchospasm and auto-PEEP

17. In a patient with ARDS, the indication to switch from volume cycled ventilation to pressure cycled ventilation is:
    A. Peak pressure of 35 cm water or greater
    B. Lung compliance less than 35 mL/cm water
    C. Plateau pressure of 35 cm water or greater
    D. Peak pressure and plateau pressure total 35 cm water

18. A 70-kg (154-lb) patient with a stroke is being mechanically ventilated in the A/C mode with the following settings:
Minute ventilation, 8.4 L
I:E ratio, 1:2
Fio_2, 0.35
Rate, 12
Mechanical dead space, 150 mL

His ABG results are as follows:
pH, 7.30
$Paco_2$, 51 torr
HCO_3^-, 24 mEq/L
Pao_2, 107 torr
On the basis of this information, it would be most
appropriate to recommend:
A. Decreasing the Fio_2
B. Decreasing the minute ventilation
C. Increasing the respiratory rate
D. Decreasing the mechanical dead space

19. The chest radiograph of a patient receiving
mechanical ventilation reveals atelectasis in both
bases. In addition, the patient's breath sounds are
diminished bilaterally, and she has a low-grade fever.
Which of the following ventilator adjustments
should the respiratory therapist recommend?
A. Increasing the flow rate
B. Lengthening the expiratory time
C. Increasing the ventilator frequency
D. Increasing the ventilator sigh volume

20. When permissive hypercapnia is being used to help
manage a patient with ARDS, the following should
be remembered:
I. Bicarbonate may be given to increase the pH
if needed.
II. The carbon dioxide level is allowed to increase
in a controlled manner.
III. The pH should be kept between 7.45 and 7.35.
IV. The pH should be kept greater than 7.25.
V. The $Paco_2$ should be kept between 40 and 50 torr.
A. I, II, and IV
B. III and V
C. II and IV
D. II and V

21. Your patient has the desire to breathe spontaneously
and has a tidal volume that is 4 mL/kg of ideal body
weight. Because of facial trauma from an automobile
accident, she has an endotracheal tube that is
smaller than the ideal size. She also had lung
contusions in the crash. Her Pao_2 is 63 torr on 55%
oxygen. What ventilator mode(s) would you
recommend for her?
A. A/C with flow-by for triggering the ventilator
B. Low level pressure support ventilation with
PEEP
C. SIMV with low level pressure support and PEEP
D. SIMV with high level pressure support (PSV_{max})

22. An apneic 60-kg (132-lb) patient is being ventilated
with the PC mode. Her ventilator settings are:
Tidal volume, 700 mL
Rate, 10/min
Oxygen, 60%
Mechanical dead space, 100 mL
Her ABG shows:

Pao_2, 66 torr
$Paco_2$, 55 torr
pH, 7.32
Base excess, 0
Considering this information, all of the following
individual ventilator adjustments would improve
her ABG values *except*:
A. Increase the respiratory rate to 14/min
B. Increase the tidal volume to 800 mL
C. Change to an SIMV mode with a rate of 10/min
D. Remove the mechanical dead space

23. Indications that the patient is tolerating SIMV
include all of the following *except*:
A. The respiratory rate is increased.
B. The heart rate is stable.
C. The blood gas results are stable.
D. Accessory muscles of ventilation are not being
used.

24. Your 55-kg (120-lb) female patient is being
ventilated with an SIMV rate of 10, tidal volume of
600 mL, 10 cm water of therapeutic PEEP, and 35%
inspired oxygen. She has an 8.0-mm inner diameter
tracheostomy tube. Her spontaneous tidal volume is
350 mL, and the rate is 10/min. The most recent
ABG shows Pao_2 95, $Paco_2$ 42, and pH 7.40. What
would you recommend?
A. Reduce the SIMV rate to 3.
B. Reduce the PEEP to 7 cm water.
C. Increase the SIMV rate to 12.
D. Add 10 cm of pressure support.

25. Five adult patients are being weaned from
mechanical ventilation. Their bedside spirometry
values are shown below.

	f	$\dot{V}_E$ (L)	V_T (mL)	FEV_1 (mL/kg)	MIP (cm water)
Patient 1	7	2.45	350	5	−35
Patient 2	12	5.44	501	0	−30
Patient 3	15	8.25	550	15	−20
Patient 4	37	11.1	300	13	−15
Patient 5	40	17.0	425	7	−15

Which of the following patients may be ready for
extubation?
A. Patients 1 and 2
B. Patients 1 and 4
C. Patients 2 and 3
D. Patients 3 and 5

26. The measurements below are obtained on a patient
while he is being mechanically ventilated:

	6 PM	8 PM
Total respiratory rate	14	14
PEEP (cm water)	8	8
P plateau (cm water)	15	15
P peak (cm water)	30	45
Compliance (mL/cm water)	40	40

In this situation, the most appropriate action would be to:
A. Increase therapeutic PEEP.
B. Administer a bronchodilating agent.
C. Administer a diuretic agent.
D. Administer a paralyzing agent.

27. When working with a patient who recently had a bowel resection and is receiving a paralyzing medication to prevent fighting against the ventilator, it is important to:
A. Give the patient caffeine as a central nervous system stimulant.
B. Give the patient a sedative medication for pain.
C. Give the patient a narcotic medication for pain.
D. Talk quietly because the patient is probably sleeping.

28. If your ventilator dependent patient has a large amount of thick tracheal secretions, it is best to:
A. Use a cascade-type humidifier warmed to body temperature.
B. Use an HME for his or her humidity needs.
C. Use no humidification system so that the secretions will dry out to some extent.
D. Either B or C is acceptable.

29. All of the following are needed to assemble a free-standing CPAP system *except:*
A. An exhaled volume spirometer
B. A low pressure or disconnect alarm
C. Water traps in the inspiratory and expiratory tubing
D. A device to create the CPAP pressure

30. A patient with a closed head injury and increased ICP is being mechanically ventilated in the A/C mode with an FiO_2 of 0.3, a rate of 12, and a tidal volume of 700 mL. Her ABG results are shown:
pH, 7.44
$PaCO_2$, 35 torr

PaO_2, 295 torr
The physician orders a $PaCO_2$ of 25 torr for the patient. What should the respiratory therapist change on the ventilator to accomplish this?
A. Add 100 mL of mechanical dead space.
B. Increase the tidal volume by 100 mL.
C. Change to the PC mode.
D. Decrease the ventilator rate to 10/min.

31. Expiratory retard is indicated in the ventilator management of a patient with:
A. Pulmonary edema
B. Bronchospasm and air trapping
C. Pleural effusion
D. Pneumothorax

32. An 80-kg (176-lb) man with bilateral pneumonia is being ventilated in the PC mode. The following data are available:

	8 AM	**12 PM**
Set respiratory rate	12/min	12/min
Total respiratory rate	16/min	26/min
Exhaled tidal volume	800 mL	600 mL
Inspiratory pressure	28 cm water	28 cm water

What is the most appropriate thing to do at this time?
A. Sedate the patient.
B. Increase the set respiratory rate.
C. Add 5 cm PEEP.
D. Increase the inspiratory pressure.

33. A 17-year-old girl has been admitted with status asthmaticus and placed on a Drager Evita 4 ventilator. The physician wants to know if she has any auto-PEEP. Which ventilator waveform would be best for determining whether the patient has any auto-PEEP?
A. Maximum voluntary ventilation tracing
B. Flow/volume loop
C. Flow/time
D. Pressure/time

ANSWER KEY

1. **D.** Rationale: ARDS results in stiff lungs that are at risk of volutrauma if too large a tidal volume is forced into them. PCIRV is used with these patients because the peak pressure is limited to a safe level. The long inspiratory time used with PCIRV helps to oxygenate the patient. Asthma and chronic bronchitis are noted for high airway resistance, not stiffness of the lungs. These patients need a long expiratory time for complete exhalation. PCIRV would likely cause more air trapping because of the long inspiratory time and short expiratory time. A pulmonary contusion is a lung bruise from trauma. It is neither helped or hindered by PCIRV.

2. **C.** Rationale: Mean airway pressure is the average pressure throughout the breathing cycle. It is found by

determining a series of inspiratory pressure and expiratory pressure points during short time intervals through a patient's breath cycle. See Fig. 15-28 for an example. P_{peak} minus the plateau pressure gives a general indication of airway resistance. P_{peak} divided by inspiratory time is used as a respiratory care calculation. Tidal volume divided by peak pressure is used to calculate dynamic compliance. See question 12 for an example.

3. **C.** Rationale: Pulmonary edema, pulmonary fibrosis, and ARDS are all conditions in which the lungs become stiff. This results in decreased lung compliance and increased WOB. Emphysema is caused by the loss of connective tissue within the lungs and results in

increased lung compliance. As a result, the lungs are overinflated.

4. **A.** Rationale: MMV ventilation is used to provide a secure minimum minute volume to unstable patients. Often, these patients have an unstable respiratory drive because of a stroke or brain injury. MMV is a variation on SIMV; it does not allow the patient to trigger each breath like the A/C mode does. MMV is not like CPAP because MMV delivers mandatory tidal volume breaths.

5. **B.** Rationale: Near-drowning patients are traditionally ventilated with the A/C or SIMV mode with a constant volume. HFV has been shown effective in ventilating patients with airway procedures such as laryngoscopy and bronchoscopy. HFO has been shown effective in patients with a bronchopleural fistula because the small tidal volumes and low driving pressures do not force gas out through the lung tear. This allows the tissues to heal.

6. **D.** Rationale: Review the indications for ventilatory support in Box 15-1. These indications include a rapid, shallow breathing index of more than 105, Pa_{CO_2} of more than 55 torr, and cardiac dysrhythmias. The patient is not dangerously hypoxic with a PaO_2 of 70 torr.

7. **A.** Rationale: Because the patient's left lung has been removed, he or she should have a delivered tidal volume that is about half of normal for two lungs. Giving a normal or larger than normal tidal volume for two lungs is likely to overdistend the patient's one remaining lung.

8. **A.** Rationale: ARDS is characterized by very stiff lungs. A negative-pressure ventilator is unable to generate enough pressure to adequately ventilate any patient with low lung compliance. Also, an iron lung does not offer any modes other than Control and cannot add PEEP. The other three conditions (neuromuscular defects, kyphoscoliosis, and COPD in acute failure) are not as challenging to ventilate. These patients are not intubated and require only assisted ventilation for a short period. Negative-pressure ventilation has been used with these patients successfully.

9. **B.** Rationale: Review Box 15-4 and Fig. 15-17 for information on the evaluation of an optimal PEEP study. As PEEP establishes the patient's FRC, the pulmonary compliance should improve. Ventilation better matches perfusion, so that shunt will decrease and PaO_2 will increase. In addition, the patient's pulmonary vascular resistance (PVR) decreases as the lungs are properly ventilated and blood flow through them is normalized. If too much PEEP is applied, the lungs will be overstretched. This causes the PVR to increase and cardiac output to decrease as venous return to the lungs and heart is decreased. As a result,

the patient's blood pressure decreases, and heart rate increases.

10. **D.** Rationale:

$$Cst = \frac{Exhaled\ tidal\ volume - Compressed\ volume}{plateau\ pressure - PEEP}$$

In this situation, use the corrected tidal volume because the compressed volume has already been subtracted from the exhaled tidal volume. The following equation results:

$$Cst = \frac{600\ mL}{48 - 12}$$
$$= \frac{600\ mL}{36}$$
$$Cst = 17\ mL/cm\ water$$

11. **D.** Rationale: Static compliance (Cst) is calculated as follows:

$$Cst = \frac{Exhaled\ tidal\ volume - Compressed\ volume}{plateau\ pressure - PEEP}$$

Compressed volume =
Compliance factor × Plateau pressure (4 mL/cm water × 25 cm water) = 100 mL

$$Cst = \frac{700\ mL - 100\ mL}{25 - 6}$$
$$= \frac{600\ mL}{19}$$

$$Cst = 32\ mL/cm\ water$$

12. **B.** Rationale: Dynamic compliance (Cdyn) is calculated as follows:

$$Cdyn = \frac{Exhaled\ tidal\ volume - Compressed\ volume}{peak\ pressure - PEEP}$$

Compressed volume =
Compliance factor × Peak pressure (4 mL/cm water × 35 cm water) = 140 mL

$$Cdyn = \frac{700\ mL - 140\ mL}{35 - 6}$$
$$= \frac{560\ mL}{29}$$
$$Cdyn = 19\ mL/cm\ water$$

13. **A.** Rationale: HFJV involves the delivery of very small tidal volume breaths at a very high rate. It is impractical to try to measure these very small tidal volumes. The other three listed items plus a high pressure air source, suitable patient circuit, and the ventilator itself are needed for HFJV.

14. **C.** Rationale: An increased airway resistance (caused by bronchospasm or airway secretions) causes the peak pressure to increase. A decrease in lung compliance (caused by pulmonary edema, pneumonia, or pleural effusion) causes the plateau pressure to increase. This, in turn, drives up the peak pressure. Without having both the peak and plateau pressures, there is no way to know more specifically what has

caused the peak pressure to increase. If either the lung compliance had increased or the airway resistance had decreased, the peak pressure would have decreased.

15. **D.** Rationale: Therapeutic PEEP increases a patient's FRC. This increased lung volume enables better ventilation and perfusion matching. As a result, intrapulmonary shunting past underventilated alveoli is reduced. Increasing inspiratory time and sigh volume improves alveolar filling and may help to increase oxygenation. However, they do not increase FRC and, therefore, do not reduce shunting.

16. **A.** Rationale: A 200-mL air leak through the pleural chest tube would explain the difference in delivered and returned tidal volumes. If the patient had a deflated endotracheal tube cuff, the delivered tidal volume would be decreased. The selected ventilator is microprocessor driven and has the ability to monitor itself. A warning of a system failure such as a miscalibrated spirometer would have occurred. No indication is noted that the patient has asthma or any condition causing bronchospasm. This ventilator has the ability to monitor auto-PEEP, and none is indicated.

17. **C.** Rationale: Recent research has shown that alveolar overstretching and damage can occur when the plateau pressure is 35 cm water or greater. Therefore the patient should be switched from volume cycled ventilation to pressure cycled ventilation (pressure control) with a peak pressure of no higher than 35 cm water. A high peak pressure may be caused by high airway resistance or lung stiffness. Lung compliance is calculated from tidal volume divided by plateau pressure. There is no direct connection between calculated lung compliance and alveolar overstretching. Both peak pressure and plateau pressure should be monitored. However, the combination has no direct connection to alveolar overstretching.

18. **D.** Rationale: Interpretation of the patient's ABG results indicates hypercarbia and resulting respiratory acidosis. The best solution to the problem is to remove the 150 mL of mechanical dead space. There is no urgent need to decrease the patient's 35% oxygen because this is not a toxic amount. Decreasing the patient's minute volume further raises the carbon dioxide level and lowers the pH. Although increasing the respiratory rate would help to blow off some carbon dioxide, the best solution is to remove the dead space. After another set of ABGs is drawn and analyzed, the rate can be increased if still needed to blow off CO_2.

19. **D.** Rationale: Atelectasis is best treated by giving the patient a larger sigh volume. This should help to open up alveoli that have collapsed or are prone to collapsing. Changing flow rate, expiratory time, and ventilator frequency have no impact on lung volume.

20. **A.** Rationale: Permissive hypercapnia involves the gradual increasing of a patient's carbon dioxide level such that the pH does not become overly acidotic. It may be necessary to give the patient intravenous bicarbonate to keep the pH greater than 7.25. During permissive hypercapnia, the patient's $Paco_2$ can increase well above 50 torr, and the pH will probably decrease below the normal range of 7.35.

21. **C.** Rationale: SIMV allows the patient to breathe spontaneously when she wants to while still receiving support from the ventilator. A low level of pressure support should help to reduce her added WOB from the small endotracheal tube. Therapeutic PEEP is justified because of her PaO_2 measurement of only 63 torr on 55% oxygen. The A/C mode does not allow her to take any totally spontaneous tidal volume breaths. In addition, she would benefit from some therapeutic PEEP. A high level of pressure support (PSV_{max}) does not offer her the "safety net" of support offered by SIMV at this stage of her recovery. Some therapeutic PEEP is needed.

22. **C.** Rationale: Interpretation of the patient's ABG values shows an increased carbon dioxide level with resulting respiratory acidosis. An SIMV rate of 10/min does not increase the patient's baseline minute volume from the PC rate of 10. Because the patient is apneic, she will not be adding to the minute volume total. The patient's minute volume will be increased by both a higher respiratory rate and a larger tidal volume. Removing the mechanical dead space will prevent the patient from rebreathing her own carbon dioxide. All three of these options result in a lower $Paco_2$ and correction of the low pH.

23. **A.** Rationale: Review Box 15-3 for indications of SIMV tolerance/intolerance if needed. An increased respiratory rate (usually accompanied by a decreasing tidal volume) indicates that the patient is fatigued and needs more ventilator support. Review the rapid, shallow breathing index calculation shown in Box 15-1 if needed. Stable vital signs and blood gas values indicate good tolerance of the WOB. Lack of accessory muscle use indicates that the diaphragm is strong enough to ventilate the patient.

24. **B.** Rationale: ABG results show adequate oxygenation; therefore the PEEP level can be safely reduced from 10 to 7 cm water. A decrease in SIMV rate from 10 to 3 is too large. A smaller rate of decrease from 10 to about 6 is more reasonable at this stage in the patient's recovery. ABG results show adequate ventilation. No need is seen to increase the SIMV rate at this time. No indication is present that the patient has an increased airway resistance problem that would justify the addition of pressure support. Her tracheostomy tube is the appropriate size, and her spontaneous rate and tidal volume are adequate.

25. **C.** Rationale: Review Box 15-5 for indications of the ability to wean. Only patients 2 and 3 have all parameters within the normal ranges listed. Patient 1 has a low respiratory rate, tidal volume, and forced expiratory volume in 1 second (FEV_1). Patient 4 has a fast respiratory rate, low tidal volume, and low MIP. Patient 5 has a fast respiratory rate, low FEV_1, and low MIP.

26. **B.** Rationale: The only patient parameter that has changed significantly is the increase in P peak from 30 to 45 cm water. This can be caused only by an increase in airway resistance. Although several things can cause this (bronchospasm, secretions, biting or kinking of the endotracheal tube), the only option that fits is giving a bronchodilating agent. Increasing PEEP has no effect on airway resistance. A diuretic agent (such as furosemide [Lasix]) would help to eliminate pulmonary edema and lower a patient's plateau pressure (P plateau). However, this value is unchanged, so no worsening is indicated. A paralyzing agent will not affect any of the recorded patient values.

27. **C.** Rationale: Even though the patient is paralyzed and cannot request a medication for pain relief, the patient can feel the surgical pain. Paralyzing medications do not block touch (pain) or the other senses. A narcotic medication (morphine) is justified for pain relief. Caffeine does not have a role in the care of a patient who has been pharmacologically paralyzed. A sedative medication may be given to relieve any anxiety the patient may have, but it would not affect the patient's pain. Unfortunately, there is no easy way to tell when the paralyzed patient is awake or sleeping. Regardless, it is important to talk normally to the patient so that he or she knows what medical care is being given.

28. **A.** Rationale: An AARC Clinical Practice Guideline recommends the use of a cascade-type humidifier warmed to body temperature to help liquify thick secretions. An HME should be used only if the patient has few secretions. The secretions should not be allowed to dry out. If they did, it would be very difficult to remove them by suctioning.

29. **A.** Rationale: A spirometer is not needed because the patient's tidal volumes cannot be accurately measured while on the CPAP system. If a spirometer were incorporated into the CPAP system, it would register continuous flow rather than patient volumes. An alarm system is needed for patient safety, and water traps are used to keep the tubing clear. A pressure-generating device must be added to set and maintain the CPAP level.

30. **B.** Rationale: Increasing the tidal volume from 700 to 800 mL will decrease the patient's $Paco_2$ toward the goal. Another ABG sample should be taken in 15 minutes to see if the ordered $Paco_2$ of 25 torr has been achieved. Adding 100 mL of mechanical dead space will increase, rather than decrease, the patient's carbon dioxide level. Changing to the PC mode with the same settings will maintain the same minute volume and same $Paco_2$ as at present. Decreasing the ventilator rate from 12 to 10/min results in a higher, rather than lower, carbon dioxide level.

31. **B.** Rationale: Expiratory retard acts like pursed lips breathing in a patient with bronchospasm to put backpressure on the small airways. This results in a more complete exhalation. None of the other conditions is helped by expiratory retard. It is possible that the pneumothorax would be worsened by the added pressure, causing more air to leak through the torn lung tissue.

32. **D.** Rationale: The decrease in patient tidal volume is significant. Probably the patient's lung compliance has worsened. The patient has increased his respiratory rate to make up for the lost minute volume. The best solution is to increase the pressure control inspiratory pressure to produce the previous tidal volume of 800 mL. Sedating the patient will result in a dramatic decrease in minute volume with resulting hypercarbia and hypoxia. Increasing the set respiratory rate will deliver a higher minute volume and relieve the patient of some of the burden of triggering the ventilator. However, it will not correct the main problem—a decreased tidal volume. Without blood gas results to document hypoxia, no indication is found to add PEEP.

33. **C.** Rationale: The flow/time tracing enables any auto-PEEP to be detected. See Fig. 15-2 for the graphic. The maximum voluntary ventilation tracing is done in the pulmonary function laboratory to evaluate a patient's overall breathing ability. It is not useful for detecting auto-PEEP. A flow/volume loop can be done on many microprocessor ventilators and is helpful in evaluating flow at the end of exhalation. However, the flow/time tracing is the best detector of auto-PEEP. A pressure/time tracing (see Fig. 15-1, *top graphic*) is not helpful in detecting auto-PEEP.

16 Mechanical Ventilation of the Neonate

Note 1: The National Board for Respiratory Care (NBRC) has released the *RRT Examination Matrix* (covering the testable items on the Written Registry Exam) and the *CSE Examination Matrix* (covering the testable items on the Clinical Simulation Exam). Turn to the appendices at the back of this book for both publications in their original formats. This book is intended to cover all of the testable items in these two publications. This chapter (and all others) uses the abbreviation "WRE" for the coded items testable on the Written Registry Exam *and* Clinical Simulation Exam. The listed difficulty (R, Recall; Ap, Application; An, Analysis) relates to the question difficulty on the Written Registry Exam. The abbreviation "CSE" is used for the coded items testable on *only* the Clinical Simulation Exam. Because no question difficulty level is given for this exam, be prepared for anything.

Note 2: A review of the most recent Written Registry Examinations has shown an average of two questions (2% of the exam) that cover the application of continuous positive airway pressure (CPAP) or mechanical ventilation of the neonate. The Clinical Simulation Exam is comprehensive and may include everything that should be known or performed by an advanced level respiratory therapist. Of the 10 scenarios presented in the Clinical Simulation Examination, expect one neonatal and one pediatric patient. CPAP or mechanical ventilation or both may be involved in both situations. Be sure to review neonatal assessment in Chapter 1.

MODULE A

Perform continuous positive airway pressure and continuous mechanical ventilation to achieved adequate artificial ventilation and/or recommend modifications in ventilatory support based on the patient's response

1. Initiate and adjust continuous positive airway pressure breathing (WRE code: IIID2b) [Difficulty: An]

a. Physiologic effects

Continuous positive airway pressure (CPAP) and positive end-expiratory pressure (PEEP) increase the patient's functional residual capacity (FRC). In neonates, the most common cause of a decreased FRC is infant respiratory distress syndrome (RDS). This condition is caused by the lack of surfactant in the lungs of the premature neonate. The neonate with RDS has relatively airless lungs that are prone to atelectasis. This results in hypoxemia. In addition, each tidal volume breath requires a greater-than-normal inspiratory effort (Fig. 16-1). The restoration of FRC in the neonate increases PaO_2, decreases the percentage of shunt, narrows the alveolar to arterial difference in oxygen, and reduces work of tidal volume breathing. CPAP must be used with caution in neonates with persistent pulmonary hypertension of the newborn (PPHN). An excessive amount of pressure in the alveoli compresses the capillary bed. This decreases pulmonary blood flow, which in turn increases blood flow through the patent ductus arteriosus and worsens the problem.

b. Indications, contraindications, and hazards

CPAP is indicated for any condition that results in an unacceptably low PaO_2 secondary to a decreased FRC. Some neonates respond so well to CPAP that mechanical ventilation is not needed. In addition, CPAP has been used to keep open the airways of infants with tracheal malacia or other conditions in which the airways collapse abnormally. In general, contraindications include any CPAP-related condition that results in a worsening of the patient's original status. Some neonates cannot tolerate CPAP and progressively hypoventilate as the pressure level is increased. Clinical judgment is needed to decide how high the $PaCO_2$ should be allowed to increase before discontinuing the CPAP and beginning mechanical ventilation. In general, the $PaCO_2$ should not be greater than 50 torr as long as the pH is at least 7.25. An absolute contraindication is apnea resulting in hypoxemia and hypotension. These infants should be mechanically ventilated. Box 16-1 gives a complete listing of indications, contraindications, and hazards.

c. Initiation

Before starting CPAP, a set of baseline arterial blood gas values should be taken. Transcutaneous oxygen

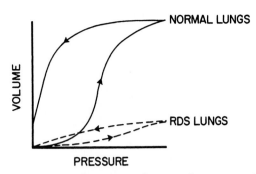

Fig. 16-1 Pressure/volume curves for normal neonate and for one with infant respiratory distress syndrome (RDS). Normal neonate's lungs inhale a relatively large tidal volume at low pressure. Note that when the same pressure is placed against the lungs of an infant with RDS, the tidal volume is much smaller. To get a normal tidal volume, the RDS infant must generate a much greater negative pressure. *(From Carlo WA, Martin RJ: Principles of neonatal assisted ventilation,* Pediatr Clin North Am *33:221, 1986.)*

BOX 16-1   Indications, Contraindications, and Hazards of CPAP Therapy

INDICATIONS

Infant respiratory distress syndrome (RDS)

Atelectasis

Pulmonary edema

Apnea of prematurity

Tracheal malacia

Recent extubation

Transient tachypnea of the newborn

Physical examination shows some, if not all, of the following:

Respiratory rate 30%–40% greater than normal

Substernal and suprasternal retractions

Nasal flaring

Expiratory grunting

Cyanosis

Chest radiograph shows atelectasis or pulmonary edema

Arterial blood gases showing:

PaO_2 < 50 torr on 60% or more oxygen

Adequate ventilation with a $PaCO_2$ < 50 torr and pH > 7.25

Weaning from mechanical ventilation when the intermittent mandatory ventilation (IMV) rate is about 4–12/min, the pulmonary condition is improved, blood gases show acceptable $PaCO_2$, and there is acceptable PaO_2 on PEEP. The CPAP level is set to match the level of PEEP used on the ventilator.

CONTRAINDICATIONS

Prolonged apnea leading to hypoxemia and hypotension (begin mechanical ventilation)

Untreated pneumothorax or other evidence of a pulmonary gas leak

Unstable cardiovascular status such as bradycardia and hypotension

Inadequate ventilation with a $PaCO_2$ > 50 torr and pH < 7.25

Unilateral pulmonary problem: untreated congenital diaphragmatic hernia

Nasal CPAP should not be used on a patient with cleft palate, choanal atresia, or tracheoesophageal fistula

HAZARDS

Persistent pulmonary hypertension of the newborn (PPHN)

Increased intracranial pressure that can cause intraventricular hemorrhage

Decreased cardiac output

CPAP may be ineffective if the neonate weighs < 1000–1200 g

---

monitoring or pulse oximetry may be substituted in some clinical situations if oxygenation is the only parameter that must be measured. The neonate's vital signs should also be recorded. Assemble the CPAP circuit and pressure device. The decision must be made whether to apply the CPAP above the epiglottis (Figs. 16-2 and 16-3) or to intubate the infant and apply the CPAP within the trachea. Nasal CPAP (NCPAP) and nasopharyngeal tube CPAP (NP-CPAP) are both widely used to apply pressure from above the epiglottis. The neonate or infant must have an endotracheal tube placed to apply CPAP within the trachea. Among the factors to be considered are the neonate's gestational age and weight, the amount of secretions that need to be suctioned, the pulmonary problem, and the

Fig. 16-2 Nasal continuous positive airway pressure devices for infants. **A**, Jackson-Reese tubes. **B**, Argyle nasal cannula (prongs). **C**, Endotracheal tube cut shorter for nasopharyngeal insertion (NP tube). *(From Blodgett D: Manual of pediatric respiratory care procedures, Philadelphia, 1982, JB Lippincott.)*

Exam Hint

Questions on the Written Registry Examination typically ask about the indications to start CPAP, the initial CPAP setting, CPAP adjustment, and when to switch from CPAP to mechanical ventilation.

Fig. 16-3 An assembly for supporting nasal continuous positive airway pressure prongs in an infant. *(Modified from advertisement of Stayflex tubing system from Ackrad; from Sills JR: Respiratory care registry guide, ed 1, St Louis, 1994, Mosby.)*

TABLE 16-1	Commonly Recommended Blood Gas Goals for CPAP and Mechanical Ventilator Therapy	
	Age of Neonate	
	Less than 72 hours	More than 72 hours
PaO_2 (torr)	60–70	50–70
$PtcO_2$ (torr)	>50,* <90*	>40,* <90*
SpO_2	92%–96%	92%–96%
$PaCO_2$ (torr)	35–45†	45–55
$PtcCO_2$ (torr)	May be used after correlation with $PaCO_2$ as discussed in Chapter 3	
pH	7.25–7.45	7.25–7.45

*$PtcO_2$ values may be used after they have been shown to correlate within 15% of the PaO_2 from an arterial blood gas.
†With CPAP, this value may be increased to 50–55 torr as long as the pH is ≥ 7.25.
NOTE: Keep the PaO_2 ≤ 80 torr in the premature neonate to reduce the risk of retinopathy of prematurity.

likelihood of mechanical ventilation eventually becoming necessary. More mature and larger infants with few secretions and relatively stable pulmonary conditions will most likely have CPAP applied above the epiglottis by nasal prongs or nasopharyngeal tube. In contrast, less mature and smaller infants (less than 1000 to 1200 g) who need suctioning and have relatively unstable pulmonary conditions will probably be intubated. Mechanical ventilation can then be easily started if needed.

CPAP is usually started at about 4 to 5 cm water pressure, whether the pressure is applied above or below the epiglottis. The inspired oxygen percentage is usually kept at the previously set level. It is important to make only one change at a time so that each adjustment in care can be evaluated for its own effect. For example, if you simultaneously increased the oxygen percentage by 10% and started 5 cm water of CPAP, it would not be known whether the increase in PaO_2 was from the additional oxygen, the CPAP, or both. Usually the long-term inspired oxygen is limited to 40% to 50% because of concern of the possibility of pulmonary oxygen toxicity.

d. Adjustment and weaning

Blood gases and vital signs must be evaluated at the starting CPAP level. The heart rate, blood pressure, and respiratory rate should be stable or improved. Blood gases should be measured in about 10 minutes. See Table 16-1 for the recommended blood gas limits. In general, the PaO_2 should be kept between 60 and 70 torr, $PaCO_2$ less than 50 to 55 torr, and pH at least 7.25. If the PaO_2 is too

low and the patient's vital signs are acceptable, the CPAP may be increased in a step of 2 cm water. The vital signs and blood gases should then be reevaluated. If necessary, the process of adding CPAP and reassessing the patient can be continued. It is rare to find that more than 10 cm water CPAP is necessary. The maximum CPAP level in a neonate is generally held to be 12 cm water; the maximum CPAP level in an infant is generally held to be 15 cm water.

Mechanical ventilation is usually indicated if more than these maximum CPAP pressures are needed to correct hypoxemia. Depending on the patient, even levels less than these maximum CPAP pressures may not be well tolerated. The infant may become exhausted from exhaling against the backpressure of the CPAP system. That is seen clinically as decreased chest movement from the smaller tidal volume. The $PaCO_2$ will probably increase. It may be necessary to place the infant on mechanical ventilation to decrease the work of breathing and then add PEEP to maintain the FRC. When nasal prongs or a nasopharyngeal tube is used, CPAP pressures of greater than 8 cm water may cause the infant's mouth to open. This results in the loss of CPAP. A crying infant also opens its mouth and loses the CPAP. In either case, the CPAP pressure gauge decreases to zero or fluctuates below the set pressure.

As the patient improves, it is necessary to reduce the CPAP level so as not to cause pulmonary barotrauma. The pressure level can be reduced in steps of about 2 cm water. The vital signs and blood gases should be reassessed after each step. The apparatus is usually removed when the CPAP level is down to 2 to 4 cm water.

The infant is then placed into an oxyhood at the same oxygen percentage as before or 5% to 15% higher. If the infant has an endotracheal tube that is needed for suctioning or a secure airway, the pressure is usually left at 2 to 4 cm water. After extubation, the infant is placed into an oxyhood as before.

If the infant was breathing more than 50% oxygen while on the CPAP, it may be more important to reduce the oxygen before decreasing the CPAP level. The following guidelines may prove helpful when deciding whether to lower the oxygen percentage or the CPAP level first:

a. If the patient has been breathing more than 50% oxygen for more than 48 hours and has stable vital signs without any pulmonary barotrauma, decrease the oxygen first. Lower the inspired oxygen in 5% to 15% steps, and check the oxygenation level after each reduction. Attempt to get the oxygen down to 40%, if possible. Then decrease the CPAP level.

b. If the patient is breathing 50% oxygen or less and has unstable vital signs or pulmonary barotrauma, decrease the CPAP first. After the CPAP is reduced (or removed entirely) and the patient is stable, reduce the inspired oxygen percentage.

2. Mechanical ventilation

a. Change the type of ventilator to be used on the patient (WRE code: IIIG3i) [Difficulty: An]

Most neonatal patients requiring life support receive time-triggered, pressure-limited, time cycled mechanical ventilation (TPTV). These ventilators are pneumatically powered with electrical controls and alarm systems. They are used in the intermittent mandatory ventilation (IMV) mode and feature a continuous flow of gas. They are pressure limited to prevent an excessive peak airway pressure and can have therapeutic PEEP added. Furthermore, they are capable of reaching the Food and Drug Administration (FDA) limited rate of 150 breaths/min. The majority of neonatal and small pediatric patients can be effectively ventilated on these types of units.

High frequency ventilation (HFV) with a small tidal volume has been approved by the FDA for use in the rescue of neonates with RDS and a bronchopulmonary fistula or pulmonary interstitial emphysema (PIE) for whom conventional TPTV ventilation fails. HFV also has been used in the short-term support of neonates with a congenital diaphragmatic hernia until corrective surgery can be performed.

A volume cycled ventilator can be used on an infant who weighs more than 10 kg (22 lb). Any conventional volume cycled ventilator can be used if it can be set to deliver a tidal volume as small as 50 mL. Volume-oriented ventilation can also be performed with a neonatal TPTV-type ventilator if the patient is apneic. This technique is discussed later.

When selecting a ventilator, it is important to choose one that offers the features needed to ventilate the patient. For example, if real-time graphics are needed to evaluate the patient's response to a ventilator adjustment, the proper unit will be needed. Any selected ventilator must be able to meet the typical tidal volume goal for a neonatal or small pediatric patient of 6 to 8 mL/kg. A patient receiving HFV for an FDA-approved pulmonary problem has a smaller tidal volume goal.

b. Initiate and adjust different combinations of ventilatory techniques (e.g., assist/control, intermittent mandatory ventilation, synchronous intermittent mandatory ventilation, therapeutic positive end-expiratory pressure, pressure support, pressure control ventilation, inverse ratio ventilation, inspiratory hold) (WRE code: IIID2e) [Difficulty: An]

With traditional neonatal TPTV, a set tidal volume is not ordered and cannot be measured. With volume cycled ventilation of a pediatric patient, the tidal volume is ordered just as it is with an adult patient. Typically the therapist is expected to set the following ventilator controls based on a protocol or the patient's condition and response to the ventilator: sensitivity, flow, inspiratory/expiratory (I:E) ratio, alarms, and humidified gas temperature.

1. Sensitivity

No sensitivity control is found on traditional continuous flow TPTV-type neonatal ventilators. The IMV mode is used with these units. Newer ventilators have the ability to sense a neonate's respiratory effort and trigger a machine delivered breath. Some units sense a change in flow through the ventilator circuit when the neonate inspires. Other ventilators make use of electrocardiogram-type leads on the neonate's chest to sense a change in electrical impedance (skin resistance) when the neonate makes an inspiratory effort. A child on a volume cycled ventilator should have the sensitivity set at about −1 to −2 cm water pressure. No matter which method the ventilator uses to sense the patient's respiratory effort, the neonate or child should not have to work very hard to trigger a machine tidal volume.

2. Flow

Flow is adjusted to set the inspiratory time and I:E ratio or to meet the patient's needs or both. The flow should be increased if the patient appears to be attempting to inhale faster than the ventilator is delivering the tidal volume.

3. I:E ratio

The I:E ratio is adjusted to ensure that the patient can inhale in as physiologically appropriate a manner as possible and can completely exhale the inspired tidal volume.

A ventilator with real-time graphics can reveal the presence of auto-PEEP (incomplete exhalation).

4. Alarms

Alarm systems are different for each type of ventilator. Generally speaking, they are set with a safety margin of ±10% from the patient's normal ventilator settings. A variation of greater than 10% results in an audible or visual alarm condition.

5. Humidified gas temperature

The goal for most patients is to minimize their humidity deficit by giving gas that is humidified and warmed to near body temperature. It is common to have the gas warmed to 90°F to 95°F/35°C. It should be measured in the inspiratory limb of the circuit as close to the patient as possible.

A review of the literature dealing with neonatal critical care shows that few universally accepted strategies exist for the use and modification of CPAP/PEEP and mechanical ventilation. What is presented here is an attempt to describe widely accepted approaches to neonatal TPTV and related therapy. The approach used in this discussion focuses on adjusting the ventilator and treating a neonate based on its pathologic problem.

3. Indications for mechanical ventilation

All authors agree that apnea is an absolute indication for mechanical ventilation. A general indication is any condition that causes respiratory failure. This is usually documented by unacceptable arterial blood gases. Box 16-2 lists indications for mechanical ventilation.

BOX 16-2   Common Indications for the Initiation of Mechanical Ventilation

RESPIRATORY FAILURE
Pao_2 < 50 torr despite maximal CPAP therapy (10–12 cm water) and 60% or more inspired oxygen
$Paco_2$ > 60 torr and pH < 7.25

NEUROLOGIC
Complete apnea
Apneic periods leading to hypoxemia and bradycardia
Intracranial hemorrhage
Drug depression

PULMONARY CONDITIONS
Infant respiratory distress syndrome (RDS)
Diffuse pneumonia
Pulmonary edema
Meconium aspiration
Diaphragmatic hernia
Prophylactic use
Cyanotic congenital cardiac defect
Persistent pulmonary hypertension of the newborn (PPHN)
Postoperatively after major thoracic or abdominal surgery

MATH REVIEW

Time constants of ventilation. NOTE: This concept has not been directly tested by the NBRC. It is hoped that understanding the concept of time constants as used here and in the earlier text will help the reader understand lung pathology and why certain ventilator adjustments are made.

It is important in any patient requiring mechanical ventilation to consider both the patient's lung/thoracic compliance and airway resistance when setting inspiratory and expiratory times. This is especially important in neonates because, in comparison with adults, they are less compliant and have greater resistance. In addition, neonates are usually ventilated at faster rates. As a review, the respective lung/thoracic compliances (C_{LT}) and airway resistances (Raw) of normal adults and infants are shown here:

Adult lung/thoracic compliance: 100 mL/cm water pressure (0.1 L/cm water pressure)
Neonatal lung/thoracic compliance: 5 mL/cm water pressure (.005 L/cm water pressure; about 20 times stiffer than in an adult)
Adult airway resistance: 2 cm water/L/sec
Neonatal airway resistance: 20 to 40 cm water/L/sec (about 10 to 20 times more resistance to airflow than in an adult)

The placement of an endotracheal tube to facilitate mechanical ventilation will result in a total pulmonary resistance ranging from 50 to 150 cm water/L/sec. The time constant of ventilation (Tc or time constant of the respiratory system, T_{RS}) is calculated as the product of compliance and resistance:

Time constant in seconds = compliance (L/cm water) × resistance (cm water/L/sec)

For example, using these values for a spontaneously breathing normal neonate, its time constant is calculated as:

Tc = compliance (0.005 L/cm water) × resistance (30 cm water/L/sec)
= 0.005 × 30 seconds
= 0.15 seconds

Although it is technically impractical to measure the time constant of ventilation at the bedside, the concept is important because it relates to two important clinical considerations during mechanical ventilation. First, it relates to the pressure that develops at the alveolar level as the tidal volume is delivered. For each time constant, progressively more of the peak inspiratory pressure (PIP) is applied within the alveoli (Fig. 16-4). As can be seen, at three time constants, 95% of the PIP is applied to the alveoli. At five time constants, virtually the entire PIP is applied at the alveolar level. Second, the time constant relates to how rapidly the lung recoils to baseline (FRC) during an exhalation. As shown in Fig. 16-4, it will takes

Fig. 16-4 Graphic presentation of the percentage of inspiratory and expiratory volume and pressure in comparison with time constants of ventilation. *(From Chatburn RL: Principles and practice of neonatal and pediatric mechanical ventilation,* Respir Care 36:569, 1991.)

BOX 16-3   Common Mechanical Ventilator Parameters for Neonates with Normal Lungs

Delivered tidal volume: 6–8 mL/kg (This may be estimated by calculation if the neonate is apneic and the pressure limit is not reached until the end of the inspiratory time.)

Pressure limit (peak inspiratory pressure or PIP): 10–20 cm water

Frequency: 10–20/min

I:E ratio: 1:2 to 1:10

Inspiratory time (T_I): ≥0.4 sec

Expiratory time (T_E): ≥0.5 sec

PEEP: none unless 2–4 cm water is added to replace "epiglottal PEEP"

Inspiratory flow: sufficient to see the chest move and hear bilateral breath sounds during the inspiration; 5–8 L/min commonly used; or start with at least twice the infant's estimated minute volume (respiratory rate × estimated tidal volume of 7 mL/kg). Check the blood gases for the $PaCO_2$.

Oxygen percentage: 40%

---

three time constants to exhale 95% and five time constants to exhale completely.

The clinical significance of this relates directly to the pulmonary condition of the patient. Infants with stiff lungs and normal resistance, as found in RDS, have a short time constant. Alveolar pressure quickly increases to match the PIP. The lungs then rapidly recoil during exhalation so that there is little chance of air trapping. Infants with normal compliance and increased resistance, as found in meconium aspiration, have a long time constant. It takes a relatively long time for the alveolar pressure to reach the PIP. A relatively long time is needed for the exhalation to be complete. Because of this, these infants are at risk for air trapping and auto-PEEP.

4. Initiation and adjustments based on the patient's condition
a. Patients with normal cardiopulmonary function

Patients with normal cardiopulmonary function may need mechanical ventilation because of apnea from anesthesia, paralysis, or a neurologic condition. The initial TPTV ventilator parameters for this type of patient are listed in Box 16-3. Once mechanical ventilation is established, it is important to evaluate the patient's blood gases, vital signs, breath sounds, and any other pertinent clinical information before changing any ventilator parameters.

As the patient recovers and begins to breathe spontaneously, it will probably be necessary to reduce the ventilator delivered minute volume. This encourages the child to breathe more because the final goal is to wean and extubate the patient completely. The most accepted way to reduce the ventilator delivered minute volume is to

reduce the ventilator rate. A reduction of about 10% is a good starting place but must be tailored to meet the patient's needs. The tidal volume is maintained as originally set. Obtain a set of blood gases in 10 to 20 minutes (or monitor the transcutaneous or pulse oximetry values) and check the patient's vital signs to see how well the adjustment is tolerated.

If the blood gases show an elevated $PaCO_2$, the ventilator delivered minute volume must be increased. This can be done by increasing either the alveolar ventilation or respiratory rate. Alveolar ventilation can be increased by increasing either the inspiratory flow or pressure limit (if it has been reached) to increase the tidal volume. The ventilator rate may be increased if the flow and pressure limit cannot be increased. An increase of about 10% is a good starting place but must be tailored to meet the patient's needs. As before, blood gases and vital signs should be monitored after every change to see if the increase is well tolerated and accomplishing what was intended.

If the blood gases show that the $PaCO_2$ is lower than desired, the ventilator delivered minute volume must be decreased. The first parameter to adjust is usually the rate. Try decreasing the rate by about 10%, and check another set of blood gas values. If other parameters must be reduced, try decreasing the inspiratory flow or inspiratory time about 10% to decrease the tidal volume. Again, check the blood gas values after every adjustment.

If the blood gases show that the PaO_2 is higher or lower than necessary, the oxygen percentage must be adjusted. An increase or decrease of about 5% is a good starting place but must be adjusted as needed. If the patient does not respond to the increased oxygen as expected, the patient should be reevaluated. It may be necessary to reclassify him or her into one of the following categories.

MATH REVIEW

Calculation of estimated tidal volume during TPTV mechanical ventilation. The NBRC examination content outline does not specifically list estimated tidal volume calculations. However, the information may be useful in understanding concepts presented later in the text.

If the neonatal patient receiving TPTV is apneic and neither assisting nor fighting against the ventilator delivered breath, it is possible to calculate an approximate tidal volume. This is referred to as volume-oriented ventilation by some authors. The following formula is used:

$$\text{Calculated tidal volume} = (T_I \times \dot{V}) - Vc$$

In which:

T_I = inspiratory time (It is important that either the pressure limit is not reached or the pressure limit is reached at the same time inspiratory time is completed. If the pressure limit is reached before the inspiratory time limit is reached, part of the inspiratory time is spent as an inflation hold, and no additional tidal volume is delivered.)

$\dot{V}$ = inspiratory flow rate on the ventilator in mL/sec

Vc = volume compressed in the circuit and ventilator (This is found by multiplying the peak inspiratory pressure by the manufacturer's stated compliance factors for the circuit and ventilator.)

For example, estimate the delivered tidal volume for an apneic 5-kg infant. The ventilator parameters are: inspiratory flow of 5.5 L/min, frequency of 20/min, I:E ratio of 1:3, inspiratory time of 0.75 seconds, and expiratory time of 2.25 seconds. PIP is 15 cm water. The internal compliance of the ventilator is 0.4 mL/cm water, and the circuit compliance factor is 1.6 mL/cm water.

$$\text{Calculated tidal volume} = (T_I \times \dot{V}) - Vc$$

In which:

T_I = 0.75 seconds

$\dot{V}$ = 5.5 L/min (This is converted to mL/sec by dividing the flow in L/min by 60 seconds. So 5.5 L/min = 0.092 L/sec or 92 mL/sec.)

V_c = 0.4 + 1.6 mL/cm water = 2 mL/cm water = 2 mL/cm water × 15 cm water PIP = 30 mL

Therefore

Calculated tidal volume = (0.75 sec × 92 mL/sec) − 30 mL
= (69 mL) − 30 mL
= 39 mL (This is within the ideal tidal volume range of 30 to 40 mL [based on 5-kg weight × 6 to 8 mL/kg].)

It must be emphasized that this is only a calculated tidal volume. Leaks in the system, a decrease in the patient's compliance, or an increase in the patient's resistance decreases the true tidal volume. Conversely, an increase in

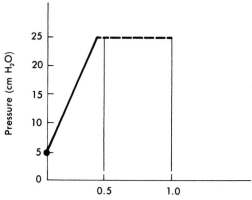

Fig. 16-5 Pressure/time curve seen with pressure limit set at 25 cm water and inspiratory time being increased from 0.5 to 1 second. Pressure limit is reached when inspiratory time is about 0.5 second. As inspiratory time is increased to 1 second (or greater), the pressure limit is held at 25 cm water, resulting in a "square wave" pressure curve. *(From Betis P, Thompson JE, Benjamin PK:* Mechanical ventilation. *In Koff PB, Eitzman DV, Neu J, editors:* Neonatal and pediatric respiratory care, *ed 2, St Louis, 1993, Mosby.)*

the patient's compliance or a decrease in the patient's resistance increases the true tidal volume. If the pressure limit is reached before the inspiratory time is completed, less volume than expected will be delivered. This is because part of the inspiratory time is spent as an inflation hold, and no additional tidal volume is delivered (Fig. 16-5). Finally, the infant must be completely passive during the delivery of the breath.

b. Patients with decreased lung compliance and normal airway resistance such as those with infant respiratory distress syndrome

Although RDS is the most common cause of decreased lung compliance and normal airway resistance, it is seen in other lung conditions including pneumonia and pulmonary edema (Fig. 16-6). The greatest challenge presented in the care of these infants is to oxygenate them without causing oxygen toxicity or pulmonary barotrauma. Common recommendations for the initial ventilator settings are listed in Box 16-4. As discussed earlier, blood gases, vital signs, and so forth must be monitored after the infant is placed on the ventilator. Any further adjustments can then be determined and evaluated by another set of blood gases and vital signs.

The issue of time constants of ventilation helps to clarify the various options available for adjusting the ventilator. As presented earlier, the time constant of ventilation (Tc or time constant of the respiratory system, T_{RS}) is calculated as the product of compliance and resistance. For example, using the following values for a

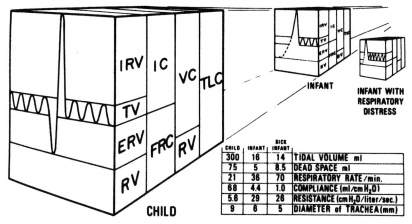

Fig. 16-6 Comparison of the lung volumes and capacities of a 6-year-old child, normal infant, and an infant with infant respiratory distress syndrome (RDS). Note relatively high compliance and low resistance of a normal child compared with an infant, and an infant with RDS compared with normal infant. *(From Chatburn RL, Lough MD: Mechanical ventilation. In Lough MD, Doershuk CF, Stern RC, editors:* Pediatric respiratory therapy, *ed 3, St Louis, 1985, Mosby.)*

mechanically ventilated neonate with RDS, time constant is calculated as

Tc = compliance (0.001 L/cm water because the lungs are less compliant) × Resistance (100 cm water/L/sec because the infant is intubated) Simplify as follows:
= 0.001 × 100 seconds
= 0.1 seconds (Compare this with a Tc of .15 for a normal, spontaneously breathing neonate.)

Neonates with RDS have a relatively short time constant; therefore the tidal volume and ventilating pressure

---

BOX 16-4   Common Mechanical Ventilator Parameters for Neonates with Low Compliance and Normal Resistance

Delivered tidal volume: 6-8 mL/kg
Pressure limit: 20-25 cm water (This may need to be increased up to 35-40 cm water.)
Frequency: 30-60/min (This may need to be increased to 150/min.)
I:E ratio: 1:2 (This may eventually need to be altered to an inverse I:E ratio.)
Inspiratory time (T_I): between 0.4 and 0.7 sec (This may need to be increased.)
Expiratory time (T_E): ≥0.5 sec (This may need to be decreased.)
PEEP: 2-4 cm water initially (This may need to be increased up to 8-10 cm water.)
Inspiratory flow: sufficient to see the chest move and hear bilateral breath sounds during the inspiration; 5-8 L/min commonly used. As a general rule, the faster the rate, the higher the flow must be to deliver an adequate tidal volume. Check the blood gases for the Pa_{CO_2}.
Oxygen percentage: 40% (This may need to be increased to keep the Sp_{O_2} >92%.)

---

are delivered rather quickly to the lungs. However, because the lungs are so stiff, there is usually no problem with the tidal volume being fully exhaled as long as five time constants are allowed. An expiratory time of at least 0.5 seconds is usually set initially. The various options available for increasing oxygenation are discussed on the following pages.

1. Administer oxygen, as needed, on the ventilator to prevent hypoxemia (WRE code: IIID4b) [Difficulty: An]

Up to 100% oxygen can be given to the neonate in the short term. Hypoxemia cannot be tolerated, and supplemental oxygen is usually the best way to correct it. See Chapter 15 for equations that can be used to predict the oxygen percentage change needed to correct the patient's hypoxemia. Although hypoxemia cannot be tolerated, several limiting factors exist. First, it is commonly held that giving more than 50% oxygen for more than 48 to 72 hours increases the risk of pulmonary oxygen toxicity. Second, if more than 80% oxygen is given, some poorly ventilated alveoli will have all of the oxygen absorbed from them, leading to denitrogenation absorption atelectasis. Third, keep the neonate's Pa_{O_2} below 80 torr to minimize the risk of retinopathy of prematurity (ROP). Fourth, if the hypoxemia is caused by a decreased FRC because of the lack of surfactant and small lung volumes, increasing the oxygen will not markedly increase the Pa_{O_2}. Other solutions, such as those discussed later, must be used.

2. Increased inspiratory flow

Increasing the flow increases the tidal volume until the pressure limit is reached. Increasing the tidal volume should result in an increased Pa_{O_2} and is likely to reduce the Paco$_2$. If the pressure limit is reached, the delivered tidal volume is held in the lungs for the duration of the inspiratory time. This acts as an inflation hold and should also increase the Pao$_2$. The mean airway pressure is increased by increasing the flow. (See Fig. 16-7 for the pressure waveforms seen during low flow and high flow conditions.) Under high flow conditions, the pressure waveform takes on a characteristic square shape (square wave) because the pressure limit is reached. This pattern of ventilation is currently widely used with these types of patients.

3. Increased inspiratory time, leading to inverse ratio ventilation

As with increasing the flow, increasing the inspiratory time increases the tidal volume until the pressure limit is reached. If the pressure limit is reached, any increased inspiratory time acts as inflation hold. This also increases the mean airway pressure and should result in an increased Pao$_2$. (See Fig. 16-5 for the pressure waveform change as the inspiratory time is increased.)

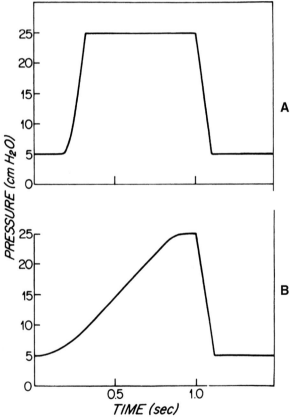

Fig. 16-7 Comparison of pressure/time curves showing influence of inspiratory flow when the pressure limit is set at 25 cm water pressure. **A**, Curve at high flow rate. Pressure limit is reached very early in the inspiratory time with resulting "square wave" flow pattern. **B**, Curve at low flow rate. Pressure limit is not reached until inspiratory time is almost 1 second. *(From Chatburn RL, Lough MD: In Lough MD, Doershuk CF, Stern RC, editors:* Pediatric respiratory therapy, *ed 3, St Louis, 1985, Mosby.)*

Some authors have advocated an increased inspiratory time as an important way to improve oxygenation. This has led to the use of inverse I:E ratios of up to 3:1 (0.33) or 4:1 (0.25) to produce an adequate Pao$_2$. The inspiratory time should be increased in small time increments and followed in 10 to 20 minutes with a blood gas to determine whether the desired improvement in oxygenation was achieved. Inspiratory time is increased only as long as necessary to result in a satisfactory Pao$_2$. Great care must be taken to adjust expiratory time, respiratory rate, or both when a prolonged inspiratory time is used. Obviously, expiratory time must be reduced to keep the same rate as the inspiratory time is increased, or the rate must be reduced as the inspiratory time is increased if the expiratory time cannot be reduced. Care must be taken to ensure that the tidal volume is fully exhaled to avoid auto-PEEP.

As the neonate's lung compliance improves, the inspiratory time must be decreased for two reasons. First, the alveolar pressure is more readily transmitted throughout the lungs and may decrease venous return to the heart. That results in a decreased cardiac output. Second, the more normal lungs are more prone to barotrauma or volutrauma. The inspiratory time should be decreased in small time increments and followed with a set of blood gases to be sure that the neonate is not hypoxemic.

4. Increased positive end-expiratory pressure

Increased PEEP has the greatest effect on improving the patient's FRC and is probably the most effective at increasing the Pao$_2$. As discussed in regard to CPAP therapy, the pressure is usually started out at 4 to 5 cm water. A blood gas is then checked and, if necessary, PEEP is added in 2- to 3-cm water increments. Commonly, between 4 and 7 cm is needed; it is rare for more than 10 cm of PEEP to be needed. Another blood gas should be checked for Pao$_2$ after every addition of pressure. PEEP has the greatest impact on increasing the mean airway pressure of all the options presented here. Excessive PEEP may cause a decreased venous return to the heart and decreased cardiac output. It also may cause barotrauma, resulting in PIE, pneumothorax, or pneumomediastinum. Care must be taken to evaluate the patient carefully after each increase in PEEP. Watch for a sudden deterioration in the patient's condition as a sign of a pulmonary air leak. As the patient's Pao$_2$ improves, the PEEP level should be reduced in steps of about 2 to 3 cm water. As always, recheck the blood gases with each adjustment.

5. Increased pressure limit

To deliver a larger tidal volume, it may become necessary to increase the pressure limit when it is reached by the PIP. It may also be necessary to increase the pressure limit to restore the original tidal volume after the addition of PEEP. This is because the original tidal volume is reduced

Fig. 16-8 Pressure/time curve showing effect of addition of positive end-expiratory pressure (PEEP) on tidal volume. Initially, tidal volume is delivered by pressure difference of 30 cm water (difference between 0 and 30 cm water pressure). With addition of 5 cm water PEEP, pressure difference is reduced to 25 cm water (difference between 5 and 30 cm water pressure). This results in less tidal volume being delivered. *(From Burgess WR, Chernik V: Respiratory therapy in newborn infants and children, ed 2, New York, 1986, Thieme.)*

when PEEP is added and the PIP reaches the pressure limit. This is shown in Fig. 16-8. To restore the original tidal volume, the pressure limit (and PIP) must be increased by the same amount as the added PEEP. It is important to remember that as PEEP is reduced, the pressure limit must also be reduced by the same amount. This maintains the original tidal volume.

6. Increased respiratory rate

Increasing the ventilator respiratory rate increases the minute volume and probably increases the Pao_2 and reduces the $Paco_2$. Patients with stiff lungs and short time constants of ventilation often respond well to an increased respiratory rate. To that end, some authors advocate using a rate of up to 150/min on a conventional time-triggered, pressure-limited, time cycled mechanical ventilator, if necessary. (It should be noted that the FDA has set the upper rate limit of 150/min on these units.) A rate of greater than 150/min is termed *high-frequency ventilation* (HFV) and requires a special ventilator.

7. High frequency ventilation

HFV involves the use of a ventilator respiratory rate that is much greater than commonly needed. The FDA defines HFV as a rate of more than 150/min. Because of this FDA definition of HFV, conventional neonatal TPTV ventilators are not considered high-frequency ventilators. Several manufacturers have developed ventilators capable of rates significantly greater than 150/min. One of these must be used when HFV is indicated. The FDA also has set some guidelines for the appropriate use of HFV. See Box 16-5 for the clinical indications for HFV.

Despite the FDA guidelines, many respiratory therapists consider a rate of greater than 40/min on a neonatal patient to be HFV. When a conventional TPTV ventilator is used to deliver a respiratory rate of up to 150/min, the term *high frequency positive-pressure ventilation* (HFPPV) is

used. Experience has shown that many RDS infants can be successfully managed with a conventional TPTV ventilator set to deliver a small tidal volume at a rate between 40 and 150/min. However, when these methods fail, true HFV is needed.

Ventilator manufacturers have developed two different technologies for delivering FDA-defined HFV. The first is called *high frequency jet ventilation* (HFJV). With HFJV, small jets of gas are directed down the patient's endotracheal tube. These gas jets entrain additional gas into the tube. The two combined volumes of gas make up the patient's tidal volume. The patient exhales passively because of normal lung recoil. The second method is called *high frequency oscillation* (HFO) or *high frequency oscillatory ventilation* (HFOV). With HFO, a pumping device (piston, diaphragm, or sound speaker) actively pushes a small tidal volume into the patient from a continuous flow of gas (called bias flow) passing through the circuit and by the endotracheal tube. HFO technology can deliver very high rates because the patient actively exhales the delivered tidal volume. This active exhalation is created by the backstroke of the pumping device that pulls the tidal volume out of the patient's airways and lungs. See Table 16-2 for a comparison of HFV methods and characteristics.

Initial HFV settings depend on the patient's diagnosis, clinical situation, current conventional ventilator settings, and the type of high frequency ventilator to be used. Generally speaking, the initial HFV settings include a tidal volume large enough to see chest movement and a continuation of the patient's original mean airway pressure, PEEP level, and oxygen percentage. The I:E ratio should be set at 1:2, and the high frequency rate should be between 10 and 15 Hertz (Hz), depending on the infant's body

---

BOX 16-5 Common Clinical Indications for the Use of High Frequency Ventilation in Infants and Children

Severe hypoxemia and hypercarbia unresponsive to conventional ventilation techniques
    Infant respiratory distress syndrome (RDS)
    Acute respiratory distress syndrome (ARDS)
    Pneumonia
    Aspiration syndromes
    Pulmonary hemorrhage
Conventional ventilation with a persistent pulmonary air leak
    Pneumothorax
    Bronchopleural fistula
    Pulmonary interstitial emphysema (PIE)
    Pneumomediastinum
    Pneumoperitoneum
Persistent pulmonary hypertension of the newborn (PPHN)
Pulmonary hypoplasia
Bronchoscopy, laryngoscopy, or tracheal surgery

TABLE 16-2 High Frequency Ventilation			
	HFPPV	**HFJV**	**HFO**
Rate	60–150/min	≤600/min	≤1200/min
V_T	35 mL/kg	25 mL/kg	13 mL/kg
I/E ratio	1:3–1:2	1:3–1:2	1:3–1:2
Technical application	Conventional ventilator	Special ventilator	Special ventilator
F_{IO_2}	0.2–11.0	0.2–11.0	0.2–11.0
PEEP	0–20	0–20	0–20
Expiration	Passive	Passive	Active
Gas movement	Bulk flow	Bulk flow	Diffusion

HFJV, High frequency jet ventilation; HFO, high frequency oscillation; HFPPV, high frequency positive-pressure ventilation.

weight. (One Hertz is defined as 1 respiratory cycle/sec; 60 respiratory cycles/min. For example, a rate of 600/min is 10/sec or 10 Hz.) After the patient is stabilized on HFV, an arterial blood gas sample should be drawn and analyzed, vital signs assessed, and a chest radiograph obtained. In a patient without a pulmonary air leak, a chest radiograph finding of lung expansion to T8 to T9 on the right hemidiaphragm, without intercostal bulging, is believed to show the best lung volume. Once established, the HFV rate is seldom changed. Adjustments in tidal volume are made by increasing or decreasing what is referred to as either drive pressure (with HFJV) or amplitude (with HFO). Increasing drive pressure/amplitude increases the tidal volume and decreases the carbon dioxide level. The patient's oxygenation also should improve as the mean airway pressure is increased. Decreasing drive pressure/amplitude decreases the tidal volume and increases the carbon dioxide level. If the patient's oxygenation should decrease too much, additional therapeutic PEEP may be needed. See Fig. 16-9 for a protocol on initiation and adjustment of HFO. Fig. 16-10 shows a protocol for weaning from HFO.

Exam Hint

Recent Written Registry Exams have included a question about the application or modification of HFV. Know that increasing the amplitude results in a larger tidal volume and a reduction in the patient's Pa_{CO_2}. Reducing the amplitude would have the opposite effect.

8. Instillation of exogenous surfactant

The primary problem with a premature neonate with RDS is the lack of surfactant, a phospholipid, to reduce the surface tension in the alveoli. In 1991, the FDA approved the use of exogenous surfactant that can be directly instilled into the lungs of RDS neonates. Exosurf Neonatal (a synthetic product), Survanta and Infasurf (both bovine lung extract), and Curosurf (a pig lung extract) have been successfully used clinically. These drugs have proven very beneficial to premature neonates with

inadequate natural surfactant. After the drug is administered, the patient's lung compliance improves dramatically. Usually, the drug allows rapid reductions in the ventilator delivered oxygen percentage, rate, pressure limit, and PEEP.

Exam Hint

Recent Written Registry Exams have included a question about exogenous surfactant being indicated in a neonate with RDS.

Each of the options discussed in this section has its advocates; however, it seems logical that the best possible care would come from the proper application of each option when it is best suited to the patient's condition. To that end, Chatburn, Waldemar, and Lough (1983) developed a rather comprehensive approach to the adjustment of the various ventilator parameters to optimize the care of the RDS infant. They use the initial and subsequent blood gas results to direct the various ventilator changes that have been discussed. Because of the complexity of the logic in the algorithm, it is recommended that their articles, listed in the references, be read to appreciate its use fully.

c. Patients with increased airway resistance and normal lung compliance such as meconium aspiration syndrome

Although meconium aspiration is a commonly seen cause of increased airway resistance, it also is seen in infants with excessive airway secretions or bronchospasm. These neonates usually have normal lung compliance, and their clinical problem is getting enough air into and out of the lungs. The meconium or other obstruction causes uneven airflow and results in hypoxemia, air trapping, auto-PEEP, and an increased risk of barotrauma or volutrauma. Because of these issues, two key clinical goals exist. The first is to minimize turbulence during inspiration by reducing the inspiratory flow

Fig. 16-9 Optimal lung volume high frequency oscillatory ventilation strategy flow chart. *(From Minton S, Gerstmann D, Stoddard R: Cardiopul Rev, Yorba Linda, Calif, 1995, Sensormedics Corp. PN 770118-001.)*

HFOV "Optimum" Lung Volume Strategy
Pulmonary Injury Sequence Without Air Leak
Weaning Strategy

Fig. 16-10 High frequency oscillatory ventilation flow cart for weaning from optimal lung volume strategy. *(From Minton S, Gerstmann D, Stoddard R: Cardiopul Rev, Yorba Linda, Calif, 1995, Sensormedics Corp. PN 770118-001.)*

rate as much as possible. The second is to give a long enough expiratory time to prevent air trapping. Common recommendations for the ventilator settings are listed in Box 16-6. As discussed earlier, blood gases,

---

BOX 16-6   Common Mechanical Ventilator Parameters for Neonates with Increased Airway Resistance and Normal Lung Compliance

Delivered tidal volume: 6–8 mL/kg

Pressure limit: <20 cm water

Frequency: 20–40/min

I:E ratio: 1:3 to 1:10

Inspiratory time (T_I): between 0.4 and 0.7 sec (This may need to be increased.)

Expiratory time (T_E): ≥0.5 sec (This may need to be increased.)

PEEP: 2–4 cm water if needed

Inspiratory flow: sufficient to see the chest move and hear bilateral breath sounds during the inspiration. 5–8 L/min commonly used.

Oxygen percentage: 40% (This may need to be increased to keep the SpO_2 > 92%).

---

vital signs, and so forth must be monitored after the infant is placed on the ventilator. Listen to the breath sounds to detect the end of exhalation and a pause before the start of the next inspiration. This is to ensure that the exhalation has been complete and there is no air trapping that would lead to auto-PEEP. Any further adjustments can then be determined and evaluated by another set of blood gases and vital signs.

Look again at the issue of time constants of ventilation to understand better the various options for adjusting the ventilator. Using the following values for a mechanically ventilated neonate with meconium aspiration, its time constant is calculated as follows:

Tc = compliance (0.005 L/cm water) × resistance (150 cm water/L/second because the infant is intubated and has an obstructive problem) Simplify as follows:

= 0.005 × 150 second

= 0.75 second (Compare this with a Tc of 0.15 for a normal, spontaneously breathing neonate and a Tc of 0.1 for a ventilated infant with RDS.)

This relatively long time constant means that the tidal volume and PIP are rather slowly delivered to the alveoli. Little chance occurs of causing barotrauma or volutrauma from high ventilating pressures; however, it takes a fairly long inspiratory time to deliver an adequate tidal volume. Care must be taken to provide enough expiratory time for the tidal volume to be exhaled completely. In brief then, the challenge is to deliver an adequate tidal volume to maintain acceptable blood gases at a rate slow enough to prevent air trapping on exhalation.

In general, the inspiratory flow and rate are kept low, inspiratory and expiratory times are kept relatively long, and the I:E ratio should favor a long time for complete exhalation. Furthermore, it is important to suction the airway frequently to remove meconium or secretions. Postural drainage and percussion also are provided to mobilize the secretions so that they can be suctioned out. Usually these procedures and the natural breakdown of meconium result in reduced airway resistance within a few days. Ventilatory support can then be lessened.

d. Patients with persistent pulmonary hypertension of the newborn

PPHN also is referred to as persistent pulmonary hypertension (PPH), persistent fetal circulation (PFC), or persistence of the fetal circulation. Infants with PPHN are first seen clinically with an elevated pulmonary artery pressure and a right-to-left shunt through a patent ductus arteriosus or the foramen ovale or both. Because of this, their oxygenation fluctuates greatly. The problem may be seen right after birth or up to 24 hours later. PPHN seems to result from fetal hypoxemia and acidosis. These, in turn, are caused by or associated with maternal drug addiction, infection, pre-eclampsia, abruptio placenta, post-term gestation, oligohydramnios, and meconium staining or aspiration. The following four tests are done to help confirm the diagnosis:

1. Hyperoxia test: This is the first test and is done after an arterial blood gas has shown a low PaO_2. The test involves having the patient inspire 100% oxygen for about 10 minutes and obtaining a second arterial blood gas. If the PaO_2 does not improve to more than 50 torr, a fixed right-to-left shunt is proven. The shunt may be from PPHN or a cyanotic heart defect. If the PaO_2 does go over 100 torr, the neonate probably has parenchymal lung disease and should be treated accordingly.

2. Preductal and postductal arterial blood sampling: Simultaneously draw and then analyze (a) a blood gas sample from the right radial or brachial artery to check the preductal PaO_2, and (b) a blood gas sample from the left brachial, left radial, either femoral artery, or the umbilical artery catheter to check the postductal PaO_2. Compare the results. A decrease in saturation from preductal to postductal blood of greater than 10% or a decrease in PaO_2 of greater than 15 to 20 torr indicates shunting. For example, significant shunting is indicated by a

preductal PaO_2 of 70 torr and a postductal PaO_2 of 45 torr. This same test may be performed noninvasively with either transcutaneous oxygen monitoring or pulse-oximetry monitoring. The $PtcO_2$ monitors should be placed over the right upper chest for preductal blood and left upper chest, abdomen, or either thigh for postductal blood. Pulse-oximetry monitors should be placed on the right hand for preductal blood and left hand or either foot for postductal blood. Again, a greater than 15 to 20 torr decrease in preductal to postductal $PtcO_2$ or a greater than 10% decrease in saturation in preductal to postductal SpO_2 confirms a significant shunt.

It is important to note that if the neonate has a shunt through the foramen ovale instead of the ductus arteriosus, this test will be negative. The preductal and postductal oxygen levels will be the same. Shunting through the foramen ovale is seen in as many as 50% of PPHN babies.

3. Hyperoxia/hyperventilation test: The infant is manually ventilated with 100% oxygen at a rate and pressure adequate to reduce the carbon dioxide level significantly. When this "critical $PaCO_2$" (usually between 20 and 30 torr) is reached, the pulmonary artery pressure decreases, the lungs are better perfused, and the PaO_2 improves. Although the patient's color will likely change from cyanotic to pink and the $PtcO_2$ and SpO_2 values will improve, the test is confirmed by a postductal PaO_2 of greater than 80 torr. The critical $PaCO_2$ value, ventilation rate, and manometer pressure on the manual ventilator should be recorded. These values can be used later to set the mechanical ventilator parameters.

4. Echocardiography: This procedure can be used to identify an intracardiac shunt through the foramen ovale or evidence of increased right ventricular pressure as a sign of pulmonary hypertension.

Any infant who shows signs of PPHN, such as positive results to any of these tests or the need for more than 70% oxygen to prevent hypoxemia, should be considered for hyperventilation therapy. The goal is to reduce pulmonary artery hypertension and thus reduce shunting and improve the PaO_2. This is accomplished by hyperventilating the patient to his or her critical $PaCO_2$. Box 16-7 lists common ventilator parameters used to treat persistent pulmonary hypertension. Once the proper ventilator settings are found and the blood gas goals are met, the patient is maintained at this level for 1 or more days. It is often necessary to paralyze the infant pharmacologically with pancuronium bromide (Pavulon) or a similar drug to ensure that the patient's breathing is synchronized with the ventilator. This is especially important when high ventilator rates are needed. After about 24 hours, the

BOX 16-7   Common Mechanical Ventilator Parameters to Treat a Neonate with Persistent Pulmonary Hypertension

Delivered tidal volume: 6–8 mL/kg initially; 8–10 mL/kg may be needed to hyperventilate the neonate

Pressure limit: 20–25 cm water. Use as little pressure as possible but be prepared to increase to 35 cm water to deliver an adequate tidal volume

Frequency: 60–100/min may be needed to decrease the $PaCO_2$ to the critical level of probably between 20 and 30 mm Hg. A rate of ≤ 150/min has been used.

I:E ratio: 1:2 (This depends on the respiratory rate needed to decrease the carbon dioxide level.)

Inspiratory time (T_I): between 0.4 and 0.7 sec (This must be decreased at higher respiratory rates.)

Expiratory time (T_E): ≥0.5 sec (This must be decreased at higher respiratory rates.)

PEEP: none if possible to lower the mean airway pressure and prevent crushing of the pulmonary capillary bed; 2–4 cm water may be used if needed.

Inspiratory flow: sufficient to see the chest move and hear bilateral breath sounds during the inspiration; 5–8 L/min commonly used initially. Flow must be increased at higher respiratory rates.

Oxygen percentage: ≤70%–100% to keep the postductal PaO_2 > 55 torr and ideally between 115 and 120 torr.

---

ventilator is adjusted to increase the $PaCO_2$ by 1 to 2 torr. If the PIP is greater than 45 cm water, it should be reduced first. A blood gas is drawn to see if the PaO_2 is stable and if the $PaCO_2$ increased the desired small amount. If this first reduction in support is tolerated, it may be slowly followed by further reductions. Each step back from hyperventilation should be small so that the $PaCO_2$ increases only by 1 to 2 mm Hg each time.

As this happens, the patient should be supported in every other way. The medication tolazoline (Priscoline) is a pulmonary vasodilator that has proven to be successful in about one of six neonates with PPHN. Watch for signs of pulmonary barotrauma or bronchopulmonary dysplasia from the high peak pressures and oxygen percentages required with these patients.

1. Modify special gases: inhaled nitric oxide (WRE code: IIIF5) [Difficulty: R, Ap, An]

Inhaled nitric oxide (iNO) gas has been approved for use as a pulmonary artery vasodilator in neonates with PPHN and increased pulmonary vascular resistance. Clinical improvement often occurs when a small amount of NO is inhaled by a neonate with PPHN or RDS. It is important to keep the concentration of iNO as low as possible to achieve this clinical improvement. The upper limit of a therapeutic dose of iNO is less than 20 parts per million

(ppm). This is because nitric oxide combines with oxygen to form nitrogen dioxide (NO_2). A level of nitrogen dioxide greater than 10 ppm can cause cell damage, hemorrhage, and pulmonary edema leading to death. As the NO_2 increases, it causes an increase in the patient's methemoglobin level. Therefore the serum level of this nonfunctional form of hemoglobin also must be monitored. Patients who receive iNO are usually also receiving mechanical ventilation. In addition, special iNO measurement and delivery systems are needed, and levels of inspired oxygen, nitric oxide, and nitrogen dioxide must be measured. As the patient's PPHN improves, the level of iNO can be reduced.

Exam Hint

Because recent Written Registry Exams have had a question on inhaled nitric oxide, it is recommended that related discussions be reviewed in Chapters 5 and 6.

e. Patients with bronchopulmonary dysplasia

The neonate in whom bronchopulmonary dysplasia (BPD) develops is usually born prematurely with a low birth weight. He or she is a survivor of RDS but has had serious lung damage in the process. It is controversial whether high peak pressures, high mean airway pressures, high inspired oxygen percentages, or a combination of these factors is the main cause of BPD. It is important to try to minimize all of them so that new lung tissues can grow to replace lung tissue that has been damaged. It is important to try to wean these infants as quickly as possible to avoid further ventilator-induced damage. If acceptable blood gases can be maintained with a ventilator rate of less than 15/min, the infant may be extubated. Nasal CPAP may be used to help maintain the PaO_2. See Box 16-8 for the commonly recommended ventilator settings for a BPD patient.

A number of medications are used to help optimize the patient's pulmonary function. Methylxanthines such as aminophylline or caffeine are beneficial as respiratory stimulants. Further evidence suggests that they help to strengthen the diaphragm and decrease muscle fatigue. The diuretic furosemide (Lasix) has been widely reported to improve lung compliance and airway resistance by decreasing any pulmonary edema fluid. Remember that patients receiving furosemide must be given a potassium chloride supplement to replace what is lost through the kidneys. Some authors have reported the use of corticosteroids to be helpful in weaning because of increased pulmonary compliance. This possible advantage must be balanced against the known problems associated with the prolonged use of the medication. Finally, a dietary supplement of vitamin E

BOX 16-8   Common Mechanical Ventilator Parameters for Neonates with Bronchopulmonary Dysplasia

Delivered tidal volume: 6-8 mL/kg

Pressure limit: as low as possible and not to exceed 25 cm water

Frequency: as low as possible to maintain the $Paco_2$ between 35 and 45 torr. Some authors report accepting a $Paco_2$ as high as 55 to 65 torr to minimize the need to increase peak and mean pressures.

I:E ratio: 1:2 to 1:10

Inspiratory time (T_I): between 0.3 and 0.7 sec

Expiratory time (T_E): ≥0.5 sec to allow for a complete exhalation

PEEP: ≤2-4 cm water

Inspiratory flow: sufficient to see the chest move and hear bilateral breath sounds during the inspiration; 5-8 L/min commonly used initially.

Oxygen percentage: as low as possible to keep the Pao_2 between 55 and 65 torr. Some authors report accepting a Pao_2 as low as 35 torr to minimize the need to increase peak and mean pressures. It must be noted that a Pao_2 < 55 torr increases the risk of pulmonary hypertension.

---

may increase lung healing. It is hoped that the use of surfactant replacement therapy early in the treatment of the RDS neonate will reduce the incidence of BPD.

5. Monitor the mean airway pressure to evaluate the patient's response to respiratory care (WRE code: IIIE0) [Difficulty: An]

Mean airway pressure ($P\overline{aw}$) is the average pressure over an entire breathing cycle. A number of current neonatal and adult ventilators are able to calculate the value. $P\overline{aw}$ is influenced by both the patient's lung thoracic compliance (C_{LT}) and airway resistance (Raw). If the ventilator settings are unchanged, a decrease in compliance or an increase in resistance will result in an increase in the mean airway pressure. This is because in a neonatal ventilator, the pressure limit is reached earlier and held for the duration of the inspiratory time. Conversely, if the patient's compliance increases or the resistance decreases, the $P\overline{aw}$ will decrease. It is important to evaluate the patient further when a change in $P\overline{aw}$ is noticed. This is because the new pressure by itself does not show you whether a change in compliance, resistance, or both have occurred. Any treatments that improve lung compliance and reduce airway resistance are shown by a reduced mean airway pressure.

In general, an increase in mean airway pressure increases the patient's oxygenation. This is because the alveoli are kept open longer, allowing more time for diffusion and preventing alveolar collapse. If alveolar ventilation is improved, the $Paco_2$ also will be reduced. Clinical evidence suggests that a mean airway pressure of 12 or more centimeters water pressure is associated with an increased risk of pulmonary barotrauma and decreased cardiac output. This is especially true if PEEP is increased to raise the $P\overline{aw}$. Watch the patient closely whenever a ventilator change is made that increases the $P\overline{aw}$. A sudden deterioration in cardiopulmonary function may be caused by a pneumothorax. A reduction in urine output, an increased heart rate, and decreased blood pressure are often seen when the cardiac output is reduced. The mean airway pressure should be reduced if either of these situations is seen. To prevent these complications, it is necessary to reduce the mean airway pressure whenever the patient's compliance improves.

Usually the mean airway pressure is the result of the patient's lung compliance, airway resistance, and the various ventilator settings. The initial mean airway pressure should be considered along with the ventilator settings when interpreting the first set of arterial blood gases. Based on the blood gas results, ventilator adjustments may be needed. Note the $P\overline{aw}$ at each adjustment.

A number of ventilator control adjustments influence the patient's mean airway pressure. (See Fig. 16-11 for several examples of airway pressure tracings based on ventilator control changes.) If the patient's compliance and resistance are stable, the $P\overline{aw}$ will be *increased* by the following: (1) an increased inspiratory flow, (2) an increased pressure limit (assuming the pressure limit has been previously reached), (3) an increase in PEEP, (4) an increased inspiratory time (assuming no change in ventilator rate and a decreased expiratory time), and (5) a decreased expiratory time (assuming an increased ventilator rate). These ventilator adjustments should result in an increased Pao_2 and possibly a decreased $Paco_2$. Measure blood gases to be sure of the patient's response.

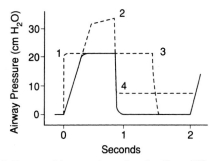

Fig. 16-11 Pressure/time tracings showing four different ventilator settings that can be used to increase mean airway pressure. *1,* Inspiratory flow is increased. *2,* Pressure limit is increased. *3,* Inspiratory time is increased. This also changes the I:E ratio by reducing expiratory time if rate is kept the same. *4,* Positive end-expiratory pressure is added. *(From Harris TR: In Goldsmith JP, Karotkin EH, editors:* Assisted ventilation of the neonate, *Philadelphia, 1981, WB Saunders.)*

If the patient's compliance and resistance are stable, the Paw will be *decreased* by the following: (1) a decreased inspiratory flow, (2) a decreased pressure limit (assuming the pressure limit has been previously reached), (3) a decrease in PEEP, (4) a decreased inspiratory time (assuming no change in ventilator rate and an increased expiratory time), and (5) an increased expiratory time (assuming a decreased ventilator rate). These ventilator adjustments may result in a decreased Pa_{O_2} and possibly an increased Pa_{CO_2}. Measure blood gases to be sure of the patient's response.

It should be noted that of all the various controls that have an influence on the mean airway pressure, PEEP has the greatest impact. Usually a one-for-one relation exists between the addition or removal of PEEP and the resulting Paw. For example, the Paw is 10 cm water when 5 cm water of PEEP is added. The resulting Paw is seen to become 15 cm water. If 2 cm of PEEP is removed, the Paw will decrease to 13 cm water.

6. Monitor the ventilator alarm systems and adjust them as needed (WRE code: IIIE9 and IIIF9a) [Difficulty: An]

All alarm systems must function properly, so test all audible and visual alarms. The respiratory therapist should be familiar with the most widely used neonatal ventilators and those that can be used with pediatric as well as adult patients. It is common practice to set most ventilator alarms at ±10% from the set value.

If the patient is on a CPAP system, the low-pressure or disconnection alarm should be set to alarm if the pressure decreases about 2 cm water below the set level. For example, if the patient is on 8 cm water CPAP, the alarm setting should be set at 6 cm water.

Many types of alarm systems have a timer that can be set to delay when the alarm sounds. For example, if the neonatal patient has a ventilator rate of 30/min, the cycling time between mandatory breaths is 2 seconds. The delay should be set so that the alarm sounds in 1 to 2 seconds after a mandatory breath fails to be delivered. If the patient is on a CPAP system, the timer may be set for no delay or a short delay after the CPAP pressure decreases below the set value. Always adjust all alarm systems to fit the clinical situation and the patient's condition.

7. Ventilator flow, volume, and pressure waveforms
a. Review existing information in the patient's chart (WRE code: IA7b) [Difficulty: An]

A patient who has been intubated and placed on a modern mechanical ventilator with a microprocessor and graphics software can have ventilator flow, volume, and pressure waveforms visualized on the monitor. Some units allow the information to be stored in memory or printed out. Look for this information and compare it with the patient's current situation.

b. Perform the procedure to measure pressure/volume and flow/volume loops (WRE code: IB7b) [Difficulty: Ap, An]

Because not every ventilator can provide waveform information, the correct unit must be selected for the patient. For example, the Drager Babylog 8000 has the monitor and graphics software built into the unit. Other neonatal ventilators, such as the VIP Bird, can be upgraded to provide graphic information. Some ventilators, such as the Hamilton Galileo, can be used with any size patient and provide waveform information. Follow the ventilator manufacturer's guidelines to direct the unit to create flow, volume, or pressure waveforms.

c. Interpret ventilator pressure/volume and flow/volume loops (WRE code: IB8j) [Difficulty: An]

Ventilator flow, volume, and pressure waveforms offer much clinically useful information. For example, expiratory flow can be monitored to look for air trapping and auto-PEEP. As discussed earlier, this is a concern if the neonate has obstructive airway disease or if a high respiratory rate is being used. Volume can be monitored as an indicator of improving or worsening lung compliance. Pressure also can be monitored as it relates to improving or worsening lung compliance. Less pressure is needed to deliver the desired tidal volume if the patient's lung compliance is improving. Conversely, more pressure is needed to deliver the desired tidal volume if the patient's lung compliance is worsening. Chapter 15 and this chapter include examples of waveform tracings.

d. Adjust ventilator settings based on ventilator graphics (WRE code: IIIG3h) [Difficulty: An]

As discussed earlier, be prepared to make adjustments in the ventilator as indicated by graphics. For example, if air trapping and auto-PEEP are observed, be prepared to increase the expiratory time, decrease the inspiratory time, or decrease the tidal volume to ensure that a complete exhalation occurs.

8. Adequately oxygenate the patient to prevent accidental hypoxemia before and after suctioning, changing the ventilator circuit, or performing other procedures during which the patient is disconnected from the ventilator (WRE code: IIID6) [Difficulty: An]

Chapter 13 discusses the suctioning procedure and steps that should be taken to prevent hypoxemia during suctioning. Children younger than 6 months should have their oxygen percentage increased by 10% to 20% for the procedure.

MODULE B
Mechanical ventilation equipment

1. Ventilators

As discussed in Chapter 15, the literature produced by the manufacturers and the descriptions used in many standard texts break the various ventilators into more categories than used by the NBRC. To avoid confusion, this text uses the NBRC's more simplified terminology. A pneumatically powered ventilator is defined here as powered by compressed gas. It may be electrically controlled with electrical alarm systems. Fluidic ventilators are defined here as being pneumatically powered and partially or completely controlled by fluidic methods. Fluidic controls make use of compressed gas for cycling and other ventilator functions. Both of these types of neonatal ventilators use compressed air and oxygen that go to an air/oxygen mixer (blender) to determine the inspired oxygen. The gas then goes to a flow meter where the continuous flow per minute through the ventilator circuit is set. Depending on the ventilator, either compressed air or oxygen is used to drive the other control functions in fluidic ventilators.

An electrically powered ventilator is defined here as being electrically powered and controlled. Compressed air and oxygen go to a blender where the inspired oxygen is set. A microprocessor ventilator is defined here as being controlled by a microprocessor; it may be pneumatically or electrically powered. All of these types of ventilators are limited to the 150 breaths/min maximum rate set by the FDA. A high frequency ventilator is capable of delivering a respiratory rate of more than 150/min.

a. Pneumatic ventilators
1. Get the necessary equipment for the procedure (WRE code: IIA6a) [Difficulty: An]

It is beyond the scope of this text to discuss in detail the functions of pneumatic ventilators and the following types of ventilators. Refer to the manufacturer's literature for specific information. Examples of neonatal pneumatic ventilators include the Babybird, Babybird 2, Bio-Med MPV-10, BEAR Cub BP2001, and Healthdyne 105. They are used to deliver conventional TPTV mechanical ventilation to the majority of neonatal and pediatric patients. The Bio-Med Devices MVP-10 is an example of a pediatric transport ventilator.

2. Put the equipment together and make sure that it works properly (WRE code: IIA6a) [Difficulty: An]
3. Troubleshoot any problems with the equipment (WRE code: IIA6a) [Difficulty: An]

Make sure that the air and oxygen high-pressure hoses are screwed tightly into the air/oxygen blender. A gas leak is heard as a whistling or hissing sound. If either gas source is cut off to the blender, its alarm will sound.

b. Fluidic ventilators
1. Get the necessary equipment for the procedure (WRE code: IIA6a) [Difficulty: An]

The Sechrist IV-100B and IV-200 ventilators are pneumatically powered and electrically and fluidically controlled.

2. Put the equipment together and make sure that it works properly (WRE code: IIA6a) [Difficulty: An]
3. Troubleshoot any problems with the equipment (WRE code: IIA6a) [Difficulty: An]

Fluidic ventilators are prone to the same kind of problems with leaking high-pressure air and oxygen hoses as pneumatic ventilators. In addition, they are very sensitive to obstructions. Make sure that all inlet filters are intact and free of debris.

c. Electric ventilators
1. Get the necessary equipment for the procedure (WRE code: IIA6a) [Difficulty: An]

At the time of this writing, no exclusively neonatal units fit the earlier definition of an electric ventilator; however, some adult ventilators such as the Newport Breeze, Siemens Servo 300A, Siemens Servo *i*, and Drager Evita 2 Dura can deliver tidal volumes small enough for a pediatric patient.

2. Put the equipment together and make sure that it works properly (WRE code: IIA6a) [Difficulty: An]
3. Troubleshoot any problems with the equipment (WRE code: IIA6a) [Difficulty: An]

Make sure that the electrical power source is secure. Do not use a unit that does not power up or operate properly.

d. Microprocessor ventilator
1. Get the equipment necessary for the procedure (WRE code: IIA6a) [Difficulty: An]

The LifeCare PLV-102 and Nelcor Puritan Bennett Companion 2801 are microprocessor controlled and electrically powered. They are home care ventilators that can deliver tidal volumes small enough for pediatric patients (50 mL).

2. Put the equipment together, and make sure that it works properly (WRE code: IIA6a) [Difficulty: An]

Both the LifeCare PLV-102 and the Nelcor Puritan Bennett Companion 2801 must have a stable electrical supply. They also must have an oxygen source for adding to the tidal volume if more than room air is required by the patient. An oxygen analyzer should also be put inline to monitor the oxygen percentage because it varies with a changing respiratory rate or tidal volume.

3. Troubleshoot any problems with the equipment (WRE code: IIA6a) [Difficulty: An]

The Infrasonics Infant Star series, Drager Babylog 8000 Plus, VIP Bird, and VIP Bird Gold are electrically and pneumatically powered and controlled by a microprocessor. Some of the current generation of primarily adult ventilators are capable of delivering tidal volumes and rates appropriate for infants. The Hamilton Veolar is an example. Microprocessor ventilators typically come with self-diagnostic software. If a problem is detected, the unit will display it on the monitor. Little exists to repair with these units at the bedside. Occasionally a computer chip must be replaced in the department.

e. High frequency ventilators
1. Get the necessary equipment for the procedure (WRE code: IIA6a) [Difficulty: R, Ap, An]

The Bunnell Life Pulse High Frequency Ventilator provides HFJV. The SensorMedics 3100A High-Frequency Oscillatory Ventilator and Infrasonics Infant Star 950 Ventilator are examples of high frequency oscillator (HFO) ventilators.

2. Put the equipment together and make sure that it works properly (WRE code: IIA6a) [Difficulty: R, Ap, An]

Hands-on experience with these ventilators is recommended. The following are needed for proper assembly of a HFJV: (1) a pressurized oxygen source, (2) a pressurized air source, (3) an air/oxygen proportioner (blender), (4) a pressure regulator for controlling the patient's peak pressure, (5) an injector line to add the jet volume to the endotracheal tube, and (6) an intravenous infusion pump to supply a steady drip of water to the jet ventilator injector line for nebulization.

An HFO ventilator needs the following basic accessories for assembly: (1) a pressurized oxygen source, (2) a pressurized air source, (3) an air/oxygen proportioner (blender), and (4) a passover- or cascade-type humidifier.

3. Troubleshoot any problems with the equipment (WRE code: IIA6a) [Difficulty: R, Ap, An]

Make sure that gas sources are stable, all tubing connections are tight, and humidification systems are functioning properly. Because the patient's tidal volume is very small, it cannot be accurately measured. Any leaks will result in an undetectable loss of delivered tidal volume.

2. Ventilator breathing circuits
a. Get the necessary equipment for the procedure (WRE code: IIA10a) [Difficulty: Ap]

Conventional neonatal ventilators use a circuit that has all of the standard features of an adult circuit as discussed in Chapter 15. Commonly, disposable single-patient use corrugated plastic circuits are used. They are inexpensive and meet the needs of most patients. Condensation is drained out into water traps that are placed at low points in the natural draping of the inspiratory and expiratory limbs of the circuit. If excessive moisture is a problem or if the gas temperature must be maintained within a narrow range, a heated-wire circuit may be used. These types of circuits are built with a heated wire either loosely threaded through the lumen or coiled within the tubing itself. They are integrated with the humidification system and a servo unit for automatic temperature regulation. As expected, these circuits are considerably more expensive than the disposable types and may be sterilized and reused between patients.

Another possible concern with disposable, corrugated circuits is their relatively high internal resistance and compressible volume. The corrugations lead to gas turbulence that increases as the flow is increased. When the tubing is warmed, it becomes more stretchable. This results in more tidal volume lost to the circuit instead of being delivered to the patient.

When high flow rates and ventilating pressures are needed, as in HFV, a smooth bore and low compressible volume circuit is used instead of the standard disposable type. A special circuit made of noncompliant tubing is needed with the SensorMedics 3100A ventilator. In addition, to complete an HFJV circuit, a Hi-Lo Jet endotracheal tube or special endotracheal tube adapter is needed to deliver the jetted gas and add the entrained gas for the tidal volume. These are shown in Chapter 15.

b. Put the equipment together and make sure that it works properly (WRE code: IIA10a) [Difficulty: Ap]
c. Troubleshoot any problems with the equipment (WRE code: IIA10a) [Difficulty: Ap]

Conventional neonatal ventilator circuits are basically the same as adult circuits with an inspiratory limb and an expiratory limb. Water traps are usually added. An obvious difference is the smaller diameter so that less compressible volume is present. Some are smooth bore to minimize gas turbulence, and some have a heated wire running through them to keep a constant temperature and eliminate condensation. It is important that a heated-wire circuit be used only with the servo-controlled humidifier for which it is designed. Mixing circuits and humidifiers can lead to either overheating or underheating problems. Furthermore, do not cover a heated-wire circuit with a blanket. The circuit should not be allowed to touch the patient to avoid burns. If the patient is inside an incubator, the circuit's temperature probe must be kept outside.

An added feature is a third small bore tubing for measuring the proximal airway pressure. The tube runs from the patient Y to the proximal airway pressure nipple on the ventilator. Make sure that all the connections are tight to prevent gas leaks.

3. Continuous positive airway pressure devices

a. Get the necessary equipment for the procedure (WRE code: IIA10c) [Difficulty: Ap]

Nasal CPAP devices are widely used with neonates who are born prematurely and have RDS. Their immature lungs lack sufficient surfactant and need the CPAP pressure to keep the alveoli open. Often, nasal CPAP meets the patient's needs so that endotracheal intubation and mechanical ventilation can be avoided. Nasal CPAP works with neonates because they are obligate nose breathers.

Nasal CPAP is associated with the hazards of gastric distention and reflux aspiration. These occur when the airway pressure forces air into the stomach. A gastric tube is usually inserted to vent the air out. Two different devices are available for administering nasal CPAP. A nasopharyngeal tube is actually an endotracheal tube that has been cut shorter (see Fig. 16-2, C). Select a tube that is the largest that can be easily inserted into the patient. Nasal prongs come in short and long versions (see Fig. 16-2, A and B); both types involve prongs that fit into both nostrils. The prongs come in different diameters so that the proper size can be found to fit the internal diameter of the infant's nares.

b. Put the equipment together and make sure that it works properly (WRE code: IIA10c) [Difficulty: Ap]

Follow the manufacturer's instructions for assembly of the CPAP device and CPAP circuit. See Figs. 16-2 and 16-3 as well as the illustration of the CPAP circuit in Chapter 15 for general assembly guidance.

c. Troubleshoot any problems with the equipment (WRE code: IIA10c) [Difficulty: Ap]

A sudden decrease in the CPAP level to zero indicates a disconnection at the patient or somewhere in the breathing circuit. Check all connections, and reassemble the break. The patient may need to be manually ventilated while the problem is corrected.

If the CPAP level decreases more than 2 cm of water pressure during an inspiration, the flow is inadequate and should be increased. Flow also is inadequate if the patient shows an increased use of accessory muscles of respiration or appears to have an increased work of breathing. Too high a flow is seen by an inadvertently high level of CPAP or the appearance that the patient is having a difficult time exhaling. A common problem with small diameter tubes like these is mucus plugging. A plugged tube may result in a backup of gas and can increase CPAP; however, depending on the CPAP system, no change in pressure may be present. Careful patient monitoring is important. Watch for a decrease in oxygenation, an increase in the respiratory rate, or retractions as signs of airway obstruction. Suction to clear out the mucus plug or remove the tube and place a new one.

4. Continuous positive airway pressure circuit

a. Get the necessary equipment for the procedure (WRE code: IIA10c) [Difficulty: Ap]

The general discussion and an illustration related to CPAP systems were presented in Chapter 15. Free-standing neonatal systems are similar to those used with adults. All currently available neonatal ventilators offer a CPAP mode. This allows the practitioner to switch the intubated neonate easily from IMV to CPAP without the need to set up new equipment.

b. Put the equipment together and make sure that it works properly (WRE code: IIA10c) [Difficulty: Ap]

c. Troubleshoot any problems with the equipment (WRE code: IIA10c) [Difficulty: Ap]

The previous discussion about putting together and fixing problems with the CPAP device applies to the CPAP circuit.

> **Exam Hint**
>
> A sudden decrease in CPAP level indicates a disconnection within the circuit or at the patient connection.

5. Humidification equipment

a. Get the necessary equipment for the procedure (WRE code: IIA3) [Difficulty: An]

The general discussion of humidification equipment was presented in Chapters 8 and 15. See the figures there and the general discussion for setups in ventilator and CPAP breathing circuits. Both heated humidifiers and heat and moisture exchangers are used with pediatric patients. Heated passover-type humidifiers systems are preferred with neonates.

  b. **Put the equipment together and make sure that it works properly (WRE code: IIA3) [Difficulty: An]**
  c. **Troubleshoot any problems with the equipment (WRE code: IIA3) [Difficulty: An]**

Again, see Chapters 8 and 15 for assembly and troubleshooting of humidification systems. With a cascade-type or passover-type humidifier, the gas temperature is usually maintained close to the neonate's body temperature to maintain a neutral thermal environment. Make sure that the water level is kept in the recommended range to humidify the gas properly.

6. Perform quality control procedures for mechanical ventilators (WRE code: IIC4) [Difficulty: Ap, An]

Follow the manufacturer's guidelines for quality control procedures on mechanical ventilators. The microprocessor ventilators usually have a software package that performs self-diagnostic tests on the unit. If a problem is found, it is displayed on the monitor. Obviously the ventilator should deliver the volume, flow, and pressure that is set on the control. Do not use a ventilator that fails a quality control check.

MODULE C
Respiratory care plan

1. Analyze available information to determine the patient's pathophysiologic state (CSE code: IIIH1)

Refer to Chapter 1 or earlier in this chapter for a detailed discussion on neonatal assessment. The discussion of the most common neonatal pulmonary conditions was presented earlier in this chapter.

2. Determine the appropriateness of the prescribed therapy and goals for the identified pathophysiologic state (CSE code: IIIH3)

Specific recommendations for ventilatory support for the various pulmonary conditions were given earlier in the chapter.

  a. **Stop the treatment or procedure if the patient has an adverse reaction to it (CSE code: IIIF1)**
  b. **Discontinue treatment based on the patient's response (WRE code: IIIG1e) [Difficulty: An]**

Be prepared to stop a particular treatment or change in ventilator parameter if the patient has an adverse reaction to it. Physical assessment is vitally important because neonates or small children cannot communicate how they feel about their care.

An infant who is attempting to exhale when the IMV breath is being delivered is said to be "bucking" or "fighting" the ventilator. This problem is almost unavoidable because the IMV breaths cannot be synchronized on the majority of neonatal ventilators. If the asynchrony between the infant's efforts and the ventilator are too great, an increased risk of hypoxemia and barotrauma or volutrauma exists. Carefully evaluate the patient to determine whether the patient is breathing rapidly because of pain or improper adjustment of the ventilator. Make sure that the flow, rate, pressure limit, and so forth are correctly set for the patient's condition. Sedation or paralysis should be considered only after all other causes of asynchrony have been ruled out.

Antianxiety agents are not typically used with neonates. Morphine sulfate or other opiates are typically used for pain, but other less powerful medications also may be tried. If the patient must be paralyzed, pancuronium (Pavulon), atracurium (Tracrium), and vecuronium (Norcuron) are commonly used. Remember that these paralyzing agents have no effect on the patient's ability to feel pain or to be afraid of what is happening. Pain medications must be given as necessary.

3. Treat a tension pneumothorax (WRE code: III I2) [Difficulty: Ap, An]

A chest radiograph and physical examination of the neonate will reveal if abnormal air or fluid is found around the lung(s) or heart. If a patient has a tension pneumothorax, a pleural chest tube *must* be inserted to remove the air and relieve the pressure within the chest. A nontension pneumothorax of greater than 10% is often also treated by inserting a pleural chest tube. A pleural chest tube also is placed to remove blood or other fluid from the pleural space. Chapter 18 has specific information that relates to treating a pneumothorax.

A pneumomediastinum, pneumopericardium, or pneumoperitoneum that puts the patient at risk also must be treated. A chest tube is then inserted into the area where the abnormal air is found. The same chest tube also removes any abnormal collection of fluid. A chest tube is usually placed behind the heart to remove any blood that should leak out after open heart surgery.

If a neonate is being ventilated on a constant volume ventilator, the amount of air that is lost through the pleural chest tube can be calculated. This is done by subtracting the measured exhaled volume from the measured inhaled volume. For example:

Inspired tidal volume = 40 mL

Exhaled tidal volume = −30 mL

10 mL of tidal volume is lost through the pleural chest tube

It is not possible to measure tidal volume when the neonate is ventilated by any other means. In a case like this, it is possible to make only a qualitative judgment on pleural air leak. In other words, if air is seen to bubble out through the pleural drainage system, an air leak is present. When the air stops bubbling, the pleural tear has healed. See Chapter 18 for a complete discussion on pleural drainage systems.

4. Weaning from the ventilator

a. Recommend procedures for weaning from mechanical ventilation (WRE code: IIIG1d) [Difficulty: An]

b. Initiate and modify weaning procedures (CSE code: IIID5 and IIIF2j)

As the neonate's condition improves, consideration must be given as to the best weaning method. Specific steps in increasing ventilator support were discussed earlier with each of the types of common pathologic conditions and the various modes of ventilation. In general, ventilator support should be reduced in the opposite manner that it was increased. Remember to evaluate the patient's arterial blood gas values and vital signs before and after making a change in the ventilator parameters. If the patient's condition deteriorates, the ventilator setting(s) should be placed as before. General steps in weaning ventilator support in a patient receiving traditional time-triggered, pressure limited, time cycled mechanical ventilation (TPTV) include

a. Reduce the oxygen percentage in 2% to 5% steps down to 40% or less, while meeting the oxygenation goal (see Table 16-1).

b. Once the patient is receiving 40% or less oxygen, the PEEP level can be decreased in 1- to 2-cm water increments. The goal is a PEEP level of 3 to 4 cm water while meeting the oxygenation goal.

c. Next, PIP can be reduced in 1- to 2-cm water increments. The goal is a PIP of 15 to 18 cm water. The patient's arterial blood gas goals must be met (see Table 16-1).

d. The ventilator rate is now reduced in steps of 1 to 5 breaths per minute. The patient's spontaneous breathing rate should increase as the ventilator rate is reduced. The goal is a ventilator rate of less than 10/min. Arterial blood gas goals must continue to be met.

The decision to extubate with CPAP therapy or limited ventilator support is based on the neonate's return to health and toleration of these steps of reduced ventilator support. If the endotracheal tube is not needed for a suctioning route, the tube can be removed. The following additional steps are generally taken to ensure an appropriate, safe extubation:

a. Feedings should be withheld for several hours to reduce the risk of aspiration.

b. Perform an endotracheal tube "leak test" by delivering a mandatory breath and auscultating a leak at the neonate's larynx. An audible leak indicates the absence of laryngeal edema. If a leak cannot be heard, the neonate should be given a treatment of aerosolized racemic epinephrine to reduce the edema. Do not extubate a patient with laryngeal edema because it is likely that the endotracheal tube will need to be put back in.

c. Hyperoxygenate the neonate.

d. Suction the trachea and the oral pharynx.

e. Deliver a large tidal volume breath and remove the endotracheal tube when the lungs are full.

f. Suction the mouth as needed.

g. Provide supplemental oxygen by face mask or nasal cannula.

h. Follow-up arterial blood gases and frequent monitoring of vital signs and breath sounds should be done after extubation.

i. Be prepared to reintubate if the patient's condition deteriorates or a suctioning route is needed.

BIBLIOGRAPHY

AARC Clinical Practice Guideline: Application of continuous positive airway pressure to neonates via nasal prongs or nasopharyngeal tube, *Respir Care* 39:817, 1994.

AARC Clinical Practice Guideline: Application of continuous positive airway pressure to neonates via nasal prongs, nasopharyngeal tube, or nasal mask: 2004 revision and update, *Respir Care* 49(9):1100, 2004.

AARC Clinical Practice Guideline: Humidification during mechanical ventilation, *Respir Care* 37:887, 1992.

AARC Clinical Practice Guideline: Neonatal time-triggered, pressure-limited, time-cycled, mechanical ventilation, *Respir Care* 39:808, 1994.

AARC Clinical Practice Guideline: Patient-ventilator system checks, *Respir Care* 37:882, 1992.

AARC Clinical Practice Guideline: Surfactant replacement therapy, *Respir Care* 39:824, 1994.

AARC Clinical Practice Guideline: Ventilator circuit changes, *Respir Care* 39:797, 1994.

Aloan CA, Hill TV: *Respiratory care of the newborn and child,* ed 2, Philadelphia, 1997, Lippincott-Raven.

Avery ME, Tooley WH, Keller JB, et al: Is chronic lung disease in low birth weight infants preventable? A survey of eight centers, *Pediatrics* 79:26, 1987.

Barnhart SL, Czervinske MP: *Perinatal and pediatric respiratory care,* Philadelphia, 1995, WB Saunders.

Boros SJ, Matalon SV, Ewald R, et al: The effect of independent variations in inspiratory-expiratory ratio and end expiratory pressure during mechanical ventilation in hyaline membrane disease: the significance of mean airway pressure, *J Pediatr* 91:794, 1981.

Branson RD, Hess DR, Chatburn RL: *Respiratory care equipment,* ed 2, Philadelphia, 1999, Lippincott Williams & Wilkins.

Burgess WR, Chernick V: *Respiratory therapy in newborn infants and children,* ed 2, New York, 1986, Thieme.

Cairo JM, Pilbeam SP: *Mosby's respiratory care equipment,* ed 7, St Louis, 2004, Mosby.

Carlo WA, Martin RJ: *Principles of neonatal assisted ventilation,* Pediatr Clin North Am 33:221, 1986.

Cavanagh K: High frequency ventilation of infants: an analysis of the literature, *Respir Care* 35:815, 1990.

Chang DW: *Clinical application of mechanical ventilation,* ed 2, Albany, NY, 2001, Delmar.

Chatburn RL: High frequency ventilation: a report on a state of the art symposium, *Respir Care* 29:839, 1984.

Chatburn RL: Principles and practice of neonatal and pediatric mechanical ventilation, *Respir Care* 36:569, 1991.

Chatburn RL, Lough MD: Mechanical ventilation. In Lough MD, Doershuk CF, Stern RC, editors: *Pediatric respiratory therapy,* ed 3, St Louis, 1985, Mosby.

Chatburn RL, Waldemar AC, Lough MD: Clinical algorithm for pressure-limited ventilation of neonates with respiratory distress syndrome, *Respir Care* 28:1579, 1983.

Coghill CH, Haywood JL, Chatburn RL, Carlo WA: Neonatal and pediatric high-frequency ventilation: principles and practice, *Respir Care* 36:596, 1991.

Gagnon C, Simoes J: The management of the mechanically ventilated infant receiving pancuronium bromide (Pavulon), *Neonat Netw* 4:20-24, 1985.

Goldberg RN, Bancalari E: Bronchopulmonary dysplasia: clinical presentation and the role of mechanical ventilation, *Respir Care* 31:591, 1986.

Goldberg RN, Bancalari E: Therapeutic approaches to the infant with bronchopulmonary dysplasia, *Respir Care* 36:613, 1991.

Goldsmith JP, Karotkin EH: *Assisted ventilation of the neonate,* ed 2, Philadelphia, 1996, WB Saunders.

Hess DR, Kacmarek RM: *Essentials of mechanical ventilation,* New York, 1996, McGraw-Hill.

HIFI Study Group: High-frequency oscillatory ventilation compared with conventional mechanical ventilation in the treatment of respiratory failure in preterm infants, 320:88, 1989.

Jobe A: Surfactant treatment for respiratory distress syndrome, *Respir Care* 31:467, 1986.

Koff PB, Eitzman DV, Neu J: *Neonatal and pediatric respiratory care,* ed 2, St Louis, 1993, Mosby.

MacIntyre NR, Branson RD: *Mechanical ventilation,* Philadelphia, 2001, WB Saunders.

Milner AD, Hoskyns EW: High frequency positive pressure ventilation in neonates, *Arch Dis Child* 64:1, 1989.

Miyagawa CI: Sedation of the mechanically ventilated patient in the intensive care unit, *Respir Care* 32:792, 1987.

Nicks JJ, Becker MA: High-frequency ventilation of the newborn: past, present, and future, *Respir Ther* 4(4), 1991.

Pilbeam SP: *Mechanical ventilation: physiological and clinical applications,* ed 3, St Louis, 1998, Mosby.

Schmidt JM: Nitric oxide therapy in neonates: adding to the arsenal, *Respir Ther* 7:37, 1994.

Smith I: The impact of surfactant on neonatal intensive care unit management, *Respir Ther* 4(4):22-26, 1991.

Spear ML, Spitzer AR, Fox WW: Hyperventilation therapy for persistent pulmonary hypertension of the newborn, *Perinatol/Neonat* 9:27, 1985.

Tobin MJ: What should the clinician do when a patient "fights the ventilator"? *Respir Care* 36:395, 1991.

Whitaker K: *Comprehensive perinatal and pediatric respiratory care,* ed 3, Albany, NY, 2001, Delmar.

White GC: *Equipment theory for respiratory care,* ed 4, Albany, NY, 2005, Delmar.

SELF-STUDY QUESTIONS

1. A neonate younger than 72 hours old with pulmonary problems should have his PaO_2 kept in the _____ range on the lowest inspired oxygen level.
   - A. 40–45 torr
   - B. 45–50 torr
   - C. 60–70 torr
   - D. 80–90 torr

2. If CPAP is administered through an endotracheal tube, the child should be extubated when the CPAP pressure is:
   - A. 0–2 cm water
   - B. 2–3 cm water
   - C. 4–6 cm water
   - D. 6–8 cm water

3. If you observe that your patient has apnea spells leading to bradycardia, you should:
   - A. Start CPAP.
   - B. Start mechanical ventilation.
   - C. Start an aerosolized bronchodilator.
   - D. End CPAP.

4. The time to switch a patient from CPAP to mechanical ventilation is indicated by:
   - I. CPAP of 8 to 10 cm water with a resulting PaO_2 of less than 50 torr
   - II. FIO_2 of 0.8 or more resulting in a PaO_2 of less than 50 torr
   - III. $PaCO_2$ of greater than 60 torr
     - A. I
     - B. II
     - C. I and II
     - D. I, II, and III

5. Identify the rationale for the use of pressure-limiting or "square wave ventilation":
   - I. It increases the $PaCO_2$.
   - II. It reduces the peak pressure.
   - III. It decreases the PaO_2.
   - IV. It increases the patient's oxygenation.
   - V. No change is seen in the patient's $PaCO_2$.
     - A. I, II, and III
     - B. I and III
     - C. I, II, and IV
     - D. II, IV, and V

6. An actively moving neonate is receiving 8 cm water CPAP by nasal prongs with 40% oxygen at a flow

of 4 L/min. It is noticed that the CPAP pressure is variable between 4 and 8 cm water. What is the most likely cause of this?
   A. The patient is taking more shallow breaths.
   B. The patient's breathing rate has decreased.
   C. There is a leak when the neonate turns its head.
   D. Someone has accidentally changed the oxygen percentage.

7. Hyperventilation is recommended in which of the following types of patients?
   A. Meconium aspiration
   B. PPHN
   C. RDS
   D. Infant with normal lung compliance

8. Increasing the pressure limit on the ventilator increases the patient's risk of:
   A. ROP
   B. Oxygen toxicity
   C. Pneumothorax
   D. Tracheoesophageal fistula

9. You are taking care of a newborn who has aspirated meconium. You would recommend which of the following ventilator settings:
   A. I:E of 1:2
   B. I:E of 2:1
   C. I:E of 1:4
   D. I:E of 1:1

10. Given the following choices, which would you select to increase the Pao_2 in a neonate on a standard pressure-limited type ventilator?
   I. Increase inspiratory time.
   II. Increase the pressure limit if it is reached.
   III. Decrease flow.
   IV. Increase PEEP.
   V. Decrease the IMV rate.
   A. I and V
   B. II and III
   C. III and IV
   D. I, II, and IV

11. If you increase PEEP without increasing the pressure limit by the same amount, the patient's:
   A. Minute volume will increase.
   B. Tidal volume will decrease.
   C. $Paco_2$ will decrease.
   D. Tidal volume will increase.

12. A premature neonate with a low Apgar score is demonstrating hypoxemia, intercostals retractions, and expiratory grunting noises. What is the best way to correct these problems?
   A. Nebulize albuterol.
   B. Suction the neonate.
   C. Instill surfactant into the airway.
   D. Give supplemental oxygen.

13. All of the following are indications for HFV *except*:
   A. Cleft palate before surgical correction
   B. PPHN
   C. RDS unresponsive to conventional ventilation
   D. Mechanical ventilation patient with unresolved pneumothorax

14. High frequency oscillatory ventilation is being used with a neonate with RDS. The following settings are in use: 50% oxygen, rate 700/min, amplitude 10 cm water, 4 cm water PEEP. The patient's $Paco_2$ is 52 torr. What should be recommended to correct the carbon dioxide level?
   A. Increase the amplitude.
   B. Decrease the amplitude.
   C. Increase the PEEP level.
   D. Increase the inspiratory time.

15. A premature newborn is becoming progressively more hypoxic and tachypneic despite being in an oxyhood with 50% oxygen. The decision is made to begin CPAP. What initial pressure should the respiratory therapist recommend?
   A. 0–2 cm water
   B. 2–3 cm water
   C. 4–5 cm water
   D. 6–8 cm water

ANSWER KEY

1. **C.** Rationale: A Pao_2 in the range of 60 to 70 torr is adequate for a newborn infant. Less would result in unnecessary hypoxemia. A higher value is not needed. See Table 16-1 for all blood gas recommendations.

2. **B.** Rationale: Extubation is performed with a CPAP level of 2 cm water because this small amount of pressure is used to maintain the neonate's normal FRC. A lower CPAP pressure while intubated would result in loss of FRC and possibly hypoxemia. If a higher CPAP level is needed to treat a clinical problem, the patient should not be extubated.

3. **B.** Rationale: CPAP does not provide ventilation to support a patient with apnea spells. Mechanical ventilation is indicated to support the patient's breathing when apnea spells leading to bradycardia are present. An aerosolized bronchodilator does not affect a patient in a way that corrects apnea.

4. **D.** Rationale: All three listed items are indications to change from CPAP to mechanical ventilation. A neonatal patient who is receiving 8 to 10 cm water CPAP and 80% oxygen and who is still hypoxemic should have mechanical ventilation started.

5. **D.** Rationale: Pressure-limited "square wave ventilation" is widely accepted as the standard way to ventilate the majority of neonatal patients because it: (1) limits the peak pressure to a predetermined safe level, (2) increases the patient's oxygenation by maintaining the peak pressure for the duration of the inspiratory time, and (3) can be adjusted without affecting the patient's carbon dioxide level.

6. **C.** Rationale: A variable CPAP pressure indicates a leak in the system—in this case, most likely with the fit of the CPAP prongs into the neonate's nostrils. Smaller tidal volume or decreased respiratory rate should not have any effect on the CPAP level. The flow through the system should be the same without regard for the oxygen percentage set on the blender.

7. **B.** Rationale: It has been clinically shown that hyperventilation of the patient with PPHN causes pulmonary vasodilation. This improves the patient's condition by allowing more blood to pass through the pulmonary circulation to be oxygenated. Hyperventilation has not been shown to improve the other listed conditions.

8. **C.** Rationale: Increasing the pressure limit on the ventilator increases the patient's tidal volume. This increased pressure and tidal volume can increase the risk of lung tissues being torn. This can result in a pneumothorax or other types of barotrauma or volutrauma. ROP is a complex condition related to prematurity and frequent swings in the patient's arterial blood oxygen and carbon dioxide levels. Oxygen toxicity is related to the patient inhaling a high percentage of oxygen for a prolonged period. A tracheoesophageal fistula can be the result of a developmental defect or caused by tissue damage from an endotracheal tube and nasogastric tube.

9. **C.** Rationale: When meconium is aspirated, it causes a serious airway obstruction problem. Because of this, additional time is needed for the patient's tidal volume to be exhaled; therefore select the longest expiratory time possible.

10. **D.** Rationale: Increased inspiratory time keeps the alveoli open longer to improve oxygenation. If the pressure limit is increased, a larger tidal volume will be delivered, and oxygenation will be improved. Additional PEEP increases the patient's FRC and improves oxygenation. If flow is decreased, the tidal volume will be decreased. This results in the oxygen level decreasing. Decreasing the ventilator IMV rate decreases the patient's minute volume. This results in the oxygen level decreasing.

11. **B.** Rationale: The patient's tidal volume is determined by the difference between the pressure limit and PEEP level. If the PEEP is increased without increasing the pressure limit, the difference between them decreases, and the tidal volume decreases (see Fig. 16-8). Minute volume decreases, not increases, if the difference between the pressure limit and PEEP level is decreased. The patient's $PaCO_2$ increases, not decreases, if the tidal volume and minute volume decrease. Tidal volume decreases, not increases, when the difference between pressure limit and PEEP decreases.

12. **C.** Rationale: The neonate is premature with signs of respiratory distress syndrome (RDS). The best way to improve the patient's lung compliance and function is to administer exogenous surfactant. Albuterol has no effect on lung compliance. No signs are noted of secretions that need to be suctioned out. Although supplemental oxygen may help to correct the hypoxemia, it does nothing to correct the fundamental problem caused by RDS.

13. **A.** Rationale: An oral or nasal endotracheal tube is inserted into a patient's airway before a cleft palate is surgically repaired; a standard neonatal ventilator is used if needed. No special reason exists to use HFV. Patients with all of the other clinical situations have been shown to benefit by HFV.

14. **A.** Rationale: With HFO, the amplitude is directly related to the tidal volume, so increasing amplitude will increase the patient's tidal volume and reduce the $PaCO_2$. Decreasing the amplitude would have the opposite effect. Increasing PEEP would reduce the difference between the PEEP level and the amplitude (peak pressure). This would reduce the patient's tidal volume. The I:E ratio probably has little impact, in this situation, on the patient's carbon dioxide level.

15. **C.** Rationale: It is common clinical practice to begin CPAP at 4 to 5 cm water pressure. Less than this is not likely to improve the patient's condition significantly. An initial CPAP of 6 to 8 cm water may not be needed to improve oxygenation and may result in cardiopulmonary complications. It is safer to start at 4 to 5 cm water, assess the patient, and determine whether more CPAP is needed.

17

Home Care and Pulmonary Rehabilitation

Note 1: The National Board for Respiratory Care (NBRC) has released the *RRT Examination Matrix* (covering the testable items on the Written Registry Exam) and the *CSE Examination Matrix* (covering the testable items on the Clinical Simulation Exam). Turn to the appendices at the back of this book for both publications in their original formats. This book is intended to cover all of the testable items in these two publications. This chapter (and all others) uses the abbreviation "WRE" for the coded items testable on the Written Registry Exam *and* Clinical Simulation Exam. The listed difficulty (R, Recall; Ap, Application; An, Analysis) relates to the question difficulty on the Written Registry Exam. The abbreviation "CSE" is used for the coded items testable on *only* the Clinical Simulation Exam. Because no question difficulty level is given for this exam, be prepared for anything.

Note 2: A review of the most recent Written Registry Examinations has shown an average of five questions (5% of the exam) that cover home care or pulmonary rehabilitation. The Clinical Simulation Exam is comprehensive and may include everything that should be known or performed by an advanced level respiratory therapist.

MODULE A
Patient and family teaching

1. Explain the planned therapy and goals to the patient in understandable terms to achieve optimal therapeutic outcomes (WRE code: IIIK1) [Difficulty: An]

Determining the patient's ideal therapeutic goals is best done with a team approach. The patient's physician, nurse, and respiratory therapist should work together. The first consideration should be the patient's diagnosis. Next, determine whether the patient's condition is permanent, improving, or worsening. Objective information such as arterial blood gas results, pulmonary function testing results, chest radiographs, sputum production, and vital signs must be evaluated. The patient cannot be expected to do more than he or she is physically capable of. It is also important to evaluate the patient's mental state. Is he or she emotionally ready to go home and be taught about self-care or start a rehabilitation program? Each patient's therapeutic goals must be individualized. If the patient is not physically or emotionally ready to take

care of himself or herself, the family or a paid care provider is needed.

The patient and family must understand the therapeutic goals and how they are to be achieved. Effective teaching methods include the following:

a. Speak at the patient's and family's level of understanding. Medical language usually reserved for peer discussions is not understandable to people without a medical background, yet using overly simple explanations can be insulting to someone who is intelligent or well educated or both. In either case, the important information will not be perceived as intended. Give the patient written instructions as needed.

b. Frequently ask the patient and family whether they have any questions, and then answer them.

c. Have the patient and family explain back to you in their own words how they understand what you just described.

d. Have the patient and family demonstrate back to you all procedures and techniques.

e. Reteach anything that is misunderstood.

f. Retest the patient and family as needed.

g. Document in the patient's chart what has been instructed.

2. Counsel the patient and family about the importance of smoking cessation (WRE code: IIIK3) [Difficulty: An]

Absolute proof exists that smoking causes emphysema, chronic bronchitis, lung cancer, and heart disease. These conditions occur in the smoker who directly inhales the smoke as well as in the nonsmoking spouse and children from secondhand smoke. Asthmatics often find that their bronchospasm is worsened when they inhale tobacco smoke. Obviously it is important that any patient with a smoking-related cardiopulmonary disease cease smoking. The patient's family must also stop smoking. Continued exposure to tobacco smoke harms the patient.

Because the nicotine found in tobacco is highly addictive, many patients find that they cannot stop smoking without having withdrawal symptoms such as agitation and craving for a cigarette. To aid in stopping smoking, it is often helpful to meet with a group of people who also are trying to stop. This group support helps the patient feel less alone in his or her efforts to stop smoking. The patient's physician also must be involved in this process.

If the patient has been unable to stop smoking because of withdrawal symptoms, it is likely that he or she is addicted to nicotine. A nicotine replacement system that allows gradual withdrawal greatly aids in smoking cessation. Although no smoking cessation plan works in every case, the highest percentage of patients are able to stop smoking if they have a combination of psychological support and a gradual reduction in nicotine.

Several well-established nicotine replacement and reduction systems currently exist. All are available without prescription. The Commit lozenge is held in the mouth to release a controlled amount of nicotine. Nicotine polacrilex (Nicorette) is a gum that is chewed by the patient to release a dose of nicotine. The Nicotrol Inhaler allows the user to inhale nicotine through a device shaped like a cigarette. Nicotine transdermal patches are another nicotine reduction system. Prostep, Nicoderm, and Habitrol are three brands of patches that, when placed onto the skin, allow a set amount of nicotine to be absorbed. With these systems, the patient starts with a relatively high dose of the drug and, over a period of weeks, goes through a series of patches with less and less nicotine. It is critical that the patient not smoke while using one of these systems. Patients who continue to smoke run the risk of a nicotine overdose, which increases the risk of a myocardial infarction.

A third option is taking the drug Zyban (bupropion HCl). It was originally found helpful in the care of patients with depression and also acts to alter the brain's chemistry so that nicotine craving is reduced. A physician must prescribe it.

Some patients experience problems with nicotine replacement and reduction systems. The transdermal patch can cause skin irritation. If this happens, the patch should be moved to another site. Some patients report insomnia or strange dreams while taking replacement nicotine at night. Patients with this problem should remove the patch before sleeping.

Exam Hint

Most past examinations have had a question related to recommending a nicotine replacement system to a patient wishing to stop smoking or possible side effects of the nicotine system.

3. Counsel the patient and family about disease management (WRE code: IIIK2) [Difficulty: An]

The respiratory therapist should have a solid understanding of the pathophysiology of the commonly found

cardiopulmonary and cardiovascular conditions. This includes, but is not limited to asthma, emphysema, chronic bronchitis, pneumonia, pulmonary fibrosis, cystic fibrosis, right and left heart failure, stroke, and neuromuscular diseases. Be prepared to teach the patient and family about the patient's disease, its cause, and its medical management.

MODULE B
Home respiratory care services

1. Interview the patient to determine the presence of dyspnea or orthopnea or both, increased work of breathing, and sputum production (WRE code: IB4b) [Difficulty: An]

It is very likely that all of the patients receiving home respiratory care services will have at least one of these issues. Review the discussion of each in Chapter 1, as needed.

2. Interview the patient to determine what his or her family and social life is like (WRE code: IB4c) [Difficulty: An]

The home environment is an important consideration in discharge planning with the patient and family. Barriers to the patient's mobility and complete recovery must be identified so that they can be eliminated or minimized. Ideally, the patient's home environment is determined by visiting the patient's home; however, the following questions also can be asked in the hospital:

a. How many floors does your home have?
b. Do you have to go up a set of stairs to get into your home?
c. Is your bedroom on the main floor?
d. If your bedroom is upstairs, can it be relocated to a room on the main floor?
e. If your bedroom were relocated to the main floor, would it be easy for you to get to a bathroom and the kitchen?
f. Does anyone who lives with you smoke?
g. Is there anything else in or around your home that puts smoke or dust into the air?

The answers to these types of questions may lead to other questions about the patient's home environment. Think of the patient's disease or condition and the answers that are given to determine a discharge plan that minimizes any inconveniences or barriers.

The patient's family and social life is an important consideration in discharge planning with the patient and family. Whether the patient is an adult or a child, it is important to know about his or her home life. Probably no one knows more about the patient or cares more about his or her well-being than the immediate family. Very close friends can assist the family or even replace a nonexistent one. The following questions can be asked of an adult patient and family:

a. Is your spouse able to help you at home?

b. Do you have other family members who can help you at home?

c. Can neighbors or family friends help you at home?

d. Do you belong to any clubs or church? Can you get to them?

e. Do you garden, have a pet, or have any hobbies at your home?

f. Have you smoked? If yes, for how long? How many packs of cigarettes a day?

g. Have you used illegal drugs? What have you used? For how long?

The following questions can be asked of the family of a minor child:

a. Do both parents live at home? If not, with whom does the child live? Do both parents care for the child?

b. Can any siblings help care for the child?

c. Do you have other family members who can help you care for the child at home?

d. Can neighbors or family friends help you care for the child at home?

e. Does the child belong to any clubs or church? Can you get the child to them? Can they help you care for the child at home?

f. Can you get the child to and from school?

The answers to these types of questions may lead you to think of other questions about the patient's family and social life. Think of the patient's disease or condition and the answers that are given to determine a discharge plan that minimizes any disturbances in family life.

3. Examine the patient's home and recommend how it can be modified to ensure safety and meet infection control standards (CSE code: IIIF2c)

Evaluate the following aspects of the patient's home environment:

a. Does the patient live alone or have a spouse or companion to help provide care? Make sure that telephone numbers to relatives, helpful neighbors, the patient's physician, ambulance service, local hospital, pharmacy, and any other support services are posted by each telephone.

b. Make sure that all respiratory care equipment is cleaned (see Chapter 2 for suggestions on methods of disinfection) and functioning properly.

c. Check that home oxygen systems are working properly. If the patient has an oxygen concentrator, make sure that the filters are cleaned and that the alarms are set and working. Make sure that an oxygen cylinder, regulator, and oxygen delivery system are working properly as a backup system if the oxygen concentrator fails.

d. Have the patient centrally locate all necessary items for daily living. The patient should avoid unnecessary stair climbing. It might be recommended that the patient convert the living room, if it is located near the kitchen and bathroom, into a bedroom. Clothing can be modified with Velcro fasteners, snaps, or zippers if the patient cannot use buttons easily. Shoes can be put on more easily with a long-handled shoehorn. Avoid shoes with laces. A long-handled comb or brush makes grooming easier.

e. The kitchen should be modified so that all commonly used equipment is on the counter. Everyday dishes, utensils, and foods should be placed so that they can be easily reached in cabinets and drawers within an arm's reach. The patient should not have to bend over, stoop down, or climb onto a footstool to get anything that is needed.

f. The bathroom may have to have handholds added to the walls by the toilet and shower or tub for extra security when using these facilities. A shower chair can be added so that the patient can sit while bathing. A hand-held shower head might make bathing easier.

g. Check the home for airborne irritants. Smoking by the patient or anyone else in the home must be stopped. The patient should avoid contact with other forms of indoor pollution such as aerosol sprays, paints, varnishes, dust, and so forth. A high-efficiency particulate air (HEPA) filtration system is best for removing indoor airborne pollutants and irritants. Indoor kerosene-fueled space heaters should not be used because they release carbon monoxide.

h. The patient should avoid contact with any known allergens, people who smoke, or substances to which he or she has a bad reaction.

4. Modify respiratory care procedures for use in the home (CSE code: IIIF2d)

5. Monitor and maintain all respiratory care equipment used in the home (CSE code: IIIF2a)

Home care equipment is essentially the same as that found in any hospital. The same types of equipment problems can occur in the patient's home as in the hospital. Those who wish to learn more about specific brands of home care equipment are referred to the several excellent books that discuss respiratory care equipment or the manufacturer's literature. Review, if necessary, the respiratory care procedures presented in this or other respiratory care books because they can be performed in the home care setting as well as in the hospital.

BOX 17-1 Guidelines for Starting and Stopping Home Apnea Monitoring

INDICATIONS TO START HOME APNEA MONITORING

Infant has had one or more apparent life-threatening apnea events.

Infant is preterm and symptomatic of apnea.

Infant is a sibling of two or more SIDS victims.

Infant has central nervous system–based hypoventilation.

INDICATIONS TO STOP HOME APNEA MONITORING

Two to three months have passed without a significant number of alarms.

Two to three months have passed without an apnea episode.

Infant can tolerate stress of illnesses (e.g., nasopharyngitis) or immunizations (e.g., diphtheria-pertussis-tetanus [DPT]) without apnea episodes.

SIDS, Sudden infant death syndrome.

6. Apnea monitoring

a. Perform apnea monitoring (WRE code: IB7i) [Difficulty: Ap, An]

Apnea monitoring is indicated in an infant who has documented periods of apnea of prematurity resulting from an immature central nervous system. This condition is most commonly seen in infants younger than 35 weeks' gestational age. The usual monitoring guidelines include apneic periods that last longer than 20 seconds and are associated with bradycardia with a heart rate of less than 100 beats/min. Hypoxemia is often demonstrated by cyanosis, pallor, or documented desaturation through pulse oximetry. In addition, the infant may show marked limpness, choking, or gagging. Other conditions such as intracranial hemorrhage, patent ductus arteriosus, upper airway obstruction, hypermagnesemia, infection, maternal narcotic agents, and so forth should be ruled out before apnea of prematurity is confirmed. If this is the infant's problem, it is usually outgrown by the time the infant is 40 weeks' postconceptional age. Home apnea monitoring is not indicated in normal infants, in preterm infants without symptoms of apnea, or to test for sudden infant death syndrome (SIDS). See Box 17-1 for guidelines on starting and stopping home apnea monitoring.

Apnea monitors currently in use sense respiratory efforts through the changing electrical impedance measured through the chest wall as the infant breathes. Impedance is resistance to the flow of electricity through the skin and other organs. The monitor sends out a small, constant electrical current that results in a voltage across the two electrodes on the infant's chest. As the infant breathes and the chest wall expands and contracts, a resulting change in voltage occurs. This fluctuation is measured and interpreted as inhalation and exhalation. Similarly, smaller voltage changes are measured with each heart beat. This is measured and interpreted as the heart rate.

The following are desirable features on a home apnea monitor: (1) ability to store and display events for later analysis, (2) identification of breathing patterns and apnea periods, (3) identification of heart rate patterns, (4) estimation of tidal volume, and (5) identification of hypoxemia by pulse oximetry. Setting up a home apnea monitor involves placing the electrodes properly on the infant's chest, turning on the monitor, and setting the proper high and low limits for the alarms.

Two electrodes are usually placed where the greatest amount of movement occurs during breathing. Most often, this is on the infant's upper chest between the nipples and armpits (Fig. 17-1). With older infants, the electrodes might have to be placed on the sides over the lower ribs. Occasionally one electrode is placed on the chest and the other on the infant's abdomen. Some monitoring systems require that a Velcro belt be placed around the infant over the electrodes to keep them in place. (Obviously this works only if both electrodes are on the chest.) Other systems make use of electrodes with an adhesive. In either case, for best results, the infant's chest should be washed with mild soap and water and dried before the electrodes are placed. This results in the best electrical conduction. Do not use baby oils, lotions, or powders over the electrode sites. Attach the lead wires to the electrodes. These connect to the patient cable that is then connected to the monitor. Occasionally static electricity causes some interference with the signal. A third chest electrode is then added to act as a ground wire.

TRANSDUCER   CONDITIONER   DISPLAY

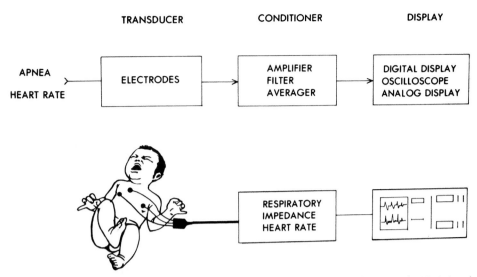

Fig. 17-1 Block diagram for impedance apnea and heart rate monitor. *(From Lough MD. In Lough MD, Williams TJ, Rawson JE, editors:* Newborn respiratory care, *St Louis, 1979, Mosby.)*

The monitor should be plugged into a working electrical outlet and turned on. Set the unit to charge the internal battery so that it can be made portable for later use. Confirm that the infant's respiratory and heart rates are being sensed and displayed. If pulse oximetry is a feature on the unit, the probe should be properly placed on the infant, and an SpO_2 value should be displayed. Set the high and low alarm values according to the physician's orders or established protocols. For example:

1. Set the apnea alarm to trigger after 20 seconds.
2. Set the low heart rate alarm to trigger if the heart rate is less than 100 beats/min.
3. If available, set the pulse oximeter alarm to trigger if the SpO_2 decreases to less than 90%.
4. If available, set the high heart rate alarm to trigger if the heart rate is greater than 150 beats/min.

Multiple alarms provide for a greater margin of patient safety. They also indicate what physiologically deteriorates first in the infant. These backup alarm systems are important because the apnea monitor senses chest wall movement, not air movement. It is possible for the infant to have an upper airway obstruction and continue to make breathing attempts; therefore the apnea monitor will not alarm because the chest wall is moving. The bradycardia or desaturation alarms will signal that the infant is in trouble.

It is critically important that the parent(s) know about the infant's medical condition. They need to understand how the monitor functions and what to do if the alarms go off. They should demonstrate their knowledge of the monitor's functions and be given written instructions on it. The parents should not be more than 10 seconds away from the infant at any time, which means that the infant will not be apneic for more than 30 seconds (20 seconds alarm delay and 10 seconds for the parents to respond).

The parents must know how to give tactile stimulation to the infant, use the manual resuscitator, call for emergency help, and perform infant cardiopulmonary resuscitation.

b. Interpret apnea monitoring results (CSE code: IB8g)

Alarm situations fall into two basic categories: patient alarms and equipment alarms. Patient alarms mean that the infant either is apneic, has a heart rate below or above an acceptable level, or is desaturated. One, any two, or all three alarms may be triggered. Other than the audible alarm, a visual alarm flashes to show the problem(s), and the recording device keeps track of the events. The parents should be instructed first to care for the infant, and then, when the infant is back to normal, the alarms can be reset.

Three types of equipment alarms are found: electrode or lead problem, low battery, or monitor failure. The unit should have different visual and audible alarms for equipment failure so that the family does not mistakenly think that the infant is in trouble. An electrode or lead problem alarm usually occurs because the electrode came off of the infant or the lead became disconnected. The family should be taught how to fix these types of problems. A low battery alarm indicates that not much time is left for the monitor to function on battery power. The family should be instructed to plug the monitor into a functioning electrical outlet, and the unit should be set to recharge the battery. A monitor failure alarm indicates a serious internal problem with the monitor. It is not functioning properly and should not be used. The family should be instructed to observe the infant continuously and call the home care company for a replacement monitor.

Apnea monitors in current use record and store the alarm situations discussed previously. The information can usually be downloaded into a computer for a visual display of breathing and heart rate patterns, equipment problems, and the dates and times of their occurrences. The therapist or physician should review all this data to determine what kinds of problems the patient had.

MODULE C
Pulmonary rehabilitation

1. Interview the patient to determine how much exercise he or she can tolerate and how active the patient is on a daily basis (WRE code: IB4b) [Difficulty: An]

The following subject areas and questions will help you to further determine the patient's exercise tolerance and activities of daily living (ADLs):

Personal grooming
  a. Do you get short of breath when dressing?
  b. What is the most difficult part of dressing?
  c. Are you able to wash your hair regularly?
  d. Are you (men) able to shave regularly?
  e. Does using extra oxygen help you to do these things without getting as short of breath?

In-home activities
  a. Can you go up and down stairs without getting short of breath?
  b. Can you walk through your home without getting short of breath?
  c. Can you cook or prepare nutritious meals?
  d. Does using extra oxygen help you to do these things without getting as short of breath?

Out-of-home activities
  a. Can you go shopping without getting short of breath?
  b. What clubs, church, and so forth do you attend regularly?
  c. Can you do yard or garden work?
  d. Do you have a pet dog that you walk through the neighborhood?
  e. Does using extra oxygen help you to do these things without getting as short of breath?

The patient with chronic and severe cardiopulmonary disease will tell you of a very restricted and limited lifestyle. Extra oxygen may have only a limited benefit. The patient with chronic, but moderate, cardiopulmonary disease is able to live a somewhat limited but full lifestyle. Extra oxygen may help greatly at times when the patient becomes short of breath. The otherwise healthy patient who has an acute cardiopulmonary disease should tell of a previously full and enjoyable lifestyle. Extra oxygen may be needed now but not on recovery.

2. Have the patient perform a 6-minute walk (CSE code: IB7f)

A 6-minute walk procedure involves the therapist having a patient walk as far as possible in 6 minutes. Before the walk is started, the therapist will instruct the patient about the procedure, assess the patient's vital signs, and check the pulse oximetry value. If supplemental oxygen is used by the patient, it will also be set up to be taken with the patient during the walk. The therapist will monitor the patient during the walk and after the 6-minute walk is competed. Often patients will need to rest, and even sit down, during the walk. After the walk is completed, the therapist will monitor the patient again. The total distance walked will be noted. All of this information is recorded in the patient's chart. As the patient makes progress in the pulmonary rehabilitation program, the 6-minute walk will be periodically repeated. An increasing 6-minute walk distance would indicate an increase in the patient's functional ability and that the rehabilitation program is succeeding. (Note: As the patient improves, the exercise goal may be changed to a 12-minute walk. The goal of the test is to determine how far the patient can walk in 12 minutes. All of the previous and following considerations apply as well.) The following information provides additional details of aspects of a pulmonary rehabilitation program.

The patient's physical condition must be evaluated before designing an exercise program. Besides chronic obstructive pulmonary disease (COPD), the patient may have other conditions that further limit his or her ability to safely participate in a rehabilitation program. See Box 17-2 for the suggested parameters to assess. If the patient is too ill or too limited in ability, he or she should not be placed into a rehabilitation program.

Although the patient's physical condition is the most important thing to evaluate from a safety point of view, other aspects of his or her life also must be reviewed. These include a nutritional evaluation, a psychosocial evaluation, and a vocational evaluation. Because these areas are beyond the scope of practice of most respiratory therapists, the physician must call in other experts. In addition, any patient who is still smoking must be enrolled in a smoking cessation program.

Similar to preparing a patient for home care, all aspects of the patient's physical condition information must be evaluated. Each patient must have an individualized program and be physically and emotionally prepared to begin the rehabilitation program. As discussed next, the patient is placed into either an open- or closed-end program format. The starting and ending points of the program are determined based on the patient's physical condition, heart rate target, and stress test results.

A graded exercise program is an individually structured sequence of events that is designed to safely increase the patient's exercise tolerance. It is a critical component of any pulmonary rehabilitation program. In 1942, the Council of Rehabilitation defined rehabilitation as "the restoration of the individual to the fullest medical, mental, emotional, social, and vocational

---

BOX 17-2 Patient Evaluation before Starting a Pulmonary Rehabilitation Program

History
Complete physical examination
Chest radiograph
Resting diagnostic electrocardiogram
Complete blood count
Serum electrolytes
Urinalysis
Arterial blood gases
Theophylline level
Sputum analysis
Pulmonary-function tests
  Spirometry
  Lung volume study
  Diffusion capacity
  Before and after bronchodilator study
Pulmonary stress test including
  Electrocardiogram
  Blood pressure
  Heart rate
  Respiratory rate
  Pulse oximetry
  Maximum ventilation
  Oxygen consumption
  Carbon dioxide production
  Respiratory quotient

See Chapter 4 for information on pulmonary function testing and Chapter 18 for information on cardiopulmonary stress testing.

BOX 17-3 Effects of Inactivity

METABOLISM
Decreased metabolic rate, decreased protein catabolism, negative nitrogen balance, decubitus ulcers, imbalance of cellular electrolytes, and gastrointestinal hypomotility

PSYCHOSOCIAL
Decreased learning ability, decreased motivation to learn, decreased retention of new material, decreased problem-solving ability, exaggerated or inappropriate emotional reactions, perceptual and motor changes, and increased somatic concerns

RESPIRATORY SYSTEM
Decreased movement of secretions, decreased use of respiratory muscles, and development of microatelectasis and infection

MUSCULAR SYSTEM
Loss of normal muscle tone, decreased muscle efficiency, increased local muscle oxygen consumption, rapid onset of fatigue, and contracture

CARDIOPULMONARY SYSTEM
Decreased cardiac output, venous stasis, thromboembolism, and pulmonary emboli

SKELETAL SYSTEM
Osteoporosis, reabsorption of calcium from the bone, and increased incidence of compression fractures

---

From May DF: *Rehabilitation and continuity of care in pulmonary disease,* St Louis, 1991, Mosby.

---

potential of which he/she is capable" (Hodgkin, 1993). In 1974, The American College of Chest Physicians' Committee on Pulmonary Rehabilitation adopted the following:

Pulmonary rehabilitation may be defined as an art of medical practice wherein an individually tailored, multidisciplinary program is formulated which through accurate diagnosis, therapy, emotional support, and education, stabilizes or reverses both the physio- and psychopathology of pulmonary diseases and attempts to return the patient to the *highest possible functional capacity* [italics added] allowed by his pulmonary handicap and overall life situation (Petty, 1975).

It further states: "In the broadest sense, pulmonary rehabilitation means providing good, comprehensive respiratory care for patients with pulmonary disease."

The patient with pulmonary disease who is inactive because of his or her condition experiences a slow deterioration in overall body function. It is well known that physical activity is important for general health. Box 17-3 lists the effects of inactivity.

The remainder of this discussion focuses on how to start a patient in a graded exercise program and to monitor his or her progress through it. (Note that the education of the patient about normal and abnormal lung function, respiratory care procedures, medications, and so forth is addressed in earlier sections of this book and in other textbooks dedicated solely to pulmonary rehabilitation.)

a. Benefits of an exercise program

The benefits of the exercise program must be stressed to the patient to gain his or her acceptance of it. If the patient does not believe that the program will make his or her life better, it will not be followed. In 1981, the American Thoracic Society Executive Committee adopted the following as principle objectives of pulmonary rehabilitation:

1. To control and alleviate as much as possible the symptoms and pathologic complications of respiratory ailments.
2. To teach the patient how to achieve optimal capability for carrying out his or her ADLs.

Most authors agree with the following general therapeutic goals:

1. The primary goal is to increase the patient's functional ability as much as possible. This can best be

determined by finding out what the patient wants to be able to do with his or her life on a daily basis. From this list of ADLs, a series of short- and long-term goals can be developed. One of the primary short-term goals should be that the patient feels better. He or she should be able to control or reduce any symptoms. This alone improves the patient's quality of life. Make sure that the patient's goals are realistic and can be reached. The family must be involved with any major decision making. Often it is helpful to break a large goal down into several smaller tasks so that the patient and family receive frequent positive feedback.

2. Improve the patient's self-image. This should follow when goal number one is reached. The patient should experience less anxiety and depression and also feel better about himself or herself.

3. Increase the patient's ability to exercise. This may depend on the level of the patient's disability. In general, the worse the patient's lung disease is, the less able the patient is to increase his or her exercise level.

4. Decrease the frequency and length of any hospitalizations.

5. Prolong the patient's life by the proper use of oxygen and other respiratory care modalities.

Note that the benefits did not list an improvement in the patient's cardiopulmonary condition. Numerous studies have documented that pathologic changes seen in COPD do *not* improve despite the patient being in a rehabilitation program. It is important that the therapist correct any misunderstanding of this.

Exam Hint

Past examinations have included one or two questions related to identifying the goals or benefits or both of a pulmonary rehabilitation program.

---

b. Individualized graded exercise program

The program format and features may vary considerably. Minimally, the patient's physician should specify four parts to the exercise prescription: mode, intensity, duration, and frequency. The following program formats and suggestions are typical of what might be ordered.

c. Program format

There are two basic types of formats. Each has its own advantages and disadvantages depending on what the patient's limitations and preferences may be. The *open-end format* allows the patient to enter and progress through the program at his or her own pace. Because each patient's goals are individualized, the time of their accomplishment is relatively unimportant as long as progress is being made. The program facilitator (often a respiratory

therapist) acts as a coordinator. This may include making sure that educational materials are available for the patient, exercise equipment is available, and the patient's questions are answered. The patient may stay in the program until the last goal is achieved. The advantages of this program are that it is self-directed and can be adjusted if the patient has a schedule conflict. The disadvantage of this program is that no group support or involvement with other people who have COPD is included.

The *closed-end format* involves the program facilitator setting up a formal schedule of educational topics and exercise sessions. These group events commonly last from 1 to 3 hours and may occur from 1 to 3 times per week. The whole program can vary in length from 8 to 16 weeks, depending on the content. These events are attended by a group of patients who share a common problem and have common goals to cope with. One major advantage of this program is that most patients do better when they have peers to call on for emotional support. The facilitator will probably find that it is easier to schedule speakers when a sure time frame can be set. The disadvantages of this program relate to the loss of individual goals and attention. If a patient misses a session, he or she will have to wait for the topic to be repeated at the next program. If the group is too large, the facilitator may not have time to help a patient with an individual goal.

d. Strength training

Many patients are so weak from years of relative inactivity that they must regain muscle strength before working on increased endurance. The specific muscle groups that need strengthening can be determined by physical examination. In general, the large muscle groups of the legs and arms and inspiratory muscles must be strengthened.

Before beginning strength training, the patient must perform calisthenics for about 10 minutes as a "warm-up." It is important to stretch the muscles and joints and increase circulation before starting more vigorous activity. See Fig. 17-2, groups 1 to 7, for a series of progressively more demanding calisthenic exercises. All patients should at least be able to perform the calisthenics shown in groups 1 and 2 for a warm-up. The patient must focus on breath control (pursed-lips breathing) during the warm-up period to avoid dyspnea.

Arm and leg strengthening can be done in a variety of ways for about 10 minutes. Typically, a 1- or 2-lb weight is used. Barbell weights can be held as the arms are moved to the back, front, sides, and overhead to strengthen the arms, shoulders, and chest and back muscles. Ankle weights can be strapped on. The legs are then moved to the back, front, sides, and the legs lifted with knees bent, or the initial calisthenics can be repeated with added weight. The abdominal muscles can be strengthened by having the patient lie on his or her back and placing a 2-lb weight on the abdomen. The patient

Group 1 Exercises

Fig. 17-2 Modified calisthenic exercises. In all groups, the figure to the left is the starting point. The figures to the right show the sequence of steps in the exercise. The patient can adjust the pace of exercises to either increase or decrease the energy that is spent. In general, most patients choose 10 to 15 repetitions per minute. Exercises shown in groups 1 and 2 are useful during the warm-up period of either a strength or endurance program. Exercises shown in groups 3 and 4 are more demanding and can be used for muscle reconditioning by many patients in an endurance program. The most demanding exercises are those shown in groups 5, 6, and 7. Patients with only moderate disability may be able to progress to this level for further muscle conditioning. *(From May DF: Rehabilitation and continuity of care in pulmonary disease, St Louis, 1991, Mosby.)*

then concentrates on maintaining breath control against the added weight.

Inspiratory muscle strengthening is done in two ways. First, the patient is told to take in a deep sigh and hold it for a brief time. This both stretches the rib cage and increases the work load of the primary and secondary inspiratory muscles. The deep sigh should be repeated several times. Second, the patient uses a specific inspiratory muscle training device. The PFLEX device is popular because it is inexpensive and can be gradually adjusted to increase the work load as the patient improves. Review the discussion in Chapter 7 and see Fig. 7-1.

Finally, the patient should spend about 10 minutes in "cool-down" activities. This may involve more light calisthenics or slow walking. The cool-down period allows the body to return to a slower metabolic rate while still maintaining good circulation to the arms and legs. This helps to eliminate any lactic acid that might have built up in the muscles during the more vigorous exercise. Increased lactic acid may cause some muscle aches after exercise. Inform the patient that some muscle soreness may be felt the next day. It can be relieved by taking an anti-inflammatory medication such as aspirin if the physician approves. See Box 17-4 for specific guidelines for a strength training program.

Group 2 Exercises

Fig. 17-2, cont'd

It is helpful, but not necessary, for the patient to have access to professional body building equipment found in many gymnasiums. In addition, a physical therapist is helpful in designing a training program.

e. Endurance training

Endurance training is designed to build up the patient's stamina to perform essential ADLs. It does this by improving the functioning of the patient's cardiopulmonary and cardiovascular systems. When these systems are functioning better, they can meet the patient's need for increased oxygen delivery to and carbon dioxide removal from exercising muscles.

Endurance training must be preceded by the patient performing calisthenics for about 10 minutes as a warm-up. Just as in strength training, it is important to stretch the muscles and joints and increase circulation before starting more vigorous activity. See Fig. 17-2, groups 1 through 7, for a series of progressively more demanding calisthenic exercises. All patients should be able to at least perform the calisthenics shown in groups 1 and 2 for a warm-up.

Patients who can perform the activities shown in groups 3 and 4 gain some endurance training as well. Some very debilitated patients may not be able to perform at this higher level. Some less debilitated patients will eventually be able to advance to the highest levels. The patient must focus on breath control (pursed-lips breathing) during the warm-up period to avoid dyspnea.

The actual endurance exercise that is selected must meet the patient's needs. He or she can walk, use a treadmill, ride a bicycle ergometer, swim, or do a combination of these. The method that is selected must be both practical and fun for the patient. For this reason, walking is usually the main activity; however, the upper body should not

Group 3 Exercises

Fig. 17-2, cont'd

be ignored. An arm ergometer, rowing machine, or barbell weights can be used for upper-body endurance.

A key concept of the endurance program is that the patient must exercise at a level great enough to increase the heart rate to a predetermined level. The increased heart rate (HR) reflects the increased metabolic rate and work being performed by the patient. The target heart rate must be maintained for 20 to 30 minutes to have any muscle training effect. Exercising at a lower heart (and metabolic) rate is not as beneficial. Exercising at a higher heart rate may be dangerous to the patient. Karvonen's formula is used to determine the target heart rate for endurance training:

Target heart rate (HR) = (% intensity [maximum HR − resting HR]) + resting HR

In which:

Target HR = the target HR for the exercise period
% intensity = 60% to 80%

Maximum HR = maximum HR determined by either of the following formulas:
  a. Maximum HR = 220 − age of the patient
  b. Maximum HR = 210 − (age of the patient × 0.65)
  Resting HR = the patient's resting HR

EXAMPLE

Determine the target HR for a 50-year-old patient (of either sex) who is enrolled in an endurance training program. The patient has a resting HR of 80 beats/min. The

Group 4 Exercises

Fig. 17-2, cont'd

patient's maximum heart rate is 170 (220 − 50 for the patient's age = 170).

Target HR = (% intensity [maximum HR − resting HR]) + resting HR

Lowest target HR = (0.60 [170 − 80]) + 80

= 0.60 [90]) + 80

= (54) + 80

= 134 beats/min

Highest target HR = (0.80 [170 − 80]) + 80

= (0.80 [90]) + 80

= (72) + 80

= 152 beats/min

The range of target HRs for this patient is 134 to 152 beats/min. The patient must monitor his or her HR during the exercise period to make sure that it stays within this range. This is most easily accomplished by feeling the radial or carotid pulse and counting heartbeats for a 15-second period, and then multiplying by 4 to find the HR for 1 minute.

Finally, as in strength training, the patient should spend about 10 minutes in "cool-down" activities. This may involve light calisthenics or slow walking. As discussed earlier, the cool-down period allows the body to return to a slower metabolic rate while still maintaining good circulation to the arms and legs. This helps to eliminate any lactic acid that may have built up in the

Group 5 Exercises

Fig. 17-2, cont'd

muscles during the endurance exercise. See Box 17-4 for specific guidelines for an endurance training program.

f. Assessment of the patient's progress in the program

The following indicate that the patient is making progress:

1. The patient subjectively feels that he or she is doing as well as can be expected. The patient is motivated to try new things.
2. Symptoms are reduced or at least under control.
3. Cardiopulmonary function tests and blood gases show improvement. Even a slowing in the patient's former rapid rate of decline is a good sign.
4. The patient reports an increase in the distance that can be walked at his or her own pace.
5. The patient reports an increase in the 6-minute (or 12-minute) walk distance. The 6-minute (or 12-minute) walk is a measurement of how far a person can maximally walk in the given time period.

The following indicate that the patient's health is deteriorating:

1. He or she subjectively feels worse. The patient is afraid to try new things.
2. Symptoms are worse. The patient feels dyspneic at less exertion than before.
3. The sputum has changed. It may be thick and harder to cough out or have changed color to yellow or green. The patient may be coughing out more than before or less if it cannot be brought up.
4. Cardiopulmonary function tests and blood gases are worse. The patient may need more oxygen, an aerosolized bronchodilator, or other cardiopulmonary medications.

Group 6 Exercises

Fig. 17-2, cont'd

5. The patient cannot walk or perform as much work as before without having the symptoms worsen.

MODULE D
Respiratory care plan

1. **Analyze available information to determine the patient's pathophysiologic state (CSE code: IIIH1)**

Review the common cardiopulmonary conditions, as needed, in the previous chapters of this book or a specific pathology book.

2. **Determine the appropriateness of the prescribed therapy and goals for the identified pathophysiologic state (CSE code: IIIH3)**
   a. **Review the interdisciplinary patient and family care plan (WRE code: IIIH1b) [Difficulty: An]**
   b. **Review the planned therapy to establish the therapeutic plan (WRE code: IIIH1a) [Difficulty: An]**
   c. **Recommend changes in the therapeutic plan if supportive data exist (WRE code: IIIH2) [Difficulty: An]**

Group 7 Exercises

Fig. 17-2, cont'd

Review the appropriate discussion in the earlier chapters of this book or others.

d. Conduct disease management education programs (WRE code: IIIK2) [Difficulty: An]

The therapist should be able to implement a patient's disease management program. For example, the patient may have a home care program to manage emphysema, asthma, cystic fibrosis, or congestive heart failure. In addition, the therapist should monitor the patient's compliance with the program. For example, is the patient faithfully following the smoking cessation program, or has he or she "cheated"? Is the patient following the asthma control program by monitoring his or her peak flow and adjusting inhaled medications according to the physician's order?

BOX 17-4   Guidelines for Strength and Endurance Training

STRENGTH TRAINING

This involves a low number of repetitions of a high-intensity activity, such as lifting weights

Warm-up period involving calisthenics for about 10 min

The following strengthening program should last about 10 min:

  Three sets of 10 to 15 repetitions of an activity

  Each set is followed by a rest period of a few minutes

  The patient should work at 85% to 90% of the maximum capacity of the muscles being exercised

Cool-down period involving calisthenics for about 10 min

The patient should exercise every other day (for example, Monday, Wednesday, and Thursday)

This program may precede or be done simultaneously with an endurance program

It takes 4 to 8 weeks for improved strength to be realized

ENDURANCE TRAINING

This involves a high number of repetitions of a relatively low-intensity activity, such as walking

Warm-up period involving calisthenics for about 10 min

The patient should do the following:

  Exercise continuously for about 20 to 30 min

  Exercise at a level that results in the target heart rate being maintained

  Cool-down period involving calisthenics for about 10 min

The patient should exercise every other day (for example, Tuesday, Thursday, and Saturday)

This program may follow or be done simultaneously with a strength program

It takes 4 to 8 weeks for improved endurance to be realized

Modified from May DF: *Rehabilitation and continuity of care in pulmonary disease*, St Louis, 1991, Mosby.

---

e. Stop the treatment or procedure if the patient has an adverse reaction to it (CSE code: IIIF1)

The respiratory therapist should know the complications and hazards of any patient care activity that is performed. These were discussed in the previous chapters. Be prepared to stop the treatment or procedure if the patient has an adverse reaction to it. Additionally, be prepared to recommend to the physician that the treatment or procedure be discontinued if it is likely to result in additional adverse reactions.

f. Discontinue treatment based on the patient's response (WRE code: IIIG1e) [Difficulty: An]

Be prepared to recommend that a treatment or procedure be discontinued. See the previous chapters for discussion on when care procedures should be stopped.

3. Develop the outcomes of respiratory care protocols (WRE code: IIIH4b) [Difficulty: An]
4. Apply respiratory care protocols to patient care situations (WRE code: IIH6) [Difficulty: Ap]
5. Monitor the outcomes of respiratory care protocols (WRE code: IIIH5) [Difficulty: An]

Respiratory care protocols may be used at home as well as in the hospital. An oxygen therapy protocol can be implemented that uses the patient's pulse-oximetry values to adjust the oxygen percentage or flow up or down. For example, keep the patient's SpO_2 less than 95% but greater than 85%. A second protocol may be using inhaled sympathomimetic bronchodilators based on the patient's peak flow results.

The patient's physical condition must be evaluated before designing a home care or rehabilitation program. Besides the primary diagnosis, the patient may have other conditions that further limit his or her ability to participate safely. If the patient is too ill or too limited in ability, he or she should not be placed into a home care or rehabilitation program.

Although the patient's physical condition is the most important thing to evaluate from a safety point of view, other aspects of his or her life also must be reviewed. These include a nutritional evaluation, a psychosocial evaluation, and a vocational evaluation. Because these areas are beyond the scope of practice of most respiratory therapists, the physician must call in other experts.

Be prepared to evaluate the patient's condition and make suggestions for changing goals, methods, and so forth. The therapist must have a thorough understanding of the patient's condition and individual goals to evaluate his or her progress toward meeting them. Objectively consider the patient's physical, emotional, and social condition. The therapist also must listen to the patient's subjective opinion about his or her situation. Be prepared to make recommendations to the patient and attending physician for modifying the goals depending on the patient's changing condition.

6. Communicate the outcomes of therapy and change the therapy based on the protocol (WRE code: IIIA5) [Difficulty: An]

Inform the patient's nurse or physician and the supervising therapist if any serious question or problem occurs with the patient. Routine communication should occur as needed between these people and any other caregiver.

7. Record and evaluate the patient's response to the treatment(s) or procedure(s), including the following:
a. Record and interpret the following: heart rate and rhythm, respiratory rate, blood pressure, body temperature, and pain level (WRE code: IIIA1b, IIIA1c) [Difficulty: An]

b. **Record and interpret the patient's breath sounds (WRE code: IIIA1a) [Difficulty: An]**

c. **Record and interpret the type of cough the patient has and the nature of the sputum (WRE code: IIIA1a) [Difficulty: An]**

d. **Recheck any math work and make note of incorrect data (WRE code: IIIA2) [Difficulty: An]**

Review the previous chapters for relevant information on assessment as needed.

8. **Communicate information relevant to coordinating patient care and discharge planning (e.g., scheduling, avoiding conflicts, and sequencing of therapies) (WRE code: IIIA3) [Difficulty: An]**

Before the patient is discharged, it is vital that there be effective coordination between the hospital and the home care company. Typically, the discharge plan would include the following:

1. Patient evaluation that determines the patient is ready for discharge. The patient needs to have recovered sufficiently to leave the hospital.

2. Determination of the best place for the patient to go for further recovery and the necessary patient care resources. It must be determined whether the patient can go home or should go to an extended care facility. If the patient is to go home, it must be determined whether the family can provide the necessary care. If not, home care respiratory therapists and nurses will have to be arranged for.

3. Determination that the patient's financial resources are adequate. If not, social services will have to be contacted to work with the patient's insurance company or other financial support agencies.

BIBLIOGRAPHY

American Association for Respiratory Care: Clinical Practice Guideline: Oxygen therapy in the home or extended care facility, *Respir Care* 37:918, 1992.

American Association for Respiratory Care: Clinical Practice Guideline: Discharge planning for the respiratory care patient, *Respir Care* 40:1308, 1995.

American Association for Respiratory Care: Clinical Practice Guideline: Long-term invasive ventilation in the home, *Respir Care* 40:1313, 1995.

American Association for Respiratory Care: Clinical Practice Guideline: Providing patient and caregiver training, *Respir Care* 41:658, 1996.

American Association for Respiratory Care: Clinical practice guideline: Pulmonary rehabilitation, *Respir Care* 47(5):617, 2002.

American Association for Respiratory Care: Clinical Practice Guideline: Suctioning the patient in the home, *Respir Care* 44:99, 1999.

Bell CW, Blodgett D, Goike C, et al: *Home care and rehabilitation in respiratory medicine,* Philadelphia, 1984, Lippincott.

Belman MJ, Wasserman K: Exercise training and testing in patients with chronic obstructive pulmonary disease, *Basics Respir Dis* 10(2):1-6, 1981.

Branson RD, Hess DR, Chatburn RL: *Respiratory care equipment,* ed 2, Philadelphia, 1999, Lippincott Williams & Wilkins.

Cairo JM, Pilbeam, SP: *Mosby's respiratory care equipment,* ed 7, St Louis, 2004, Mosby.

Christopher KL: At-home administration of oxygen. In Kacmarek RM, Stoller JK, editors: *Current respiratory care,* Toronto, 1988, BC Decker.

Connors G, Hilling L, editors: *American Association of Cardiovascular and Pulmonary Rehabilitation: guidelines for pulmonary rehabilitation programs,* Champaign, Ill, 1993, Human Kinetics.

Des Jardins T, Burton GG: *Clinical manifestations and assessment of respiratory disease,* ed 4, St Louis, 2002, Mosby.

Dunlevy CL: Patient education and health promotion. In Scanlan CL, Wilkins RL, Stoller JK, editors: *Egan's fundamentals of respiratory care,* ed 7, St Louis, 1999, Mosby.

Edge RS: Infection control. In Barnes TA, editor: *Respiratory care practice,* St Louis, 1988, Mosby.

Eubanks DH, Bone RC: *Comprehensive respiratory care,* ed 2, St Louis, 1990, Mosby.

Farzan S, Farzan D: *A concise handbook of respiratory disease,* ed 4, Stamford, Conn, 1997, Appleton & Lange.

Gilmartin M: Transition from the intensive care unit to home: patient selection and discharge planning, *Respir Care* 39:456, 1994.

Gourley DA: Respiratory home care. In Wyka KA, Mathews PJ, Clark WF, editors: *Foundations of respiratory care,* Albany, NY, 2002, Delmar.

Heuer AJ, Scanlan CL: Respiratory care in alternate settings. In Wilkins RL, Stoller JK, Scanlan CL, editors: *Egan's fundamentals of respiratory care,* ed 8, St Louis, 2003, Mosby.

Hodgkin JE: Home care and pulmonary rehabilitation. In Kacmarek RM, Stoller JK, editors: *Current respiratory care,* Toronto, 1988, BC Decker.

Hodgkin JE, Celli BR, Connors GL: *Pulmonary rehabilitation: guides to success,* ed 3, Philadelphia, 2000, Lippincott Williams & Wilkins.

Hodgkin JE, Connors GA: Pulmonary rehabilitation. In Burton GG, Hodgkin JE, Ward JJ, editors: *Respiratory care: a guide to clinical practice,* ed 4, Philadelphia, 1997, JB Lippincott.

Holden DA, Stelmach KD, Curtis PS, et al: The impact of a rehabilitation program on functional status of patients with chronic lung disease, *Respir Care* 35:332, 1990.

Kwiatkowski CA, Tougher-Decker R, O'Sullivan-Maillet J: Nutritional aspects of health and disease. In Scanlan CL, Wilkins RL, Stoller JK, editors: *Egan's fundamentals of respiratory care,* ed 7, St Louis, 1999, Mosby.

Lewis ML, Hagarty EM, Lawlor B: Home respiratory care. In Fink JB, Hunt GE, editors: *Clinical practice in respiratory care,* Philadelphia, 1999, Lippincott Williams & Wilkins.

Lucas J, Golish JA, Sleeper G, et al: *Home respiratory care,* Norwalk, Conn, 1988, Appleton & Lange.

MacIntyre NR: Pulmonary rehabilitation. In Hess DR, MacIntyre NR, Mishoe SC, et al, editors: *Respiratory care principles and practices,* Philadelphia, 2002, WB Saunders.

May DF: *Rehabilitation and continuity of care in pulmonary disease,* St Louis, 1991, Mosby.

McInturff SL, O'Donohue WJ Jr: Respiratory care in the home and alternate sites. In Burton GG, Hodgkin JE, Ward JJ, editors: *Respiratory care: a guide to clinical practice,* ed 4, Philadelphia, 1997, JB Lippincott.

Mulligan SC, Masterson JG, Devane JG, et al: Clinical and pharmacokinetic properties of a transdermal nicotine patch, *Clin Pharmacol Ther* 47:331, 1990.

Nett LM: The physician's role in smoking cessation, *Chest Suppl* 97(2):28s, 1990.

Petty TL: Pulmonary rehabilitation, *Basics Respir Dis* 1975.

Petty TL: Pulmonary rehabilitation: better living with new technology, *Respir Care* 30:98, 1985.

Petty TL, Nett LM: *Enjoying life with emphysema,* Philadelphia, 1987, Lea & Febiger.

Pulmonary rehabilitation: official American Thoracic Society statement, *Am Rev Respir Dis* 124:663, 1981.

Rennard SI, Daughton D: Transdermal nicotine for smoking cessation, *Respir Care* 38:290, 1993.

Scanlan CL, Heuer A, Wyka KA: Respiratory care in alternate sites. In Scanlan CL, Wilkins RL, Stoller JK, editors: *Egan's fundamentals of respiratory care,* ed 7, St Louis, 1999, Mosby.

Sobush D, Dunning M, McDonald K: Exercise prescription components for respiratory muscle training: past, present, and future, *Respir Care* 30:34, 1985.

Taylor C, Lillis C, LeMond P: *Fundamentals of nursing: the art and science of nursing care,* ed 2, Philadelphia, 1993, JB Lippincott.

White GC: *Equipment theory for respiratory care,* ed 3, Albany, NY, 1999, Delmar.

Wilkins RL, Dexter JR: *Respiratory disease: a case study approach to patient care,* ed 2, Philadelphia, 1998, FA Davis.

Wyka KA: Cardiopulmonary rehabilitation. In Wilkins RL, Stoller JK, Scanlan CL, editors: *Egan's fundamentals of respiratory care,* ed 8, St Louis, 2003, Mosby.

Wyka KA: Pulmonary rehabilitation. In Wyka KA, Mathews PJ, Clark WF, editors: *Foundations of respiratory care,* Albany, NY, 2002, Delmar.

SELF-STUDY QUESTIONS

1. The therapeutic goals of a rehabilitation program include all the following *except:*
   A. Decreased hospitalizations
   B. Reversal of lung disease
   C. Increase the patient's energy level
   D. Increase the patient's ability to perform ADLs

2. A home care patient calls to say that he cannot feel any oxygen coming out of the nasal cannula. The oxygen concentrator is making odd cycling noises. What should the respiratory therapist recommend?
   A. Reset the circuit breaker on the concentrator and call back in an hour.
   B. Switch the cannula to a liquid oxygen system at a higher flow rate than the concentrator.
   C. Switch the cannula to an oxygen cylinder at the same flow rate as the concentrator.
   D. Disassemble the concentrator, and clean out the air filter.

3. An open-end-format exercise program should be recommended to a patient who has an unpredictable work and social schedule because of the following:
   I. Members of the exercise group can offer support to each other.
   II. It is self-directed by the patient.
   III. The facilitator can easily plan group activities.
   IV. The patient can adjust the schedule of activities if necessary.
   A. II and IV
   B. I and III
   C. IV
   D. II and III

4. All of the following are indications for monitoring infant apnea at home *except:*
   A. Surgically repaired cleft palate
   B. Apnea periods lasting 25 seconds
   C. Two older siblings died of SIDS
   D. Premature infant with apnea periods and bradycardia

5. The components of a strength training program include:
   I. Cool-down period
   II. Strengthening exercises performed daily
   III. Warm-up period
   IV. Strengthening exercises performed every other day
   V. Exercises performed for 20 to 30 minutes continuously
   A. I and II
   B. III, IV, and V
   C. II, III, and V
   D. I, III, and IV

6. You are supervising a patient who is participating in an endurance training rehabilitation program. Her target heart rate is between 130 and 150 beats/min. She is exercising on a bicycle ergometer, and her heart rate is 167 beats/min. What would you advise her to do?
   A. Exercise only until she begins to perspire.
   B. Continue exercising if she feels that she can handle the workload.
   C. Exercise a maximum of 10 minutes each day.
   D. Slow down on the ergometer until her heart rate decreases to the target level.

7. Home apnea monitoring can usually be stopped when all the following conditions exist *except:*
   A. The infant has gone 30 days without an apnea episode.

B. The infant has had a diphtheria-pertussis-tetanus (DPT) immunization without any consequences.

C. Three months have passed without any alarms sounding.

D. Two months have passed without an apnea episode.

8. A pulmonary rehabilitation patient is ordered to perform a 6-minute walk to improve her endurance. The patient should be instructed to:

A. Ride a bicycle ergometer for 6 minutes, and note the distance pedaled.

B. Walk as quickly as possible for 3 minutes, and double the distance covered.

C. Walk as far as possible in 6 minutes, and note the distance.

D. Walk as far as possible in 1 minute, and multiply the distance by six.

9. The respiratory therapist is working with a group of COPD patients who need to begin a pulmonary rehabilitation program. A closed-end program would be best for the group for all of the following reasons *except:*

A. Group members can offer emotional support to each other.

B. The program facilitator can direct group activities.

C. Learning activities can be optimally sequenced.

D. Each patient can easily adjust activities if a scheduling conflict arises.

10. A COPD patient who is trying to quit smoking is using a nicotine patch. He complains of skin irritation on his arm where the patch is placed and difficulty sleeping. The respiratory therapist should recommend the following:

I. Apply a topical cortisone cream to the irritated skin.

II. Move the patch to another area.

III. Take a sleeping pill.

IV. Remove the patch before going to bed.

V. Drink a beer or a glass of wine before going to bed.

    A. IV and V

    B. II and IV

    C. I, III, and IV

    D. I, II, IV, and V

11. A patient receiving public aid is being discharged. The physician has ordered 2 L/min of home oxygen as needed for shortness of breath. Which of the following should be set up in the home?

A. A bank of H tanks and simple oxygen mask

B. Liquid oxygen system with air entrainment mask

C. Oxygen concentrator with oxygen-conserving cannula

D. A portable, shoulder bag oxygen tank and a regular nasal cannula

12. A 50-year-old patient with COPD is a participant in an exercise program. Which of the following are expected benefits of the program?

I. Improved pulmonary function studies

II. Increased strength

III. More exercise tolerance

IV. Reversal of lung disease

    A. I and II only

    B. II and III only

    C. I, II, and III only

    D. I, II, III, and IV

ANSWER KEY

1. **B.** Rationale: Research has shown that lung disease cannot be reversed by a patient attending a rehabilitation program. However, a rehabilitation program can be expected to decrease a patient's number of hospitalizations, increase the patient's energy level, and increase the patient's ability to perform activities of daily living (ADLs). These are all worthy goals that will improve the quality of the patient's life.

2. **C.** Rationale: The oxygen concentrator has failed. The patient should switch the cannula to an oxygen cylinder at the same flow rate as the concentrator. This delivers the needed oxygen supply to the patient until the therapist can repair the unit. It is not the patient's responsibility to perform equipment repairs such as resetting the circuit breaker on the concentrator or disassembling the concentrator to clean out the air filter. In addition, the patient should not have to run the risk of not having the ordered oxygen while waiting an hour to call the therapist back for an equipment update or to ask for further assistance. The patient should not be told to increase the flow of oxygen through a liquid oxygen system above that which has been ordered by the physician.

3. **A.** Rationale: An open-end exercise program offers these two advantages: (1) it is self-directed by the patient, and (2) the patient can adjust the schedule of activities if necessary. A closed-end exercise program offers these two advantages: (1) members of the exercise group can offer support to each other, and (2) the facilitator can easily plan group activities.

4. **A.** Rationale: A surgically repaired cleft palate has no connection with infant apnea. Apnea periods lasting 25 seconds, death of two or more older siblings from sudden infant death syndrome (SIDS), and a premature infant with apnea periods and bradycardia are all serious enough situations that apnea monitoring is indicated. See Box 17-1 if needed.

5. **D.** Rationale: These three steps are needed in a strengthening program: (1) warm-up period, (2) strengthening exercises performed every other day, and (3) cool-down period after the strengthening exercises. Strengthening exercises should not be performed daily because the muscles that have been worked need a day to recover before exercising again. Endurance exercises should be performed for 20 to 30 minutes continuously, *not* strengthening exercises.

6. **D.** Rationale: It would be safer to have the patient slow down on the ergometer until her heart rate decreases to the target level. The patient's target heart rate range is based on her age and physical conditioning. If the patient exercised only until she began to perspire, she would probably not gain any exercise benefit. As previously stated, the target heart rate range is based on the patient's age and physical conditioning. She should not continue exercising at this elevated heart rate even if she feels that she can handle the workload. The patient gains little benefit from exercising for a maximum of 10 minutes each day. Current guidelines dictate that a person should exercise for 20 to 30 continuous minutes.

7. **A.** Rationale: Current guidelines dictate that an infant must go at least 2 to 3 months without an apnea episode, *not* 30 days without an apnea episode, to discontinue apnea monitoring. An infant can have apnea monitoring stopped if the other listed options are met. See Box 17-1 if necessary.

8. **C.** Rationale: A 6-minute walk test requires that the patient walk as far as possible in 6 minutes and note the distance. It is hoped that as the patient's conditioning improves, her distance walked will increase. The patient must walk, rather than ride a bicycle ergometer, for 6 minutes.

9. **D.** Rationale: It is only in an open-end-format rehabilitation program that each patient can easily adjust activities if a scheduling conflict arises. In a closed-end-format rehabilitation program, all group members do the same thing at the same time. This way they can offer emotional support to each other, and the program facilitator can direct group activities and optimally sequence learning activities.

10. **B.** Rationale: Moving the patch to another area of skin allows the irritated area to heal. Removing the patch before going to bed removes the stimulating nicotine that has been preventing sleep. A physician, not a respiratory therapist, should make the recommendation to apply a topical cortisone cream to the irritated skin. Only a physician should make the recommendation that the patient take a sleeping pill. Although a patient may choose to drink a beer or a glass of wine before going to bed to help induce sleep, the respiratory therapist should not make this recommendation. If nicotine is preventing the patient from sleeping at night, it is best to remove the patch. Sleeping pills and alcohol can probably be avoided if the nicotine patch is removed at night.

11. **C.** Rationale: An oxygen concentrator and oxygen-conserving cannula economically provides the necessary oxygen to the patient. A bank of H tanks is expensive to set up and takes up more space than a concentrator. In addition, a nasal cannula is preferred over a simple oxygen mask to deliver 2 L/min of oxygen to a patient going home. A liquid oxygen system is more expensive to set up than a concentrator for a patient who will be using the system only during periods of shortness of breath. In addition, an air entrainment mask order must specify the patient's oxygen percentage (24%, 28%, and so on). A portable oxygen tank does not provide a long enough duration of flow to the cannula if the patient has prolonged shortness of breath. An oxygen-conserving cannula is more economical than a regular cannula.

12. **B.** Rationale: Studies have shown that patients who complete a rehabilitation program can expect benefits of increased strength and more exercise tolerance. Unfortunately, the patient cannot expect to experience clinically significant improvement in pulmonary function studies. This is because the lung damage COPD patients have is not reversible.

18 Special Procedures

Note 1: The National Board for Respiratory Care (NBRC) has released the *RRT Examination Matrix* (covering the testable items on the Written Registry Exam) and the *CSE Examination Matrix* (covering the testable items on the Clinical Simulation Exam). Turn to the appendices at the back of this book for both publications in their original formats. This book is intended to cover all of the testable items in these two publications. This chapter (and all others) uses the abbreviation "WRE" for the coded items testable on the Written Registry Exam *and* Clinical Simulation Exam. The listed difficulty (R, Recall; Ap, Application; An, Analysis) relates to the question difficulty on the Written Registry Exam. The abbreviation "CSE" is used for the coded items testable on *only* the Clinical Simulation Exam. Because no question difficulty level is given for this exam, be prepared for anything.

Note 2: A review of the most recent Written Registry Examinations has shown an average of six questions (6% of the exam) that cover the following mix of special procedures that do not belong with the topics in the previous chapters. The Clinical Simulation Exam is comprehensive and may include everything that should be known or performed by an advanced level respiratory therapist.

MODULE A

Patient transportation

1. **Participate in intrahospital patient transport (WRE code: III I3b) [Difficulty: An]**
2. **Participate in land or air patient transport outside of the hospital (WRE code: III I3a) [Difficulty: Ap, An]**

Be prepared to perform, during patient transport, all the respiratory care practices and procedures that have been described in this and other texts. It is extremely important that all equipment and supplies be accounted for before leaving the patient's room for the next location. This is especially true if the patient is being moved to another hospital. Obviously, with interhospital transport, once under way, it is not possible to obtain something that was forgotten. To help ensure that this does not happen, it is wise to have a checklist of everything that may be needed. In addition, all equipment must be checked for proper function. Calculate the duration of the oxygen cylinders at expected liter flows. Make sure that batteries and light bulbs work and have spare batteries and light bulbs.

If mechanical ventilation will be needed, select a unit that is lightweight, portable, and has solid-state circuitry. For intrahospital transport, many respiratory care departments use pneumatically powered units. Typically, for interhospital transport, an electrically powered unit is selected. Make sure that it can be powered by both alternating current (AC) and direct current (DC) from batteries. If the ventilator will be used for helicopter or unpressurized cabin fixed-wing aircraft, it must be able to deliver an intermittent mandatory ventilation (IMV)/synchronous intermittent mandatory ventilation (SIMV) mode through a demand valve rather than through a reservoir system. The ventilator controls should not be adversely affected by changes in atmospheric pressure during ascent and landing.

Exam Hint

Usually one question on the examination deals with the effects of increased altitude when flying in an unpressurized helicopter or airplane. Remember that as altitude increases, barometric pressure (P_B) decreases. Decreased barometric pressure directly leads to a decrease in the alveolar pressure of oxygen (P_{AO_2}) that results in a decrease in the patient's arterial pressure of oxygen (Pa_{O_2}). In addition, as barometric pressure decreases at increased altitude, gases within the patient (stomach and intestine, pneumothorax, and lung) expand. The air within the endotracheal tube cuff expands, and the delivered tidal volume increases. This requires adjustments in the ventilator settings. Later, when the aircraft descends to land, the increased barometric pressure results in a decrease in the cuff volume, the tidal volume, and the patient's internal gas volumes. Be prepared to adjust the ventilator again.

---

3. Participate in disaster management (CSE code: III I3c)

Respiratory therapists are an important group of health care professionals who take part in disaster planning. Be prepared to perform any and all respiratory care practices and procedures listed in this book or in other respiratory care textbooks.

MODULE B

Assist the physician who is performing the following procedures

1. Cardioversion (CSE code: IIIJ3)

Cardioversion (or countershock) refers to deliberately sending a direct current (DC) electrical shock through the patient's heart. Its purpose is to suppress an abnormal heartbeat so that the normal pacemaker at the sinoatrial (SA) node takes over. This is accomplished if a great enough electrical current is sent through the chest wall to cause the depolarization of a critical mass of myocardial cells. After this, the SA node should take over as the pacemaker, provided that the heart muscle is oxygenated and not too acidotic. Two different types of cardioversion exist: defibrillation (also called unsynchronized cardioversion) and synchronized cardioversion. Both were introduced in Chapter 11 for the treatment of specific arrhythmias.

Defibrillation is performed in an emergency situation (see Fig. 11-41). Patients who need to be defibrillated include those in ventricular tachycardia or ventricular flutter (see Figs. 11-38 and 11-39) when they are pulseless, unresponsive, hypotensive or have pulmonary edema and ventricular fibrillation (see Fig. 11-40). Because the fastest possible action is needed, no attempt is made to synchronize the defibrillation shock with the heart's rhythm. While cardiopulmonary resuscitation (CPR) is being performed, the defibrillator unit is prepared. The defibrillating paddles (large positive and negative electrodes) are placed on the patient's right anterior and left lateral chest wall. The physician or other qualified person (respiratory therapist, registered nurse, or paramedic) performing the defibrillation should call out, "Stand clear." All other medical personnel should stand back from the patient and the bed and not touch anything that is electrically grounded. When the buttons on the paddles are pushed, the shock is administered. If it is successful, the patient's heartbeat returns to normal sinus rhythm. If the initial shock is unsuccessful, CPR is continued. The defibrillator is then recharged for another attempt as quickly as possible. Box 18-1 shows the sequence of increasingly more powerful countershocks that can be given.

Synchronized cardioversion is similar in some ways to defibrillation. An electrical shock is sent by two paddles through the heart to suppress paroxysmal atrial tachycardia, atrial flutter, atrial fibrillation, or hemodynamically

---

BOX 18-1 Wattage Used in Synchronous Cardioversion and Defibrillation

SYNCHRONIZED CARDIOVERSION OF AN INFANT
0.5-1.0 J (watt-seconds) per kg
Stepwise increases in energy should be used if the initial shock fails to convert the rhythm.

SYNCHRONIZED CARDIOVERSION OF AN ADULT
Atrial flutter and paroxysmal atrial tachycardia: 50-100 J
Stepwise increases in energy should be used if the initial shock fails to convert the rhythm: 200, 300, 360.

ATRIAL FIBRILLATION
Stepwise increases in energy should be used if the initial shock fails to convert the rhythm: 200, 300, 360.

VENTRICULAR TACHYCARDIA WITH A REGULAR FORM AND RATE WITH OR WITHOUT A PULSE
100 J
Stepwise increases in energy should be used if the initial shock fails to convert the rhythm: 200, 300, 360.

VENTRICULAR TACHYCARDIA WITH AN IRREGULAR FORM AND RATE
200 J
Stepwise increases in energy should be used if the initial shock fails to convert the rhythm: 300, 360.

DEFIBRILLATION
INFANT:
2 J/kg
4 J/kg for second and succeeding attempts

ADULT
200 J on first attempt
200-300 J on second attempt
Up to 360 J on third and succeeding attempts

J, Joules. 1 Joule = 1 watt-second of power.

---

stable ventricular tachycardia (see Figs. 11-25, 11-26, and 11-27) so that the SA node takes over. Its major difference from defibrillation is that the electrical shock is administered automatically by the defibrillator after an R wave is recognized by the electrocardiogram (ECG) monitor (see Fig. 11-5). The ECG electrodes must be in place and the best lead (often lead II) selected to show a clear, strong, upright R wave. The defibrillator unit is set for synchronized cardioversion. The physician holds the paddles on the patient's right anterior and left lateral chest wall. When the discharge buttons are pushed on the paddles, the shock is sent after the next R wave and is identified by the ECG monitor.

Cardioversion is not considered an emergency; however, it is performed as quickly as possible so that the patient does not stay in the abnormal rhythm any longer than necessary. Synchronized cardioversion is performed only if medical treatment with antiarrhythmia drugs or carotid artery massage has no effect. Because these patients are usually conscious, they should be sedated with diazepam (Valium), midazolam (Versed), or a similar medication. Patients who are hypotensive or already unconscious should not be sedated.

The respiratory therapist's role in cardioversion may include

    a. Making sure that the ECG electrodes are properly positioned for either monitoring or diagnosing the rhythm, as the physician requires.

    b. Making sure that the ECG monitor and electrocardiograph are working properly.

    c. Making sure that the ECG lead that results in a strong R wave is selected; usually the R wave is upright in lead II.

    d. Charging the defibrillator to the power level ordered by the physician.

    e. Adding the electrode cream to the electrode paddles to decrease the skin's resistance to electricity.

    f. Being prepared to keep a patent airway, manually ventilate the patient, or begin chest compressions, if necessary.

2. Bronchoscopy

a. Assist with the bronchoscopy procedure (WRE code: IIIJ1) [Difficulty: An]

Bronchoscopy is a procedure that involves looking directly into the patient's tracheobronchial airways. The physician can perform a number of diagnostic and therapeutic tasks under direct vision. (See Box 18-2 for uses, limitations, and risks of bronchoscopy.)

Typical duties of the respiratory therapist during bronchoscopy may include the following:

1. Inform the patient of the procedure and have him or her sign the medical release form.
2. Have a sedative such as midazolam (Versed) or (diazepam) Valium administered for conscious sedation, if needed.
3. Nebulize a topical anesthetic, such as 4% lidocaine (Xylocaine), to the airway.

BOX 18-2   **Uses, Limitations, and Risks of Bronchoscopy**

RIGID BRONCHOSCOPY

DIAGNOSTIC USE:

Biopsy of tumors within the main airway

THERAPEUTIC USES:

Treatment of massive hemoptysis by cold-saline lavage or placement of a Fogarty catheter to occlude the airway
Removal of foreign body in infants and small children
Aspiration of inspissated secretions and mucus plugs

LIMITATIONS:

Cannot be used for observing or treating problems beyond the left or right main-stem bronchus
Cannot be used with patients with disease or trauma of the cervical spine who cannot hyperextend their necks
Cannot be used with patients with disease or trauma of the jaw who cannot open their mouths wide enough to pass the tube

FIBEROPTIC BRONCHOSCOPY

DIAGNOSTIC USES:

Search for the origin of a positive sputum cytology
Evaluate lung lesions and perform transbronchial biopsy of lung tissue (should be done only under fluoroscopic control)
Stage lung cancer preoperatively
Investigate unexplained hemoptysis, unexplained cough, localized wheeze, or stridor
Search for the cause of unexplained paralysis of a vocal cord or hemidiaphragm
Search for the cause of superior vena cava syndrome, chylothorax, or unexplained pleural effusion
Assess airway patency and investigate suspected bronchial tear or other injury after thoracic trauma

Investigate a suspected tracheoesophageal fistula
Investigate problems related to an endotracheal tube such as tracheal damage, airway obstruction, or tube placement
Obtain mucus for identification of pathogens
Investigate suspected injury secondary to inhaled superheated gas and smoke from an enclosed fire
Investigate suspected injury secondary to the aspiration of gastric contents
Perform bronchoalveolar lavage

THERAPEUTIC USES:

Remove secretions or mucus plugs that cannot be cleared by other methods
Remove small foreign bodies
Remove abnormal endobronchial tissue or foreign material by forceps or laser techniques

INCREASED RISKS RELATED TO RIGID OR FIBEROPTIC BRONCHOSCOPY:

Recent myocardial infarction or unstable angina
Unstable cardiac arrhythmia
Partial tracheal obstruction
Unstable bronchial asthma
Severe hypoxemia
Hypercarbia
Pulmonary hypertension (risk of hemorrhage after biopsy)
Bleeding disorder (risk of hemorrhage after biopsy)
Lung abscess (airway may be flooded with purulent material)
Pulmonary infection from contaminated equipment
Pneumothorax from transbronchial biopsy
Respiratory failure requiring mechanical ventilation of the patient

4. Check the fiberoptic unit for proper function: working light source, working thumb control to flexible tip, working adjustable eyepiece focus, and patency of the suction and biopsy channel.
5. Check the functioning of the biopsy brush and forceps.
6. Set up and monitor the patient's ECG.
7. Monitor the patient's vital signs.
8. Place and monitor the pulse oximeter on the patient.
9. Administer oxygen via a nasal catheter or the suction and biopsy channel on the unit.
10. Collect all suctioned material or other specimens for culture and sensitivity.
11. Perform biopsies and brushings for cytology.
12. Operate any photographic equipment.
13. If the patient is being mechanically ventilated during fiberoptic bronchoscopy, perform the following:
    a. Place a bronchoscopy adapter between the endotracheal tube and Y of the circuit. This keeps a seal around the bronchoscopy tube to minimize any decrease in tidal volume.
    b. Watch for an increase in the peak pressure from the increased resistance caused by the bronchoscopy tube.
    c. Be prepared to make adjustments in inspired oxygen rate, flow, and tidal volume.
    d. Be prepared to switch from conventional volume ventilation to high frequency jet ventilation if needed.
14. Tend to the patient's comfort.
15. Use a glutaraldehyde disinfecting solution (Cidex) on the equipment between patients.

Fig. 18-1 Rigid tube bronchoscope being inserted into patient's trachea. Note how head and neck must be hyperextended. *(From Simmons KF: In Scanlan CL, Spearman CB, Sheldon RL, editors: Egan's fundamentals of respiratory care, ed 5, St Louis, 1990, Mosby.)*

> ### Exam Hint
>
> **U**sually one question on the examination asks about indications for bronchoscopy or hazards related to the procedure.

b. Select a bronchoscope for the planned procedure (WRE code: IIA22) [Difficulty: R, Ap, An]

The rigid bronchoscope is a straight, hollow, stainless steel tube (Fig. 18-1). It has a distal light source so that the airway can be seen and a side port for providing oxygen or mechanical ventilation to the patient. The right and left mainstem bronchi can be observed by passing a mirror through the main channel. A hook or net can be passed through the main channel into the trachea or either bronchus to remove a foreign body. The rigid bronchoscope is preferred for the treatment of massive hemoptysis or to remove a foreign body.

Flexible fiberoptic bronchoscopy (FFB) uses a smaller diameter flexible tube with two sets of fiberoptic bundles that shine light into the airway and allow viewing of the airway. It has gained wide popularity because it is better tolerated by the patient and allows for better visualization and collection of specimens from smaller bronchi (Figs. 18-2 and 18-3). The adult bronchoscopy tube is about 5 to 6 mm outer diameter (OD), and the pediatric tube is about 3 mm OD. The small diameter and ability to guide the catheter allow the operator to look into the bronchus to each lung segment (segmental bronchi). The fiberoptic bronchoscope is preferred over the rigid one when the patient is being mechanically ventilated or has disease or trauma to the skull, jaw, or cervical spine. As shown in Fig. 18-2, a photo connection allows the assistant either to take still photographs of pulmonary anatomy or to videotape the entire procedure.

A limitation of the pediatric unit is that there is no channel outlet for suctioning purposes. This is because of its small size. If a patient has an obstructing bronchial tumor, a special laser fiberoptic bronchoscope is used to burn away part of it. This enables the patient to breathe more easily, but this procedure is not a cure for the cancer.

c. Put the fiberoptic bronchoscope together, make sure that it works properly, and identify any problems (WRE code: IIA22) [Difficulty: R, Ap, An]

The fiberoptic bronchoscope comes preassembled (see Fig. 18-2 for its primary features). If photographing or videotaping is planned, the camera must be attached at the photo connection. Have a central or portable suctioning

Fig. 18-2 Flexible fiberoptic bronchoscopy with its components and special features. *(From Simmons KF: In Scanlan CL, Spearman CB, Sheldon RL, editors: Egan's fundamentals of respiratory care, ed 5, St Louis, 1990, Mosby.)*

Fig. 18-3 Flexible fiberoptic bronchoscopy procedure being performed on patient. *(From Williams SF, Thompson JM: Respiratory disorders, St Louis, 1990, Mosby.)*

system set up with suctioning tubing. In addition, the following steps must be used to check for proper functioning:

1. Make sure the light source shines through to the distal end of the bronchoscope.
2. Look through the eyepiece. Point the distal end of the bronchoscope at a close object, and adjust the lens to bring it into focus.
3. Adjust the thumb control to bend the distal tip.

4. Pass biopsy forceps or brush through the channel port to the outlet.
5. Make sure the suctioning tubing connects to the channel port.

d. Fix any problems with the equipment (WRE code: IIA22) [Difficulty: R, Ap, An]

If the light source does not work, you must check the manufacturer's equipment manual to help determine if the problem could be something simple such as a burned-out light bulb or a more serious problem. Similarly, problems with the camera equipment can be resolved by checking the manufacturer's equipment manual.

Failure to pass a biopsy forceps or brush through the channel port probably means that an obstruction such as dried blood or tissue is present. Try applying suction through the channel port to clear out the debris. It also may be helpful to squirt sterile distilled water from a syringe through the channel. Try suctioning again or pushing the biopsy forceps through the channel. If alternating suction, instilling water, and pushing the forceps through the channel does not dislodge the debris, the unit cannot be used. Try soaking the bronchoscope in water to soften the debris before repeating these processes. If the channel cannot be cleared, the unit must be sent back to the manufacturer for repairs.

3. Review the patient's chart for information on pleural fluid (WRE code: IA3) [Difficulty: Ap, An]

Thoracentesis (also called thoracocentesis) is the surgical puncture of the chest wall and pleural space with a needle to aspirate pleural fluid for therapeutic or diagnostic purposes. Thoracentesis is performed as a therapeutic procedure to remove air or fluid that has accumulated in the pleural space and is causing the patient pain, dyspnea, hypoxemia, or a combination of these. Thoracentesis also is performed as a diagnostic procedure to get a fluid sample for analysis to diagnose the cause of a pleural effusion. Pleural fluid may be a *transudate* that results from congestive heart failure, cirrhosis, nephrotic syndrome, or hypoproteinemia. Pleural fluid may also be an *exudate* that results most often from inflammatory, infectious, or neoplastic diseases of the pleura or lung. Other causes of an exudate include pulmonary infarction, chest trauma, drug hypersensitivity, and collagen vascular disease.

Look in the patient's chart for information on the nature of the fluid. If assisting with the removal of the fluid, compare the previously removed fluid with the fluid being removed at this time. Evaluate the gross appearance of the fluid that has just been removed. A *transudate* is found when the fluid is clear, serous, or light yellow. It contains few cells of any kind. This is most commonly found in patients with congestive heart failure and pulmonary edema. A *chylothorax* is found when the fluid is opalescent or pearly white in color. Chyle is lymphatic fluid that drains into the pleural cavity when the thoracic duct is blocked. This could be caused by injury to the neck or a tumor that invades the thoracic duct. A *hemothorax* is found when the pleural fluid is bloody (sanguineous or serosanguineous). Chest wall injury or puncture is the usual cause. An *empyema* is found when the fluid is thick and puslike with a foul odor. The patient usually has a lung infection, and infected fluid has entered the pleural space. In all cases, the collected pleural fluid sample should be sent to the laboratory for detailed analysis.

4. Treat a tension pneumothorax (WRE code: III I2) [Difficulty: Ap, An]

In an emergency when the patient has a tension pneumothorax and rapidly worsening vital signs, the pleural air must be rapidly removed from the chest. This is done by placing a large bore needle (16 gauge or larger) through the second or third intercostal space in the midclavicular line of the affected lung. The intrapleural air leaves the chest, allowing the lung to expand. A pleural chest tube is then inserted for a long-term solution to the problem.

A chest tube (also called tube thoracostomy) may be inserted into either one or both pleural spaces around the lungs, the mediastinal space, or pericardial space around the heart. This procedure is indicated when air or fluid or both in any of these spaces interferes with normal lung or heart function. Box 18-3 lists the indications for the insertion of a chest tube.

In addition to this, the patient is often given 100% oxygen by a nonrebreather mask for two reasons. First, treat the patient for hypoxemia. Second, if pure oxygen were to enter the pleural space through a tear in lung tissue, it would be quickly absorbed into the blood. This would allow the lung to expand faster than if the patient were breathing a lower percentage of oxygen.

General steps in inserting a pleural chest tube follow:

1. Check the patient's chest radiograph for the location of the air or fluid in the pleural space and its relation to the ribs and other tissues.

BOX 18-3   Indications for the Insertion of a Chest Tube

PLEURAL SPACE (See Fig. 18-5, *D*)
Tension pneumothorax
Greater than a 10% to 20% simple pneumothorax
Hemothorax
Empyema
Pleural effusion
Chylothorax

MEDIASTINAL SPACE
Free air
Free blood or other fluid

PERICARDIAL SPACE (See Fig. 18-6)
Cardiac tamponade
Pneumopericardium

2. Prepare the patient as described in the thoracentesis procedure. The patient is usually positioned to lie on his or her back or with the lung of the unaffected side down on the bed.
3. The physician anesthetizes the tube insertion site as shown in Fig. 18-4, *A* and *B*.
4. The physician creates an opening into the patient's chest wall to place the chest tube (Fig. 18-5). A tube to remove *air* is placed into one of two places and then advanced toward the apex of the lung. With a midclavicular approach, the tube is placed over the top edge of a rib into the second to fourth intercostal space. With a midaxillary approach (preferred site),

the tube is placed over the top edge of a rib into the fourth to sixth intercostal space. A tube to remove *fluid* is placed over the top edge of the rib into the sixth to eighth intercostal space. It is inserted at the midaxillary line and advanced toward the posterior base of the lung. Mediastinal or pericardial tubes are placed via an opening below the xiphoid process and placed posterior to the heart (Fig. 18-6). This is most commonly done during open heart surgery.
5. The tube is secured by sutures covered by a sterile 4 × 4-inch gauze pad and tape.
6. The other end of the tube is connected to the drainage system (discussed later).

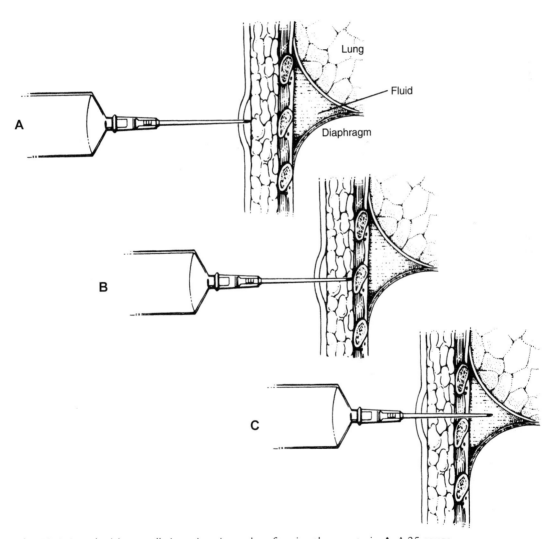

Fig. 18-4 Anesthetizing needle insertion site and performing thoracentesis. **A**, A 25-gauge needle is used to inject lidocaine (Xylocaine) into thoracentesis puncture site until skin is raised. **B**, A 22-gauge needle is used to inject lidocaine into periosteum of rib and surrounding tissues. The properly anesthetized patient should feel no pain during thoracentesis. **C**, A 22- or larger-gauge aspirating needle is pushed through numbed tissues, over top edge of rib, and into pleural space. Fluid sample can now be aspirated. *(From Martin L: Pulmonary physiology in clinical practice: the essentials for patient care and evaluation, St Louis, 1987, Mosby.)*

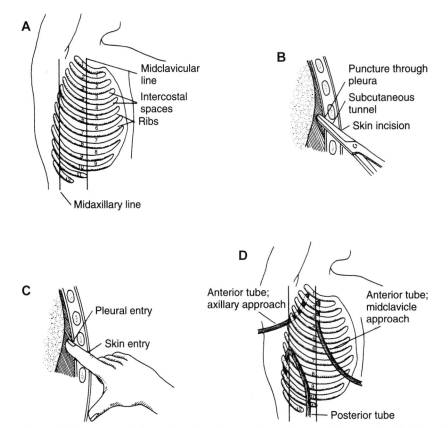

Fig. 18-5 Technique for inserting pleural chest tube. **A**, Anatomic landmarks. **B**, Dissecting through tissues with hemostat. **C**, Using finger to widen opening and ensure that lung has not been punctured. **D**, Proper tube placement. Air is removed by tube that is placed toward the apex of the lung. Fluid is removed by tube placed toward the posterior base of the lung. *(Modified from Anderson HL, Bartlett RH: Respiratory care of the surgical patient. In Burton GG, Hodgkin JE, Ward JJ, editors:* Respiratory care: a guide to clinical practice, *ed 3, Philadelphia, 1991, JB Lippincott.)*

Fig. 18-6 Pericardiocentesis with needle and syringe. Pericardial or mediastinal chest tube also is inserted by substernal approach. *(From Sproul CW, Mullanney PJ, editors:* Emergency care: assessment and interventions, *St Louis, 1974, Mosby.)*

7. Place the patient with his or her back against the bed or with the unaffected side down on the bed. The physician may want the head of the bed elevated or flat.

8. Observe the patient for dizziness, cyanosis, and changes in heart rate and respiratory rate. (See Box 18-4 for the most commonly seen complications.)

Exam Hint

Every past examination has had at least one question that relates to identifying a patient having a tension pneumothorax, requiring the insertion of a large bore needle or a pleural chest tube. Know the indications of a tension pneumothorax, including sudden deterioration of vital signs and hypoxemia, decreased breath sounds over the affected lung, decreased chest wall movement over the affected lung, hyper-resonant percussion note over the affected lung, and shift of the mediastinal structures away from the affected lung. See Fig. 1-2 for a chest radiograph showing a pneumothorax.

5. Pleural drainage system

a. Select a pleural drainage system (CSE code: IIA23)

Modern drainage systems consist of either three or four chambers or sections designed to regulate the vacuum level, hold any drained fluids, prevent any outside air from entering the patient's thorax, and act as a pressure relief valve in case the vacuum regulator should fail. Argyle and Pleurovac are two well-known manufacturers. The systems for draining the pleural space are discussed here, but the principles are the same for draining the mediastinal and pericardial spaces.

b. Put a pleural drainage system together, make sure that it works properly, and identify any problems with it (CSE code: IIA23)

Refer to Fig. 18-7 for the assembly and operation of the three-chamber drainage system. The four-chamber drainage system is shown in Fig. 18-8 and is discussed concurrently.

Vacuum level. The operation of the wall or central vacuum systems was discussed in Chapter 13. It is common practice to set a partial vacuum of −15 to −20 cm water pressure to the pleural space.

Suction control. The suction control chamber is dry when the unit is unpacked. Follow the manufacturer's instructions for adding the correct amount of water. The proper water level is generally 15 to 20 cm high and results in that level of vacuum being applied to the patient's pleural space.

It is normal to have room air drawn into the opening on top and bubbling through the water column. This corresponds to bottle or chamber C in Fig. 18-8. The constant air bubbling causes the water level to gradually decrease from evaporation. Water must be added occasionally.

Water seal. The water-seal chamber, which corresponds to chamber B in Fig. 18-8, is a safety feature. It is dry when unpacked. Follow the manufacturer's directions as to the amount of water to add. Typically, the water-seal tube should have about 2 cm of water in it for any patient

Fig. 18-7 Three-chamber pleural drainage systems. **A,** Homemade three-chamber drainage system. The depth at which the suction column tube is placed under water determines the level of vacuum that will be applied against patient's pleural space. **B,** Schematic drawing of a modern manufactured three-chamber drainage system. *(From Shapiro BA, Kacmarek RM, Cane RD, et al: Clinical application of respiratory care, ed 4, St Louis, 1991, Mosby.)*

air to bubble through. As indicated by the arrows, it is designed to permit air to leave the patient's chest cavity. (Air also will be seen bubbling through when fluid enters the drainage collection chamber and displaces some of its air.) However, room air cannot be drawn "backward" through the water to enter the chest if the vacuum fails or is disconnected.

The water-seal chamber must be checked regularly to see if any air is bubbling through from the patient's chest. If so, the patient has an active air leak. If the chest tube has been placed into the pleural space, it shows that the patient has an unhealed pneumothorax or bronchopleural

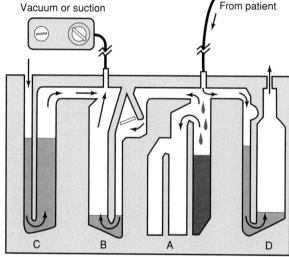

Fig. 18-8 Four-chamber pleural drainage systems. **A,** Homemade four-chamber drainage system. The depth at which the suction column tube in chamber C is placed under water determines the level of vacuum that will be applied against patient's pleural space. **B,** Schematic drawing of modern manufactured four-chamber drainage system. Chamber D acts to vent high-pressure air if vacuum should be turned off or malfunction. *(Modified from Pilbeam SP, Deshpande VM: Curr Rev Respir Ther 5:151, 1983.)*

fistula. If the chest tube has been placed into the mediastinum or pericardium, it indicates that air is leaking through a tear in the lung structures to these areas. When the air leak stops, it indicates that the tissues have healed over the tear.

Drainage collection. The drainage collection chamber, which corresponds to bottle or chamber A in Fig. 18-8, is designed to hold any fluid that is removed from the pleural space. It is divided into several sections that are marked off for volume measurement. The volume that has accumulated in the chamber should be recorded each hour. A sudden, significant increase in

the amount of drainage should be called to the physician's attention. This is especially important if the patient is losing blood. Note the color of the drainage. Blood is obviously red, chyle is white, pus from an empyema is yellow or green, and pleural effusion fluid is a straw-yellow color. The whole drainage system must be replaced when the drainage collection chamber becomes filled.

Pressure relief valve on the four-chamber system. This additional chamber is a safety feature and is seen on four-chamber systems such as those shown in Fig. 18-8, chamber D. Its purpose is to act as an escape route for any gas leaking from the patient if the vacuum system is accidentally turned off or disconnected. Without the relief valve, air pressure from a pneumothorax might increase to a dangerous level. Instead, the air and pressure are released. In three-chamber systems, the pressure has to build up to the point that water in the suction control chamber "geysers" out before the pressure is relieved.

c. Fix any problems with the pleural drainage system (CSE code: IIA23)

A number of problems can occur with chest drainage systems. The practitioner must understand how the systems are designed to work and how to recognize and correct the situation. See Table 18-1 for examples of problems and their correction. Fig. 18-9 lists important considerations when assessing the patient on chest drainage.

Exam Hint

Remember that a pleural drainage system is operating properly when air leaking from a pneumothorax is seen bubbling through the water seal. Most examinations have a question concerning this or some other aspect of managing a patient with a pleural drainage system.

---

6. Intubation (WRE code: IIIJ3) [Difficulty: An]

The procedure for a therapist performing oral endotracheal intubation was discussed in Chapter 12. The following discussion is limited to assisting an anesthesiologist or other trained physician in performing a nasal endotracheal intubation. Most commonly, the respiratory therapist is the assistant. See Box 18-5 for indications and contraindications and Box 18-6 for complications of nasal endotracheal intubation. Two different procedures are used for passing an endotracheal tube by the nasal route: blind nasotracheal intubation and direct vision nasotracheal intubation.

TABLE 18-1	Troubleshooting Problems with Chest Drainage Systems
Problem	**Corrective Action**
Drainage system is cracked open or drainage tubing is permanently disconnected from the drainage system	If the patient has a leaking pneumothorax: Leave the tube open to room air so the pleural air can be vented out. As quickly as possible, place the distal end of tubing into a glass of water to create a water seal. If the patient does not have a leaking pneumothorax, clamp the distal end of the tube to prevent room air from being drawn into the pleural space. In either case, attach the tube to a new drainage system as soon as possible.
No bubbling through the suction control chamber	Increase the vacuum pressure. Correct any leak in the system.
Water is spouting out of the suction control chamber (three-bottle system)	Turn on the vacuum. Remove obstruction inside tubing between vacuum and drainage system.
Air leak through the water-seal chamber	Check the patient for a pneumothorax; report a new air leak to the physician. Check for a leaking seal between the drainage tube and the patient's chest. Check for a hole in the drainage tube, a loose connection between the tube and the drainage system, or if a fenestration in the tubing has pulled out of the chest wall.
Fluid has filled a dependent loop in the tubing	Drape the tubing so that no loops or kinks are present
No change in drainage	Check for loops or kinks in tube. Milk the tube to remove any clots. No action if drainage has ceased.
Drainage-collection chamber is full	Prepare another unit, clamp the tube while making the exchange, and unclamp the tube after the new unit is functioning.

Fig. 18-9 Assessing a patient on chest drainage. *(From Erickson RS: Mastering the ins and outs of chest drainage, Nursing 19:47, 1989.)*

BOX 18-5　Indications and Contraindications for Nasal Endotracheal Intubation

GENERAL INDICATIONS FOR ENDOTRACHEAL INTUBATION

Provide a secure, patent airway
Provide a route for mechanical ventilation
Prevent aspiration of stomach or mouth contents
Provide a route for suctioning the lungs
General anesthesia

INDICATIONS FOR NASAL INTUBATION

Patient has a cervical spine abnormality or injury
Use of muscle relaxants may cause a complete loss of the airway
Limited movement of the cervical spine or mandible
Lower facial injury or surgery

CONTRAINDICATIONS FOR NASAL INTUBATION

Basilar skull fracture
Nasal tumors
Deviated nasal septum
Severe coagulation disorder

BOX 18-6　Complications of Nasal Endotracheal Intubation

GENERAL COMPLICATIONS

Reflex laryngospasm
Perforation of the esophagus or pharynx
Esophageal intubation
Bronchial intubation
Reflex bradycardia
Tachycardia or other arrhythmias from hypoxemia
Hypotension
Bronchospasm
Aspiration of tooth, blood, gastric contents, laryngoscope bulb
Laceration of pharynx or larynx
Nosocomial infection
Vocal cord injury
Laryngeal or tracheal injury from the tube or the excessive cuff pressure
Mucosal bleeding
Trauma to the larynx during an attempted blind intubation
Sinusitis

COMPLICATIONS AFTER EXTUBATION

Reflex laryngospasm
Aspiration of stomach contents or oral secretions
Sore throat
Hoarseness
Laryngeal edema (postintubation croup)

Blind nasotracheal intubation. Be prepared to assist in blind nasotracheal intubation by positioning the patient properly, providing supplemental oxygen or manual ventilation to the patient, and getting and preparing the endotracheal tube or other equipment. A stylet is not indicated. Often, the physician orders the patient to be prepared by having 1% phenylephrine sprayed into the nares. This medication constricts the blood vessels, which dilates the nasal passages, making intubation easier and also reducing the risk of bleeding. Often, 4% lidocaine (Xylocaine) is sprayed into the nares for its local anesthetic effect. The distal end of the endotracheal tube is usually also covered with sterile lidocaine ointment.

This procedure is done without the aid of a laryngoscope to visualize the patient's anatomy and expose the trachea. The general procedure is to place the patient in the sniffer's position, advance the tube to the oropharynx, and then continue to advance it on inspiration only. Changing the patient's head position, feeling for air movement through the tube or pressure over the larynx, or pulling on the tongue may be needed to help guide the tube into the trachea.

In addition, several different devices can aid in this intubation. The physician may choose to place a so-called *trigger tube* into the patient. This special endotracheal tube has a wire placed into it along the inside curve to the tip (see Fig. 12-20). The wire is pulled when the tube is near the larynx to bend the tip more anterior to aim it into the trachea. A *lighted stylet* can be passed through the tube so that the light source is at the distal tip. The light shines through the skin over the larynx. When this is seen, the tube is advanced and the stylet is removed. A *fiberoptic bronchoscope* can be placed through the tube and guided into the patient's trachea. The tube is then advanced, and the bronchoscope removed. Another choice is the *intubation guide.* This is a stylet with a flexible tip that can be bent by the physician through a proximal handle (Fig. 18-10). The intubation guide is passed through and beyond the distal end of the endotracheal tube. When the guide is in the oropharynx, the tip can be bent in an anterior direction and directed into the trachea. The tube is then advanced over the guide and into the trachea. The guide is then removed.

Direct vision nasotracheal intubation. The respiratory therapist assists with direct vision nasotracheal intubation and prepares the patient and endotracheal tube as with blind endotracheal intubation. This procedure is different from the previous procedure in that intubation equipment is used to visualize the patient's anatomy and see the glottis. Prepare a laryngoscope handle, the physician's choice of either a straight or curved blade, and Magill forceps.

The lubricated tube is advanced to the oropharynx. The laryngoscope blade is then placed into the mouth and

Fig. 18-10 Intubation guide stylet. Flexible tip can be guided by pulling or pushing on ring attached to wire running to distal end. Once the end of the guide is directed into trachea, the endotracheal tube is slipped over it. After intubation, the guide is withdrawn. *(Modified from Heffner JE: Managing difficult intubations in critically ill patients, Respir Manage 19(3):53, 1989.)*

Fig. 18-11 Direct vision nasotracheal intubation. Note that Magill forceps and laryngoscope and blade are both used. Magill forceps is used to grasp tip of endotracheal tube and pull it anterior into trachea. *(From Shapiro BA, Harrison RA, Cane RD: Clinical application of respiratory care, ed 4, St Louis, 1991, Mosby.)*

used to expose the glottis. The Magill forceps is then placed into the mouth. It is used to grasp the endotracheal tube and guide it into the trachea (Fig. 18-11). Care must be taken not to place the pinchers over the cuff to avoid tearing it.

With either method, the tube must be properly positioned so that the cuff is in the trachea beyond the vocal cords (Fig. 18-12). The cuff is then inflated, its pressure adjusted to a safe level, the tube secured in place by tape, and a radiograph taken of the chest and neck.

7. Tracheostomy (WRE code: IIIJ2) [Difficulty: An]

A *tracheostomy* is a surgical opening in the anterior tracheal wall. The opening is usually placed below the cricoid cartilage and through the second, third, or fourth ring of tracheal cartilage (Fig. 18-13, *A*). The term *tracheotomy* is used to describe the surgical procedure itself (the two terms are often used interchangeably).

Commonly, the tracheostomy is created in the operating room under sterile conditions. When the respiratory therapist is called to assist, it is usually because of a patient emergency. The emergency situation commonly involves an upper airway obstruction such as facial trauma or surgery in which an endotracheal tube cannot

be placed by either the oral or nasal route. Because of time constraints, the full sterile technique may be skipped over in favor of a clean technique. The physician's preference and the situation itself dictate how the procedure is performed. The respiratory therapist also may be called to assist in the procedure when the patient is already

Fig. 18-12 Properly placed nasotracheal tube. *(From Shapiro BA, Harrison RA, Cane RD: Clinical application of respiratory care, ed 4, St Louis, 1991, Mosby.)*

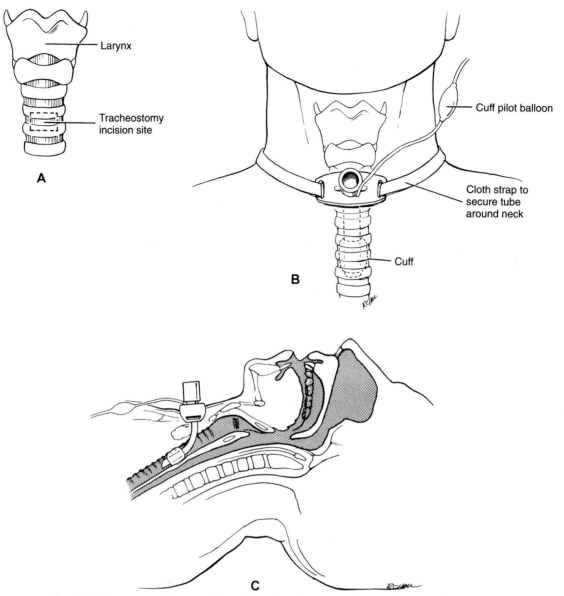

Fig. 18-13 Anatomy of larynx and insertion of tracheostomy tube. **A,** Close-up of larynx and tracheostomy incision site. **B,** Anterior cut-away view of tracheostomy tube after its insertion. **C,** Lateral cut-away view of tracheostomy tube after its insertion. *(From Eubanks DH, Bone RC: Comprehensive respiratory care: a learning system, ed 2, St Louis, 1990, Mosby.)*

intubated. Usually this involves an unstable patient who requires long-term mechanical ventilation. Because of the patient's critical condition, the physician makes the decision to perform the tracheostomy at the bedside rather than in the operating room. The respiratory therapist may be responsible for preparing the patient, disinfecting the tracheostomy site, setting up the sterile field around the site, and setting up the equipment and supplies. Each hospital or physician may have a prescribed way that this is done. The general steps are listed here:

1. Inform the patient of the procedure, and have him or her sign the medical release form if time permits.

2. Have a sedative or pain-relieving agent administered if needed.

3. If necessary, trim or shave the insertion site clear of body hair.

4. Put on a sterile mask, cap, gown, and gloves according to protocol.

5. Disinfect the insertion site with an iodine (Betadine) soaked sterile 4 × 4-inch gauze pad. Place the pad at the center of the insertion site, and move it in a widening spiral away from the center. This step should be repeated with a second sterile gauze pad. Let the iodine dry.

TABLE 18-2	Common Complications of a Tracheostomy
Complication	**Approximate Time of Onset**
Bleeding	During and after surgery for up to 24 hr; if possible, do not replace the first tube for 2 to 3 days
Pneumothorax	During the procedure
Infection of the stoma or lungs	Usually seen after second day
Subcutaneous or mediastinal emphysema	May be seen during the procedure or at any later time

6. Protect the area around the insertion site with a sterile fenestrated surgical drape.
7. Prepare the sterile field with the tracheostomy tube, scalpel, supplies, and so forth. Have a local anesthetic such as lidocaine (Xylocaine) available in a syringe with needle. The physician injects this into the insertion site.
8. Assist the physician into his or her sterile mask, cap, gown, and gloves.
9. Get the proper size tracheostomy tube (see Table 12-1).
10. Assist the physician with the procedure as needed. If the patient is already intubated, withdraw the endotracheal tube after the tracheostomy has been created and the physician is ready to place the tracheostomy tube into the opening.
11. Make any adjustments in the patient's respiratory care equipment as needed.
12. Dispose of any used supplies and so forth after the procedure is completed.
13. Tend to the patient's comfort.

See Chapter 12 for further discussion on the indications for the various airway routes and when to routinely change a tracheostomy tube. Table 18-2 lists the common complications of a tracheostomy.

MODULE C
Sleep-disordered breathing

1. Overnight pulse oximetry
a. Perform overnight pulse oximetry (WRE code: IB7j) [Difficulty: An]

A sleep apnea study (cardiopulmonary sleep study or polysomnography) is performed to determine whether the patient has sleep-disordered breathing. Furthermore, it can help to determine the type of disorder and monitor the patient's response to treatment. Box 18-7 lists the indications for a polysomnography sleep study. The following procedures are usually performed before the sleep study:

BOX 18-7   Indications for a Cardiopulmonary Sleep Study

Patient with COPD whose awake PaO_2 is > 55 torr but who has pulmonary hypertension, right heart failure (cor pulmonale), or polycythemia

Patient whose awake PaO_2 is < 55 torr without continuous supplemental oxygen and who must have the proper oxygen flow rate set for sleeping at night. Overnight sleep ear oximetry should be performed.

Patient with restrictive ventilatory impairment secondary to chest wall or neuromuscular disturbances who also has chronic hypoventilation, polycythemia, pulmonary hypertension, disturbed sleep, morning headaches, or daytime somnolence and fatigue

Patient with awake $PaCO_2$ > 45 torr who also has polycythemia, pulmonary hypertension, disturbed sleep, morning headaches, or daytime somnolence and fatigue

Patient with snoring, obesity, and other symptoms indicating disturbed sleep pattern

Patient with excessive daytime sleepiness or sleep-maintenance insomnia

Patient with nocturnal cyclic bradytachyarrhythmias, atrioventricular conduction abnormalities while asleep, or increased abnormal ventricular beats compared with those when awake

---

1. History of the problem from both the patient's and the bed partner's viewpoint
2. Physical examination including neck, upper airway, blood pressure, heart rate, and respiratory rate and pattern
3. Arterial blood gas (ABG) results or pulse-oximetry results
4. Hemoglobin
5. Thyroid function
6. Chest and upper airway radiograph examinations; may include a computed axial tomographic scan of the upper airway if obstructive sleep apnea is suspected
7. ECG

The following physiologic parameters are usually measured during a polysomnography sleep study:

1. Pulse oximetry for O_2 saturation. An ear or bridge-of-nose oximetry probe is recommended. Finger oximetry is not recommended because the unit may fall off during patient movement.
2. Sleep stages through an electroencephalographic (EEG) recording of brain wave activity and electro-oculographic (EOG) recording of eye movements.
3. Inspiratory and expiratory airflow by nasal thermistor, pneumotachograph, or end-tidal CO_2 analyzer.
4. Inspiratory and expiratory effort by respiratory inductive plethysmography. (Some may prefer to

have the patient swallow a transducer to measure esophageal pressure changes.)

5. Body position related to normal and abnormal breathing patterns.
6. Periodic arm and leg movements.
7. ECG for monitoring heart rate and arrhythmias.

Because of the cost involved in a polysomnography study, overnight pulse oximetry (OPO) has been studied as a less expensive way to determine desaturation from sleep apnea. OPO can be performed in the patient's home or in the hospital setting. The respiratory therapist may be responsible for preparing the patient and setting up the equipment and supplies. Each hospital or physician may have a prescribed procedure. The general steps are listed here:

1. Inform the patient of the procedure, and have him or her sign the medical release form.
2. Attach the pulse oximeter, ECG leads, and other monitoring equipment to the patient.
3. Calibrate the equipment, and make sure it is working properly.
4. Record the patient's parameters during the course of a 6-hour or longer sleep period. The patient also may be recorded by videotape and audiotape during the sleep period.
5. Make any adjustments in the patient's respiratory care equipment as needed.
6. Dispose of any used supplies after the procedure is completed.
7. Tend to the patient's comfort.

b. Interpret the results of overnight pulse oximetry (WRE code: IB8g) [Difficulty: An]

Apnea is the cessation of breathing for 10 seconds or longer. Sleep apnea is diagnosed when a patient experiences at least 30 apneic periods during 6 hour of sleep. Numerous studies have shown that OPO can be used to screen patients with moderate to severe sleep apnea. These patients will have had a least 10 apnea episodes per hour in which their SpO_2 decreased at least 4% from baseline to less than 90%. In cases where the OPO results were difficult to interpret, polysomnography was called for.

During polysomnography, the EEG tracing should confirm that the apneic periods occur during both of the major sleep stages. The first stage is called *non–rapid eye movement* (non-REM) sleep and starts soon after the person loses consciousness. The second stage is called *rapid eye movement* (REM) sleep and follows after the non-REM stage. Normally people cycle through both stages about every 1 to 1.5 hours during the night. This normal cycle of sleep is important for both mental and physical health. People with disturbed sleep do not dream as they should and are not physically rested when they awaken. Whether the patient was evaluated by OPO or polysomnography, the results lead to one of the following classifications for sleep apnea.

Obstructive sleep apnea. Obstructive sleep apnea results when the patient's upper airway is obstructed despite continued breathing efforts (Figs. 18-14 and 18-15). Patients with this problem often exhibit the following symptoms:

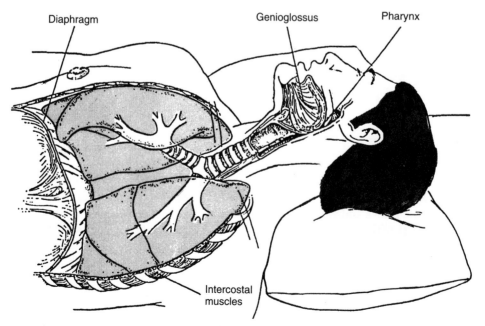

Fig. 18-14 Obstructive sleep apnea. These patients often obstruct when lying supine and genioglossus muscle of the tongue fails to oppose the negative force on the airway during inspiration. *(From Des Jardins TL: Clinical manifestations of respiratory disease, ed 2, St Louis, 1990, Mosby.)*

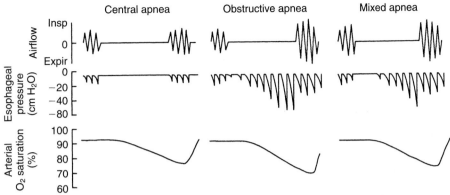

Fig. 18-15 Typical patterns of airflow, esophageal pressure (or respiratory inductive plethysmography) showing respiratory effort, and arterial oxygen saturation produced by central, obstructive, and mixed sleep apnea. Central apnea shows lack of respiratory effort resulting in no airflow. Obstructive apnea shows continued respiratory effort but no airflow because of airway obstruction. Mixed apnea starts with initial lack of respiratory effort (central apnea). Later, breathing efforts are made, but no airflow occurs because of airway obstruction (obstructive apnea). Arterial desaturation results from all three types of apnea. When desaturation becomes great enough and the carbon dioxide level high enough, the patient (we hope) awakens enough to breathe again. *(From Des Jardins TL: Clinical manifestations and assessment of respiratory disease, ed 3, St Louis, 1995, Mosby.)*

loud snoring (reported by the bed partner), morning headache, excessive daytime sleepiness, depression or other personality changes, decreased intellectual ability, sexual dysfunction, bed-wetting (nocturnal enuresis), or abnormal limb movements during sleep.

Obstructive sleep apnea is associated with the following: middle-age men, obesity, short neck, hypothyroidism, testosterone administration, myotonic dystrophy, temporomandibular joint disease, narrowed upper airway from excessive pharyngeal tissue, enlarged tongue (macroglossia), enlarged tonsils or adenoids, deviated nasal septum, recessed jaw (micrognathia), goiter, laryngeal stenosis or web, or pharyngeal neoplasm. Management of patients with obstructive sleep apnea may include any of the following:

1. Weight reduction
2. Sleeping on either side or the abdomen; do not sleep in the supine position
3. Continuous positive-airway pressure (CPAP) mask or BiPAP mask
4. Surgery to open the airway: mandibular advancement, palatopharyngoplasty, or tracheostomy
5. Protriptyline (Triptil, Vivactil) to decrease REM sleep (when most obstructive episodes occur)
6. Have the patient wear a tongue-retaining device to prevent it from obstructing the pharynx

Exam Hint

There is often a question about the use of CPAP to treat obstructive sleep apnea.

7. Have the patient wear a neck collar to keep the head and neck aligned with the body

Central sleep apnea. Central sleep apnea is diagnosed when the respiratory center of the medulla fails to signal the respiratory muscles for breathing to occur. The patient makes no respiratory effort, and no air movement occurs (see Fig. 18-15). Patients with this problem often exhibit normal weight, mild snoring, insomnia, and lesser levels of daytime sleepiness, depression, or sexual dysfunction than does the obstructive sleep apnea patient.

Central sleep apnea is associated with primary alveolar (idiopathic) hypoventilation (Ondine's curse), muscular dystrophy, bilateral cervical cordotomy, bulbar poliomyelitis, encephalitis, brainstem infarction or neoplasm, spinal surgery, or hypothyroidism. Management of patients with central sleep apnea may include the following:

1. Negative pressure ventilation for sleeping
2. Intubation or tracheostomy and positive pressure ventilation if the patient has acute ventilatory failure
3. Phrenic nerve pacemaker

Mixed sleep apnea. Mixed sleep apnea is diagnosed when the patient shows evidence of both central and obstructive apnea. The patient usually first stops all breathing efforts (central apnea). After some time, the patient makes attempts to breathe but cannot because the upper airway is blocked (obstructive apnea) (see Fig. 18-15). Patients with mixed sleep apnea may show a variety of symptoms and traits from those listed earlier. Clinical management may include any of the treatments mentioned that prove to be effective.

Whatever the cause of the sleep apnea, it must be treated. If the apnea is left to continue its pathologic course, a number of problems may develop, such as pulmonary hypertension, cor pulmonale, polycythemia, cardiac arrhythmias, and even unexplained nocturnal death. At the very least, the patient's personal, family, and social life will suffer.

> ## Exam Hint
>
> **K**now how to differentiate between the clinical signs of obstructive and central sleep apnea. Usually a question is asked about identifying that a patient has obstructive sleep apnea. The key is to recognize that the patient will not be moving any air despite making breathing efforts. Nasal CPAP should be used to treat the patient's condition.

MODULE D
Respiratory care plan

1. Analyze available information to determine the patient's pathophysiologic state (CSE code: IIIH1)

See the previous topics for discussion of the patient's disease state.

2. Determine the appropriateness of the prescribed therapy and goals for the identified pathophysiologic state (CSE code: IIIH3)
a. Stop the treatment or procedure if the patient has an adverse reaction to it (CSE code: IIIF1)

Patient safety should always be an important consideration during the treatment or procedure. Specific concerns were discussed with each of the topics in this chapter. Be prepared to stop the treatment or procedure if the patient has an adverse reaction to it. In addition, be prepared to recommend to the physician that the treatment or procedure be discontinued if it is likely to result in additional adverse reactions.

b. Discontinue treatment based on the patient's response (WRE code: IIIG1e) [Difficulty: An]

There are typically three reasons for a patient's treatment to be discontinued. First, the patient has recovered and no longer needs the treatment or procedure. It is expensive and wasteful to perform unnecessary treatments. Second, the patient has had an adverse reaction and is likely to have an adverse reaction every time the treatment or procedure is repeated. Third, the patient's condition is terminal, and the patient or responsible family member wants all treatment to be stopped.

MODULE E
Quality assurance and quality control

1. Develop the outcomes of quality improvement programs (WRE code: IIIH4a) [Difficulty: An]

The broad concept of quality assurance (QA) can be viewed as a personal and departmental philosophy that ensures constant improvement in production and service. A number of ways exist to approach the subject. A key to QA is understanding what the respiratory care department should do for the patients, the physicians, the nurses, and other allied health professionals, as well as for the hospital. Once these objectives are determined, the QA program can be instituted. Minimally, the following can be done:

1. Make sure that all respiratory care equipment is working properly or, if malfunctioning, is repaired.
2. Audit the patient's medical records to find out if all ordered services were performed. If not, find out why.
3. Communicate with patients during their hospitalization and after discharge to find out their impressions of the care they received.
4. Communicate with the physicians, nurses, and so forth to find out if their needs for optimizing patient care are being met.
5. Work with the hospital administration to find ways to contain unnecessary costs, expand into new areas as opportunities arise, and so forth.

2. Perform respiratory care quality assurance (WRE code: IIIH3) [Difficulty: Ap]
3. Record and monitor the outcomes of quality assurance programs by using accepted statistical methods (WRE code: IIC6) [Difficulty: Ap]

Be able to calculate *mean* (average), *median* (middle value in a series of numbers), and *mode* (most common value). Consult a math book to review these calculations, if necessary.

4. Perform quality control procedures for blood gas analyzers, CO-oximeters, blood gas sampling devices, oxygen analyzers, pulmonary function equipment, noninvasive (transcutaneous) monitors, and mechanical ventilators (WRE code: IIC1,2,3,4,5) [Difficulty: Ap, An]

Quality improvement (QI) refers to the processes used to identify areas for improvement in patient care services. QA refers to any evaluation of services provided and the results achieved as compared with accepted standards.

These standards are developed through a process called *benchmarking* in which agreement is reached on fair and reasonable patient care criteria and outcomes. Previous chapters contain information on quality control procedures in the NBRC areas listed earlier.

5. Verify all computations and note erroneous data (WRE code: IIIA2) [Difficulty: An]

Exam Hint

Usually one question deals with the general concept of QA. The question could relate to gathering the appropriate information to determine whether a respiratory care procedure is making a difference in patient care. For example, is a change in the aerosolized bronchodilator protocol improving patient compliance or resulting in fewer patient days in the hospital.

BIBLIOGRAPHY

AARC Clinical Practice Guideline: Fiberoptic bronchoscopy assisting, *Respir Care* 38:1173, 1993.

AARC: Clinical Practice Guideline: In-hospital transport of the mechanically ventilated patient: 2002 revision and update, *Respir Care* 47(6):721, 2002.

AARC Clinical Practice Guideline: Management of airway emergencies, *Respir Care* 40:749, 1995.

AARC Clinical Practice Guideline: Polysomnography, *Respir Care* 40:1236, 1995.

Anderson HL, Bartlett RH: Respiratory care of the surgical patient. In Burton GG, Hodgkin JE, Ward JJ, editors: *Respiratory care: a guide to clinical practice,* ed 3, Philadelphia, 1991, JB Lippincott.

Barnes TA, editor: *Core textbook of respiratory care practice,* ed 2, St Louis, 1994, Mosby.

Branson RD, Hess DR, Chatburn RL, editors: *Respiratory care equipment,* ed 2, Philadelphia, 1999, Lippincott Williams & Wilkins.

Brutinel WM, Cortese DA: Fiberoptic bronchoscopy. In Burton GC, Hodgkin JE, Ward JJ, editors: *Respiratory care: a guide to clinical practice,* ed 4, Philadelphia, 1997, Lippincott-Raven.

Cairo JM: Assessment of physiologic function. In Cairo JM, Pilbeam SP, editors: *Mosby's respiratory care equipment,* ed 6, St Louis, 1999, Mosby.

Chavis AD, Grum CM: Fiberoptic bronchoscopy with mechanical ventilation, *Choices Respir Manage* 21:4, 1991.

Chavis AD, Grum CM: Pulmonary procedures during mechanical ventilation, *Choices Respir Manage* 21:29, 1991.

Coppolo DP, Brienza LT, Pratt DS, May JJ: A role for the respiratory therapist in flexible fiberoptic bronchoscopy, *Respir Care* 30:323, 1985.

Deshpande VM, Pilbeam SP, Dixon RJ: *A comprehensive review in respiratory care,* East Norwalk, Conn, 1988, Appleton & Lange.

Des Jardins TL: *Clinical manifestations and assessment of respiratory disease,* ed 4, St Louis, 2000, Mosby.

Epstein LJ, Dorlac GR: Cost-effectiveness analysis of nocturnal oximetry as a method of screening for sleep apnea-hypoventilation syndrome, *Chest* 113:97, 1998.

Erickson RS: Mastering the ins and outs of chest drainage: I, *Nursing* 19:37, 1989.

Erickson RS: Mastering the ins and outs of chest drainage: II, *Nursing* 19:47, 1989.

Eubanks DH, Bone RC: *Comprehensive respiratory care: a learning system,* ed 2, St Louis, 1990, Mosby.

Guidelines for fiberoptic bronchoscopy, *ATS News* 12:14, 1986.

Howard TP: Foreign body extraction by means of combined rigid and flexible bronchoscopy: a case report, *Respir Care* 33:786, 1988.

Johnson MD: Noninvasive monitoring. In Aloan CA, Hill TV, editors: *Respiratory care of the newborn and child,* ed 2, Philadelphia, 1997, Lippincott-Raven.

Kendall Hospital Products, Curity Thoracentesis Tray (package insert), Boston, Mass.

Khoury JB, Radtke RA: Sleep assessment. In Hess DR, MacIntyre NR, Mishoe SC, et al, editors: *Respiratory care principles and practices,* Philadelphia, 2002, WB Saunders.

Kilkenny LA, Fernandes KS, Strollo PJ Jr: Disorders of sleep. In Wilkins RL, Stroller JK, Scanlan CL, editors: *Egan's fundamentals of respiratory care,* ed 8, St Louis, 2003, Mosby.

Lewis CA, Eaton TE, Fergusson W, et al: Home overnight pulse oximetry in patients with COPD: more than one recording may be needed, *Chest* 123:1127, 2003.

Lough MD: Newborn respiratory care procedures. In Lough MD, Williams TJ, Rawson JE, editors: *Newborn respiratory care,* St Louis, 1979, Mosby.

Mims BC: You can manage chest tubes confidently, *RN* 48:39, 1985.

Netzer N, Eliasson AH, Netzer C, Kristo DA: Overnight pulse oximetry for sleep-disordered breathing in adults, *Chest* 120:625–633, 2001.

Peters RM: Chest trauma. In Moser KM, Spragg RG, editors: *Respiratory emergencies,* ed 2, St Louis, 1982, Mosby.

Plevak DJ, Ward JJ: Airway management. In Burton GC, Hodgkin JE, Ward JJ, editors: *Respiratory care: a guide to clinical practice,* ed 4, Philadelphia, 1997, Lippincott-Raven.

Podnos SD, Chappell TR: Hemoptysis: a clinical update, *Respir Care* 30(11):977–985, 1985.

Sachs S: Fiberoptic bronchoscopy. In Hess DR, MacIntyre NR, Mishoe SC, et al, editors: *Respiratory care principles and practices,* Philadelphia, 2002, WB Saunders.

Shapiro BA, Kacmarek RM, Cane RD, et al: *Clinical application of respiratory care,* ed 4, St Louis, 1991, Mosby.

Smalling T, Valente J: Examining laser surgery, *J Respir Care Pract* 11:93, 1998.

Whitaker K: *Comprehensive perinatal and pediatric respiratory care,* ed 2, Albany, NY, 1997, Delmar.

Williams SF, Thompson JM: *Respiratory disorders,* St Louis, 1990, Mosby.

SELF-STUDY QUESTIONS

1. All the following should be done when preparing to helicopter transport an adult patient requiring mechanical ventilation *except:*
   A. Select a heated cascade-type humidification system.
   B. Calculate the duration of the oxygen cylinder that will be used.
   C. Select a ventilator that uses a demand valve IMV system rather than one with an external reservoir IMV system.
   D. Select a lightweight and portable ventilator.

2. A 60-year-old patient with a smoking history and recurrent bouts of left lung pneumonia has a persistent chest radiograph shadow in the left lower lobe area. Despite 2 days of postural drainage with percussion and incentive spirometry, the haziness has not cleared. What should be recommended next?
   A. Nebulize a bronchodilator medication
   B. Rigid tube bronchoscopy
   C. Flexible fiberoptic bronchoscopy
   D. Nebulize hypertonic saline to induce a cough

3. Which of the following conditions is first treated by placing a large bore needle at the midclavicular line through the second or third intercostal space?
   A. 5% Pneumothorax
   B. Pleural effusion
   C. Hemothorax
   D. Tension pneumothorax

4. Which of the following should the respiratory therapist evaluate to determine whether a patient's chest drainage system is functioning properly and removing pleural air?
   A. Fluid is present in the collection chamber.
   B. The vacuum level is set at −15 cm water.
   C. Air is bubbling in the water-seal chamber.
   D. Air is bubbling in the suction control chamber.

5. An intubated patient receiving mechanical ventilation will be transported from Chicago to Denver by an airplane with an unpressurized cabin. A pressure-cycled transport ventilator will be used. The patient should be monitored for which during the flight?
   I. Increased cuff volume
   II. Decreased tidal volume
   III. Hypoxemia
   IV. Increased tidal volume
   V. Fluid retention

   A. I, III, and IV
   B. II, III, and V
   C. II and III
   D. I and IV

6. A mechanically ventilated patient is having a central venous line inserted by the subclavian vein route. He coughs vigorously. Within a minute the peak pressure on the ventilator increases significantly, and the Spo$_2$ value is progressively decreasing. Chest percussion demonstrates a hyper-resonant sound over the right side of the chest, and breath sounds are diminished on the right side. What is the most important thing to do at this time?
   A. Complete the insertion of the central venous pressure (CVP) line.
   B. Insert a pleural chest tube on the right side.
   C. Get a chest radiograph.
   D. Compare the peak and plateau pressures on the ventilator.

7. A conscious adult patient with atrial fibrillation is being prepared for synchronous cardioversion. Which of the following should be recommended?
   I. Administer midazolam (Versed) before starting.
   II. Administer flumazenil (Romazicon) before starting.
   III. Charge the defibrillator to 100 J.
   IV. Charge the defibrillator to 360 J.
   V. Set the ECG machine to lead II.
   VI. Have a manual resuscitator on standby.

   A. II and III
   B. I, II, and IV
   C. I, III, and V
   D. I, III, V, and VI

8. All of the following may be done by a respiratory therapist during a tracheostomy procedure *except:*
   A. Insert the tracheostomy tube into the new stoma.
   B. Disinfect the surgical site.
   C. Check for proper functioning of the tracheostomy tube.
   D. Withdraw the endotracheal tube when the stoma is ready for the tracheostomy tube.

9. A respiratory therapist is assisting an anesthesiologist in a direct vision nasotracheal intubation of a patient. All of the following equipment will be needed *except:*
   A. Magill forceps
   B. Laryngoscope handle with blade
   C. Sterile, water-soluble lubricant
   D. Lubricated stylet

ANSWER KEY

1. **A.** Rationale: A heated cascade-type humidification system is inappropriate because the water will splash through the ventilator circuit and into the patient because of the constant motion during transport. A heat and moisture exchanger should be used instead. The oxygen cylinder duration should be calculated to be sure that it lasts long enough for the trip. A demand valve IMV system should be chosen because it is not affected by altitude changes. A lightweight and portable ventilator is needed because the helicopter has a weight limit for equipment and passengers, and the chosen ventilator should be designed to tolerate the rough motion that can occur during a transport.

2. **C.** Rationale: A flexible fiberoptic bronchoscopy is indicated for two reasons. First, the patient has a history of smoking and recurrent bouts of pneumonia of the left lung. Second, other treatment procedures have failed to produce improvement in the patient's chest radiograph. These things should make one suspicious of a lung tumor. It is very doubtful that nebulizing a bronchodilator medication or hypertonic saline will make any difference in this patient's condition. No indication of bronchospasm or retained secretions is noted. A rigid tube bronchoscope cannot be used to look into the left lower lobe bronchus because it is not flexible. It can be used only to view the trachea and right and left main stem bronchi.

3. **D.** Rationale: A tension pneumothorax can be immediately treated by placing a large bore (often 16 gauge) needle through the second or third intercostal space at the midclavicular line on the affected side. Later, a pleural chest tube should be inserted. Although a 5% pneumothorax is abnormal, it is probably not life threatening. Sometimes the patient is given supplemental oxygen as needed and monitored. The pneumothorax gas may be reabsorbed into the tissues, and no other treatment may be necessary. A pleural effusion or hemothorax requires a thoracentesis procedure to remove the fluid. This would probably be done through the lower area of the patient's back because the fluid is gravity dependent.

4. **C.** Rationale: If air is seen to bubble in the water-seal chamber, it is known that vacuum is applied to the drainage system and the patient has pleural air (pneumothorax) that is being removed. The presence of fluid in the collection chamber confirms that the patient has pleural fluid that is being removed. It does not confirm that pleural air is being removed. A vacuum level of -15 cm water is normal and should result in air being seen to bubble in the suction control chamber. However, it does not confirm that pleural air is being removed. See Figs. 18-7 and 18-8.

5. **A.** Rationale: According to Boyle's law, pressure and volume are inversely proportional. Therefore as barometric pressure decreases at increased altitude, the volume of gas in the patient's endotracheal tube cuff increases and the tidal volume increases. Despite the increased tidal volume, the patient is likely to become hypoxic because the alveolar pressure of oxygen (P_{AO_2}) decreases and therefore the arterial pressure of oxygen (Pa_{O_2}) decreases as the barometric pressure decreases. The patient's tidal volume should be monitored and adjusted during the flight, and pulse-oximetry value should be monitored to look for hypoxemia and the need to increase the inspired oxygen percentage. No link exists between fluid retention and change in barometric pressure.

6. **B.** Rationale: All of the stated signs point to a tension pneumothorax. Because the patient's condition is rapidly deteriorating, it is most important to insert a pleural chest tube on the right side. Because it is very likely that the CVP needle pierced the lung and caused the pneumothorax, the procedure should be stopped at this time. Although a chest radiograph would be indicated if the patient's condition were stable, getting one now will unnecessarily delay inserting the needed chest tube. Nothing of clinical value is to be gained at this time by comparing the peak and plateau pressures on the ventilator. They will both increase because of the tension pneumothorax. This information only reinforces the previous signs, and doing this procedure now delays the needed chest tube.

7. **D.** Rationale: Before a conscious patient undergoes a cardioversion procedure, he or she should be given a sedative. The drug midazolam (Versed) is given intravenously for conscious sedation. The proper initial power setting for the first attempt at cardioversion of an adult patient with atrial fibrillation is 100 J (see Box 18-1). Set the ECG machine to lead II so that an upright R wave is detected by the unit. On occasion, the medication midazolam and shock from the cardioversion can cause a patient to stop breathing temporarily. For this reason, the respiratory therapist should have a manual resuscitator on standby and be ready to assist the patient's breathing. The drug flumazenil (Romazicon) is given intravenously *after* the procedure is finished to reverse the sedating effect of the midazolam. A defibrillator charge of 360 J is the maximum used to defibrillate a patient. It is far too high for a first attempt at cardioversion (see Box 18-1).

8. **A.** Rationale: The surgeon should insert the first tracheostomy tube into the stoma in case there is a problem. A respiratory therapist may replace a tracheostomy tube after the stoma is well established. The therapist may assist with the procedure by disinfecting the surgical

site, checking the tube cuff, and withdrawing the endo-tracheal tube when the surgeon has created the stoma and is ready to insert the tracheostomy tube.

9. **D.** Rationale: A stylet (lubricated or not) is not put through an endotracheal tube during a nasotracheal intubation procedure. This is because the tube should be kept flexible to follow the natural contours of the patient's airway anatomy. A stylet makes the endotracheal tube stiff and causes damage to the nasal passage. A Magill forceps is used to lift the tip of the tube for insertion into the trachea. A laryngoscope handle with blade is used as during an oral intubation procedure (see Fig. 18-11). The tip of the endotracheal tube is lubricated so that it slides easily through the patient's nasal passage.

Registry Examination Matrix and Detailed Content Outline for Advanced Respiratory Therapy (RRT)

Registry Examination for Advanced Respiratory Therapists (RRT)

RRT Examination Matrix

Content Area	Cognitive Level			Number of Items
	Recall	Application	Analysis	
I. Patient data evaluation and recommendations	**6**	**2**	**12**	**20**
A. Review existing data in the patient record	0	1	3	4
B. Collect and evaluate additional pertinent clinical information	2	4	8	14
C. Recommend procedures to obtain additional data	0	1	1	2
II. Equipment application and cleanliness	**2**	**5**	**11**	**18**
A. Select, assemble, use, and troubleshoot equipment	2	4	9	15
B. Ensure infection control	0	0	1	1
C. Perform quality control procedures for blood gas analyzers, co-oximeters, and sampling devices; oxygen analyzers; pulmonary function equipment; mechanical ventilators; noninvasive monitors [e.g., transcutaneous]; record and monitor qc data using accepted statistical methods	0	1	1	2
III. Therapeutic procedure initiation and modification	**3**	**7**	**52**	**62**
A. Maintain records and communicate information	0	1	4	5
B. Maintain a patent airway including the care of artificial airways	0	0	3	3
C. Remove bronchopulmonary secretions	0	0	3	3
D. Achieve adequate respiratory support	0	1	5	6
E. Evaluate and monitor patient's objective and subjective responses to respiratory care	1	1	7	9
F. Independently modify treatment techniques based on the patient's response	1	1	9	11
G. Recommend modifications in the respiratory care plan based on the patient's response	1	1	10	12
H. Determine the appropriateness of the prescribed respiratory care plan and recommend modifications when indicated	0	1	4	5
I. Initiate, conduct, or modify respiratory care techniques in an emergency setting	0	1	3	4
J. Act as an assistant to the physician performing special procedures	0	0	2	2
K. Initiate and conduct pulmonary rehabilitation and home care within the prescription	0	0	2	2
Totals	**7**	**18**	**75**	**100**

	Recall	Application	Analysis

Open cells show an examination could include items from indicated cognitive levels. Shaded cells prevent appearance of items on examinations.

I. Patient Data Evaluation and Recommendations

	Recall	Application	Analysis
I.	2	6	12

A. Review Existing Data in the Patient Record Including

	Recall	Application	Analysis
A.	0*	1*	3*

1. Patient history [e.g., present illness, admission notes, respiratory care orders, progress notes, diagnoses, DNR status] . . . .
2. Physical examination relative to the cardiopulmonary system [e.g., vital signs, physical findings] . . . .
3. Lab data [e.g., CBC, chemistries/electrolytes, coagulation studies, Gram-stain, culture and sensitivities, urinalysis, pleural fluid] . . . .
4. Pulmonary function results. . . . .
5. Blood gas results . . . .
6. Imaging studies [e.g., radiographic, CT, MRI, PET, V/Q scan angiogram] . . . .
7. Monitoring data
   a. pulmonary mechanics [e.g., maximum inspiratory pressure, vital capacity] . . . .
   b. respiratory monitoring [e.g., rate, tidal volume, minute volume, I:E, inspiratory and expiratory pressures; airway graphics] . . . .
   c. pulmonary compliance, airways resistance, work of breathing . . . .
   d. noninvasive monitoring [e.g., V_D/V_T, capnography, pulse oximetry, transcutaneous O_2/CO_2]. . . . .
8. Maternal and perinatal/neonatal history and data [e.g., Apgar scores, gestational age, L/S ratio, pre/post-ductal oxygenation studies] . . . .

B. Collect and Evaluate Additional Pertinent Clinical Information

	Recall	Application	Analysis
B.	2	4	8

1. Assess patient's overall cardiopulmonary status by **inspection** to determine
   a. general appearance [e.g., muscle wasting, venous distention, peripheral edema, diaphoresis, clubbing, cyanosis, capillary refill, chest configuration, evidence of diaphragmatic movement, breathing pattern, accessory muscle activity, asymmetrical chest movement, intercostal and/or sternal retractions, nasal flaring] . . . .
   b. cough, amount and character of sputum
   c. transillumination of chest, Apgar score, gestational age
2. Assess patient's overall cardiopulmonary status by **palpation** to determine
   a. heart rate, rhythm, and force . . . .
   b. asymmetrical chest movements, tactile fremitus, crepitus, tenderness, secretions in the airway, tracheal deviation . . . . .
3. Assess patient's overall cardiopulmonary status by **auscultation** to determine presence of
   a. breath sounds [e.g., normal, abnormal] . . . .
   b. heart sounds and rhythms [e.g., normal, abnormal]. . . . . . .
   c. blood pressure. . . . .
4. Interview patient to determine
   a. level of consciousness/sedation, orientation to time, place and person, emotional state, ability to cooperate, level of pain
   b. presence of dyspnea and/or orthopnea, work of breathing, sputum production, exercise tolerance and activities of daily living
   c. social history [e.g., smoking, substance abuse]. . . . .
   d. advance directives [e.g., DNR status]. . . . .
5. Assess patient's learning needs . . . .
6. Review chest radiograph to determine
   a. quality of imaging [e.g., patient identification, positioning, exposure] . . . .
   b. position of endotracheal or tracheostomy tube. . . . .
   c. presence of or change in pneumothorax or subcutaneous emphysema, other extrapulmonary air, consolidation and/or atelectasis, pulmonary infiltrates . . . .
   d. position of chest tube(s), nasogastric and/or feeding tube, pulmonary artery catheter, pacemaker, and other catheters. . . . .
   e. presence and position of foreign bodies. . . . .
   f. position of or change in hemidiaphragms, hyperinflation, pleural fluid, pulmonary edema, mediastinal shift, patency and size of major airways . . . .
7. Perform procedures including
   a. 12-lead ECG. . . . .
   b. pulse oximetry, capnography. . . . .
   c. tidal volume, minute volume, peak flow, vital capacity . . . . .
   d. bedside spirometry [e.g., FVC, FEV_1] . . . .
   e. arterial sampling – percutaneous or line . . . .
   f. blood gas/hemoximetry analysis. . . . .
   g. lung mechanics [e.g., MIP, MEP, pulmonary compliance, plateau pressure, airways resistance]. . . . .

* The number in each column is the number of items in that content area and cognitive level contained in each examination. For example, in category I.A., no items will be asked at the recall level, one item at the application level and three items at the analysis level. The items could be asked relative to any tasks listed (1-8) under category I.A.

	Recall	Application	Analysis
h. ventilator pressure-volume and flow-volume loops	▓		
i. apnea monitoring	▓		
j. overnight pulse oximetry	▓		
k. tracheal tube cuff pressure and/or volume	▓		▓
l. tracheal intubation	▓		
m. pulmonary function laboratory studies [e.g., flows, volumes, diffusion studies, pre- and post-bronchodilator]	▓		
n. auto-PEEP detection			▓

8. Interpret procedure results including
	Recall	Application	Analysis
a. transcutaneous O_2/CO_2 monitoring	▓		▓
b. pulse oximetry, capnography	▓	▓	
c. tidal volume, minute volume, peak flow, vital capacity	▓		
d. bedside spirometry [e.g., FVC, FEV_1]	▓		
e. blood gas/hemoximetry analysis	▓		
f. lung mechanics [e.g., MIP, MEP, pulmonary compliance, plateau pressure, airways resistance]	▓	▓	
g. overnight pulse oximetry	▓		
h. tracheal tube cuff pressure and/or volume	▓		
i. pulmonary function laboratory studies [e.g., flows, volumes, diffusion studies, pre- and post-bronchodilator]	▓	▓	
j. ventilator pressure-volume and flow-volume loops	▓		
k. auto-PEEP			

	Recall	Application	Analysis
C. Recommend Procedures to Obtain Additional Data Including	**0**	**1**	**1**
1. Radiographic and other imaging studies		▓	
2. Lung mechanics [e.g., pulmonary compliance, airways resistance, work of breathing]			▓
3. Blood gas analysis, pulse oximetry, transcutaneous O_2/CO_2 monitoring			
II. Equipment Application and Cleanliness	**2**	**5**	**11**
A. Select, Assemble, Use, and Troubleshoot Equipment Including	**2**	**4**	**9**
1. Oxygen administration devices	▓		
a. low-flow devices [e.g., nasal cannula]	▓		▓
b. high-flow devices [e.g., air entrainment mask]	▓		
2. CPAP devices – mask, nasal, or bi-level	▓		
3. Humidifiers [e.g., bubble, passover, cascade, wick, heat moisture exchanger]	▓		
4. Pneumatic aerosol generator (nebulizer)	▓		
5. Resuscitation devices [e.g., manual resuscitator (bag-valve), mouth-to-valve mask resuscitator]	▓		▓
6. Ventilators			
a. pneumatic, electric, fluidic, microprocessor	▓		▓
b. noninvasive positive pressure	▓		
c. high frequency	▓		
7. Artificial airways	▓		
a. oro- and nasopharyngeal airways	▓		
b. endotracheal tubes	▓		
c. tracheostomy tubes and buttons	▓		
d. intubation equipment [e.g., laryngoscope and blades, fiberoptic devices, exhaled CO_2 detection devices]	▓		▓
8. Suctioning devices [e.g., suction catheters, specimen collectors, oropharyngeal suction devices]	▓		▓
9. Gas delivery, metering, and clinical analyzing devices			
a. gas cylinders, regulators, reducing valves, connectors and flowmeters, air/oxygen blenders	▓		▓
b. oxygen concentrators, air compressors, portable liquid oxygen systems			▓
10. Patient breathing circuits	▓		
a. continuous mechanical ventilation	▓		
b. IPPB	▓		
c. CPAP, PEEP valve assembly	▓		
d. non-invasive ventilation	▓		
11. Aerosol (mist) tents	▓		▓
12. Incentive breathing devices	▓		
13. Percussors and vibrators	▓		
14. High Frequency Chest Wall Oscillation (HFCWO) [e.g., ThAIRapy Vest®]	▓		
15. He/O_2 therapeutic gas	▓		
16. ECG machines (12-lead)	▓		▓
17. Arterial catheters	▓		
18. Oximetry monitoring devices [e.g., pulse oximeter, transcutaneous]	▓		▓
19. Metered dose inhalers (MDI), MDI spacers	▓		▓
20. Dry powder inhalers	▓		▓
21. CO, He, O_2 and specialty gas analyzers	▓		
22. Bronchoscopes	▓		

	Recall	Application	Analysis

23. Select, assemble, and use speaking tubes and valves ....
24. Troubleshoot speaking tubes and valves ....

B. Ensure Infection Control — Recall 0, Application 0, Analysis 1

1. Assure selected equipment cleanliness [e.g., select or determine appropriate agent and technique for disinfection and/or sterilization, perform procedures for disinfection and/or sterilization, monitor effectiveness of sterilization procedures] .....
2. Assure proper handling of biohazardous materials..

C. Perform Quality Control Procedures For — Recall 0, Application 1, Analysis 1

1. Blood gas analyzers, co-oximeters, and sampling devices ....
2. Oxygen analyzers...
3. Pulmonary function equipment ....
4. Mechanical ventilators ....
5. Noninvasive monitors [e.g., transcutaneous]...
6. Record and monitor QC data using accepted statistical methods.....................................

III. Therapeutic Procedure Initiation and Modification — Recall 3, Application 7, Analysis 52

A. Maintain Records and Communicate Information — Recall 0, Application 1, Analysis 4

1. Record therapy and results using conventional terminology as required in the health care setting and/or by regulatory agencies by noting and interpreting patient's response to therapy including
   a. auscultatory findings, cough and sputum production and characteristics...........................
   b. vital signs [e.g., heart rate, respiratory rate, blood pressure, body temperature, pain level].....
   c. pulse oximetry, heart rhythm, capnography ....
2. Verify computations and note erroneous data...
3. Communicate information relevant to coordinating patient care and discharge planning [e.g., scheduling, avoiding conflicts, sequencing of therapies] ....
4. Apply computer technology to
   a. document patient management..
   b. monitor workload assignments ....
5. Communicate results of therapy and alter therapy per protocol(s)...................................
6. Explain planned therapy and goals to patient in understandable terms to achieve optimal therapeutic outcome ....

B. Maintain a Patent Airway Including the Care of Artificial Airways — Recall 0, Application 0, Analysis 3

1. Insert oro- and nasopharyngeal airways..
2. Perform endotracheal intubation ....
3. Maintain
   a. proper cuff inflation ....
   b. adequate humidification...
4. Perform extubation procedure ....

C. Remove Bronchopulmonary Secretions — Recall 0, Application 0, Analysis 3

1. Perform
   a. postural drainage and percussion and/or vibration ....
   b. nasotracheal suctioning...
2. Suction artificial airways...
3. Administer aerosol therapy, administer prescribed agents [e.g., bronchodilators, corticosteroids, saline, mucolytics] ......
4. Instruct and encourage bronchopulmonary hygiene techniques ....

D. Achieve Adequate Respiratory Support — Recall 0, Application 1, Analysis 5

1. Instruct in
   a. proper breathing technique, encourage deep breathing, instruct and monitor techniques of incentive spirometry......
   b. inspiratory muscle training techniques ....
2. Initiate and adjust
   a. IPPB therapy ....
   b. continuous mechanical ventilation settings..
   c. noninvasive ventilation ....
   d. elevated baseline pressure [e.g., CPAP, PEEP]..
   e. combinations of ventilatory techniques [e.g., SIMV, PEEP, PS, PCV, IRV, inspiratory hold].............
3. Select ventilator graphics [e.g., waveforms, scales] ....
4. Administer
   a. aerosolized drugs [e.g., bronchodilators, corticosteroids, mucolytics]............................
   b. oxygen – on or off a ventilator ....
5. Position patient to minimize hypoxemia...
6. Prevent procedure-associated hypoxemia [e.g., oxygenate before and after suctioning and equipment changes].........
7. Adhere to infection control policies and procedures [e.g., Standard Precautions] ....

	Recall	Application	Analysis
E. Evaluate and Monitor Patient's Objective and Subjective Responses to Respiratory Care	1	1	7
1. Recommend and review chest radiograph			
2. Obtain a blood gas sample			
a. by puncture			
b. from an arterial or pulmonary artery catheter			
c. from arterialized capillary blood			
3. Perform			
a. pulse oximetry			
b. blood gas and co-oximetry analyses			
c. capnography			
4. Interpret blood gas and co-oximetry results			
5. Observe changes in sputum characteristics			
6. Observe for signs of patient-ventilator dysynchrony			
7. Measure and record vital signs, monitor cardiac rhythm, evaluate fluid balance – intake and output			
8. Perform spirometry, determine vital capacity, measure pulmonary compliance and airways resistance, interpret airway graphics, measure peak flow			
9. Monitor mean airway pressure, adjust and check alarm systems, measure tidal volume, respiratory rate, airway pressures, I:E, and maximum inspiratory pressure			
10. Measure F_IO_2 and/or liter flow			
11. Monitor endotracheal or tracheostomy tube cuff pressure			
12. Auscultate chest and interpret changes in breath sounds			
F. Independently Modify Treatment Techniques Based on the Patient's Response	1	1	9
1. IPPB [e.g., volume, flow, pressure, F_IO_2, mouthpiece/mask]			
2. Incentive breathing devices			
3. Aerosol therapy			
a. modify patient breathing patterns			
b. change type of equipment, change aerosol output			
c. change dilution of medication, adjust temperature of the aerosol			
4. Oxygen therapy			
a. change mode of administration, adjust flow, and F_IO_2			
b. set up or change an O_2 blender			
c. set up an O_2 concentrator or liquid O_2 system			
5. Specialty gas [e.g., He/O_2, NO] therapy [e.g., change mode of administration, adjust flow, adjust gas concentration]			
6. Bronchial hygiene therapy [e.g., alter patient position and duration of treatment and techniques; coordinate sequence of therapies such as chest percussion, postural drainage, and PEP therapy]			
7. Management of artificial airways			
a. change type of humidification equipment			
b. initiate suctioning			
c. inflate and/or deflate the cuff			
d. perform tracheostomy care			
8. Suctioning			
a. alter frequency and duration of suctioning			
b. change size and type of catheter			
c. alter negative pressure			
d. instill irrigating solutions			
9. Mechanical ventilation			
a. monitor and adjust alarm settings			
b. change mechanical dead space			
G. Recommend Modifications in the Respiratory Care Plan Based on the Patient's Response	1	1	10
1. Recommend			
a. institution of bronchopulmonary hygiene procedures			
b. sedation and/or use of muscle relaxant(s)			
c. insertion or change of artificial airway [e.g., endotracheal tube, LMA, tracheostomy]			
d. procedures for weaning from mechanical ventilation			
e. discontinuing treatment based on patient response			
2. Recommend changes in			
a. patient position			
b. aerosol drug dosage or concentration			
c. F_IO_2 and oxygen flow			
3. Recommend changes in mechanical ventilation to			
a. improve patient synchrony [e.g., sensitivity, mode]			
b. enhance oxygenation [e.g., F_IO_2, PEEP/CPAP level, inspiratory time]			

	Recall	Application	Analysis

c. improve alveolar ventilation [e.g., tidal volume, rate]. . . . .
d. adjust I:E settings. . . . .
e. modify ventilator techniques [e.g., pressure support, pressure control]. . . . .
f. adjust noninvasive positive pressure ventilation . . . .
g. monitor and adjust alarm settings . . . .
h. adjust ventilator settings based on ventilator graphics . . . .
i. change type of ventilator, change patient breathing circuitry. . . . .
j. alter mechanical dead space . . . .
k. modify ventilator settings to
   1) eliminate auto-PEEP. . . . .
   2) reduce plateau pressure . . . .

4. Recommend use of pharmacologic interventions including
a. bronchodilators [e.g., adrenergics, anticholinergics, theophyllines]. . . . .
b. antiinflammatory drugs [e.g., leukotriene modifiers, corticosteroids, NSAID, cromolyn sodium]. . . . .
c. mucolytics/proteolytics [e.g., acetylcysteine, RhDNAse] . . . .
d. sedatives . . . .
e. analgesics . . . .
f. diuretics . . . .
g. surfactants . . . .

H. Determine the Appropriateness of the Prescribed Respiratory Care Plan and Recommend Modifications When Indicated — Recall: 0, Application: 1, Analysis: 4

1. Review
a. planned therapy to establish therapeutic plan . . . .
b. interdisciplinary patient and family plan . . . .
2. Recommend changes in therapeutic plan when indicated based on data . . . .
3. Perform respiratory care quality assurance. . . . .
4. Develop outcomes of
a. quality improvement programs . . . .
b. respiratory care protocols . . . .
5. Monitor outcomes of respiratory care protocols . . . .
6. Apply respiratory care protocols . . . .
7. Conduct disease management education. . . . .

I. Initiate, Conduct, or Modify Respiratory Care Techniques in an Emergency Setting — Recall: 0, Application: 1, Analysis: 3

1. Treat cardiopulmonary collapse according to
a. BCLS . . . .
b. ACLS . . . .
c. Pediatric Advanced Life Support (PALS) . . . .
d. Neonatal Resuscitation Program (NRP). . . . .
2. Treat tension pneumothorax. . . . .
3. Participate in
a. land/air patient transport outside the hospital. . . . .
b. intra-hospital patient transport. . . . .

J. Act as an Assistant to the Physician Performing Special Procedures Including — Recall: 0, Application: 0, Analysis: 2

1. Bronchoscopy . . . .
2. Tracheostomy . . . .
3. Intubation . . . .

K. Initiate and Conduct Pulmonary Rehabilitation and Home Care Within the Prescription — Recall: 0, Application: 0, Analysis: 2

1. Explain planned therapy and goals to patient in understandable terms to achieve optimal therapeutic outcome . . . .
2. Educate patient and family in disease management . . . .
3. Counsel patient and family concerning smoking cessation . . . .

	Recall	Application	Analysis
TOTALS	7	18	75

CSE Examination Matrix and Detailed Content Outline

CSE Examination Matrix

I. Patient Data Evaluation and Recommendations

  A. Review Existing Data in the Patient Record Including

  B. Collect and Evaluate Additional Pertinent Clinical Information

  C. Recommend Procedures to Obtain Additional Data Including

II. Equipment Application and Cleanliness

  A. Select, Assemble, Use, and Troubleshoot Equipment Including

  B. Ensure Infection Control

  C. Perform Quality Control Procedures For

III. Therapeutic Procedure Initiation and Modification

  A. Maintain Records and Communicate Information

  B. Maintain a Patient Airway Including the Care of Artificial Airways

  C. Remove Bronchopulmonary Secretions

  D. Achieve Adequate Respiratory Support

  E. Evaluate and Monitor Patient's Objective and Subjective responses to respiratory Care

  F. Independently Modify Therapeutic Procedures Based on the Patient's Response

  G. Recommend Modifications in the Respiratory Care Plan based on the Patient's Response

  H. Determine the Appropriateness of the Prescribed Respiratory Care Plan and Recommend Modifications When Indicated.

  I. Initiate, Conduct, or Modify Respiratory Care Techniques in an Emergency Setting

  J. Act as an Assistant to the Physician Performing Special Procedures Including

  K. Initiate and Conduct Pulmonary rehabilitation and Home Care Within the Prescription

---

I. PATIENT DATA EVALUATION AND RECOMMENDATIONS

A. Review Existing Data in the Patient Record Including

1. Patient history [e.g., present illness, admission notes, respiratory care orders, progress notes, diagnoses, DNR status]
2. Physical examination relative to the cardiopulmonary system [e.g., vital signs, physical findings]
3. Lab data [e.g., CBC, chemistries/electrolytes, coagulation studies, Gram-stain, culture and sensitivities, urinalysis, pleural fluid]
4. Pulmonary function results
5. Blood gas results
6. Imaging studies [e.g., radiographic, CT, MRI, PET, $\dot{V}/\dot{Q}$ scan, angiogram]
7. Monitoring data
    a. pulmonary mechanics [e.g., maximum inspiratory pressure, vital capacity]
    b. respiratory monitoring [e.g., rate, tidal volume, minute volume, I:E, inspiratory and expiratory pressures; airway graphics]
    c. pulmonary compliance, airways resistance, work of breathing
    d. noninvasive monitoring [e.g., V_D/V_T, capnography, pulse oximetry, transcutaneous O_2/CO_2]
8. Maternal and perinatal/neonatal history and data [e.g., Apgar scores, gestational age, L/S ratio, pre/post-ductal oxygenation studies]

B. Collect and Evaluate Additional Pertinent Clinical Information

1. Assess patient's overall cardiopulmonary status by **inspection** to determine
    a. general appearance [e.g., muscle wasting, venous distention, peripheral edema,

diaphoresis, clubbing, cyanosis, capillary refill, chest configuration, evidence of diaphragmatic movement, breathing pattern, accessory muscle activity, asymmetrical chest movement, intercostal and/or sternal retractions, nasal flaring]
   b. cough, amount and character of sputum
   c. transillumination of chest, Apgar score, gestational age
2. Assess patient's overall cardiopulmonary status by **palpation** to determine
   a. heart rate, rhythm, and force
   b. asymmetrical chest movements, tactile fremitus, crepitus, tenderness, secretions in the airway, tracheal deviation
3. Assess patient's overall cardiopulmonary status by **auscultation** to determine presence of
   a. breath sounds [e.g., normal, abnormal]
   b. heart sounds and rhythms [e.g., normal, abnormal]
   c. blood pressure
4. Interview patient to determine
   a. level of consciousness/sedation, orientation to time, place and person, emotional state, ability to cooperate, level of pain
   b. presence of dyspnea and/or orthopnea, work of breathing, sputum production, exercise tolerance and activities of daily living
   c. social history [e.g., smoking, substance abuse]
   d. advance directives [e.g., DNR status]
5. Assess patient's learning needs
6. Review chest radiograph to determine
   a. quality of imaging [e.g., patient identification, positioning, exposure]
   b. position of endotracheal or tracheostomy tube
   c. presence of or change in pneumothorax or subcutaneous emphysema, other extrapulmonary air, consolidation and/or atelectasis, pulmonary infiltrates
   d. position of chest tube(s), nasogastric and/or feeding tube, pulmonary artery catheter, pacemaker, and other catheters
   e. presence and position of foreign bodies
   f. position of or change in hemidiaphragms, hyperinflation, pleural fluid, pulmonary edema, mediastinal shift, patency and size of major airways
7. Perform procedures including
   a. 12-lead ECG
   b. pulse oximetry, capnography
   c. tidal volume, minute volume, peak flow, vital capacity
   d. bedside spirometry [e.g., FVC, FEV_1]
   e. arterial sampling – percutaneous or line
   f. 6-minute walk
   g. blood gas/hemoximetry analysis
   h. lung mechanics [e.g., MIP, MEP, pulmonary compliance, plateau pressure, airways resistance]
   i. ventilator pressure-volume and flow-volume loops
   j. apnea monitoring
   k. overnight pulse oximetry
   l. tracheal tube cuff pressure and/or volume
   m. tracheal intubation

n. pulmonary function laboratory studies [e.g., flows, volumes, diffusion studies, pre- and post-bronchodilator]
   o. auto-PEEP detection
8. Interpret procedure results including
   a. transcutaneous O_2/CO_2 monitoring
   b. pulse oximetry, capnography
   c. tidal volume, minute volume, peak flow, vital capacity
   d. bedside spirometry [e.g., FVC, FEV_1]
   e. blood gas/hemoximetry analysis
   f. lung mechanics [e.g., MIP, MEP, pulmonary compliance, plateau pressure, airways resistance]
   g. apnea monitoring
   h. overnight pulse oximetry
   i. tracheal tube cuff pressure and/or volume
   j. pulmonary function laboratory studies [e.g., flows, volumes, diffusion studies, pre- and post-bronchodilator]
   k. ventilator pressure-volume and flow-volume loops
   l. auto-PEEP

C. **Recommend Procedures to Obtain Additional Data Including**
   1. Radiographic and other imaging studies
   2. Lung mechanics [e.g., pulmonary compliance, airways resistance, work of breathing]
   3. Blood gas analysis, pulse oximetry, transcutaneous O_2/CO_2 monitoring

II. **EQUIPMENT APPLICATION AND CLEANLINESS**
   A. **Select, Assemble, Use, and Troubleshoot Equipment Including**
      1. Oxygen administration devices
         a. low-flow devices [e.g., nasal cannula]
         b. high-flow devices [e.g., air entrainment mask]
      2. CPAP devices – mask, nasal, or bi-level
      3. Humidifiers [e.g., bubble, passover, cascade, wick, heat moisture exchanger]
      4. Pneumatic aerosol generator (nebulizer)
      5. Resuscitation devices [e.g., manual resuscitator (bag-valve), mouth-to-valve mask resuscitator]
      6. Ventilators
         a. pneumatic, electric, fluidic, microprocessor
         b. noninvasive positive pressure
         c. high frequency
      7. Artificial airways
         a. oro- and nasopharyngeal airways
         b. endotracheal tubes
         c. tracheostomy tubes and buttons
         d. intubation equipment [e.g., laryngoscope and blades, fiberoptic devices, exhaled CO_2 detection devices]
      8. Suctioning devices [e.g., suction catheters, specimen collectors, oropharyngeal suction devices]
      9. Gas delivery, metering, and clinical analyzing devices

a. gas cylinders, regulators, reducing valves, connectors and flowmeters, air/oxygen blenders

b. oxygen concentrators, air compressors, portable liquid oxygen systems

10. Point-of-care blood gas analyzers
11. Patient breathing circuits
   a. continuous mechanical ventilation
   b. IPPB
   c. CPAP, PEEP valve assembly
   d. non-invasive ventilation
12. Aerosol (mist) tents
13. Incentive breathing devices
14. Percussors and vibrators
15. High Frequency Chest Wall Oscillation (HFCWO) [e.g., ThAIRapy Vest®]
16. Positive expiratory pressure (PEP) devices
17. Vibratory PEP [e.g., Flutter®] mucous clearance devices
18. He/O_2 therapeutic gas
19. Manometers [e.g., water, mercury, and aneroid]
20. Respirometers [e.g., flow-sensing devices (pneumotachometer)]
21. ECG machines (12-lead)
22. Arterial catheters
23. Vacuum systems [e.g., pumps, regulators, collection bottles, pleural drainage devices]
24. Oximetry monitoring devices [e.g., pulse oximeter, transcutaneous]
25. Metered dose inhalers (MDI), MDI spacers
26. Dry powder inhalers
27. Spirometry screening equipment for bedside
28. Speaking tubes and valves
29. CO, He, O_2 and specialty gas analyzers
30. Bronchoscopes

B. Ensure Infection Control

1. Assure selected equipment cleanliness [e.g., select or determine appropriate agent and technique for disinfection and/or sterilization, perform procedures for disinfection and/or sterilization, monitor effectiveness of sterilization procedures]
2. Assure proper handling of biohazardous materials

C. Perform Quality Control Procedures For

1. Blood gas analyzers, co-oximeters, and sampling devices
2. Oxygen analyzers
3. Pulmonary function equipment
4. Mechanical ventilators
5. Gas metering devices [e.g., flowmeter]
6. Noninvasive monitors [e.g., transcutaneous]
7. Record and monitor QC data using accepted statistical methods

III. THERAPEUTIC PROCEDURE INITIATION AND MODIFICATION

A. Maintain Records and Communicate Information

1. Record therapy and results using conventional terminology as required in the health care setting and/or by regulatory agencies

a. specify therapy administered, date, time, frequency of therapy, medication, and ventilatory data

b. note and interpret patient's response to therapy including
   1) effects of therapy, adverse reactions, patient's subjective and attitudinal response to therapy
   2) auscultatory findings, cough and sputum production and characteristics
   3) vital signs [e.g., heart rate, respiratory rate, blood pressure, body temperature, pain level]
   4) pulse oximetry, heart rhythm, capnography

c. verify computations and note erroneous data

2. Communicate information
   a. regarding patient's clinical status to appropriate members of the health care team
   b. relevant to coordinating patient care and discharge planning [e.g., scheduling, avoiding conflicts, sequencing of therapies]
3. Apply computer technology to
   a. document patient management
   b. monitor workload assignments
4. Communicate results of therapy and alter therapy per protocol(s)
5. Explain planned therapy and goals to patient in understandable terms to achieve optimal therapeutic outcome
6. Counsel patient and family concerning smoking cessation and disease management education

B. Maintain a Patent Airway Including the Care of Artificial Airways

1. Properly position patient
2. Insert oro- and nasopharyngeal airways
3. Perform endotracheal intubation
4. Identify tube placement by available means
5. Change tracheostomy tubes
6. Maintain
   a. proper cuff inflation
   b. adequate humidification
7. Perform extubation procedure

C. Remove Bronchopulmonary Secretions

1. Perform
   a. postural drainage and percussion and/or vibration
   b. nasotracheal suctioning
   c. oropharyngeal suctioning
2. Suction artificial airways
3. Administer aerosol therapy, administer prescribed agents [e.g., bronchodilators, corticosteroids, saline, mucolytics]
4. Instruct and encourage bronchopulmonary hygiene techniques

D. Achieve Adequate Respiratory Support

1. Instruct in
   a. proper breathing technique, encourage deep breathing, instruct and monitor techniques of incentive spirometry
   b. inspiratory muscle training techniques

2. Initiate and adjust
   a. IPPB therapy
   b. continuous mechanical ventilation settings
   c. noninvasive ventilation
   d. elevated baseline pressure [e.g., CPAP, PEEP]
   e. combinations of ventilatory techniques [e.g., SIMV, PEEP, PS, PCV, IRV, inspiratory hold]
3. Select ventilator graphics [e.g., waveforms, scales]
4. Administer
   a. aerosolized drugs [e.g., bronchodilators, corticosteroids, mucolytics]
   b. oxygen – on or off a ventilator
5. Initiate and modify weaning procedures
6. Position patient to minimize hypoxemia
7. Prevent procedure-associated hypoxemia [e.g., oxygenate before and after suctioning and equipment changes]
8. Adhere to infection control policies and procedures [e.g., Standard Precautions]

E. Evaluate and Monitor Patient's Objective and Subjective Responses to Respiratory Care

1. Recommend and review chest radiograph
2. Obtain a blood gas sample
   a. by puncture
   b. from an arterial or pulmonary artery catheter
   c. from arterialized capillary blood
3. Perform
   a. pulse oximetry
   b. blood gas and co-oximetry analyses
   c. capnography
4. Interpret blood gas and co-oximetry results
5. Observe changes in sputum characteristics
6. Observe for signs of patient-ventilator dysynchrony
7. Measure and record vital signs, monitor cardiac rhythm, evaluate fluid balance – intake and output
8. Perform spirometry, determine vital capacity, measure pulmonary compliance and airways resistance, interpret airway graphics, measure peak flow
9. Monitor mean airway pressure, adjust and check alarm systems, measure tidal volume, respiratory rate, airway pressures, I:E, and maximum inspiratory pressure
10. Measure F_IO_2 and/or liter flow
11. Monitor endotracheal or tracheostomy tube cuff pressure
12. Auscultate chest and interpret changes in breath sounds

F. Independently Modify Therapeutic Procedures Based on the Patient's Response

1. Terminate treatment based on patient's response to therapy
2. Modify treatment techniques including
   a. IPPB [e.g., volume, flow, pressure, F_IO_2, mouthpiece/mask]
   b. Incentive breathing devices
   c. aerosol therapy
      1) modify patient breathing patterns
      2) change type of equipment, change aerosol output

   3) change dilution of medication, adjust temperature of the aerosol
   d. oxygen therapy
      1) change mode of administration, adjust flow, and F_IO_2
      2) set up or change an O_2 blender
      3) set up an O_2 concentrator or liquid O_2 system
   e. specialty gas [e.g., He/O_2, NO] therapy [e.g., change mode of administration, adjust flow, adjust gas concentration]
   f. bronchial hygiene therapy [e.g., alter patient position and duration of treatment and techniques; coordinate sequence of therapies such as chest percussion, postural drainage, and PEP therapy]
   g. management of artificial airways
      1) reposition or change endotracheal or tracheostomy tube
      2) change type of humidification equipment
      3) initiate suctioning
      4) inflate and/or deflate the cuff
      5) perform tracheostomy care
   h. suctioning
      1) alter frequency and duration of suctioning
      2) change size and type of catheter
      3) alter negative pressure
      4) instill irrigating solutions
   i. mechanical ventilation
      1) improve patient synchrony [e.g., sensitivity, mode]
      2) enhance oxygenation [e.g., F_IO_2, PEEP/CPAP level, inspiratory time]
      3) improve alveolar ventilation [e.g., tidal volume, rate]
      4) adjust I:E settings
      5) modify ventilator techniques [e.g., pressure support, pressure control]
      6) adjust noninvasive positive pressure ventilation
      7) monitor and adjust alarm settings
      8) adjust ventilator settings based on ventilator graphics
      9) change type of ventilator, change patient breathing circuitry
      10) change mechanical dead space
   j. procedures for weaning from mechanical ventilation

G. Recommend Modifications in the Respiratory Care Plan Based on the Patient's Response

1. Recommend
   a. institution of bronchopulmonary hygiene procedures
   b. sedation and/or use of muscle relaxant(s)
   c. insertion or change of artificial airway [e.g., endotracheal tube, LMA, tracheostomy]
   d. procedures for weaning from mechanical ventilation
   e. extubation
   f. discontinuing treatment based on patient response

2. Recommend changes in
   a. patient position
   b. aerosol drug dosage or concentration
   c. F_IO_2 and oxygen flow
3. Recommend changes in mechanical ventilation to
   a. improve patient synchrony [e.g., sensitivity, mode]
   b. enhance oxygenation [e.g., F_IO_2, PEEP/CPAP level, inspiratory time]
   c. improve alveolar ventilation [e.g., tidal volume, rate]
   d. adjust I:E settings
   e. modify ventilator techniques [e.g., pressure support, pressure control]
   f. adjust noninvasive positive pressure ventilation
   g. monitor and adjust alarm settings
   h. adjust ventilator settings based on ventilator graphics
   i. change type of ventilator, change patient breathing circuitry
   j. alter mechanical dead space
   k. modify ventilator settings to
      1) eliminate auto-PEEP
      2) reduce plateau pressure
4. Recommend use of pharmacologic interventions including
   a. bronchodilators [e.g., adrenergics, anticholinergics, theophyllines]
   b. antiinflammatory drugs [e.g., leukotriene modifiers, corticosteroids, NSAID, cromolyn sodium]
   c. mucolytics/proteolytics [e.g., acetylcysteine, RhDNAse]
   d. sedatives
   e. analgesics
   f. diuretics
   g. surfactants

H. Determine the Appropriateness of the Prescribed Respiratory Care Plan and Recommend Modifications When Indicated

1. Analyze available data to determine pathophysiological state
2. Review
   a. planned therapy to establish therapeutic plan
   b. interdisciplinary patient and family plan
3. Determine appropriateness of prescribed therapy and goals for identified pathophysiological state
4. Recommend changes in therapeutic plan when indicated based on data
5. Perform respiratory care quality assurance
6. Develop outcomes of
   a. quality improvement programs
   b. respiratory care protocols
7. Monitor outcomes of
   a. quality improvement programs
   b. respiratory care protocols
8. Apply respiratory care protocols
9. Conduct disease management education

I. Initiate, Conduct, or Modify Respiratory Care Techniques in an Emergency Setting

1. Treat cardiopulmonary collapse according to
   a. BCLS
   b. ACLS
   c. Pediatric Advanced Life Support (PALS)
   d. Neonatal Resuscitation Program (NRP)
2. Treat tension pneumothorax
3. Participate in
   a. land/air patient transport outside the hospital
   b. intra-hospital patient transport
   c. disaster management

J. Act as an Assistant to the Physician Performing Special Procedures Including

1. Bronchoscopy
2. Tracheostomy
3. Cardioversion
4. Intubation

K. Initiate and Conduct Pulmonary Rehabilitation and Home Care Within the Prescription

1. Explain planned therapy and goals to patient in understandable terms to achieve optimal therapeutic outcome
2. Educate patient and family in disease management
3. Counsel patient and family concerning smoking cessation
4. Instruct patient and family to assure safety and infection control

Index

Note: Page numbers followed by f indicate figures; those followed by t indicate tables; those followed by b indicate boxed material.